An Introduction to
Community
Sixth Edition
Health

James F. McKenzie, PhD, MPH, CHES
Robert R. Pinger, PhD
Jerome E. Kotecki, HSD
Department of Physiology and Health Science
Ball State University

JONES AND BARTLETT PUBLISHERS
Sudbury, Massachusetts
BOSTON   TORONTO   LONDON   SINGAPORE

World Headquarters

Jones and Bartlett Publishers
40 Tall Pine Drive
Sudbury, MA 01776
978-443-5000
info@jbpub.com
www.jbpub.com

Jones and Bartlett Publishers Canada
6339 Ormindale Way
Mississauga, Ontario L5V 1J2
Canada

Jones and Bartlett Publishers
  International
Barb House, Barb Mews
London W6 7PA
United Kingdom

Jones and Bartlett's books and products are available through most bookstores and online booksellers. To contact Jones and Bartlett Publishers directly, call 800-832-0034, fax 978-443-8000, or visit our website www.jbpub.com.

Substantial discounts on bulk quantities of Jones and Bartlett's publications are available to corporations, professional associations, and other qualified organizations. For details and specific discount information, contact the special sales department at Jones and Bartlett via the above contact information or send an email to specialsales@jbpub.com.

Production Credits

Chief Executive Officer: Clayton Jones
Chief Operating Officer: Don W. Jones, Jr.
President, Higher Education and Professional Publishing: Robert W. Holland, Jr.
V.P., Design and Production: Anne Spencer
V.P., Manufacturing and Inventory Control: Therese Connell
V.P., Sales and Marketing: William J. Kane
Acquisition Editor: Jacqueline Ann Geraci
Associate Editor: Amy L. Flagg
Associate Editor: Patrice Mailloux Andrews
Senior Production Editor: Julie Champagne Bolduc
Marketing Manager: Wendy Thayer
Marketing Associate: Meagan Norlund
Interactive Technology Manager: Dawn Mahon Priest
Composition: Publishers' Design and Production Services, Inc.
Cover Design: Hannus Design Associates
Photo Research Manager/Photographer: Kimberly Potvin
Associate Photo Researcher/Photographer: Christine McKeen
Printing and Binding: Malloy, Inc.
Cover Printing: John Pow Company

Library of Congress Cataloging-in-Publication Data

McKenzie, James F.
    An introduction to community health / James F. McKenzie, Robert R. Pinger,
Jerome E. Kotecki. — 6th ed.
        p. ; cm.
    Includes bibliographical references and index.
    ISBN 978-0-7637-4634-6 (alk. paper)
    1. Community health services—United States.   2. Public health—United
States.   3. Medical care—United States.   4. Environmental health—United
States.   I. Pinger, R. R.   II. Kotecki, Jerome Edward.   III. Title.
    [DNLM: 1. Community Health Services—United States.   2. Delivery of
Health Care—United States.   3. Environmental Health—United States.
4. Public Health—United States.   WA 546 AA1 M47i 2008]
    RA445.M29 2008
    362.12—dc22

                                                        2007030763

6048

Additional photographic credits appear on page 638, which constitutes a continuation of the copyright page.

Printed in the United States of America
11 10 09 08 07   10 9 8 7 6 5 4 3 2 1

CONTENTS

CHAPTER 6   **THE SCHOOL HEALTH PROGRAM:
A COMPONENT OF COMMUNITY HEALTH**   145

UNIT FOUR
ENVIRONMENTAL HEALTH AND SAFETY   445

PREFACE
For the Sixth Edition

As its title suggests, *An Introduction to Community Health* was written to introduce students to community health. It is a textbook that combines the power of today's electronic technology, via the Internet, with the traditional textbook presentation. We believe that your students will find *An Introduction to Community Health* easy to read, understand, and use. If they read the chapters carefully and make an honest effort to answer the review questions and to complete some of the activities, we are confident that students will gain a good understanding of the realm of community health. *An Introduction to Community Health* incorporates a variety of pedagogical elements that assist and encourage students to understand complex community health issues. Each chapter of the book includes (1) chapter objectives, (2) a scenario, (3) an introduction, (4) content, (5) marginal definitions of key terms, (6) a chapter summary, (7) a scenario analysis and response, (8) review questions, (9) activities, (10) information about Web activities, and (11) references. In addition, many figures, tables, boxes, and photos have been presented to clarify and illustrate the concepts presented in the text. Select content in each chapter is dedicated to the *Healthy People 2010* goals and objectives and, when available, their midcourse review updates. In the back of the book you will find four appendixes (calculation of an odds ratio, operational definitions used to classify federal data on race and ethnicity, and a self-assessment checklist for cultural diversity and cultural competency), a glossary of key terms used throughout the text, and a complete subject and person index.

Chapter Objectives

The chapter objectives identify the content and skills that should be mastered through reading the chapters, answering the end-of-chapter questions, and completing the activities. To use the objectives effectively, they should be reviewed before and after reading the chapters. This review will help your students focus on the major points in each chapter and facilitate answering the questions and completing the activities at the end of each chapter.

Scenarios

Short scenarios are presented at the beginning of each chapter. The purpose of these scenarios is to bridge the gap between your students' personal experiences and ideas discussed within the chapter. The chapter content will enable your students to propose solutions to the community health problem posed in the scenario.

Introduction

Each chapter begins with a brief introduction that informs the reader of the topics to be presented and explains how these topics relate to others in the book.

Marginal Definitions

Key terms are introduced in each chapter of the textbook. These terms are important to the understanding of the chapter. Such terms are presented in boldface type within each chapter, and the definitions are presented in the margins (marginal definitions). Before reading the chapter, it is suggested that the student skim the chapters, paying particular attention to the key terms. This should provide greater understanding of the content. The boldfaced terms, including those defined in the margin, appear in the glossary at the end of the book. In addition, some words in the textbook have been italicized for emphasis, and are often key terms that have been defined either in another chapter or the glossary.

Content

Although each chapter in the textbook could be expanded and, indeed, there are entire books written on many of the topics we cover, we believe each chapter contains the essential material needed to introduce your students to the issues related to community health. To enhance and facilitate learning, the chapters are organized in four units: Foundations of Community Health, The Nation's Health, Health Care Delivery, and Environmental Health and Safety.

Chapter Summary

At the end of each chapter, the reader will find several bulleted points that review the major concepts contained in each chapter.

Scenario: Analysis and Response

Following the chapter summary, students are provided with an opportunity to respond to the scenario presented earlier in the chapter. The content presented in the chapter will help the students to formulate their responses or solutions.

Review Questions

The purpose of the questions at the end of each chapter is to provide the readers with feedback regarding their mastery of the chapter's content. The questions reinforce the chapter objectives and key terms.

Activities

The activities at the end of each chapter provide an opportunity for students to apply their new knowledge in a meaningful way. The activities, which are presented in a variety of formats, should appeal to the varying learning styles of your students.

Community Health on the Web

The Internet contains a wealth of information about community and public health. The Web activities are presented to encourage students to further explore the chapter's content by visiting relevant Web sites. These activities recap three concepts or issues from the text in each chapter. The starting point for these activities is Jones and Bartlett's own exclusive Community Health Web page (http://health.jbpub.com/book/communityhealth/6e).

Once students have connected to the designated community health link through the Jones and Bartlett Community Health home page, they will be provided with activity instructions for further exploration of the Web site. Animated flashcards, an interactive glossary, and crossword puzzles are also available online. When more up-to-date information becomes available at an assigned site, the authors are able to immediately edit the exercise to reflect the most recent material.

The Web activities bring to life the content and theory presented in the text, thus giving students a real-world context for understanding community health concepts and issues. The intent of including Web activities in the textbook is to inspire the students, in real time, to authentically assess and to critically think about what they have just read in the text by asking them thought-provoking questions related to the assigned Web site. By integrating the Web into the text, we have created a dynamic learning environment that is as up-to-date as today's newspaper.

What Is New to This Edition?

Although the format of this edition is similar to the previous edition, much has changed. First, the content and statistics throughout the book have been reviewed and updated with the latest information. New tables, figures, boxes, and photographs have been added. Second, the *Healthy People 2010* boxes that were a part of each chapter in the previous edition of the textbook now include, where available, data that show the status of each objective with regard to meeting the 2010 target figure. Third, an emphasis was placed on making changes to the content that was requested by reviewers of the previous edition of the text. Specifically, information on disasters—natural and humanmade (including bioterrorism)—and historical timelines were added to Chapter 1. Chapter 3 now includes information about bird flu. Updated tables and revised definitions of key epidemiological terms now reflect the most current understanding and usage. Chapter 5 has been expanded to include three additional models for community organizing and building: Healthy Cities/Healthy Communities, Planned Approach to Community Health (PATCH), and Mobilizing for Action through Planning and Partnerships (MAPP). The school health education chapter—Chapter 6—includes the new National Health Education Standards and the Health Education Standards for School Health Educators. The scenario in Chapter 11—Mental Health—has been revised to portray community mental health issues more effectively. The section on stress management has been revisited and expanded to include the latest research. The history of mental health care has been revised to provide students with a more accessible description. This section now includes discussions of mental health care in the prison system and access to mental health care for military personnel returning from combat zones. Chapter 12 features an in-depth discussion of underage and pathological drinking. Chapter 14 has been expanded to include more information on Medicare Parts C and D, and on consumer-driven health care, specifically health savings accounts (HSAs). And finally, Chapters 15 and 16—Environmental Concerns and the Impact of the Environment on Human Health—have been extensively reorganized, revised, and updated to reflect the progress that has been made in the past few years. Specifically, Chapter 15 takes a more health-oriented focus than in the previous editions to show the relationship between the stewardship of our environment and the healthiness of our communities. In both chapters, we have provided information to connect students to resources and solutions available on the Internet and bring them in line with much that has happened in the past few years.

Accompanying Ancillaries

Repetition is often the key to learning; in the sixth edition we offer the *Student Note-Taking Guide,* which allows students to revisit key topics discussed in the text. This edition is also accompanied by an Instructor's ToolKit CD-ROM, which includes a lecture outline and Power-Point presentation for each chapter as well as a computerized TestBank and Image Bank. These products are available free to adopters of the text. For more information about these ancillary products, please contact your sales representative at Jones and Bartlett Publishers.

ACKNOWLEDGMENTS

A project of this nature could not be completed without the assistance and understanding of a number of individuals. First, we would like to thank those individuals who have brought their expertise to the writing team. Jacquie Rainey, DrPH, CHES, Associate Dean, College of Health and Behavioral Sciences at the University of Central Arkansas, provided revisions for Chapter 2 (Organizations that Help Shape Community Health). Denise M. Seabert, PhD, CHES, Assistant Professor in the Department of Physiology and Health Science at Ball State University, completed revisions for Chapter 6 (The School Health Program: A Component of Community

Health) and Chapter 8 (Adolescents, Young Adults, and Adults). David A. Haber, PhD, the John and Janice Fisher Distinguished Professor and Associate Director of the Fisher Institute for Wellness and Gerontology at Ball State University, was responsible for the revisions to Chapter 9 (Elders). Jarmila Popovicova, PhD, Assistant Professor in the Department of Natural Resources and Environmental Management at Ball State University, completed the revisions for Chapters 15 (Environmental Concerns: Wastes and Pollution) and 16 (The Impact of Environment on Human Health). Their expertise is both welcomed and appreciated.

Second, we would like to thank several colleagues for their contributions. They include Dale B. Hahn, PhD, Department of Physiology and Health Science, Ball State University, for encouraging us to take on this project; Fariba Mirzaei, MD, MPH, Doctoral Student, Harvard School of Public Health, Harvard University, and James F. Howell, DVM, Epidemiologist, Epidemiology Resource Center, Indiana State Department of Health, for their review of and suggestions for Chapters 3 and 4; David V. Perkins, PhD, Professor, Department of Psychological Sciences, Ball State University, for his review of and suggestions for Chapter 11; the staff members of the High Library at Elizabethtown College, Elizabethtown, PA, for their assistance in making the project possible; and Billie Kennedy and Ruth Ann Duncan for their support and friendship.

Third, we would like to express our appreciation to those professionals who took the time and effort to review and provide feedback for this edition. They include Elizabeth G. Calamidas, The Richard Stockton College of New Jersey; Fran Henton, Nebraska Methodist College; Harold Horn, Lincoln Land Community College; John Janowiak, Appalachian State University; Justine Pawlukewicz, New York City College of Technology; Fred R. Pearson, Brigham Young University-Idaho; Kerry J. Redican, Virginia Polytechnic Institute and State University; Wanda Reygaert, Oakland University; Patricia Rhynders, Touro University International and Texas Woman's University; Joanne Sommers, Bowling Green State University; Cynthia Stone, Indiana University; and Maria Theresa Wessel, James Madison University.

Fourth, we would like to thank all of the employees of Jones and Bartlett Publishers. Their hard work, support, guidance, and confidence in us has been most helpful in creating this and all previous editions of this text. Specifically, we would like to thank: Jacqueline Geraci, Acquisitions Editor; Julie Bolduc, Production Editor; Patrice Andrews, Associate Editor; Wendy Thayer, Marketing Manager; Meagan Norlund, Marketing Associate; and Anne Spencer, Vice President of Design and Production.

Finally, we would like to thank our families for their love, support, encouragement, and tolerance of all the time that writing takes away from family activities.

James F. McKenzie, PhD, MPH, CHES
Robert R. Pinger, PhD
Jerome E. Kotecki, HSD

UNIT ONE

FOUNDATIONS OF COMMUNITY HEALTH

Chapter I

Community Health: Yesterday, Today, and Tomorrow

Chapter Outline

Chapter Objectives

After studying this chapter, you will be able to:

1 Accurately define the terms *health, community, community health, population health, public health,* and *public health system.*

2 Briefly describe the five major determinants of health.

3 Explain the difference between personal and community health activities.

4 List and discuss the factors that influence a community's health.

5 Briefly relate the history of community/public health, including the recent U.S. history of community and public health in the twentieth century.

6 Provide a brief overview of the current health status of Americans.

7 Describe the status of efforts to improve world health and list some plans for the future.

8 Describe the purpose of the *Healthy People 2010* goals and objectives as they apply to the planning process of the health of Americans.

9 Briefly describe the impact terrorism has on community/public health.

SCENARIO

Amy and Eric are a young working couple who are easing into a comfortable lifestyle. They have good-paying jobs, drive nice cars, are buying a home in a good neighborhood, and have two healthy preschool children. When Amy picked her children up from day care earlier in the day she learned from the head teacher that another parent had reported that his child was diagnosed with hepatitis. This news frightened Amy and made her begin to question the quality of the day care center. Amy told Eric of this situation when he got home from work. As the couple discussed whether or not they should take their children to day care as usual the following day, they discovered that they have many unanswered questions. How serious is hepatitis? What is the likelihood that their children will be at serious risk for getting the disease? What steps are being taken to control the outbreak? Is any state or local agency responsible for standardizing health practices at private day care centers in the community? Does the city, county, or state carry out any type of inspection when they license these facilities? And, if the children do not attend day care, which parent will stay home with them?

INTRODUCTION

In reflecting on the twentieth century, it is easy to point to the tremendous progress that was made in the health and life expectancy of those in the United States (see Box 1.1) and of many people of the world. Infant mortality dropped, many of the infectious diseases have been brought under control, and better family planning became available. However, there is still room for improvement! Individual health behaviors, such as the use of tobacco, poor diet, and physical inactivity, have given rise to an unacceptable number of cases of illness and death from noninfectious diseases such as cancer, diabetes, and heart disease. New and emerging infectious diseases, such as pandemic influenza (also referred to as "pan flu" and H5N1) and those caused by drug-resistant pathogens, are stretching resources available to control them. And the events stemming from the terrorist attacks on the United States on September 11, 2001 (referred to as 9/11), and the subsequent anthrax mailings have caused us to refocus our priorities. Those events "disturbed the sense of complacency many people felt about the health and safety of their living conditions."[1] In addition, those events revealed the vulnerability of the United States' ability to respond to such circumstances and highlighted the need for improvements in emergency response and the infrastructure of the public health system. Even with all that has happened in recent years in the United States and around the world, the achievement of good health remains a worldwide goal of the twenty-first century. Governments, private organizations, and individuals throughout the world are working to improve health. Although individual actions to improve one's own personal health certainly contribute to the overall health of the community, organized community actions are often necessary when health problems exceed the resources of any one individual. When such actions are not taken, the health of the entire community is at risk.

This chapter introduces the concepts and principles of community health, explains how community health differs from personal health, and provides a brief history of community health. Some of the key health problems facing Americans are also described, and an outlook for the twenty-first century is provided.

BOX 1.1

A LOOK BACK ON THE TWENTIETH CENTURY IN THE UNITED STATES

As the twentieth century came to a close, the overall health status and life expectancy in the United States were at all-time highs. Since 1900, the average lifespan of people in the United States had lengthened by more than 30 years; 25 of these years have been attributed to advances in public health.[2] There were many public health achievements that can be linked to this gain in life expectancy, however. The Centers for Disease Control and Prevention (CDC), the U.S. government agency charged with protecting the public health of the nation, singled out the "Ten Great Public Health Achievements" in the United States between 1900 and 1999. Some of these achievements will be discussed in greater detail in other chapters of this book where they are more relevant to the content being presented. Here is the entire list:[3]

1. *Vaccination.* Vaccines are now available to protect children and adults against 15 life-threatening or debilitating diseases. Rates of all vaccine-preventable diseases are down more than 97% from peak levels before vaccines were available.[4]
2. *Motor vehicle safety.* A number of advances over the years, including safety belts, air bags, safer cars and roads, and enforcement of drunk driving and other laws, have saved many lives.[4]
3. *Safer workplaces.* A number of voluntary and mandatory practices in the workplace have created a much safer work environment. In the early 1900s, the work-related death rate was about 21 per 100,000. By the mid-1990s, that number had dropped to about 4 per 100,000.[5]
4. *Control of infectious diseases.* At the beginning of the century, the leading causes of death were infectious diseases, but by mid-century many of these

diseases were under control. This control can be attributed to cleaner water, improved sanitation, and antibiotics.
5. *Decline of deaths from coronary heart disease and stroke.* While these remain the leading causes of death, significant progress has been made in reducing the death rates since 1950. This progress can be attributed to the identification and modification of risk factors such as smoking and high blood pressure, and the improved access to early detection and better treatment.
6. *Safer and healthier foods.* Over the century much of the microbial contamination of food has been significantly reduced, and the nutritional value of foods has been greatly enhanced.
7. *Healthier mothers and babies.* Infant and maternal mortality rates have decreased 90% and 99%, respectively. This can be attributed to advances in hygiene, nutrition, antibiotics, medical technology, and access to health care.
8. *Family planning.* Advances in family planning and contraceptive services have provided for greater health benefits for mothers and babies, and have reduced the transmission of several sexually transmitted diseases.
9. *Fluoridation of drinking water.* Though fluoridation of water only began in mid-century, it has played an important role in the reduction of both tooth decay and tooth loss.
10. *Recognition of tobacco use as a health hazard.* Recognition of tobacco as the single most preventable cause of death in the United States has saved the lives and suffering of millions of people in this country.

Definitions

The word *health* means different things to different people. Similarly, there are other words that can be defined in various ways. Some basic terms we will use in this book are defined in the following paragraphs.

Health

The word *health* is derived from *hal,* which means "hale, sound, whole." When it comes to the health of people, the word *health* has been defined in a number of different ways—often in its social context, as when a parent describes the health of a child or when an avid fan defines the health of a professional athlete. The most widely quoted definition of health was the one created by the World Health Organization (WHO) in 1946. That definition states that "health is a state of complete physical, mental, and social well-being and not merely the absence of disease and infirmity."[6] More recently, the WHO has also indicated that health is "a cumulative state, to be promoted throughout life in order to ensure that the full benefits are enjoyed in later years."[7] Good health is vital for maintaining an acceptable quality of life.[7] Others have stated that health cannot be defined as a state because it is ever changing. Therefore, we have chosen to define **health** as a *dynamic* state or condition of the human organism that is multidimensional (i.e., physical, emotional, social, intellectual, spiritual, and occupational) in nature, a resource for living, and results from a person's interactions with and adaptations to his or her environment. Therefore, it can exist in varying degrees and is specific to each individual and his or her situation. "For example, a person can be healthy while dying, or a person who is a quadriplegic can be healthy in the sense that his or her mental and social well-being are high and physical health is as good as it can be."[8]

A person's health status is dynamic in part because of the many different factors that determine one's health. It is widely accepted that health status is determined by the interaction of five domains: gestational endowments (i.e., genetic makeup), social circumstances (e.g., education, employment, income, poverty, housing, crime, and social cohesion), environmental conditions where people live and work (i.e., toxic agents, microbial agents, and structural hazards), behavioral choices (e.g., diet, physical activity, substance use and abuse), and the availability of quality medical care.[9] "Ultimately, the health fate of each of us is determined by factors acting not mostly in isolation but by our experience where domains interconnect. Whether a gene is expressed can be determined by environmental exposures or behavioral patterns. The nature and consequences of behavioral choices are affected by social circumstances. Our genetic predispositions affect the health care we need, and our social circumstances affect the health care we receive."[10]

Community

Traditionally, a community has been thought of as a geographic area with specific boundaries—for example, a neighborhood, city, county, or state. However, in the context of community health, a **community** is "a group of people who have common characteristics; communities can be defined by location, race, ethnicity, age, occupation, interest in particular problems or outcomes, or common bonds."[11] Communities are characterized by the following elements:

> (1) membership—a sense of identity and belonging; (2) common symbol systems—similar language, rituals, and ceremonies; (3) shared values and norms; (4) mutual influence—community members have influence and are influenced by each other; (5) shared needs and commitment to meeting them; and (6) shared emotional connection—members share common history, experiences, and mutual support.[12]

Examples of communities include the people of the city of Columbus (location), the Asian community of San Francisco (race), the Hispanic community of Miami (ethnicity), seniors in the church (age), the business or the banking communities (occupation), the homeless of Indiana (specific problem), those on welfare in Ohio (particular outcome), or local union members (common bond). A community may be as small as the group of people who live on a residence hall floor at a university or as large as all of the individuals who make up a nation. "A healthy community is a place where people provide leadership in assessing their own resources and needs, where public health and social infrastructure and policies support health, and where essential public health services, including quality health care, are available."[13]

Public, Community, and Population Health

Prior to defining the three terms *public health*, *community health*, and *population health*, it is important to note that often the terms are used interchangeably by both laypeople and professionals who work in the various health fields. When the terms are used interchangeably, most people are referring to the collective health of those in society and the actions or activities taken to obtain and maintain that health. The definitions provided here for the three terms more precisely define the group of people in question and the origin of the actions or activities.

Of the three terms, *public health* is the most inclusive. The Institute of Medicine (IOM) defined **public health** in 1988 in its landmark report *The Future of Public Health* as "what we as a society do collectively to assure the conditions in which people can be healthy."[14] The **public health system**, which has been defined as "activities undertaken within the formal structure of government and the associated efforts of private and voluntary organizations and individuals,"[14] is the organizational mechanism for providing such conditions. Even with these formal definitions, some still see public health activities as only those efforts that originate in federal, state, and local governmental public health agencies such as the Centers for Disease Control and Prevention and local (i.e., city and county) health departments.

Community health refers to the health status of a defined group of people and the actions and conditions to promote, protect, and preserve their health. For example, the health status of the people of Muncie, Indiana, and the private and public actions taken to promote, protect, and preserve the health of these people would constitute community health.

The term *population health,* which is similar to *community health,* has emerged in recent years. The primary difference between these two terms is the degree of organization or identity of the people. **Population health** refers to the health status of people who are not organized and have no identity as a group or locality and the actions and conditions to promote, protect, and preserve their health. Men younger than 50, adolescents, prisoners, and white-collar workers are all examples of populations.[15]

Personal Health versus Community Health

To further clarify the definitions presented in this chapter, it is important to distinguish between the terms *personal health activities* and *community health activities.*

Personal Health Activities

Personal health activities are individual actions and decision making that affect the health of an individual or his or her immediate family members. These activities may be preventive or curative in nature but seldom directly affect the behavior of others. Choosing to eat wisely, to regularly wear a safety belt, and to visit the physician are all examples of personal health activities.

Community Health Activities

Community health activities are activities that are aimed at protecting or improving the health of a population or community. Maintenance of accurate birth and death records, protection of the food and water supply, and participating in fund drives for voluntary health organizations such as the American Lung Association are examples of community health activities.

Within this book, you will be introduced to the many community health activities and to the organizations that are responsible for carrying them out. The following are some of the key topics that are covered in this text:

- Organizations that contribute to community health
- How communities measure health, disease, injury, and death
- Control of communicable and noncommunicable diseases
- How communities organize to solve health problems
- Community health in schools
- Community health needs of people at different stages of life
- Community health needs of special populations
- Community mental health
- Abuse of alcohol, tobacco, and other drugs

public health
things that society does collectively to assure the conditions in which people can be healthy

public health system
the organizational mechanism of those activities undertaken within the formal structure of government and the associated efforts of private and voluntary organizations and individuals

community health
the health status of a defined group of people and the actions and conditions to promote, protect, and preserve their health

population health
the health status of people who are not organized and have no identity as a group or locality and the actions and conditions to promote, protect, and preserve their health

- The health care delivery system
- Environmental health problems
- Intentional and unintentional injuries
- Occupational safety and health

Factors That Affect the Health of a Community

There are a great many factors that affect the health of a community. As a result, the health status of each community is different. These factors may be physical, social, and/or cultural. They also include the ability of the community to organize and work together as a whole as well as the individual behaviors of those in the community (see Figure 1.1).

Physical Factors

Physical factors include the influences of geography, the environment, community size, and industrial development.

Geography

A community's health problems can be directly influenced by its altitude, latitude, and climate. In tropical countries where warm, humid temperatures and rain prevail throughout the year, parasitic and infectious diseases are a leading community health problem (see Figure 1.2). In many tropical countries, survival from these diseases is made more difficult because poor soil conditions result in inadequate food production and malnutrition. In temperate climates with fewer parasitic and infectious diseases and a more than adequate food supply, obesity and heart disease are important community health problems.

Environment

The quality of our environment is directly related to the quality of our stewardship over it. Many experts believe that if we continue to allow uncontrolled population growth and continue to deplete nonrenewable natural resources, succeeding generations will inhabit communities that are less desirable than ours. Many feel that we must accept responsibility for this stewardship and drastically reduce the rate at which we foul the soil, water, and air.

Community Size

The larger the community, the greater its range of health problems and the greater its number of health resources. For example, larger communities have more health professionals and better health facilities than smaller communities. These resources are often needed because communicable diseases can spread more quickly and environmental problems are often more severe in densely populated areas. For example, the amount of trash generated by the approximately 8+ million people in New York City is many times greater than that generated by the entire state of Wyoming, with its population of about 515,000.

It is important to note that a community's size can have both a positive and negative impact on that community's health. The ability of a community to effectively plan, organize, and utilize its resources can determine whether its size can be used to good advantage.

Industrial Development

Industrial development, like size, can have either positive or negative effects on the health status of a community. Industrial development provides a community with added resources for community health programs, but it may bring with it environmental pollution and occupational illnesses. Communities that experience rapid

FIGURE 1.1

Factors that affect the health of a community.

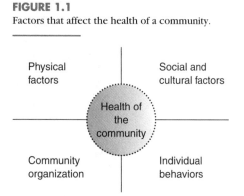

Physical factors

Social and cultural factors

Health of the community

Community organization

Individual behaviors

industrial development must eventually regulate the way in which industries (1) obtain raw materials, (2) discharge by-products, (3) dispose of wastes, (4) treat and protect their employees, and (5) clean up environmental accidents. Unfortunately, many of these laws are usually passed only after these communities have suffered significant reductions in the quality of their life and health.

Social and Cultural Factors

Social factors are those that arise from the interaction of individuals or groups within the community. For example, people who live in urban communities, where life is fast-paced, experience higher rates of stress-related illnesses than those who live in rural communities, where life is more leisurely. On the other hand, those in rural areas may not have access to the same quality or selection of health care (i.e., hospitals or medical specialists) that is available to those who live in urban communities.

Cultural factors arise from guidelines (both explicit and implicit) that individuals "inherit" from being a part of a particular society. Culture "teaches us what to fear, what to respect, what to value, and what to regard as relevant in our lives."[16] Some of the factors that contribute to culture are discussed in the following sections.

Beliefs, Traditions, and Prejudices

The beliefs, traditions, and prejudices of community members can affect the health of the community. The beliefs of those in a community about such specific health behaviors as exercise and smoking can influence policy makers on whether or not they will spend money on bike trails and no-smoking ordinances. The traditions of specific ethnic groups can influence the types of food, restaurants, retail outlets, and services available in a community. Prejudices of one specific ethnic or racial group against another can result in acts of violence and crime. Racial and ethnic disparities will continue to put certain groups, such as black Americans or certain religious groups, at greater risk.

Economy

Both national and local economies can affect the health of a community through reductions in health and social services. An economic downturn means lower tax revenues (fewer tax dollars) and fewer contributions to charitable groups. Such actions will result in fewer dollars being available for programs such as welfare, food stamps, community health care, and other community services. This occurs because revenue shortfalls cause agencies to experience budget cuts. With less money, these agencies often must alter their eligibility guidelines, thereby restricting aid to only the neediest individuals. Obviously, many people who had been eligible for assistance before the economic downturn become ineligible.

Employers usually find it increasingly difficult to provide health benefits for their employees as their income drops. The unemployed and underemployed face poverty and deteriorating health. Thus, the cumulative effect of an economic downturn significantly affects the health of the community.

Politics

Those who happen to be in political office, either nationally or locally, can improve or jeopardize the health of their community by the decisions they make. In the most general terms, the argument is over greater or lesser governmental participation in health issues. For example, there has been a long-standing discussion in the United States on the extent to which the government should involve itself in health care. Historically, Democrats have been

FIGURE 1.2

In tropical countries, parasitic and infectious diseases are leading community health problems.

in favor of such action while Republicans have been against it. However, as the cost of health care continues to grow, both sides see the need for some kind of increased regulation. Local politicians also influence the health of their communities each time they vote on health-related measures brought before them, such as a nonsmoking ordinance.

Religion

A number of religions have taken a position on health care and health behaviors. For example, some religious communities limit the type of medical treatment their members may receive. Some do not permit immunizations; others do not permit their members to be treated by physicians. Still others prohibit certain foods. For example, Kosher dietary regulations permit Jews to eat the meat only of animals that chew cud and have cloven hooves and the flesh only of fish that have both gills and scales, while still others, like the Native American Church of the Morning Star, use peyote, a hallucinogen, as a sacrament.

Some religious communities actively address moral and ethical issues such as abortion, premarital intercourse, and homosexuality. Still other religions teach health-promoting codes of living to their members. Obviously, religion can affect a community's health positively or negatively (see Figure 1.3).

Social Norms

The influence of social norms can be positive or negative and can change over time. Cigarette smoking is a good example. During the 1940s, 1950s, and 1960s, it was socially acceptable to smoke in most settings. As a matter of fact, in 1960, 53% of American men and 32% of American women smoked. Thus, in 1960 it was socially acceptable to be a smoker, especially if you were male. Now, early in the twenty-first century, those percentages have dropped to 23.4% (for males) and 18.5% (for females), and in most public places it has become socially unacceptable to smoke.[17] The lawsuits against tobacco companies by both the state attorneys general and private citizens provide further evidence that smoking has fallen from social acceptability. Because of this change in the social norm, there is less secondhand smoke in many public places, and in turn the health of the community has improved.

FIGURE 1.3
Religion can affect a community's health either positively or negatively.

Unlike smoking, alcohol consumption represents a continuing negative social norm in America, especially on college campuses. The normal expectation seems to be that drinking is fun (and almost everyone wants to have fun). Despite the fact that most college students are too young to drink legally, approximately 85% of college students drink.[18] It seems fairly obvious that the American alcoholic-beverage industry has influenced our social norms.

Socioeconomic Status

"In both the United States and Western Europe, the gap in health status and mortality between those commanding, and those who lack, economic power and social resources continues to widen. These parallel trends—of growing economic inequalities and growing social inequalities in health—reflect, in part, the relationship between people's socioeconomic position as consumers and employers or employees and their social, biological, and mental well-being."[19] That is, those in the community with the lowest socioeconomic status (SES) also have the poorest health and the most difficulty in gaining access to health care. The point of entry into the health care system for most Americans is the family doctor. The economically disadvantaged seldom have a family doctor. For them, the point of entry is the local hospital emergency department. In addition to health care access, higher incomes enable people to afford better housing, live in safer neighborhoods, and increase the opportunity to engage in health-promoting behaviors.[20]

Community Organizing

The way in which a community is able to organize its resources directly influences its ability to intervene and solve problems, including health problems. **Community organizing** "is a process through which communities are helped to identify common problems or goals, mobilize resources, and in other ways develop and implement strategies for reaching their goals they have collectively set."[21] It is not a science but an art of building consensus within a democratic process.[22] If a community can organize its resources effectively into a unified force, it "is likely to produce benefits in the form of increased effectiveness and productivity by reducing duplication of efforts and avoiding the imposition of solutions that are not congruent with the local culture and needs."[13] For example, many communities in the United States have faced community-wide drug problems. Some have been able to organize their resources to reduce or resolve these problems, whereas others have not. (See Chapter 5 for a full explanation of community organizing.)

Individual Behavior

The behavior of the individual community members contributes to the health of the entire community. It takes the concerted effort of many—if not most—of the individuals in a community to make a program work. For example, if each individual consciously recycles his or her trash each week, community recycling will be successful. Likewise, if each occupant would wear a safety belt, there could be a significant reduction in the number of facial injuries and deaths from car crashes for the entire community. In another example, the more individuals who become immunized against a specific disease, the slower the disease will spread and the fewer people will be exposed. This concept is known as **herd immunity.**

A BRIEF HISTORY OF COMMUNITY AND PUBLIC HEALTH

The history of community and public health is almost as long as the history of civilization. This brief summary provides an account of some of the accomplishments and failures in community and public health. It is hoped that a knowledge of the past will enable us to better prepare for future challenges to our community's health.

Earliest Civilizations

In all likelihood, the earliest community health practices went unrecorded. Perhaps these practices involved taboos against defecation within the tribal communal area or near the source of drinking water. Perhaps they involved rites associated with burial of the dead. Certainly, the use of herbs for the prevention and curing of diseases and communal assistance with childbirth are practices that predate archeological records.

Ancient Societies (Before 500 B.C.)

Excavations at sites of some of the earliest known civilizations have uncovered evidence of community health activities (see Figure 1.4). Archeological findings from the Indus Valley of northern India,

---

community organizing
a process through which communities are helped to identify common problems or goals, mobilize resources, and in other ways develop and implement strategies for reaching their goals they have collectively set

---

herd immunity
the resistance of a population to the spread of an infectious agent based on the immunity of a high proportion of individuals

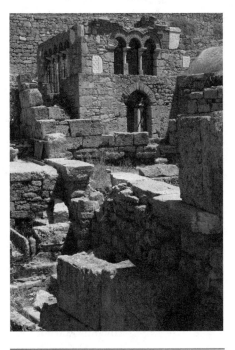

FIGURE 1.4
Archeological findings reveal community health practices of the past.

FIGURE 1.5

The Code of Hammurabi included laws
pertaining to physicians and health practices.

dating from about 2000 B.C., provide evidence of bathrooms and drains in homes and sewers below street level. Drainage systems have also been discovered among the ruins of the Middle Kingdom of ancient Egypt (2700–2000 B.C.). The Myceneans, who lived on Crete in 1600 B.C., had toilets, flushing systems, and sewers.[23] Written medical prescriptions for drugs have been deciphered from a Sumerian clay tablet dated at about 2100 B.C. By 1500 B.C. more than 700 drugs were known to the Egyptians.[24]

Perhaps the earliest written record concerning public health is the Code of Hammurabi, the famous king of Babylon, who lived 3,900 years ago. Hammurabi's code of conduct included laws pertaining to physicians and health practices (see Figure 1.5). The Bible's Book of Leviticus, written about 1500 B.C., provides guidelines for personal cleanliness, sanitation of campsites, disinfection of wells, isolation of lepers, disposal of refuse, and the hygiene of maternity.[25]

Classical Cultures (500 B.C.–A.D. 500)

During the thirteenth and twelfth centuries B.C., the Greeks began to travel to Egypt and continued to do so over the next several centuries. Knowledge from the Babylonians, Egyptians, Hebrews, and other peoples of the eastern Mediterranean was included in the Greeks' philosophy of health and medicine.[24] During the "Golden Age" of ancient Greece (in the sixth and fifth centuries B.C.), men participated in physical games of strength and skill and swam in public facilities. There is little evidence that this emphasis on fitness and on success in athletic competition was imparted equally to all members of the community.[26] Participation in these activities was not encouraged or even permitted for women, the poor, or slaves.

The Greeks were also active in the practice of community sanitation. They supplemented local city wells with water supplied from mountains as far as 10 miles away. In at least one city, water from a distant source was stored in a cistern 370 feet above sea level.[23]

The Romans improved upon the Greek engineering and built aqueducts that could transport water for many miles. Evidence of some 200 Roman aqueducts remains today, from Spain to Syria and from northern Europe to northern Africa. The Romans also built sewer systems and initiated other community health activities, including the regulation of building construction, refuse removal, and street cleaning and repair.[25]

The Roman Empire was the repository for Greek medical ideas, but with few exceptions, the Romans did little to advance medical thinking. However, they did make one important contribution to medicine and health care—the hospital. Although the first hospitals were merely infirmaries for slaves, before the end of the Roman era, Christians had established public hospitals as benevolent charitable organizations.[24] When the Roman Empire eventually fell in A.D. 476, most of the public health activities ceased.

Middle Ages (A.D. 500–1500)

The period from the end of the Roman Empire in the West to about 1500 has become known as the Middle Ages. The Eastern Roman Empire (the Byzantine Empire), with its capital in Constantinople, continued until 1453. While the Greco-Roman legacy of society was largely preserved in the Eastern Roman Empire, it was lost to most of western Europe. Most of what knowledge remained was preserved only in the churches and monasteries.

The medieval approach to health and disease differed greatly from that of the Roman Empire. During this time, there was a growing revulsion for Roman materialism and a growth of spirituality. Health problems were considered to have both spiritual causes and spiritual solutions.[23] This was especially true at the beginning of the Middle Ages, during a period known as the Dark Ages (500–1000). Both pagan rites and Christian beliefs blamed disease on supernatural causes. St. Augustine, for example, taught that diseases were caused by demons sent to torment the human spirit, and most Christians generally believed that disease was a punishment for sins.[24]

The failure to take into account the role of the physical and biological environment in the causation of communicable diseases resulted in the failure to control the unrelenting epidemics during this **spiritual era of public health.** These epidemics were responsible for the suffering and death of millions. One of the earliest recorded epidemic diseases was leprosy. It has been estimated that by 1200, there were 19,000 leper houses and leprosaria in Europe.[23]

The deadliest of the epidemic diseases of the period was the plague. It is hard for us, living here in the twenty-first century, to imagine the impact of plague on Europe. Three great epidemics of plague occurred: The first began in A.D. 543, the second in 1348, and the last in 1664. The worst epidemic occurred in the fourteenth century, when the disease became known as the "black death." An estimated 25 million people died in Europe alone. This is more than the total number of people who live in the states of Ohio and Pennsylvania today. Half of the population of London was lost, and in some parts of France only 1 in 10 survived.[25]

The Middle Ages also saw epidemics of other recognizable diseases, including smallpox, diphtheria, measles, influenza, tuberculosis, anthrax, and trachoma. Many other diseases, unidentifiable at the time, took their toll. The last epidemic disease of this period was syphilis, which appeared in 1492. This, like the other epidemics, killed thousands.

> **spiritual era of public health**
> a time during the Middle Ages when the causation of communicable disease was linked to spiritual forces

Renaissance and Exploration (1500–1700)

The Renaissance period was characterized by a rebirth of thinking about the nature of the world and of humankind. There was an expansion of trade between cities and nations and an increase in population concentrations in large cities. This period was also characterized by exploration and discovery. The travels of Columbus, Magellan, and many other explorers eventually ushered in a period of colonialism. The effects of the Renaissance on community health were substantial. A more careful accounting of disease outbreaks during this period revealed that diseases such as the plague killed saints and sinners alike. There was a growing belief that diseases were caused by environmental, not spiritual, factors. For example, the term *malaria,* meaning bad air, is a distinct reference to the humid or swampy air that often harbors mosquitoes that transmit malaria.

More critical observations of the sick led to more accurate descriptions of symptoms and outcomes of disease. These observations led to the first recognition of whooping cough, typhus, scarlet fever, and malaria as distinct and separate diseases.[23]

Epidemics of smallpox, malaria, and plague were still rampant in England and throughout Europe. In 1665, the plague took 68,596 lives in London, which at the time had a population of 460,000 (a population loss of almost 15%). Explorers, conquerors, and merchants and their crews spread disease to colonists and indigenous people throughout the New World. Smallpox, measles, and other diseases ravaged the unprotected natives.

The Eighteenth Century

The eighteenth century was characterized by industrial growth. In spite of the beginnings of recognition of the nature of disease, living conditions were hardly conducive to good health. Cities were overcrowded, and water supplies were inadequate and often unsanitary. Streets

FIGURE 1.6
Prior to the elimination of smallpox, millions died or were severely disfigured by the disease.

were usually unpaved, filthy, and heaped with trash and garbage. Many homes had unsanitary dirt floors.

Workplaces were unsafe and unhealthy. A substantial portion of the workforce was made up of the poor, which included children, who were forced to work long hours as indentured servants. Many of these jobs were unsafe or involved working in unhealthy environments, such as textile factories and coal mines.

One medical advance made at the end of the eighteenth century deserves mention because of its significance for public health. In 1796, Dr. Edward Jenner successfully demonstrated the process of vaccination as a protection against smallpox. He did this by inoculating a boy with material from a cowpox (*Vaccinia*) pustule. When challenged later with material from a smallpox (*Variola*) pustule, the boy remained healthy.

Dr. Jenner's discovery remains as one of the great discoveries of all time for both medicine and for public health. Prior to Dr. Jenner's discovery, millions died or were severely disfigured by smallpox (see Figure 1.6). The only known prevention had been "variolation," inoculation with smallpox material itself. This was a risky procedure because people sometimes became quite ill with smallpox. Nonetheless, during the American Revolution, General George Washington ordered the Army of the American Colonies "variolated." He did this so that he could be sure an epi-

---

A. Early Civilizations
   1. Ancient Societies (prior to 500 B.C.)
      a. Prior to 2000 B.C.: archeological findings provide evidence of sewage disposal and written medical prescriptions for drugs
      b. Ca. 1900 B.C.: Code of Hammurabi created; includes laws for physicians and health practices
      c. Ca. 1500 B.C.: Book of Leviticus written; includes guidelines for personal cleanliness and sanitation
   2. Classical Cultures (500 B.C.–A.D. 500)
      a. Fifth and sixth centuries B.C.: Evidence that Greek men participated in physical games
      b. Greeks involved in public sanitation
      c. Romans built aqueducts and created hospitals

B. Middle Ages (A.D. 500–1500)
   1. A.D. 500–1000 (Dark Ages): most thought health problems and solutions were spiritual in nature
   2. Epidemics a concern (e.g., plague epidemics in A.D. 543 and 1348)
   3. A.D. 1200: over 19,000 leper houses
   4. A.D. 1492: syphilis epidemic was last epidemic of period

C. Renaissance and Exploration (1500–1700)
   1. Belief that disease was caused by environmental, not spiritual, factors
   2. Epidemics (e.g., smallpox, malaria, and plague) still rampant

D. Eighteenth Century (1700s)
   1. Period characterized by industrial growth; workplaces were unsafe and unhealthy
   2. 1790: first U.S. census
   3. 1793: yellow fever epidemic in Philadelphia
   4. 1796: Dr. Edward Jenner successfully demonstrated smallpox vaccination
   5. 1798: Marine Hospital Service (forerunner to U.S. Public Health Service) was formed
   6. By 1799: several of America's largest cities, including Boston, Philadelphia, New York, and Baltimore, had municipal boards of health

E. First Half of Nineteenth Century (1800–1848)
   1. U.S. government's approach to health is laissez faire
   2. 1813: first visiting nurse in United States

FIGURE 1.7
Brief history of community and public health prior to the modern era of public health (ca. 1850).

demic of smallpox would not wipe out his colonial forces.[23] Interestingly enough, the average age at death for one living in the United States during this time was 29 years.

Following the American Revolution, George Washington ordered the first U.S. census for the purpose of the apportionment of representation in the House of Representatives. The census, first taken in 1790, is still conducted every 10 years and serves as an invaluable source of information for community health planning.

As the eighteenth century came to a close, a young United States faced numerous disease problems, including continuing outbreaks of smallpox, cholera, typhoid fever, and yellow fever. Yellow fever outbreaks usually occurred in port cities such as Charleston, Baltimore, New York, and New Orleans, where ships arrived to dock from tropical America. The greatest single epidemic of yellow fever in America occurred in Philadelphia in 1793, where there were an estimated 23,000 cases, including 4,044 deaths in a population estimated at only 37,000.[27]

In response to these continuing epidemics and the need to address other mounting health problems, such as sanitation and protection of the water supply, several governmental health agencies were created. In 1798, the Marine Hospital Service (forerunner to the U.S. Public Health Service) was formed to deal with disease that was occurring onboard water vessels. By 1799, several of America's largest cities, including Boston, Philadelphia, New York, and Baltimore, also had founded municipal boards of health.

The Nineteenth Century

During the first half of the nineteenth century, few remarkable advancements in public health occurred (see Figure 1.7). Living conditions in Europe and England remained unsanitary, and industrialization led to an even greater concentration of the population within cities. However, better agricultural methods led to improved nutrition for many.

During this period, America enjoyed westward expansion, characterized by a spirit of pioneering, self-sufficiency, and rugged individualism. The federal government's approach to health problems was characterized by the French term *laissez faire,* meaning noninterference. There were also few health regulations or health departments in rural areas. Health quackery thrived; this was truly a period when "buyer beware" was good advice.

Epidemics continued in major cities in both Europe and America. In 1854, another cholera epidemic struck London. Dr. John Snow studied the epidemic and hypothesized that the disease was being caused by the drinking water from the Broad Street pump. He obtained permission to remove the pump handle, and the epidemic was abated (see Figure 1.8). Snow's action was remarkable because it predated the discovery that microorganisms can cause disease. The predominant theory of contagious disease at the time was the "miasmas theory." According to this theory, vapors, or miasmas, were the source of many diseases. The miasmas theory remained popular throughout much of the nineteenth century.

In the United States in 1850, Lemuel Shattuck drew up a health report for the Commonwealth of Massachusetts that outlined the public health needs for the state. It included recommendations for the establishment of boards of health, the collection of vital statistics, the implementation of sanitary measures, and research on diseases. Shattuck also recommended health education and controlling exposure to alcohol, smoke, adulterated food, and nostrums (quack medicines).[25] Although some of his recommendations took years to

FIGURE 1.8

In London, England, 1854, John Snow helped interrupt a cholera epidemic by having the handle removed from this pump, located on Broad Street.

reform phase (1900–1920), the 1920s, the Great Depression and World War II, and the postwar years.

The Reform Phase (1900–1920)

By the beginning of the twentieth century, there was a growing concern about the many social problems in America. The remarkable discoveries in microbiology made in the previous years had not dramatically improved the health of the average citizen. By 1910, the urban population had grown to 45% of the total population (up from 19% in 1860). Much of the growth was the result of immigrants who came to America for the jobs created by new industries (see Figure 1.9). Northern cities were also swelling from the northward migration of black Americans from the southern states. Many of these workers had to accept poorly paying jobs involving hard labor and low wages. There was also a deepening chasm between the upper and lower classes, and social critics began to clamor for reform.

The years 1900 to 1920 have been called the **reform phase of public health.** The plight of the immigrants working in the meat packing industry was graphically depicted by Upton Sinclair in his book *The Jungle*. Sinclair's goal was to draw attention to unsafe working

reform phase of public health the years of 1900–1920, characterized by social movements to improve health conditions in cities and in the workplace

11164-U. S. Inspectors examining eyes of immigrants, Ellis Island, New York Harbor.   Copyright Underwood & Underwood. U-97328

FIGURE 1.9

Ellis Island immigration between 1860 and 1910 resulted in dramatic increases in the urban population in America.

conditions. What he achieved was greater governmental regulation of the food industry through the passage of the Pure Food and Drugs Act of 1906.

The reform movement was broad, involving both social and moral as well as health issues. Edward T. Devine noted in 1909 that "Ill health is perhaps the most constant of the attendants of poverty."[28] The reform movement finally took hold when it became evident to the majority that neither the discoveries of the causes of many communicable diseases nor the continuing advancement of industrial production could overcome continuing disease and poverty. Even by 1917, the United States ranked fourteenth of sixteen "progressive" nations in maternal death rate.[28]

Although the relationship between occupation and disease had been pointed out 200 years earlier in Europe, occupational health in America in 1900 was an unknown quantity. However, in 1910 the first International Congress on Occupational Diseases was held in Chicago.[29] That same year, the state of New York passed a tentative Workman's Compensation Act, and over the next 10 years most other states passed similar laws.[20] Also in 1910, the U.S. Bureau of Mines was created and the first clinic for occupational diseases was established in New York at Cornell Medical College.[28] By 1910, the movement for healthier conditions in the workplace was well established.

This period also saw the birth of the first national-level volunteer health agencies. The first of these agencies was the National Association for the Study and Prevention of Tuberculosis, which was formed in 1902. It arose from the first local voluntary health agency, the Pennsylvania Society for the Prevention of Tuberculosis, organized in 1892.[30] The American Cancer Society, Inc., was founded in 1913. That same year, the Rockefeller Foundation was established in New York. This philanthropic foundation has funded a great many public health projects, including work on hookworm and pellagra, and the development of a vaccine against yellow fever.

Another movement that began about this time was that of public health nursing. The first school nursing program was begun in New York City in 1902. In 1918, the first School of Public Health was established at Johns Hopkins University in Baltimore. This was followed by establishment of another school at Harvard University in 1923. Also in 1918 was the birth of school health instruction as we know it today.

These advances were matched with similar advances by governmental bodies. The Marine Hospital Service was renamed the Public Health and Marine Hospital Service in 1902 in keeping with its growing responsibilities. In 1912, it became the U.S. Public Health Service.[25]

By 1900, 38 states had state health departments. The rest followed during the first decades of the twentieth century. The first two local (county) health departments were established in 1911, one in Guilford County, North Carolina, and the other in Yakima County, Washington.

The 1920s
In comparison with the preceding period, the 1920s represented a decade of slow growth in public health, except for a few health projects funded by the Rockefeller and Millbank foundations. Prohibition resulted in a decline in the number of alcoholics and alcohol-related deaths. While the number of county health departments had risen to 467 by 1929, 77% of the rural population still lived in areas with no health services.[30] However, it was during this period in 1922 that the first professional preparation program for health educators was begun at Columbia University by Thomas D. Wood, M.D., whom many consider the father of health education. The life expectancy in 1930 had risen to 59.7 years.

The Great Depression and World War II
Until the Great Depression (1929–1935), individuals and families in need of social and medical services were dependent on friends and relatives, private charities, voluntary agencies, com-

munity chests, and churches. By 1933, after three years of economic depression, it became evident that private resources could never meet the needs of all the people who needed assistance. The drop in tax revenues during the Depression also reduced health department budgets and caused a virtual halt in the formation of new local health departments.[30]

Beginning in 1933, President Franklin D. Roosevelt created numerous agencies and programs for public works as part of his New Deal. Much of the money was used for public health, including the control of malaria, the building of hospitals and laboratories, and the construction of municipal water and sewer systems.

The Social Security Act of 1935 marked the beginning of the government's major involvement in social issues, including health. This act provided substantial support for state health departments and their programs, such as maternal and child health and sanitary facilities. As progress against the communicable diseases became visible, some turned their attention toward other health problems, such as cancer. The National Cancer Institute was formed in 1937.

America's involvement in World War II resulted in severe restrictions on resources available for public health programs. Immediately following the conclusion of the war, however, many of the medical discoveries made during wartime made their way into civilian medical practice. Two examples are the antibiotic penicillin, used for treating pneumonia, rheumatic fever, syphilis, and strep throat, and the insecticide DDT, used for killing insects that transmit diseases.

During World War II, the Communicable Disease Center was established in Atlanta, Georgia. Now called the Centers for Disease Control and Prevention (CDC), it has become the premier epidemiological center of the world.

The Postwar Years

Following the end of World War II, there was still concern about medical care and the adequacy of the facilities in which that care could be administered. In 1946, Congress passed the National Hospital Survey and Construction Act (the Hill-Burton Act). The goal of the legislation was to improve the distribution of medical care and to enhance the quality of hospitals. From 1946 through the 1960s, hospital construction occurred at a rapid rate with relatively little thought given to planning. Likewise, attempts to set national health priorities or to establish a national health agenda were virtually nonexistent.

The two major health events in the 1950s were the development of a vaccine to prevent polio and President Eisenhower's heart attack. The latter event helped America to focus on its Number 1 killer, heart disease. When the president's physician suggested exercise, some Americans heeded his advice and began to exercise on a regular basis.

Period of Social Engineering (1960–1973)

The 1960s marked the beginning of a period when the federal government once again became active in health matters. The primary reason for this involvement was the growing realization that many Americans were still not reaping any of the benefits of 60 years of medical advances. These Americans, most of whom were poor or elderly, either lived in underserved areas or simply could not afford to purchase medical services.

In 1965, Congress passed the Medicare and Medicaid bills (amendments to the Social Security Act of 1935). **Medicare** assists in the payment of medical bills for the elderly and certain people with disabilities, and **Medicaid** assists in the payment of medical bills for the poor. These pieces of legislation helped provide medical care for millions who would not otherwise have received it, and this legislation also improved standards in health care facilities. Unfortunately, the influx of federal dollars accelerated the rate of increase in the cost of health care for everyone. As a result, the 1970s, 1980s, and the 1990s saw repeated attempts and failures to bring the growing costs of health care under control.

Medicare
government health insurance for the elderly and those with certain disabilities

Medicaid
government health insurance for the poor

Period of Health Promotion (1974–present)

By the mid-1970s, it had become apparent that the greatest potential for saving lives and reducing health care costs in America was to be achieved through means other than health care.

> Most scholars, policymakers, and practitioners in health promotion would pick 1974 as the turning point that marks the beginning of health promotion as a significant component of national health policy in the twentieth century. That year Canada published its landmark policy statement, *A New Perspective on the Health of Canadians*.[31] In [1976] the United States, Congress passed PL 94-317, the Health Information and Health Promotion Act, which created the Office of Health Information and Health Promotion, later renamed the Office of Disease Prevention and Health Promotion.[32]

In the late 1970s, the Centers for Disease Control conducted a study that examined premature deaths (defined then as deaths prior to age 65, but now as deaths prior to age 75) in the United States in 1977. That study revealed that approximately 48% of all premature deaths could be traced to one's lifestyle or health behavior—choices that people make. Lifestyles characterized by a lack of exercise, unhealthy diets, smoking, uncontrolled hypertension, and the inability to control stress were found to be contributing factors to premature mortality.[33] This led the way for the U.S. government's publication *Healthy People: The Surgeon General's Report on Health Promotion and Disease Prevention*.[34] "This document brought together much of what was known about the relationship of personal behavior and health status. The document also presented a 'personal responsibility' model that provided Americans with the prescription for reducing their health risks and increasing their chances for good health."[35]

Healthy People was then followed by the release of the first set of health goals and objectives for the nation, called *Promoting Health/Preventing Disease: Objectives for the Nation*.[36] These goals and objectives, now in their third edition called ***Healthy People 2010***,[20] have defined the nation's health agenda and guided its health policy since their inception (see Figure 1.10).

Healthy People 2010 the third set of health goals and objectives for the U.S that defines the nation's health agenda and guides its health policy

Community Health in the Early 2000s

Early in the new millennium, it is widely agreed that while decisions about health are an individual's responsibility to a significant degree, society has an obligation to provide an environment in which the achievement of good health is possible and encouraged. Furthermore, many recognize that certain segments of our population whose disease and death rates exceed the general population may require additional resources, including education, in order to achieve good health.

The American people face a number of serious public health problems. These problems include the continuing rise in health care costs, growing environmental concerns, the ever-present lifestyle diseases, emerging and re-emerging communicable diseases, serious substance abuse problems, and disasters, both natural and humanmade. In the paragraphs that follow, we have elaborated on each of these problems briefly because they seem to represent a significant portion of the community health agenda for the years ahead.

Health Care Delivery

Arguably, health care delivery continues to be the single greatest community health challenge in the United States. The exorbitant cost of health care is affecting the entire economy in America. Even though the annual growth rate in national health expenditure slowed during the late 1990s due primarily to the advent of managed care, the United States continues to spend more money on health care than any other industrialized country. In 2006, health care expenditures made up approximately 16.2% of America's gross domestic product, up from 10.2% in 1985. Also in 2006, national health care expenditures totaled $2.2 trillion,

A. Second Half of 19th Century (1848-1900)
 1. 1849,1854: London cholera epidemics
 2. 1850: Modern era of public health begins
 3. 1850: Shattuck's report
 4. 1854: Snow has pump handle removed from Broad Street pump
 5. 1863: Pasteur proposed germ theory
 6. 1872: American Public Health Association founded
 7. 1875-1900: Bacteriological period of public health
 8. 1876: Koch established relationship between a particular microbe and a particular disease.
 9. 1900: Reed announced that yellow fever was transmitted by mosquitos

B. Twentieth Century
 1. Health Resources Development Period (1900-1960)
   a. The Reform Phase (1900-1920)
     • 1902: First national-level voluntary health agency created
     • 1906: Sinclair's *The Jungle* published
     • 1910: First International Congress on Occupational Diseases
     • 1910: 45% of U.S. population was in the cities
     • 1911: First local health department established
     • 1913: American Cancer Society founded
     • 1917: United States ranked 14th of 16 in maternal death rate
     • 1918: Birth of school health instruction
     • 1918: First school of public health established in United States
 2. 1920s
   a. 1922: Wood created first professional preparation program for health educators
   b. 1930: Life expectancy in the United States was 59.7 years
 3. The Great Depression and WWII
   a. 1933: New Deal; included unsuccessful attempt at national health care program
   b. 1935: Social Security Act passed
   c. 1937: National Cancer Institute formed
 4. Postwar Years
   a. 1946: National Hospital Survey and Construction (Hill-Burton) Act passed
   b. 1952: Development of polio vaccine
   c. 1955: Eisenhower's heart attack

C. Period of Social Engineering (1960-1973)
 1. 1965: Medicare and Medicaid bills passed

D. Period of Health Promotion (1974-present)
 1. 1974: Nixon's unsuccessful attempt at national health care program
 2. 1974: *A New Perspective on the Health of Canadians* published
 3. 1976: Health Information and Health Promotion Act passed
 4. 1979: *Healthy People* published
 5. 1980: *Promoting Health/Preventing Disease: Objectives of the Nation* published
 6. 1990: *Health People 2000* published
 7. 1997: Clinton's unsuccessful attempt at a national health care program
 8. 2000: *Health People 2010* published

FIGURE 1.10
Brief history of community and public health from 1848 to 2000.

an average of more than $7,129 per person.[37] If left unchecked, it is estimated that the cost of health care will continue to rise faster than the rate of inflation. It was estimated that total health care expenditures would reach $4 trillion in 2015 and consume 20% of the gross domestic product.[37]

If the costs of health care were not enough, there is still a significant portion of the U.S. population without health care insurance. In 2005, the proportion of the population without health care insurance (either public or private) was approximately 16%. In other words, more than 46.6 million Americans were uninsured throughout 2005. Millions more lacked health insurance coverage for shorter periods during that year.[38]

Environmental Problems

Millions of Americans live in communities where the air is unsafe to breathe, the water is unsafe to drink, or solid waste is disposed of improperly. With a few minor exceptions, the rate at which we pollute our environment continues to increase. Many Americans still believe that our natural resources are unlimited and that their individual contributions to the overall pollution are insignificant. In actuality, we must improve upon our efforts in resource preservation and energy conservation if our children are to enjoy an environment as clean as ours. These environmental problems are compounded by the fact the world population continues to grow; it is now over 6.6 billion people and expected to reach 7.2 billion by the year 2015.[39]

Lifestyle Diseases

The leading causes of death in the United States today are not the communicable diseases that were so feared 100 years ago but chronic illnesses resulting from unwise lifestyle choices. "The prevalence of obesity and diseases like diabetes are increasing."[6] The four leading causes of death in the early 2000s are heart disease, cancer, stroke, and chronic lower respiratory diseases.[40] Although it is true that everyone has to die from some cause sometime, too many Americans die prematurely because of their unhealthy lifestyles. In the latter part of the twentieth century, it was known that better control of behavioral risk factors alone—such as lack of exercise, poor diet, use of tobacco and drugs, and alcohol abuse—could prevent between 40% and 70% of all premature deaths, one-third of all acute disabilities, and two-thirds of chronic disabilities.[41] As we begin the twenty-first century, behavior patterns continue to "represent the single most prominent domain of influence over health prospects in the United States."[10] (See Table 1.1.)

Communicable Diseases

Although communicable (infectious) diseases no longer constitute the leading causes of death in the United States, they remain a concern for several reasons. First, they are the primary reason for days missed at school or at work. The success in reducing the life-threatening

Table 1.1
Comparison of Most Common Causes of Death and Actual Causes of Death

Most Common Causes of Death, United States, 2004	Actual Causes of Death, United States, 2000
1. Diseases of the heart	1. Tobacco
2. Malignant neoplasms (cancers)	2. Poor diet and physical inactivity
3. Cerebrovascular diseases (stroke)	3. Alcohol consumption
4. Chronic lower respiratory diseases	4. Microbial agents
5. Unintentional injuries (accidents)	5. Toxic agents
6. Diabetes mellitus	6. Motor vehicles
7. Alzheimer's disease	7. Firearms
8. Influenza and pneumonia	8. Sexual behavior
9. Nephritis, nephrotic syndrome, and nephrosis	9. Illicit drug use
10. Septicemia	

Sources: Miniño, A. M, M. P. Heron, and B. L. Smith (2006). "Deaths: Preliminary Data for 2004." *National Vital Statistics Reports*, 54(19); Mokdad, A. H., J. S. Marks, D. F. Stroup, and J. L. Gerberding (2004). "Actual Causes of Death, in the United States, 2000." *Journal of the American Medical Association*, 291(10): 1238–1245; and Mokdad, A. H., J. S. Marks, D. F. Stroup, and J. L. Gerberding (2005). "Correction: Actual Causes of Death, in the United States, 2000." *Journal of the American Medical Association*, 293: 293–294.

nature of these diseases has made many Americans complacent about obtaining vaccinations or taking other precautions against contracting these diseases. With the exception of smallpox, none of these diseases has been eradicated although several should have been, such as measles.

Second, as new communicable diseases continue to appear, old ones such as tuberculosis re-emerge, sometimes in drug-resistant forms, demonstrating that communicable diseases still represent a serious community health problem in America. Legionnaires' disease, toxic shock syndrome, Lyme disease, acquired immunodeficiency syndrome (AIDS), and severe acute respiratory syndrome (SARS) are diseases that were unknown only 30 years ago. The first cases of AIDS were reported in June 1981.[42] By August 1989, 100,000 cases had been reported,[43] and it took only an additional two years to report the second 100,000 cases.[44] By June 2006, over a million cases of the disease had been reported to the CDC.[45] (See Figure 1.11.) Also, diseases that were once only found in animals are now crossing over to human populations and causing much concern and action. Included in this group of diseases are avian flu, *Escherichia coli* O157:H7, hantavirus, mad cow disease, and SARS.[1]

Third, and maybe the most disturbing, is the use of communicable diseases for bioterrorism. **Bioterrorism** involves "the threatened or intentional release of biological agents (virus, bacteria, or their toxins) for the purpose of influencing the conduct of government or intimidating or coercing a civilian population to further political or social objectives. These agents can be released by way of the air (as aerosols) food, water or insects."[11] Concern in the United States over bioterrorism was heightened after 9/11 and the subsequent intentional distribution of *Bacillus anthracis* spores through the U.S. postal system (the anthrax mailings). The anthrax mailings resulted in 22 people developing anthrax, 5 of whom died. In addition, thousands more were psychologically affected, and between 10 and 20 thousand people were advised to take postexposure prophylactic treatment because they were at known or potential risk for inhalational anthrax.[46]

FIGURE 1.11
AIDS is one of the most feared communicable diseases today.

bioterrorism
the threatened or intentional release of biological agents for the purpose of influencing the conduct of government or intimidating or coercing a civilian population to further political or social objectives

Alcohol and Other Drug Abuse

"Abuse of legal and illegal drugs has become a national problem that costs this country thousands of lives and billions of dollars each year. Alcohol and other drugs are often associated with unintentional injuries, domestic violence, and violent crimes."[47] Federal, state, and local governments as well as private agencies are attempting to address the supply and demand problems associated with the abuse of alcohol and other drugs, but a significant challenge remains for America.

Disasters

Disasters can be classified into two primary categories—natural (or conventional) and humanmade (or technological disasters).[1,48] Whereas *natural disasters* are the result of the combination of the forces of nature (e.g., hurricane, flood, blizzard, tornado, earthquake, landslide) and human activities,[49] *humanmade disasters* result from either unintentional (e.g., spill of a toxic substance into the environment) or intentional (e.g., bioterrorism) human activities, often associated with the use or misuse of technology. Both types of disasters have the potential to cause injury, death, disease, and damage to property on a large scale.[1] In recent years, the United States has felt the large-scale impact of both types of disasters via 9/11 and Hurricanes Katrina and Rita. Each of these events showed us that the preparation for such disasters was not adequate.

FIGURE 1.12
Terrorism has become a concern thoughout the world.

Even though the causes of the two categories of disasters are different, preparedness for them has many common elements. It has been noted that preparedness for natural disasters is the foundation for preparedness for humanmade disasters.[48] That is, in preparing for natural disasters, the basic components of an adequate disaster response system have been defined, and the steps necessary to build disaster preparedness capacity have been established.[48] What needs to be added are specific steps to deal with the peculiarity of the humanmade disasters. An example of this would be the need for decontamination following exposure to a biological agent.

Even given the devastating consequences of natural disasters, such as Hurricanes Katrina and Rita or the forest fires that consume many thousands of acres of woodlands each year (see Chapter 16 for more on natural disasters), it has been the intentional humanmade disasters—specifically terrorism—that have occupied much of our attention in recent years (see Figure 1.12).

Mention was made earlier of the use of a communicable disease as part of terrorism. However, in fact there are a number of agents that could be used as part of terrorism. Since the anthrax mailings, community and public health professionals have focused on the possibility that future terrorism could include chemical, nuclear/radiological, and/or biological (CNB) agents, resulting in mass numbers of casualties. Such concern led to an evaluation of community and public health emergency preparedness and response. "Determining the level of state and local health departments' emergency preparedness and response capacities is crucial because public health officials are among those, along with firefighters, emergency medical personnel, and local law enforcement personnel, who serve on 'rapid response' teams when large-scale emergency situations arise."[13] Results of that evaluation showed that the public health infrastructure was not where it should be to handle large-scale emergencies, as well as a number of more common public health concerns.

> The . . . public health infrastructure has suffered from political neglect and from the pressure of political agendas and public opinion that frequently override empirical evidence. Under the glare of a national crisis, policy makers and the public became aware of vulnerable and outdated health information systems and technologies, an insufficient and inadequately trained public health workforce, antiquated laboratory capacity, a lack of real-time surveillance and epidemiological systems, ineffective and fragmented communications networks, incomplete domestic preparedness and emergency response capabilities, and communities without access to essential public health services.[13]

Based on the results of several different evaluations that exposed many weaknesses in emergency preparedness in general and in the public health infrastructure more specifically, investment in public health preparedness has increased since September 11, 2001. Those federal departments that have been responsible for most of the effort have been the Departments of Homeland Security (DHS) and Health and Human Services (DHHS). The DHS has the responsibility of protecting America, whereas the DHHS, through the Centers for Disease Control and Prevention and the Health Resources and Services Administration, has worked to improve public health preparedness. The money has been "used for planning, training, improving communication and coordination, strengthening hospitals and laboratories, and improving epidemiology and disease surveillance in state and local areas."[1] Though much of the funding was distributed specifically to improve public health preparedness activities, there was a spillover effect on traditional public health activities. For example, even though funds may have been used to improve laboratory capacity and hire epidemiologists, these same labs and personnel have improved public health capabilities in general, not just for bioterrorism.[50] What must be recognized now is that much of the money that was spent was used for one-time capital invest-ments—such as lab equipment, communications systems, and decontamination equipment—yet there will be an ongoing need for funds to maintain these preparedness efforts.[50]

Even with all the emphasis that has been placed on preparedness since 9/11, both for emer-gencies in general and public health, there is still much to do. In December 2006, the Trust for America's Health (TFAH), a nonprofit, nonpartisan organization, released its report on the state of public health preparedness in the United States.[51] The report, titled *Ready or Not? Pro-tecting the Public's Health from Disease and Bioterrorism, 2006*, contained preparedness scores for all 50 states and the District of Columbia based on 10 key indicators to assess health emergency preparedness capabilities. Half of the states scored 6 or lower, and Oklahoma was the only state to score a 10.[51] Key findings from the report included the following:[51]

- Only 15 states are rated at the highest preparedness level to provide emergency vaccines, antidotes, and medical supplies from the Strategic National Stockpile.
- Twenty-five states would run out of hospital beds within two weeks of a moderate pan-demic flu outbreak.
- Forty states face a shortage of nurses.
- Rates for vaccinating seniors for the seasonal flu decreased in 13 states.
- Eleven states and D.C. lack sufficient capabilities to test for biological threats.
- Four states do not test year-round for the flu, which is necessary to monitor for a pandemic outbreak.
- Six states cut their public health budgets from fiscal year 2005 to 2006; the median rate for state public health spending is $31 per person per year.

The executive director of the TFAH summed up the report by saying, "The nation is nowhere near as prepared as we should be for bioterrorism, bird flu, and other health disasters. We con-tinue to make progress each year, but it is limited. As a whole, Americans face unnecessary and unacceptable levels of risk."[51]

OUTLOOK FOR COMMUNITY HEALTH IN THE TWENTY-FIRST CENTURY

So far in this chapter we have discussed community health, past and present. Now we will describe what community health leaders in the United States and elsewhere in the world hope to achieve in the coming years.

World Planning for the Twenty-First Century

World health leaders recognized the need to plan for the twenty-first century at the thirtieth World Health Assembly of the World Health Organization, held in 1977. At that assembly, del-egations from governments around the world set as a target "that the level of health to be attained by the turn of the century should be that which will permit all people to lead a socially and economically productive life."[52] This target goal became known as "Health for All by the Year 2000." The following year in Alma-Ata, U.S.S.R., the joint WHO/UNICEF (United Nations Children's Fund) International Conference adopted a Declaration on Primary Health Care as the key to attaining the goal of Health for All by the Year 2000. At the thirty-fourth World Health Assembly in 1981, delegates from the member nations unanimously adopted a Global Strategy for Health for All by the Year 2000. That same year, the United Nations

General Assembly endorsed the Global Strategy and urged other international organizations concerned with community health to collaborate with the WHO. The underlying concept of Health for All by the Year 2000 was that health resources should be distributed in such a way that essential health care services are accessible to everyone.

As we now know, the lofty goal of health for all around the world by the year 2000 was not reached. That does not mean that the goal was abandoned. With the passing into a new century, the program was renamed Health for All (HFA). HFA continues to seek "to create the conditions where people have, as a fundamental human right, the opportunity to reach and maintain the highest level of health. The vision of a renewed HFA policy builds on the WHO Constitution, the experience of the past and the needs for the future."[53]

As one might expect with all of the unrest worldwide, the progress to HFA is slow. Yet, some progress has been made. Life expectancy has increased by between six and seven years globally in the last 30 years, due primarily to (1) social and economic development, (2) the wider provision of safe water and sanitation facilities, and (3) the expansion of national health services.[54] However, all do not share in this increased life expectancy. "There are widening health inequities between and within countries, between rich and poor, between men and women, and between different ethnic groups. More than a billion of the world's poorest people are not benefiting from the major advances in health care and several countries, particularly in sub-Saharan Africa, have seen a decline in life expectancy due in part to the HIV/AIDS epidemic."[54]

Although much of the widening health gap is the result of the continuing impact of communicable diseases, global increases in noncommunicable diseases (especially from tobacco use, unhealthy diets, physical inactivity, and alcohol abuse) and unintentional injuries (primarily from road traffic crashes) also play a part. "Chronic noncommunicable diseases, including mental disorders, already represent 60% of the current global disease burden. One quarter of all chronic disease deaths occur in people under 60 years of age."[54] Further, "road traffic incidents kill an estimated 1.2 million people annually, injuring as many as 5.2 million. Over 70% of road traffic fatalities are under 45 years of age. Projections indicate that the number of road traffic casualties will increase by about 65% over the next 20 years unless there is a new commitment to prevention."[54]

The 2006 World Health Report of the WHO, *Working Together for Health*, provides a good summary of current global health:

> In this first decade of the 21st century, immense advances in human well-being coexist with extreme deprivation. In global health we are witnessing the benefits of new medicines and technologies. But there are unprecedented reversals. Life expectancies have collapsed in some of the poorest countries to half the level of the richest—attributable to the ravages of HIV/AIDS in parts of sub-Saharan Africa and to more than a dozen "failed states". These setbacks have been accompanied by growing fears, in rich and poor countries alike, of new infectious threats such as SARS and avian influenza and "hidden" behavioural conditions such as mental disorders and domestic violence.[55]

In other words, there is still much to do, and in some situations the challenges are daunting (see Table 1.2 for titles and summaries of recent World Health Reports). Nonetheless, WHO has outlined its work ahead (2006–2015) in the *11th General Programme of Work*. The WHO constitution requires that the executive board of WHO submit a general program of work for its governing body to consider. In the eleventh report, five areas have been identified as those from which the work priorities will come:

a. **Providing support to countries in moving to universal coverage with effective public health interventions.** This applies particularly to areas such as communicable and noncommunicable disease prevention and control and research; sexual and reproductive health; infant,

Table 1.2
World Health Reports

The World Health Report 2006: Working Together for Health

This report contains an expert assessment of the current crisis in the global health workforce and ambitious proposals to tackle it over the next 10 years, starting immediately. The report reveals an estimated shortage of almost 4.3 million doctors, midwives, nurses, and support workers worldwide. The shortage is most severe in the poorest countries, especially in sub-Saharan Africa, where health workers are most needed. Focusing on all stages of the health workers' career lifespan from entry to health training, to job recruitment through to retirement, the report lays out a 10-year action plan in which countries can build their health workforces, with the support of global partners.

The World Health Report 2005: Make Every Mother and Child Count

This year almost 11 million children under 5 years of age will die from causes that are largely preventable. Among them are 4 million babies who will not survive the first month of life. At the same time, more than half a million women will die in pregnancy, childbirth, or soon after. The report says that reducing this toll in line with the Millennium Development Goals depends largely on every mother and every child having the right to access to health care from pregnancy through childbirth, the neonatal period, and childhood.

The World Health Report 2004: Changing History

The 2004 report calls for a comprehensive HIV/AIDS strategy that links prevention, treatment, care, and long-term support. At a crucial moment in the pandemic's history, the international community has an unprecedented opportunity to alter its course and simultaneously fortify health systems for the enduring benefit of all.

The World Health Report 2003: Shaping the Future

The 2003 report examines the global health situation and some of the major threats to health in today's world. Drawing on many examples, the report suggests that major improvements in health for everybody are within reach, and that progress depends on collaboration among governments, international institutions, the private sector, and civil society to build stronger health systems.

The World Health Report 2002: Reducing Risks, Promoting Healthy Life

The 2002 report describes the amount of disease, disability, and death in the world today that can be attributed to a selected number of the most important risks to human health. It also shows how much this burden could be lowered in the next 20 years if the same risk factors were reduced.

The World Health Report 2001: Mental Health—New Understanding, New Hope

The 2001 report focuses on the fact that mental health—neglected for far too long—is crucial to the overall well-being of individuals, societies, and countries. The report advocates policies that are urgently needed to ensure that stigma and discrimination are broken down and that effective prevention and treatment are put in place.

Source: World Health Organization (2007). *The World Health Report.* Available at http://www.who.int/whr/2006/en/index.html and http://www.who.int/whr/previous/en/index.html.

child, adolescent and maternal health and the health of older persons; environment-related health problems, and effective responses in times of crisis.

b. **Strengthening global health security.** This should further support an integrated approach to a society-wide response to emerging and acute threats to health, including disaster and conflict situations, and incorporate preparedness planning for such threats.

c. **Generating and sustaining action across sectors to modify the behavioural, social, economic and environmental determinants of health.** This will focus on minimizing lifestyle-related risk factors, advocating action on the broad social and economic determinants of ill health, and promoting healthier and safer physical environments, better nutrition, food safety, and food security.

d. **Increasing institutional capacities to deliver core public health functions under the strengthened governance of ministries of health.** This area covers support for the development of health systems, including human resources for health, that promote equitable health gains and better respond to men's and women's different needs; that improve quality, norms, efficacy and safety; that have effective leadership and governance; and that extend social protection through fair, adequate and sustainable financing.

e. Strengthening WHO's leadership at global and regional levels and by supporting the work of governments at country level. The secretariat will strengthen its ability to take forward its core functions through its reform process around results-based management, through strengthening WHO's work in countries, monitoring norms and standards in countries, improving its mechanisms for knowledge management, investing in staff development, and ensuring sustainable sources of financing. Externally it will strengthen its work on partnerships and engage more deeply in the United Nations reform process, with a view to strengthening the response to the global health agenda, and to improving overall efficiency.[54]

As might be inferred from these stated priority areas, much of the attention for improved world health in the twenty-first century is focused on the less developed and poorer countries of the world. The plan for tackling these global health challenges and other non-health-related global challenges of the twenty-first century is guided by the *United Nations Millennium Declaration,*[56] which was adopted at the United Nations' Millennium Summit in September 2000. More information about the declaration is presented in Chapter 2 in the section that discusses the WHO.

The United States' Planning for the Twenty-First Century

In addition to its participation in WHO's plans for the twenty-first century, the United States has created its own plans. The United States has decided to develop its planning process around 10-year blocks of time. The current plan is called *Healthy People 2010.*[20] As noted earlier in this chapter, *Healthy People 2010* and its two predecessor editions do in fact outline the health agenda of the nation. Some have referred to the *Healthy People* documents as the health blueprint of the nation. Each of these documents obviously is created on the best available data at the time, but all have been structured in a similar way. All three editions have included several overarching goals and many supporting objectives for the nation's health. The goals provide a general focus and direction, while the objectives are used to measure progress within a specified period of time.[20] For example, in 2001 when the *Healthy People 2000 Final Review* document was released, it showed that 21% of the year 2000 objectives met their targets, 41% showed movement toward their targets, 11% showed mixed results, 2% showed no movement from the baseline, 15% moved away from their targets, and 10% could not be assessed because of a lack of data.[57] Based on this measured progress and other available data, the *Healthy People 2010* document was created.

Healthy People 2010 is the most sophisticated Healthy People planning document to date, which is reflective of the planning that went into creating it. The *Healthy People 2010* document is composed of three parts. *Healthy People 2010: Understanding and Improving Health,* the first part, provides a history of *Healthy People 2010* and the overall Healthy People initiative. This section also presents the Determinants of Health model (see Figure 1.13) on which Healthy People is based, describes how to use Healthy People as a systematic approach to health improvement, and defines the Leading Health Indicators (LHIs). The LHIs are new to the *Healthy People* document and were created to provide a snapshot of the health of the nation. *Healthy People 2010* identifies 10 LHIs: physical activity, overweight and obesity, tobacco use, substance abuse, responsible sexual behavior, mental health, injury and violence, environmental quality, immunization, and access to health care. The LHIs highlight major health priorities for the nation and include the individual behaviors, physical and social environmental factors, and health system issues that affect the health of individuals and communities. Each of the 10 LHIs has one or more Healthy People measures associated with it and will be used to measure progress throughout the decade.[20]

The second part of the document, *Healthy People 2010: Objectives for Improving Health,* contains the two overarching goals and detailed descriptions of 467 objectives to improve health. The two overarching goals for *Healthy People 2010* are as follows:

1. Increase quality and years of healthy life.
2. Eliminate health disparities.

The first goal is a carryover from the *Healthy People 2000* goals and has the aim to help individuals of all ages increase the quality and years of healthy life, while the second strengthens a previous goal by using the words "eliminate health disparities" instead of the previous wording of "reduce health disparities." These two goals are supported by specific objectives in 28 focus areas (see Table 1.3).

In the document, each focus area is presented as a chapter. Each chapter contains a concise goal statement that frames the overall purpose of the area, an overview of the health issue that provides the context and background for the objectives, an interim progress report on progress toward the year 2000 objectives, and the 2010 objectives. There are two types of objectives—measurable and developmental. The measurable objectives provide direction for action and include national baseline data from which the 2010 target was set. The developmental objectives provide a vision for a desired outcome or health status, but national baseline data were not available when they were written. The purpose of developmental objectives was to identify areas of emerging importance and to drive the development of data systems to measure them.

The third part of the document, *Tracking Healthy People 2010,* provides a comprehensive review of the statistical measures that will be used to evaluate progress. The purpose of this third part is to provide technical information so that others will be able to understand how the data are derived and the major statistical issues affecting the interpretation of the statistics. This is the first set of Healthy People objectives to have such a section.[20]

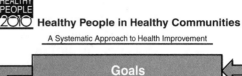

Healthy People in Healthy Communities

A Systematic Approach to Health Improvement

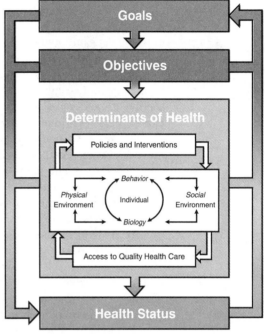

FIGURE 1.13

Healthy people in healthy communities.

Source: U.S. Department of Health and Human Services (2000). *Healthy People 2010.* Available at http://www.healthypeople.gov.

Table 1.3
Healthy People 2010 **Focus Areas**

1. Access to Quality Health Services	15. Injury and Violence Prevention
2. Arthritis, Osteoporosis, and Chronic Back Conditions	16. Maternal, Infant, and Child Health
3. Cancer	17. Medical Product Safety
4. Chronic Kidney Disease	18. Mental Health and Mental Disorders
5. Diabetes	19. Nutrition/Overweight
6. Disability and Secondary Conditions	20. Occupational Safety and Health
7. Educational and Community-Based Programs	21. Oral Health
8. Environmental Health	22. Physical Activity and Fitness
9. Family Planning	23. Public Health Infrastructure
10. Food Safety	24. Respiratory Diseases
11. Health Communication	25. Sexually Transmitted Diseases
12. Heart Disease and Stroke	26. Substance Abuse
13. HIV	27. Tobacco Use
14. Immunization and Infectious Diseases	28. Vision and Hearing

Source: U.S. Department of Health and Human Services (2000). *Healthy People 2010.* Available at http://www.healthypeople.gov.

Like the earlier versions of the Healthy People planning documents, *Healthy People 2010* had a midcourse review. Midway through the decade, the review assessed the status of the two overarching goals and national objectives. The purpose of the review was to assess the data trends for the first half of the decade, consider new science and available data, and make changes to ensure that *Healthy People 2010* remained current, accurate, and relevant, while concurrently assessing emerging public health priorities. The midcourse review was based on available data and public comments on suggested changes for objectives and subobjectives.[58]

With regard to the two overarching goals, some progress is being made, but the inability to measure the complex interactions of health, disease, disability, and early death make it difficult to quantify some of the progress. A review of the data to assess the first goal of increasing the quality and years of healthy life revealed that years of life—measured in terms of life expectancy—continue to increase. However, significant gender and racial and ethnic differences remain. Women and whites continue to live longer than their comparison groups. Although life expectancy has continued to increase, the United States continues to have lower life expectancy than many other developed nations. Data for two measures of healthy life expectancy—expected years in good or better health and expected years free of activity limitations—showed slight improvements; however, a third measure of healthy life expectancy—expected years free of selected chronic diseases—declined slightly.[59]

The midcourse review did show that there has been widespread improvements in rates for most of the populations associated with the social and demographic characteristics included in the second goal—eliminating disparities among segments of the population; however, there is little evidence of systematic reductions in disparity. Disparities—measured in terms of relative differences from the best group rate—are generally not declining. That is to say, the health gap between certain racial and ethnic groups is getting wider. Unless greater reductions occur for the populations with the highest rates, disparities will not be eliminated.[59]

The midcourse review of the objectives provided not only an opportunity to measure the progress but also to make changes to the objectives if necessary. Thus, the midcourse review yielded several changes. They included (1) establishing baselines and targets for developmental objectives, (2) changing the wording of, deleting, or adding new objectives, and (3) revising baselines and targets.[58] Of the 467 *Healthy People 2010* objectives, 28 (6%) were dropped after the midcourse review because data were not available to track them or because of a change in science; another 158 (34%) of the objectives had no data on which to track their progress. However, of this 158, it was anticipated that data would be available by the end of the decade to assess 87 of these objectives. This left 281 objectives for which progress could be assessed at midcourse (see left side of Figure 1.14). As can be seen on the right side of Figure 1.14, a total of 59% of 281 objectives either moved toward the 2010 target or met or exceeded the target.[58] However, it is clear that much work remains to be done.

When *Healthy People 2010* was written, no one envisioned what would transpire on 9/11 and in the years to follow. Thus, the threats of terrorism and bioterrorism were not specifically reflected in the original *Healthy People 2010* document.

However, the midcourse review of *Healthy People 2010* provided an opportunity to update the document based on the events of the first half of the decade. Two focus areas of *Healthy People 2010* that were influenced by these events were areas 11 (Health Communication) and 23 (Public Health Infrastructure). With regard to health communication, greater emphasis was placed on the major challenges to health communication among first responders and with the public. As noted in the midcourse review, if we are going to be appropriately prepared, both first responders and the public must have access to trusted sources and reliable information.

Concern regarding the public health infrastructure in the United States cannot be overstated. Even though the public health infrastructure was a concern when *Healthy People 2010*

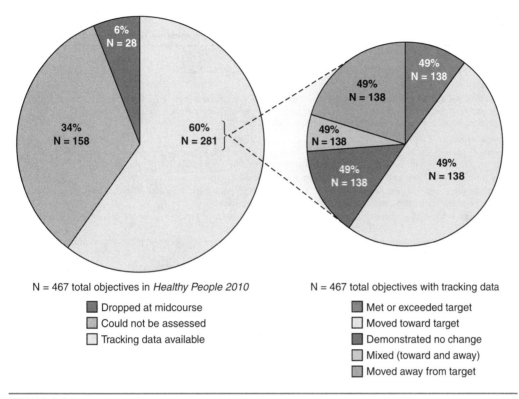

N = 467 total objectives in *Healthy People 2010*

■ Dropped at midcourse
□ Could not be assessed
□ Tracking data available

N = 467 total objectives with tracking data

■ Met or exceeded target
□ Moved toward target
■ Demonstrated no change
□ Mixed (toward and away)
■ Moved away from target

FIGURE 1.14

Healthy People 2010 objectives: status at the midcourse and summary of progress toward target attainment.

Source: U.S. Department of Health and Human Services (2006). *Healthy People 2010: Midcourse Review Executive Summary.*
Available at http://www.healthypeople.gov/data/midcourse/html/introduction.htm.

was initially published, the events of 9/11 and Hurricanes Katrina and Rita showed the public how woefully inadequate the infrastructure really was. Prior to the midcourse review, as noted earlier in the chapter, much had been done to improve the infrastructure, yet much work still remains to be completed and maintained.

Not only did the midcourse review of *Healthy People 2010* reflect a reaction to the events of 9/11, but so did the Homeland Security Act of 2002, which created the Department of Homeland Security (DHS). The DHS became the nation's fifteenth and newest cabinet department in January 2003, consolidating 22 previously disparate agencies under one unified organization.[60] It was felt that a new federal agency was needed to provide the unifying core for the vast national network of organizations and institutions involved in efforts to secure the nation (see Table 1.4 for the vision and mission statements and the strategic goals of DHS).[61] The DHS was guided during its first two years by Secretary Tom Ridge. In 2005, after Secretary Ridge stepped down, Michael Chertoff took over as the secretary. Shortly after taking office, secretary Chertoff had the DHS undergo the second-stage review, a careful study of the department's programs, policies, operations, and structure. The review was conducted "in order to recommend ways that DHS could better manage risk in terms of threat, vulnerability and consequence; prioritize policies and operational missions according to this risk-based approach; and establish a series of preventive and protective steps that would increase security at multiple levels."[62] As a result of the review, a six-point agenda for the DHS was developed and

---

Table 1.4
Vision, Mission, and Strategic Goals of the Department of Homeland Security

---

Vision
Preserving our freedoms, protecting America . . . we secure our homeland.

Mission
We will lead the unified national effort to secure America. We will prevent and deter terrorist attacks and protect against and respond to threats and hazards to the nation. We will ensure safe and secure borders, welcome lawful immigrants and visitors, and promote the free flow of commerce.

Strategic Goals
Awareness: Identify and understand threats, assess vulnerabilities, determine potential impacts, and disseminate timely information to our homeland security partners and the American public.
Prevention: Detect, deter, and mitigate threats to our homeland.
Protection: Safeguard our people and their freedoms, critical infrastructure, property, and the economy of our nation from acts of terrorism, natural disasters, or other emergencies.
Response: Lead, manage, and coordinate the national response to acts of terrorism, natural disasters, or other emergencies.
Recovery: Lead national, state, local, and private sector efforts to restore services and rebuild communities after acts of terrorism, natural disasters, or other emergencies.
Service: Serve the public effectively by facilitating lawful trade, travel, and immigration.
Organizational Excellence: Value our most important resource, our people. Create a culture that promotes a common identity, innovation, mutual respect, accountability, and teamwork to achieve efficiencies, effectiveness, and operational synergies.

Source: U.S. Department of Homeland Security (DHS) (2006). "DHS Organization." Available at http://www.dhs.gov/.

---

announced in July 2006. The six-point agenda was structured to guide the department and work toward changes that would

- Increase overall preparedness, particularly for catastrophic events;
- Create better transportation security systems to move people and cargo more securely and efficiently
- Strengthen border security and interior enforcement and reform immigration processes;
- Enhance information sharing with our partners; and
- Improve DHS financial management, human resource development, procurement, and information technology.[62]

As the DHS matures, its work and responsibilities will continue to evolve and will surely affect preparedness for all types of disasters.

As can be seen from the previous discussion, much planning and work have taken place to improve the health and safety of populations in the twenty-first century. Yet,

> The systems and the entities that protect and promote the public's health, already challenged by problems like obesity, toxic environments, a large uninsured population, and health disparities, must also confront emerging threats, such as antimicrobial resistance and bioterrorism. The social, cultural, and global contexts of the nation's health are also undergoing rapid and dramatic change. Scientific and technological advances, such as genomics and informatics, extend the limits of knowledge and human potential more rapidly than their implications can be absorbed and acted upon. At the same time, people, products, and germs migrate and the nation's demographics are shifting in ways that challenge public and private resources.[13]

Even with so much change and the many uncertainties about the future, we must stay focused on what is necessary to gain and maintain health for all. There is still much work ahead!

CHAPTER SUMMARY

- A number of key terms are associated with the study of community health, including *health, community, community health, population health, public health,* and *public health system.*

- The four factors that affect the health of a community are physical (e.g., community size), social and cultural (e.g., religion), community organization, and individual behaviors (e.g., exercise and diet).

- It is important to be familiar with and understand the history of community health in order to be able to deal with the present and future community health issues.

- The earliest community health practices went unrecorded; however, archeological findings of ancient societies (before 500 B.C.) show evidence of concern for community health. There is evidence during the time of the classical cultures (500 B.C.–A.D. 500) that people were interested in physical strength, medicine, and sanitation.

- The belief of many living during the Middle Ages (A.D. 500–1500) was that health and disease were associated with spirituality. Many epidemics were seen during this period.

- During the Renaissance period (A.D. 1500–1700), there was a growing belief that disease was caused by the environment, not spiritual factors.

- The eighteenth century was characterized by industrial growth. Science was being used more in medicine and it was during this century that the first vaccine was discovered.

- The nineteenth century ushered in the modern era of public health. The germ theory was introduced during this time, and the last fourth of the century is known as the bacteriological period of public health.

- The twentieth century can be divided into several periods. The health resources development period (1900–1960) was a time when many public and private resources were used to improve health. The period of social engineering (1960–1973) saw the U.S. government's involvement in health insurance through Medicare and Medicaid. The health promotion period began in 1974 and continues today.

- Great concern still exists for health care, the environment, diseases caused by an impoverished lifestyle, the spread of communicable diseases (such as AIDS, Legionnaires' disease, toxic shock syndrome, and Lyme disease), the harm caused by alcohol and other drug abuse, and terrorism.

- Both the WHO and the U.S. government continue to plan for the health of humanity. The planning of the United States is reflected in the *Healthy People* documents, the health agenda for the nation.

- The threat of terrorism, both in the United States and worldwide, has created many new challenges for those trying to provide improved health for all.

REVIEW QUESTIONS

1. How did the WHO define health in 1946? How has that definition been modified?
2. What is the difference between community health and public health? Community health and population health?
3. What are the five major domains that determine a person's health?

SCENARIO: ANALYSIS AND RESPONSE

The Internet has many sources of information that could help Amy and Eric with the decisions that they will have to make about the continued use of the day care center for their children. Use a search engine (e.g., Google, Yahoo!) and enter (a) hepatitis, and (b) hepatitis and day care centers. Print out the information that you find and use it in answering the following questions.

1. Based upon the information you found from the Web, if you were Amy or Eric would you take your children to the day care center the next day? Why or why not?

2. Do you feel the hepatitis problem in day care centers is a personal health concern or a community health concern? Why?

3. Which of the factors noted in this chapter that affect the health of a community play a part in the hepatitis problem faced by Amy and Eric?

4. Why does the hepatitis problem remind us of the health problems faced by people in this country prior to 1900?

5. Under which of the focus areas in the *Healthy People 2010* would hepatitis fall? Why?

4. What is the difference between personal health activities and community health activities?

5. Define the term *community*.

6. What are four major factors that affect the health of a community? Provide an example of each.

7. Identify some of the major events of community health in each of the following periods of time:

Early civilizations (prior to A.D. 500)

Middle Ages (A.D. 500–1500)

Renaissance and Exploration (A.D. 1500–1700)

The eighteenth century

The nineteenth century

8. Provide a brief explanation of the origins from which the following twentieth-century periods get their names:

Health resources development period

Period of social engineering

Period of health promotion

9. What are the major community health problems facing the United States in the twenty-first century?

10. How is the world planning for the health of people in the twenty-first century?

11. What significance do the *Healthy People* documents play in community health development in recent years?

12. What significance do you think *Healthy People 2010* will play in the years ahead?

13. How has the United States organized to deal with the threat of terrorism?

ACTIVITIES

1. Write your own definition for *health*.

2. In a two-page paper, explain how the five major determinants of health could interact to cause a disease such as cancer.

3. In a one-page paper, explain why heart disease can be both a personal health problem and a community health problem.

4. Select a community health problem that exists in your hometown; then, using the factors that affect the health of a community noted in this chapter, analyze and discuss in a two-page paper at least three factors that contribute to the problem in your hometown.

5. Select one of the following individuals (all have been identified in this chapter), go to the library and do some additional reading or find two reliable Web sites, and then write a two-page paper on the person's contribution to community health.

Edward Jenner

John Snow

Lemuel Shattuck

Louis Pasteur

Robert Koch

Walter Reed

6. Locate a copy of *Healthy People 2010.* (It is available on the Web.) Then, set up a time to talk with an administrator in your hometown health department. Find out which of the objectives the health department has been working on as priorities. Summarize in a paper what the objectives are, what the health department is doing about them, and what it hopes to accomplish by the year 2010.

COMMUNITY HEALTH ON THE WEB

The Internet contains a wealth of information about community and public health. Increase your knowledge of some of the topics presented in this chapter by accessing the Jones and Bartlett Publishers Web site at **http://health.jbpub.com/book/communityhealth/6e** and follow the links to complete the following Web activities.

• *Healthy People 2010*

• Department of Homeland Security

• The International History of Public Health

REFERENCES

1. Schneider, M.-J. (2006). *Introduction to Public Health*. Sudbury, MA: Jones and Bartlett.

2. Bunker, J. P., H. S. Frazier, and F. Mosteller (1994). "Improving Health: Measuring Effects of Medical Care." *Milbank Quarterly*, 72: 225–258.

3. Centers for Disease Control and Prevention (1999). "Ten Great Public Health Achievements—United States, 1900–1999." *Morbidity and Mortality Weekly Report*, 48(12): 241–243.

4. Koplan, J. (2000). "*21st Century Health Challenges: Can We All Become Healthy, Wealthy, and Wise?*" Available at http://www.pitt.edu/~super1/lecture/lec1361/origin.htm.

5. National Safety Council (1997). *Accident Facts, 1997 Edition*. Itasca, IL: Author.

6. World Health Organization (2007). "Frequently Asked Questions: What Is the WHO Definition of Health?" Available at http://www.who.int/suggestions/faq/en/.

7. World Health Organization (2001). *Men Ageing and Health*. Available at http://whqlibdoc.who.int/hq/2001/WHO_NMH_NPH_01.2.pdf.

8. Hancock, T., and M. Minkler (2005). "Community Health Assessment or Healthy Community Assessment." In M. Minkler, ed., *Community Organizing and Community Building for Health*, 2nd ed. New Brunswick, NJ: Rutgers University Press, 138–157.

9. McGinnis, J. M. (2001). "United States." In C. E. Koop, ed., *Critical Issues in Global Health*. San Francisco: Jossey-Bass, 80–90.

10. McGinnis, J. M., P. Williams-Russo, and J. R. Knickman (2002). "The Case for More Active Policy Attention to Health Promotion." *Health Affairs*, 21(2), 78-93.

11. Turnock, B. J. (2004). *Public Health: What It Is and How It Works*, 3rd ed. Sudbury, MA: Jones and Bartlett.

12. Israel, B. A., B. Checkoway, A. Schulz, and M. Zimmerman (1994). "Health Education and Community Empowerment: Conceptualizing and Measuring Perceptions of Individual, Organizational, and Community Control." *Health Education Quarterly*, 21(2): 149-170.

13. Institute of Medicine (2003). *The Future of the Public's Health*. Washington, DC: The National Academies Press.

14. Institute of Medicine (1988). *The Future of Public Health*. Washington, DC: The National Academies Press.

15. Green, L. W., and J. F. McKenzie (2002). "Community and Population Health." In L. Breslow, ed., *Encyclopedia of Public Health*. New York: Macmillan Reference USA.

16. Association for the Advancement of Health Education (1994). *Cultural Awareness and Sensitivity: Guidelines for Health Educators*. Reston, VA: Author.

17. American Cancer Society (2007). *Cancer Facts and Figures—2007*. Available at http://www.cancer.org.

18. American College Health Association (2006). "American College Health Association National College Health Assessment (ACHA-NCHA) Spring 2005 Reference Group Data Report (Abridged)." *Journal of American College Health*, 55(1), 5-16.

19. Moss, N., and N. Krieger (1995). "Measuring Social Inequalities in Health: Report on the Conference of the National Institutes of Health." *Public Health Reports*, 110(3): 302-305.

20. U.S. Department of Health and Human Services (2000). *Healthy People 2010*. Available at http://www.healthypeople.gov.

21. Minkler, M., and N. Wallerstein (2005). "Improving Health through Community Organizing and Community Building: A Health Education Perspective." In M. Minkler, ed., *Community Organizing and Community Building for Health*, 2nd ed. New Brunswick, NJ: Rutgers University Press, 26-50.

22. Ross, M. G. (1967). *Community Organization: Theory, Principles, and Practice*. New York: Harper & Row.

23. Rosen, G. (1958). *A History of Public Health*. New York: MD Publications.

24. Burton, L. E., H. H. Smith, and A. W. Nichols (1980). *Public Health and Community Medicine*, 3rd ed. Baltimore: Williams & Wilkins.

25. Pickett, G., and J. J. Hanlon (1990). *Public Health: Administration and Practice*, 9th ed. St. Louis, MO: Times Mirror/Mosby.

26. Legon, R. P. (1986). "Ancient Greece." *World Book Encyclopedia*. Chicago, IL: World Book.

27. Woodruff, A. W. (1977). "Benjamin Rush, His Work on Yellow Fever and His British Connections." *American Journal of Tropical Medicine and Hygiene*, 26(5): 1055-1059.

28. Rosen, G. (1975). *Preventive Medicine in the United States, 1900-1975*. New York: Science History Publications.

29. Smillie, W. G. (1955). *Public Health: Its Promise for the Future*. New York: Macmillan.

30. Duffy, J. (1990). *The Sanitarians: A History of American Public Health*. Chicago: University of Illinois Press.

31. Lalonde, M. (1974). *A New Perspective on the Health of Canadians: A Working Document*. Ottawa, Canada: Minister of Health.

32. Green, L. W. (1999). "Health Education's Contributions to the Twentieth Century: A Glimpse through Health Promotion's Rearview Mirror." In J. E. Fielding, L. B. Lave, and B. Starfield, eds., *Annual Review of Public Health*. Palo Alto, CA: Annual Reviews, 67-88.

33. U.S. Department of Health and Human Services, Public Health Service (1980). *Ten Leading Causes of Death in the United States, 1977*. Washington, DC: U.S. Government Printing Office.

34. U.S. Department of Health, Education, and Welfare (1979). *Healthy People: The Surgeon General's Report on Health Promotion and Disease Prevention* (DHEW pub. no. 79-55071). Washington, DC: U.S. Government Printing Office.

35. McKenzie, J. F., B. L. Neiger, and R. Thackeray (2009). *Planning, Implementing, and Evaluating Health Promotion Programs: A Primer*, 5th ed. San Francisco: Benjamin Cummings.

36. U.S. Department of Health and Human Services (1980). *Promoting Health/Preventing Disease: Objectives for the Nation*. Washington, DC: U.S. Government Printing Office.

37. Borger, C., S. Smith, C. Truffer, S. Keehan, A. Sisko, J. Poisal, and M. K. Clemens (2006). "Health Spending Projections through 2015: Changes in the Horizon." *Health Affairs Web Exclusive*, 25(2): 61-73.

38. DeNavas-Walt, C., B. D. Protor, and C. H. Lee (2006). *Income, Poverty, and Health Insurance Coverage in the United States: 2005* (Current Population Reports no. P60-231). Washington, DC: U.S. Government Printing Office.

39. U.S. Census Bureau (2006). *World Population Information*. Available at http://www.census.gov/ipc/www/world.html.

40. National Center for Health Statistics (2006). *Health United States, 2006 with Chartbook on Trends in Health of Americans*. Hyattsville, MD: Author.

41. U.S. Department of Health and Human Services (1990). *Prevention '89/'90*. Washington, DC: U.S. Government Printing Office.

42. Centers for Disease Control (1981). "Pneumocystis Pneumonia—Los Angeles." *Morbidity and Mortality Weekly Report*, 30: 250-252.

43. Centers for Disease Control (1989). "First 100,000 Cases of Acquired Immunodeficiency Syndrome—United States." *Morbidity and Mortality Weekly Report*, 38: 561-563.

44. Centers for Disease Control (1992). "The Second 100,000 Cases of Acquired Immunodeficiency Syndrome—United States, June 1981-December 1991." *Morbidity and Mortality Weekly Report*, 42(2):28-29.

45. Centers for Disease Control and Prevention (2006). "Twenty-five Years of HIV/AIDS—United States, 1981-2006." *Morbidity and Mortality Weekly Report*, 55(21), 585-589.

46. Gerberding, J. L., J. M. Hughes, and J. P. Koplan (2003). "Bioterrorism Preparedness and Response: Clinicians and Public Health Agencies as Essential Partners." In P. R. Lee and C. L. Estes, eds., *The Nation's Health*. Sudbury, MA: Jones and Bartlett, 305-309.

47. Pinger, R. R., W. A. Payne, D. B. Hahn, and E. J. Hahn (1998). *Drugs: Issues for Today*, 3rd ed. Boston: WCB McGraw-Hill.

48. Agency for Healthcare Research and Quality (2004). *Bioterrorism and Health System Preparedness* (Issue Brief no. 2). Available at http://www.ahrq.gov/news/ulp/btbriefs/btbrief2.htm.

49. Federal Emergency Management Agency (2007). "Are You Ready? Natural Disaster." Available at http://www.fema.gov/areyouready/natural_hazards.shtm.

50. McHugh, M., A. B. Staiti, and L. E. Felland (2004). "Trends: How Prepared Are Americans for Public Health Emergencies? Twelve Communities Weigh In." *Health Affairs*, 23(3), 201-209.

51. Trust for America's Health (2006). "Report Finds U.S. Bioterror, Bird Flu, and Health Disaster Preparedness Inadequate; Half of States Score 6 or Less Out of 10 Key Indicators [Press release]." Available at http://healthyamericans.org/newsroom/releases/release121206.pdf.

52. World Health Organization (1990). *Facts about WHO*. Geneva, Switzerland: Author.

53. World Health Organization (2003). *World Health Report 2003: Shaping the Future*. Geneva, Switzerland: Author.

54. World Health Organization (2006). *Engaging in Health: Eleventh General Programme of Work 2006-2015*. Available at http://www.who.int/gpw/GPW_En.pdf.

55. World Health Organization (2006). *The World Health Report 2006: Working Together for Health*. Available at http://www.who.int/whr/2006/en/index.html.

56. United Nations (2000). *United Nations Millennium Declaration*. New York: Author.

57. National Center for Health Statistics (2001). *Healthy People 2000 Final Review*. Hyattsville, MD: Public Health Service.

58. U.S. Department of Health and Human Services (2006). *Healthy People 2010: Midcourse Review Executive Summary*. Available at http://www.healthypeople.gov/data/midcourse/html/introduction.htm.

59. U.S. Department of Health and Human Services (2006). "Summary and Future Directions." In *Healthy People 2010: Midcourse Review Executive Summary*. Available at http://www.healthypeople.gov/data/midcourse/html/future.htm.

60. Department of Homeland Security (2005). "Homeland Security Secretary Michael Chertoff Announces Six-Point Agenda for Department of Homeland Security [Press release]." Available at http://www.dhs.gov/xnews/releases/press_release_0703.shtm.

61. U.S. Department of Homeland Security (2006). "DHS Organization." Available at http://www.dhs.gov.

62. U.S. Department of Homeland Security (2006). "Department Six-Point Agenda." Available at http://www.dhs.gov/xnews/history/editorial_0646.shtm.

Chapter 2

Organizations That Help Shape Community Health

Chapter Objectives

1 Explain the need for organizing to improve community health.

2 Explain what a governmental health organization
is and give an example of one at each of the
following levels—international, national, state,
and local.

3 Explain the role the World Health Organization
(WHO) plays in community health.

4 Briefly describe the structure and function of the
United States Department of Health and Human
Services (HHS).

5 State the three core functions of public health.

6 List the 10 essential public health services.

7 Explain the relationship between a state and local
health department.

8 Explain what is meant by the term *coordinated
school health program.*

9 Define the term *quasi-governmental* and explain
why some health organizations are classified under
this term.

10 List the four primary activities of most voluntary
health organizations.

11 Explain the purpose of a professional health
organization/association.

12 Explain how philanthropic foundations contribute
to community health.

13 Discuss the role that service, social, and religious
organizations play in community health.

14 Identify the major reason why corporations are
involved in community health and describe some
corporate activities that contribute to community
health.

SCENARIO

Mary is a hardworking senior at the local university. She is majoring in physical education and looking forward to teaching elementary physical education after graduation. Mary has always been involved in team sports and has been a lifeguard at the local swimming pool for the past four years. Mary has a fair complexion with honey-blonde hair and blue eyes. She has always tanned easily and so has not bothered very much with sunscreens. For the past few weeks, Mary has noticed a red, scaly, sharply outlined patch of skin on her forehead. She has put creams and ointments on it, but it will not go away and may be getting larger. Her roommate, Clare, sug-

gests that she should make an appointment with the campus health services office. Mary lets it go another week and then decides to see the doctor.

After looking at the patch of skin, the doctor refers Mary to a specialist, Dr. Rice, who is a dermatologist. The dermatologist suggests a biopsy be taken of the lesion to test for skin cancer. The specialist tells Mary that if it is cancer, it is probably still in its early stages and so the prognosis is good.

A potential diagnosis of cancer often raises a lot of questions and concerns. Are there any resources in the community to which Mary can turn for help?

INTRODUCTION

As noted in Chapter 1, the history of community health dates to antiquity. For much of that history, community health issues were addressed only on an emergency basis. For example, if a community faced a drought or an epidemic, a town meeting would be called to deal with the problem. It has been only in the last 100 years or so that communities have taken explicit actions to deal aggressively with health issues on a continual basis.

Today's communities differ from those of the past in several important ways. Although individuals are better educated, more mobile, and more independent than in the past, communities are less autonomous and are more dependent on state and federal funding for support. Contemporary communities are too large and complex to respond effectively to sudden health emergencies or to make long-term improvements in public health without community organization and careful planning. Better community organizing and careful long-term planning are essential to ensure that a community makes the best use of its resources for health, both in times of emergency and over the long run.

The ability of today's communities to respond effectively to their own problems is hindered by the following characteristics: (1) highly developed and centralized resources in our national institutions and organizations, (2) continuing concentration of wealth and population in the largest metropolitan areas, (3) rapid movement of information, resources, and people made possible by advanced communication and transportation technologies that eliminate the need for local offices where resources were once housed, (4) the globalization of health, (5) limited horizontal relationships between/among organizations, and (6) a system of **top-down funding** (money that comes from either the federal or state government to the local level) for many community programs.[1]

top-down funding a method of funding in which funds are transmitted from federal or state government to the local level

In this chapter, we discuss organizations that help to shape a community's ability to respond effectively to health-related issues by protecting and promoting the health of the community and its members. These community organizations can be classified as governmental, quasi-governmental, and nongovernmental—according to their sources of funding, responsibilities, and organizational structure.

GOVERNMENTAL HEALTH AGENCIES

Governmental health agencies are part of the governmental structure (federal, state, or local). They are funded primarily by tax dollars and managed by government officials. Each governmental health agency is designated as having authority over some geographic area. Such agencies exist at the four governmental levels—international, national, state, and local.

International Health Agencies

The most widely recognized international governmental health organization today is the **World Health Organization (WHO)** (see Figure 2.1). Its headquarters is located in Geneva, Switzerland, and there are six regional offices around the world. The names, acronyms, and cities and countries of location for WHO regional offices are as follows: Africa (AFRO), Brazzaville, Congo; Americas (PAHO), Washington, DC, United States; Eastern Mediterranean (EMRO), Cairo, Egypt; Europe (EURO), Copenhagen, Denmark; Southeast Asia (SEARO), New Delhi, India; and Western Pacific (WPRO), Manila, Philippines.[2]

Although the WHO is now the largest international health organization, it is not the oldest. Among the organizations (listed with their founding dates) that predate WHO are the International D'Hygiene Publique (1907), which was absorbed by the WHO; the Health Organization of the League of Nations (1919), which was dissolved when the WHO was created; the United Nations Relief and Rehabilitation Administration (UNRRA); the United Nations Children's Fund (UNICEF) (1946), which was formerly known as the United Nations International Children's Emergency Fund; and the Pan American Health Organization (PAHO) (1902), which is still an independent organization but is integrated with WHO in a regional office. Because the WHO is the largest and most visible international health agency, it is discussed at greater length in the following sections.

History of the World Health Organization

Planning for the WHO began when a charter of the United Nations was adopted at an international meeting in 1945. Contained in the charter was an article calling for the establishment of a health agency with wide powers. In 1946, at the International Health Conference, representatives from all of the countries in the United Nations succeeded in creating and ratifying the constitution of the WHO. However, it was not until April 7, 1948, that the constitution went into force and the organization officially began its work. In recognition of this beginning, April 7 is commemorated each year as World Health Day.[2]

Organization of the World Health Organization

Membership in the WHO is open to any nation that has ratified the WHO constitution and receives a majority vote of the World Health Assembly. At the beginning of 2006, 193 countries were members. The **World Health Assembly** comprises the delegates of the member nations. This assembly, which meets in general sessions annually and in special sessions when necessary, has the primary tasks of approving the WHO program and the budget for the following biennium and deciding major policy questions.[2]

The WHO is administered by a staff that includes a director-general and nine assistant directors-general. Great care is taken to ensure political balance in staffing WHO positions, particularly at the higher levels of administration.

Purpose and Work of the World Health Organization

The primary objective of the WHO as stated in the constitution is

governmental health agencies
health agencies that are part of the governmental structure (federal, state, or local) and that are funded primarily by tax dollars

World Health Organization (WHO)
the most widely recognized international governmental health organization

World Health Assembly
a body of delegates of the member nations of the WHO

FIGURE 2.1

The emblem of the World Health Organization.

Source: Courtesy of World Health Organization. Use of logo does not imply endorsement.

the attainment by all peoples of the highest possible level of health.[2] The WHO has six core functions:[2]

- Articulating consistent, ethical and evidence-based policy and advocacy positions
- Managing information by assessing trends and comparing performance; setting the agenda for, and stimulating research and development
- Catalyzing change through technical and policy support, in ways that stimulate cooperation and action and help to build sustainable national and inter-country capacity
- Negotiating and sustaining national and global partnerships
- Setting, validating, monitoring and pursuing the proper implementation of norms and standards
- Stimulating the development and testing of new technologies, tools and guidelines for disease control, risk reduction, health care management, and service delivery

The work of the WHO is financed by its member nations, each of which is assessed according to its ability to pay; the wealthiest countries contribute the greatest portion of the total budget.

Although the WHO has sponsored and continues to sponsor many worthwhile programs, an especially noteworthy one was the work of the WHO in helping to eradicate smallpox. In 1967, smallpox was active in 31 countries. During that year, 10 to 15 million people contracted the disease, and of those, approximately 2 million died and many millions of others were permanently disfigured or blinded. The last known case of smallpox was diagnosed on October 26, 1977, in Somalia.[2] In 1980, the World Health Assembly declared the global eradication of this disease. Using the smallpox mortality figures from 1967, it can be estimated that well over 40 million lives have been saved since the eradication (see Box 2.1).

As noted in Chapter 1, the current work of the WHO is guided by two documents—the *11th General Programme of Work*[2] and the United Nations Millennium Declaration, which

---

BOX 2.1 **THE KINDEST CUT**

Once I was in Geneva at the World Health Organization researching a book on communicable diseases. I met Donald Henderson, M.D., director of the smallpox eradication effort.

Not long ago, smallpox was one of the worst diseases anyone could have. About six of every ten who contracted it died. In the United States, even a single known case was regarded as an epidemic.

There is no smallpox known anywhere today. Credit the WHO smallpox vaccination effort. There is still no cure, only prevention; that is, vaccination. At that time, WHO was ready to vaccinate the world, if necessary, to eradicate the disease.

Henderson had been in one high-incidence smallpox region in South America. But few people there were coming to the WHO field station for vaccinations. The warnings about this disease were ho-hum, even though people were seeing smallpox deaths every day.

So, Henderson said, they tried bribery. Not money or goods. They substituted ordinary sewing needles for the standard stainless steel stylets, used to prick under the skin. Then the WHO people spread the word that anyone who came for immunization could keep the needle. Women wanted them for sewing and working of cloth. Men saw them as fine tips for hunting darts.

The sudden fervor and turnout for vaccination rivaled that at any Christmas Eve mass at St. Patrick's Cathedral in New York. Henderson's lesson in resourcefulness for the common good did indeed involve some low-road seduction with rewards, but it was a clear lesson, and one with merit. "Get people to come in for vaccination any way you can. But get them," he said that day in Geneva. "First get them healthy. Then there's time enough to try to educate them about staying healthy."

Source: Gallagher, R. (1993). "Resourcerer's Apprentice." *Living: The Magazine of Life,* 22(3): 12.

was adopted at the Millennium Summit in 2003.[3] Because the *11th General Programme of Work* was discussed in detail in Chapter 1, the discussion here focuses on the Millennium Declaration. The declaration set out principles and values in seven areas (peace, security, and disarmament; development and poverty eradication; protecting our common environment; human rights, democracy, and good governance; protecting the vulnerable; meeting special needs of Africa; and strengthening the United Nations) that should govern international relations in the twenty-first century.[3] Following the summit, the *Road Map* was prepared, which established goals and targets to be reached by 2015 in each of the seven areas.[4] The resulting eight goals in the area of development and poverty eradication are now referred to as the Millennium Development Goals (MDGs). More specifically, the MDGs are aimed at reducing poverty and hunger, tackling ill-health, gender inequality, lack of education, lack of access to clean water, and environmental degradation.

As can be seen from this description, the MDGs are not exclusively aimed at health, but there are interactive processes between health and economic development that create a crucial link. That is, better health is "a prerequisite and major contributor to economic growth and social cohesion. Conversely, improvement in people's access to health technology is a good indicator of the success of other development processes."[5] As such, "three of the eight goals, eight of the 18 targets required to achieve them, and 18 of the 48 indicators of progress are health-related"[5] (see Table 2.1).

To date, progress on the MDGs has been slow, and it appears that many of the targets will not be reached by 2015. Five major challenges to meeting the goals have been identified: (1) strengthening health systems, (2) ensuring health is recognized as a priority within development and economic policies, (3) developing appropriate strategies to address the diverse needs of the countries, (4) mobilizing more resources for health in the poor countries, and (5) improving the quality of health-related data in order to track progress toward the goals.[6,7] Much work lies ahead, by all people of the world, to improve the health of those most in need.

National Health Agencies

Each national government has a department or agency that has the primary responsibility for the protection of the health and welfare of its citizens. These national health agencies meet their responsibilities through the development of health policies, the enforcement of health regulations, the provision of health services and programs, the funding of research, and the support of their respective state and local health agencies.

In the United States, the primary national health agency is the Department of Health and Human Services (HHS). HHS "is the United States government's principal agency for protecting the health of all Americans and providing essential human services, especially for those who are least able to help themselves."[8] It is important to note, however, that other federal agencies also contribute to the betterment of our nation's health. For example, the Department of Agriculture inspects meat and dairy products and coordinates the Women, Infants, and Children (WIC) food assistance program; the Environmental Protection Agency (EPA) regulates hazardous wastes; the Department of Labor houses the Occupational Safety and Health Administration (OSHA), which is concerned with safety and health in the workplace; the Department of Commerce, which includes the Bureau of the Census, collects much of the national data that drives our nation's health programs; and the Department of Homeland Security (DHS) deals with all aspects of terrorism within the United States. While information about the DHS was presented in Chapter 1, each of these other departments or agencies will be discussed in greater detail in later chapters. A detailed description of the Department of Health and Human Services follows.

Table 2.1
Health-Related Millennium Development Goals, Targets, and Indicators

Goal: 1. Eradicate Extreme Poverty and Hunger
Target: 2. Halve, between 1990 and 2015, the proportion of people who suffer from hunger
    Indicator: 4. Prevalence of underweight children under five years of age
        5. Proportion of population below minimum level of dietary energy consumption[a]

Goal: 4. Reduce Child Mortality
Target: 5. Reduce by two-thirds, between 1990 and 2015, the under-five mortality rate
    Indicator: 13. Under-five mortality rate
        14. Infant mortality rate
        15. Proportion of 1-year-old children immunized against measles

Goal: 5. Improve Maternal Health
Target: 6. Reduce by three-quarters, between 1990 and 2015, the maternal mortality ratio
    Indicator: 16. Maternal mortality ratio
        17. Proportion of births attended by skilled health personnel

Goal: 6. Combat HIV/AIDS, Malaria, and Other Diseases
Target: 7. Have halted by 2015 and begun to reverse the spread of HIV/AIDS
    Indicator: 18. HIV prevalence among young people aged 15 to 24 years[b]
        19. Condom use rate of the contraceptive prevalence rate
        20. Number of children orphaned by HIV/AIDS
Target: 8. Have halted by 2015 and begun to reverse the incidence of malaria and other major diseases
    Indicator: 21. Prevalence and death rates associated with malaria
        22. Proportion of population in malaria-risk areas using effective malaria prevention and treatment measures
        23. Prevalence and death rates associated with tuberculosis
        24. Proportion of tuberculosis cases detected and cured under Directly Observed Treatment, Short-course (DOTS)

Goal: 7. Ensure Environmental Sustainability
Target: 9. Integrate the principles of sustainable development into country policies and programmes and reverse the loss of environmental resources
    Indicator: 29. Proportion of population using solid fuel
Target: 10. Halve by 2015 the proportion of people without sustainable access to safe drinking-water
    Indicator: 30. Proportion of population with sustainable access to an improved water source, urban and rural
Target: 11. By 2020 to have achieved a significant improvement in the lives of at least 100 million slum dwellers
    Indicator: 31. Proportion of urban population with access to improved sanitation

Goal: 8. Develop a Global Partnership for Development
Target: 17. In cooperation with pharmaceutical companies, provide access to affordable essential drugs in developing countries
    Indicator: 46. Proportion of population with access to affordable essential drugs on a sustainable basis

---

[a]Health-related indicator reported by the Food and Agriculture Organization only.
[b]Indicators from the MDG list reformulated by WHO and United Nations General Assembly Special Session on HIV/AIDS.

Source: World Health Organization (2003). *World Health Report 2003: Shaping the Future.* Geneva, Switzerland: Author, 28. Used with permission of the World Health Organization.

Department of Health and Human Services

The HHS is headed by the Secretary of Health and Human Services, who is appointed by the president and is a member of his or her cabinet. The Department of Health and Human Services was formed in 1980 (during the administration of president Jimmy Carter), when the Department of Health, Education, and Welfare (HEW) was divided into two new departments, HHS and the Department of Education. HHS is the department most involved with the nation's human concerns. In one way or another it touches the lives of more Americans than any other federal agency. It is literally a department of people serving people, from newborn infants to persons requiring health services to our most elderly citizens. With an annual budget in excess of approximately $698 billion (representing about 25% of the federal budget), HHS is the largest department in the federal government, and it spends approximately $195 billion more per year than the Department of Defense.[8,9]

Since its formation, HHS has undergone several reorganizations. Some of the more recent changes have been the addition of the Center for Faith-Based and Community Initiatives and an Assistant Secretary for Public Health Emergency Preparedness. Currently, the HHS is organized into 11 operating divisions (see Figure 2.2) whose heads report directly to the Secretary. In addition, the HHS has 10 regional offices (see Table 2.2). These offices serve as representatives of the Secretary of HHS in direct, official dealings with the state and local governmental organizations.

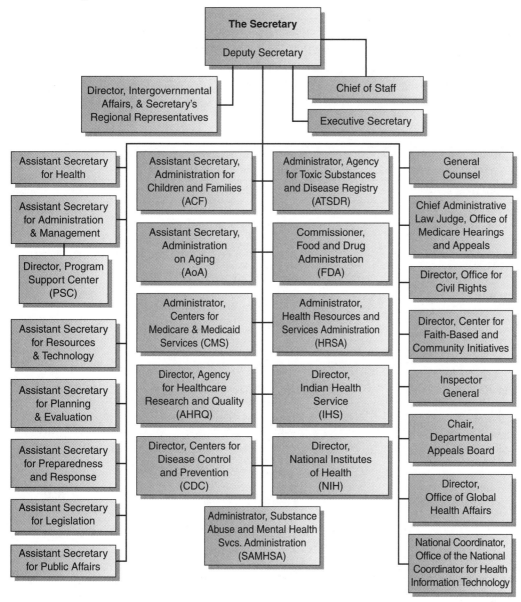

FIGURE 2.2

Organizational chart for the U.S. Department of Health and Human Services (HHS).

Source: U.S. Department of Health and Human Services (2007). Available at http://www.hhs.gov/about/orgchart.html.

Although it appears in Figure 2.2 that the Public Health Service (PHS), a long-standing federal health agency, was eliminated from HHS, this is not the case. Eight of the 11 operating divisions of HHS now constitute the PHS (AHRQ, CDC, ATSDR, FDA, HRSA, IHS, NIH, and SAMHSA). Another three operating divisions (CMS, ACF, and AoA) comprise the human services operating divisions.

Administration on Aging (AoA)

This division of the HHS is the principal agency designated to carry out the provisions of the Older Americans Act of 1965. (See Chapter 9 for more information on this act.) This agency tracks the characteristics, circumstances, and needs of older people; develops policies, plans, and programs to promote their welfare; administers grant programs to benefit older Americans; and administers training, research, demonstration programs, and protective services for older Americans. One exemplary program supported by the AoA is Meals on Wheels.

Administration for Children and Families (ACF)

The ACF is composed of a number of smaller agencies and is responsible for providing direction and leadership for all federal programs for needy children and families. One of the better-

Table 2.2
Regional Offices of the U.S. Department of Health and Human Services

Region/Areas Served	Office Address	Telephone Number
Region 1: CT, MA, ME, NH, RI, VT	John F. Kennedy Bldg. Government Center Boston, MA 02203	(617) 565-1500
Region 2: NJ, NY, Puerto Rico, Virgin Islands	Jacob K. Javits Federal Bldg. 26 Federal Plaza New York, NY 10278	(212) 264-4600
Region 3: DE, MD, PA, VA, WV, DC	Public Ledger Building 150 S. Independence Mall West Suite 436 Philadelphia, PA 19106	(215) 861-4633
Region 4: AL, FL, GA, KY, MS, NC, SC, TN	Sam Nunn, Atlanta Federal Center 61 Forsyth Street, SW Atlanta, GA 30303	(404) 562-7888
Region 5: IL, IN, MI, MN, OH, WI	233 N. Michigan Avenue Chicago, IL 60601	(312) 353-5160
Region 6: AR, LA, NM, OK, TX	1301 Young Street Dallas, TX 75202	(214) 767-3301
Region 7: IA, KS, MO, NE	Bolling Federal Building 601 East 12th Street Kansas City, MO 64106	(816) 426-2821
Region 8: CO, MT, ND, SD,UT, WY	Bryon G. Rogers Federal Office Building 1961 Stout Street Room 1076 Denver, CO 80294	(303) 844-3372
Region 9: AZ, CA, HI, NV, American Samoa, Guam, Commonwealth of the Northern Mariana Islands, Federated States of Micronesia, Republic of the Marshall Islands, Republic of Palau	Federal Office Building 50 United Nations Plaza San Francisco, CA 94102	(415) 437-8500
Region 10: AK, ID, OR, WA	Blanchard Plaza Bldg. 2201 6th Avenue Seattle, WA 98121	(206) 615-2010

known programs originating from this division is Head Start, which serves more than 900,000 preschool children. Other programs are aimed at family assistance, refugee resettlement, and child support enforcement.

Agency for Healthcare Research and Quality (AHRQ)

Prior to 1999 this division of the HHS was called the Agency for Health Care Policy and Research, but its name was changed as part of the Healthcare Research and Quality Act of 1999. AHRQ is "the Nation's lead Federal agency for research on health care quality, costs, outcomes, and patient safety."[10] AHRQ sponsors and conducts research that provides evidence-based information on health care outcomes; quality; and cost, use, and access. The information helps health care decision makers—patients and clinicians, health system leaders, and policy makers—make more informed decisions and improve the quality of health care services.

Agency for Toxic Substances and Disease Registry (ATSDR)

This agency was created by the **Superfund legislation** (Comprehensive Environmental Response, Compensation, and Liability Act) in 1980. This legislation was enacted to deal with the cleanup of hazardous substances in the environment. ATSDR's mission "is to serve the public by using the best science, taking responsive public health actions, and providing trusted health information to prevent harmful exposures and disease related to toxic substances."[11] To carry out its mission and to serve the needs of the American public, ATSDR evaluates information on hazardous substances released into the environment in order to assess the impact on public health; conducts and sponsors studies and other research related to hazardous substances and adverse human health effects; establishes and maintains registries of human exposure (for long-term follow-up) and complete listings of areas closed to the public or otherwise restricted in use due to contamination; summarizes and makes data available on the effects of hazardous substances; and provides consultations and training to ensure adequate response to public health emergencies. Although ATSDR has been responding to chemical emergencies in local communities across the country for the last 25 years, like many of the other federal health agencies its work has taken on new meaning since 9/11. For example, some of the projects the agency's staff have worked on or continue to work on include sampling dust in New York City residences after 9/11; working with New York health agencies to create a registry of people who lived or worked near the World Trade Center (WTC) on 9/11 to collect health information on those most heavily exposed to smoke, dust, and debris from the collapse of the WTC; conducting environmental sampling at anthrax-contaminated buildings; and disseminating critical information to agencies and organizations with a role in terrorism preparedness and response.[12]

> **Superfund legislation** legislation enacted to deal with the cleanup of hazardous substances in the environment

Centers for Disease Control and Prevention (CDC)

The CDC, located in Atlanta, Georgia (see Figure 2.3), "is the nation's premiere health promotion, prevention, and preparedness agency and global leader in public health."[13] The CDC serves as the national focus for developing and applying disease prevention (including bioterrorism) and control, environmental health, and health promotion and education activities designed to improve the health of the people of the United States.[13] Once known solely for its work to control communicable diseases, the CDC now also maintains records, analyzes disease trends, and publishes epidemiological reports on all types of diseases, including those that result from lifestyle, occupational, and environmental causes. Beyond its own specific responsibilities, the CDC also supports state and

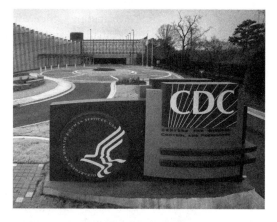

FIGURE 2.3

The Centers for Disease Control and Prevention (CDC) in Atlanta, Georgia, is one of the major operating agencies of the Department of Health and Human Services (HHS).

local health departments and cooperates with similar national health agencies from other WHO member nations.

To better meet the challenges of public health for the twenty-first century, in 2003 the CDC began a strategic planning process called the *Futures Initiative.*[13] As a part of the Futures Initiative, the CDC adopted new overarching health protection goals and a new organizational structure. The goals that were adopted included the following:

- *Preparedness:* People in all communities will be protected from infectious, environmental, and terrorist threats.
- *Health promotion and prevention of disease, injury, and disability:* All people will achieve their optimal lifespan with the best possible quality of health in every stage of life.
- *Healthy places:* The places where people live, work, learn, and play should protect and promote human health and eliminate health disparities.

The reorganization of the CDC created a structure that included the Office of the Director, the National Institute for Occupational Safety and Health (NIOSH) (see Chapter 18 for a discussion of NIOSH), and six coordinating centers/offices. The coordinating centers are as follows:

- Coordinating Center for Infectious Diseases: Includes the National Center for Immunization and Respiratory Diseases (NCIRD); the National Center for Zoonotic, Vectorborne, and Enteric Diseases (NCZVED); the National Center for HIV/AIDS, Viral Hepatitis, STD, and TB Prevention (NCHHSTP); the National Center for Preparedness, Detection, and Control of Infectious Diseases (NCPDCID); the Strategic Business Unit (SBU); and the Strategic Science and Program Unit (SSPU).
- Coordinating Center for Health Promotion: Includes the National Center for Chronic Disease Prevention and Health Promotion (NCCDPHP); the National Center for Birth Defects and Developmental Disabilities (NCBDDD); and the National Office of Public Health Genomics.
- Coordinating Center for Environmental Health and Injury Prevention: Includes the National Center for Environmental Health (NCEH)/Agency for Toxic Substances and Disease Registry (ATSDR); and the National Center for Injury Prevention and Control (NCIPC).
- Coordinating Center for Health Information and Services: Includes the National Center for Health Statistics (NCHS); the National Center for Health Marketing; and the National Center for Public Health Informatics.
- Coordinating Office for Global Health (COGH): This office provides national leadership, coordination, and support for CDC's global health activities in collaboration with CDC's global health partners.
- Coordinating Office for Terrorism Preparedness and Emergency Response (COTPER): This office has the responsibility to protect health and enhance the potential for full, satisfying, and productive living across the lifespan of all people in all communities related to community preparedness and response.

Food and Drug Administration (FDA)

The FDA touches the lives of virtually every American every day. It "is responsible for protecting the public health by assuring the safety, efficacy, and security of human and veterinary drugs, biological products, medical devices, our nation's food supply, cosmetics, and products that emit radiation. The FDA is also responsible for advancing the public health by helping to speed innovations that make medicines and foods more effective, safer, and more affordable; and helping the public get the accurate, science-based information they need to use medicines and foods to improve their health."[14] Much of this work revolves around regulatory activities and the setting of health and safety standards as spelled out in the Federal Food, Drug, and Cosmetic Act and other related laws. However, due to the complex nature of its standards and the agency's limited resources, enforcement of many FDA regulations is left to other federal agencies and to state and local agencies. For example, the Department of Agriculture is responsible for the inspection of many foods, such as meat and dairy products. Restaurants, supermarkets, and other food outlets are inspected by state and local public health agencies.

Centers for Medicare and Medicaid Services (CMS)
Established as the Health Care Financing Administration (HFCA) in 1977, the CMS is responsible for overseeing the Medicare program (health care for the elderly and the disabled), the federal portion of the Medicaid program (health care for low-income individuals), and the related quality assurance activities. Both Medicare and Medicaid were created in 1965 to ensure that the special groups covered by these programs would not be deprived of health care because of cost. In 2005, about 87 million Americans were covered by these programs.[8] In 1997, the State Children's Health Insurance Program (SCHIP) also became the responsibility of the CMS. Medicare, Medicaid, and SCHIP are discussed in greater detail in Chapter 14.

Health Resources and Services Administration (HRSA)
The HRSA is the principal primary health care service agency of the federal government that provides access to essential health care services for people who are low-income, uninsured, or who live in rural areas or urban neighborhoods where health care is scarce.[8] It "provides national leadership, program resources and services needed to improve access to culturally competent quality healthcare."[15] HRSA "helps prepare the nation's health care system and providers to respond to bioterrorism and other public health emergencies, maintains the National Health Service Corps and helps build the health care workforce through many training and education programs. HRSA administers a variety of programs to improve the health of mothers and children and serves people living with HIV/AIDS through the Ryan White CARE Act programs. HRSA also oversees the nation's organ transplantation system."[8]

Indian Health Service (IHS)
The goal of the IHS is to raise the physical, mental, social, and spiritual health of American Indians and Alaska Natives to the highest level.[16] To attain its goal, the IHS:

1. Assists tribes to develop their health programs through activities such as health management training, technical assistance, and human resource development.
2. Facilitates and assists tribes in coordinating health planning, in obtaining and using health resources available through federal, state, and local programs, and in operating comprehensive health care services and health programs.
3. Provides comprehensive health care services, including hospital and ambulatory medical care, preventive and rehabilitative services, and development of community sanitation facilities.
4. Serves as the principal federal advocate in the health field for Indians to ensure comprehensive health services for Indian people.[16]

Though health services have been provided sporadically by the United States government since the early nineteenth century, it was not until 1989 that the IHS was elevated to an agency level; prior to that time it was a division in HRSA. (See Chapter 10 for more information on the IHS.)

National Institutes of Health (NIH)
Begun as a one-room Laboratory of Hygiene in 1887, the NIH today is one of the world's foremost medical research centers, and the federal focal point for medical research in the United States.[17] The mission of the NIH "is to uncover new knowledge that will lead to better health for everyone."[17] Although a significant amount of research is carried out by NIH scientists at NIH laboratories in Bethesda and elsewhere, a much larger portion of this research is conducted by scientists at public and private universities and other research institutions. These scientists receive NIH funding for their research proposals through a competitive, peer-review

Table 2.3
Units within the National Institutes of Health (NIH)

National Cancer Institute (NCI)
National Eye Institute (NEI)
National Heart, Lung, and Blood Institute (NHLBI)
National Human Genome Research Institute (NHGRI)
National Institute on Aging (NIA)
National Institute on Alcohol Abuse and Alcoholism (NIAAA)
National Institute of Allergy and Infectious Diseases (NIAID)
National Institute of Arthritis and Musculoskeletal and Skin Diseases (NIAMS)
National Institute of Biomedical Imaging and Bioengineering (NIBIB)
National Institute of Child Health and Human Development (NICHD)
National Institute on Deafness and Other Communication Disorders (NIDCD)
National Institute of Dental and Craniofacial Research (NIDCR)
National Institute of Diabetes and Digestive and Kidney Diseases (NIDDK)
National Institute on Drug Abuse (NIDA)
National Institute of Environmental Health Sciences (NIEHS)
National Institute of General Medical Sciences (NIGMS)
National Institute of Mental Health (NIMH)
National Institute of Neurological Disorders and Stroke (NINDS)
National Institute of Nursing Research (NINR)
National Library of Medicine (NLM)
Clinical Center (CC)
Center for Information Technology (CIT)
National Center for Complementary and Alternative Medicine (NCCAM)
National Center on Minority Health and Health Disparities (NCMHD)
National Center for Research Resources (NCRR)
John E. Fogarty International Center for Advanced Study in the Health Sciences (FIC)
Center for Scientific Review (CSR)

Source: National Institutes of Health (2006). "Institutes, Centers and Offices." Available at http://www.nih.gov/icd/.

grant application process. Through this process of proposal-review by qualified scientists, NIH seeks to ensure that federal research monies are spent on the best-conceived research projects. Table 2.3 provides a listing of all the institutes and centers located in NIH.

Substance Abuse and Mental Health Services Administration (SAMHSA)
The SAMHSA is the primary federal agency responsible for ensuring that up-to-date information and state-of-the-art practice is effectively used for the prevention and treatment of addictive and mental disorders. "SAMHSA's mission is to build resilience and facilitate recovery for people with or at risk for substance abuse and mental illness."[18] Within SAMHSA, there are three centers—the Center for Substance Abuse Treatment (CSAT), the Center for Substance Abuse Prevention (CSAP), and the Center for Mental Health Services (CMHS). Each of these centers has its own set of missions that contribute to the overall mission of SAMHSA (see Chapter 11 and Chapter 12 for more information on SAMHSA).

State Health Agencies

All 50 states have their own state health departments (see Figure 2.4). Although the names of these departments may vary from state to state (e.g., Ohio Department of Health, Indiana State Department of Health), their purposes remain the same: to promote, protect, and maintain the health and welfare of their citizens. These purposes are represented in the **core functions of public health,** which include *assessment* of information on the health of the community, comprehensive public health *policy development,* and *assurance* that public health services are provided to the community.[19] These core functions have been defined further with the following 10 essential public health services.[20]

core functions of public health assessment, policy development, and assurance

1. Monitor health status to identify community health problems.
2. Diagnose and investigate health problems and health hazards in the community.
3. Inform, educate, and empower people about health issues.
4. Mobilize community partnerships to identify and solve health problems.
5. Develop policies and plans that support individual and community health efforts.
6. Enforce laws and regulations that protect health and ensure safety.
7. Link people to needed personal health services and assure the provision of health care when otherwise unavailable.
8. Ensure a competent public health and personal health care workforce.
9. Evaluate effectiveness, accessibility, and quality of personal- and population-based health services.
10. Research for new insights and innovative solutions to health problems (see Figure 2.5).

The head of the state health department is usually a medical doctor, appointed by the governor, who may carry the title of director, commissioner, or secretary. However, due to the political nature of the appointment, this individual may or may not have extensive experience in community or public health. Unfortunately, political influence sometimes reaches below the level of commissioner to the assistant commissioners and division chiefs; it is the commissioner, assistant commissioners, and division chiefs who set policy and provide direction for the state health department. Middle- and lower-level employees are usually hired through a merit system and may or may not be able to influence health department policy. These employees, who carry out the routine work of the state health department, are usually professionally trained health specialists such as microbiologists, engineers, sanitarians, epidemiologists, nurses, and health educators.

Most state health departments are organized into divisions or bureaus that provide certain standard services. Typical divisions include Administration, Communicable Disease Prevention and Control, Chronic Disease Prevention and Control, Vital and Health Statistics, Environmental Health, Health Education or Promotion, Health Services, Maternal and Child Health, Mental Health, Occupational and Industrial Health, Dental Health, Laboratory Services,

FIGURE 2.4
Each of the 50 states has its own health department.

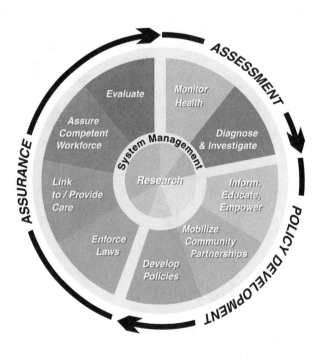

FIGURE 2.5
Core functions of public health and the 10 essential services.
Source: Office of Disease Prevention and Health Promotion (2006). "Public Health in America." Available at
http://web.health.gov/phfunctions/public.htm.

Public Health Nursing, Veterinary Public Health, and most recently, a division of Public Health Preparedness to deal with bioterrorism issues.

In promoting, protecting, and maintaining the health and welfare of their citizens, state health departments play many different roles. They can establish and promulgate health regulations that have the force and effect of law throughout the state. The state health departments also provide an essential link between federal and local (city and county) public health agencies. As such, they serve as conduits for federal funds aimed at local health problems. Federal funds come to the states as block grants. Funds earmarked for particular health projects are distributed to local health departments by their respective state health departments in accordance with previously agreed upon priorities. State health departments may also link local needs with federal expertise. For example, epidemiologists from the CDC are sometimes made available to investigate local disease outbreaks at the request of the state health department. State health departments usually must approve appointments of local health officers and can also remove any local health officers who neglect their duties.

The resources and expertise of the state health department are also at the disposal of local health departments. One particular area where the state health departments can be helpful is laboratory services; many modern diagnostic tests are simply too expensive for local health departments. Another area is environmental health. Water and air pollution problems usually extend beyond local jurisdictions, and their detection and measurement often require equipment too expensive for local governments to afford. This equipment and expertise are often provided by the state health department.

Local Health Departments

Local-level governmental health organizations, referred to as local health departments (LHDs), are usually the responsibility of the city or county governments. In large metropolitan areas, community health needs are usually best served by a city health department. In smaller cities with populations of up to 75,000, people often come under the jurisdiction of a county health department. In some rural counties where most of the population is concentrated in a single city, a LHD may have jurisdiction over both city and county residents. In sparsely populated rural areas, it is not uncommon to find more than one county served by a single health department. In 2005, there were approximately 2,864 LHDs; of that number, 62% were located in nonmetropolitan areas and 38% were in metropolitan areas (see Figure 2.6).[21]

Public Health
Prevent. Promote. Protect.

FIGURE 2.6

The common logo of public health created by the National Association of County and City Health Officials (NACCHO).

Source: National Association of County and City Health Officials (2007). "The National Identity for Local Health Departments." Available at http://www.naccho.org. Used with permission.

It is through LHDs that health services are provided to the people of the community. A great many of these services are mandated by state laws, which also set standards for health and safety. Examples of mandated local health services include the inspection of restaurants, public buildings, and public transportation systems, the detection and reporting of certain diseases, and the collection of vital statistics such as births and deaths. Other programs such as safety belt programs and immunization clinics may be locally planned and implemented. In this regard, local health jurisdictions are permitted (unless preemptive legislation is in place) to enact ordinances that are stricter than those of the state, but these jurisdictions cannot enact codes that fall below state standards. It is at this level of governmental health agencies that sanitarians implement the environmental health programs, nurses and physicians offer the clinical services, and health educators present health education and promotion programs.

Organization of Local Health Departments

Each LHD is headed by a health officer/administrator/commissioner (see Figure 2.7). In most states, there are laws that prescribe who can

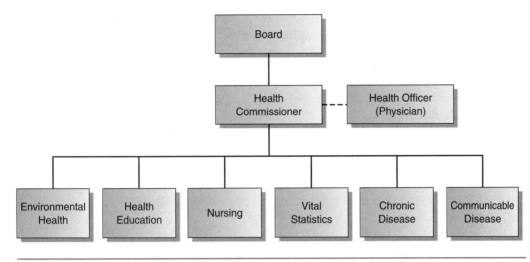

FIGURE 2.7
Organizational chart of a local public health agency.

hold such a position. Those often noted are physicians, dentists, veterinarians, or individuals with a master's or doctoral degree in public health. If the health officer is not a physician, then a physician is usually hired on a consulting basis to advise as needed. Usually, this health officer is appointed by a board of health, the members of which are themselves appointed by officials in the city or county government or, in some situations, elected by the general public. The health officer and administrative assistants may recommend which programs will be offered by the LHDs. However, they may need final approval from a board of health. Although it is desirable that those serving on the local board of health have some knowledge of community health programs, most states have no such requirement. Oftentimes, politics plays a role in deciding the make-up of the local board of health.

The local health officer, like the state health commissioner, has far-reaching powers, including the power to arrest someone who refuses to undergo treatment for a communicable disease (tuberculosis, for example) and who thereby continues to spread disease in the community. The local health officer has the power to close a restaurant on the spot if it has serious health law violations or to impound a shipment of food if it is contaminated. Because many local health departments cannot afford to employ a full-time physician, the health officer is usually hired on a part-time basis. In such cases, the day-to-day activities of the LHD are carried out by an administrator trained in public health. The administrator is also hired by the board of health based upon qualifications and the recommendation of the health officer.

Local sources provide the greatest percentage of LDH revenues (29%), followed by state funds (23%) and federal pass-through funds (13%).[21] A limited number of LHD services are provided on a fee-for-service basis. For example, there is usually a fee charged for birth and death certificates issued by the LHD. Also, in some communities, minimal fees are charged to offset the cost of providing immunizations, lab work, or inspections. Seldom do these fees cover the actual cost of the services provided. Therefore, income from service fees usually makes up a very small portion of any LHD budget. And, it is not unusual to find that many LHDs use a **sliding scale** to determine the fee for a service.

sliding scale
the scale used to determine the fee for services based on ability to pay

Coordinated School Health Programs

Few people think of public schools as governmental health organizations. Consider, however, that schools are funded by tax dollars, are under the supervision of an elected school board, and include as a part of their mission the improvement of the health of those in the school community. Because school attendance is required throughout the United States, the potential for school health programs to make a significant contribution to community health is enormous. In fact, Allensworth and Kolbe have stated that schools "could do more perhaps than any other single agency in society to help young people, and the adults they will become, to live healthier, longer, more satisfying, and more productive lives."[22] Yet coordinated school health programs have faced a number of barriers, including the following:[23]

1. Insufficient local administrative commitment
2. Inadequately prepared teachers
3. Too few school days to teach health in the school year
4. Inadequate funding
5. The lack of credibility of health education as an academic subject
6. Insufficient community/parental support
7. Concern for the teaching of controversial topics (i.e., sex education)

If communities were willing to work to overcome these barriers, the contribution of coordinated school health programs to community health could be almost unlimited.

What exactly is meant by coordinated school health? Prior to 1998, a coordinated school health program was commonly referred to as a *comprehensive school health program*. However, it was commonly confused with *comprehensive health education*. To eliminate this confusion, the term *coordinated* school health program is used. A coordinated school health program is defined as "an organized set of policies, procedures, and activities designed to protect, promote, and improve the health and well-being of students and staff, thus improving a student's ability to learn. It includes but is not limited to comprehensive school

---

BOX 2.2	PUBLIC HEALTH IN THE UNITED STATES

Governmental health agencies at the local, state, and national levels make up the backbone of the public health system. The system is there to (1) prevent epidemics and the spread of disease, (2) protect against environmental hazards, (3) prevent injuries, (4) promote and encourage healthy behaviors, (5) respond to disasters and assist communities in recovery, and (6) assure the quality and accessibility of health services.[20] It is a system that has been taken for granted by most Americans, including those who fund it. As Noreen M. Clark, Dean of the School of Public Health at the University of Michigan, stated, "often when public health works effectively, it is invisible. . . . public health is the disease you *didn't* get, the epidemic that *didn't* spread, the environmental disaster that *didn't* occur."[24]

However, the events of 9/11 "highlighted the state of the infrastructure with unprecedented clarity to the public and policy makers: outdated and vulnerable technologies; a public health workforce lacking training and reinforcements; antiquated laboratory capacity; lack of real-time surveillance and epidemiological systems; ineffective and fragmented communications networks; incomplete domestic preparedness and emergency response capabilities; and communities without access to essential public health services."[25] Yet, if the public health system is to be improved, government health agencies cannot do it alone. They will need to partner "with other organizations and sectors of society, working closely with communities and community based organizations, the health care delivery system, academia, business, and the media."[25]

Building on the vision articulated by *Healthy People 2010*—healthy people in healthy communities—the Committee on Assuring the Health of the Public in the 21st Century of the Institute for Medicine has developed 34 recommendations for assuring population health in the United States. The committee's recommendations revolve around (1) adopting a focus on population health that includes multiple determinants of health, (2) strengthening the public health infrastructure, (3) building partnerships, (4) developing systems of accountability, (5) emphasizing evidence, and (6) improving communications. More specifics about the committee's recommendations can be found at the Institute for Medicine's Web site (www.iom.edu).

health education; school health services; a healthy school environment; school counseling; pyschological and social services; physical education; school nutrition services; family and community involvement in school health; and school-site health promotion for staff."[26]

As previously stated, there are three essential components in every coordinated school health program—health education, a healthy school environment, and health services. Health instruction should be based on a well-conceived, carefully planned curriculum that has an appropriate scope (coverage of topics) and logical sequencing. Instructional units should include cognitive (knowledge), affective (attitudes), and psychomotor (behavioral) components. The healthy school environment should provide a learning environment that is both physically and mentally safe and healthy. Finally, each school's health program should provide the essential health services, from emergency care through health appraisals, to ensure that students will be healthy learners. These topics and others will be discussed in much greater detail in Chapter 6.

QUASI-GOVERNMENTAL HEALTH ORGANIZATIONS

The **quasi-governmental health organizations**—organizations that have some official health responsibilities but operate, in part, like voluntary health organizations—make important contributions to community health. Although they derive some of their funding and legitimacy from governments, and carry out tasks that may be normally thought of as government work, they operate independently of government supervision. In some cases, they also receive financial support from private sources. Examples of quasi-governmental agencies are the American Red Cross (ARC), the National Science Foundation, and the National Academy of Sciences.

quasi-governmental health organizations organizations that have some responsibilities assigned by the government but operate more like voluntary agencies

The American Red Cross

The ARC, founded in 1881 by Clara Barton (see Figure 2.8), is a prime example of an organization that has quasi-governmental status. While it has certain "official" responsibilities placed on it by the federal government, it is funded by voluntary contributions. "Official" duties of the ARC include (1) providing relief to victims of natural disasters such as floods, tornadoes, hurricanes, and fires (Disaster Services) and (2) serving as the liaison between members of the active armed forces and their families during emergencies (Services to the Armed Forces and Veterans). In this latter capacity, the ARC can assist active-duty members of the armed services in contacting their families in case of an emergency, or vice versa.

In addition to these "official" duties, the ARC also engages in many nongovernmental services. These include blood drives, safety services (including water safety, first aid, CPR, and HIV/AIDS instruction), nursing and health services, youth services, community volunteer services, and international services.

The ARC was granted a charter by Congress in 1900, and the ARC and the federal government have had a special relationship ever since. The president of the United States is the honorary chairman of the ARC. The U.S. Attorney General and Secretary of the Treasury are honorary counselor and treasurer, respectively.

The Red Cross idea was not begun in the United States. It was begun in 1863 by five Swiss men in Geneva, Switzerland, who were concerned with the treatment provided to the wounded during times of war. The group, which was called the International Committee for the Relief to the Wounded, was led by Henry Dunant. With the

FIGURE 2.8
The American Red Cross was founded by Clara Barton in 1881.

FIGURE 2.9
The red crystal: an additional emblem of the ICRC.

assistance of the Swiss government, the International Committee brought together delegates from 16 nations in 1864 to the Geneva Convention for the Amelioration of the Condition of the Wounded in Armies in the Field (now known as the first Geneva Convention) to sign the Geneva Treaty.

The efforts of Henry Dunant and the rest of the International Committee led to the eventual establishment of the International Committee of the Red Cross (ICRC). The ICRC, which still has its headquarters in Geneva and is still governed by the Swiss, continues to work today during times of disaster and international conflict. It is the organization that visits prisoners of war to ensure they are being treated humanely.[27,28]

Today, the international movement of the Red Cross comprises the Geneva-based ICRC, the International Federation of Red Cross and Red Crescent Societies (the red crescent emblem is used in Moslem countries), and the over 180 National Red Cross and Red Crescent Societies.[27] There are a number of other countries that believe in the principles of the Red Cross Movement, but have not officially joined because the emblems used by the movement are offensive. Thus, the ICRC has created a third emblem that meets all the criteria for use as a protective device and at the same time is free of any national, political, or religious connotations. The design is composed of a red frame in the shape of a square on the edge of a white background. The name chosen for this distinctive emblem was "red crystal," to signify purity. The emblem was put into use on January 14, 2007 (see Figure 2.9).[28]

Other Quasi-Governmental Organizations

Two other examples of quasi-governmental organizations in the United States are the National Science Foundation (NSF) and the National Academy of Sciences (NAS). The purpose of NSF is the funding and promotion of scientific research and the development of individual scientists. NSF receives and disperses federal funds but operates independently of governmental supervision. Chartered by Congress in 1863, the NAS acts as an advisor to the government on questions of science and technology. Included in its membership are some of America's most renowned scientists. Although neither of these agencies exists specifically to address health problems, both organizations fund projects, publish reports, and take public stands on health-related issues.

NONGOVERNMENTAL HEALTH AGENCIES

Nongovernmental health agencies are funded by private donations or, in some cases, by membership dues. There are thousands of these organizations that all have one thing in common: They arose because there was an unmet health need. For the most part, the agencies operate free from governmental interference as long as they meet Internal Revenue Service guidelines with regard to their specific tax status. In the following sections, we discuss the following types of nongovernmental health agencies—voluntary, professional, philanthropic, service, social, religious, and corporate.

voluntary health agencies nonprofit organizations created by concerned citizens to deal with a health need not met by governmental health agencies

Voluntary Health Agencies

Voluntary health agencies are an American creation. Each of these agencies was created by one or more concerned citizens who felt that a specific health need was not being met by existing governmental agencies. In a sense, these new voluntary agencies arose by themselves, in much the same way as a "volunteer" tomato plant arises in a vegetable garden. New voluntary agencies continue to be born each year. Examples of recent additions to the perhaps 100,000 agencies already in existence are the Alzheimer's Association and the First Cradle/SIDS Alliance. A discussion of the commonalities of voluntary health agencies follows.

Organization of Voluntary Health Agencies

Most voluntary agencies exist at three levels—national, state, and local. At the national level, policies that guide the agency are formulated. A significant portion of the money raised locally is forwarded to the national office, where it is allocated according to the agency's budget. Much of the money is designated for research. By funding research, the agencies hope to discover the cause of and cure for a particular disease or health problem. There have been some major successes. The March of Dimes, for example, helped to eliminate polio as a major disease problem in the United States through its funding of immunization research.

There is not always a consensus of opinion about budget decisions made at the national level; some believe that less should be spent for research and more for treating those afflicted with the disease. Another common internal disagreement concerns how much of the funds raised at the local level should be sent to the national headquarters instead of being retained for local use. Those outside the agency sometimes complain that when an agency achieves success, as the March of Dimes did in its fight against polio, it should dissolve. This does not usually occur; instead, successful agencies often find a new health concern. The March of Dimes now fights birth defects; and when tuberculosis was under control, the Tuberculosis Society changed its name to the American Lung Association in order to fight all lung diseases.

The state-level offices of voluntary agencies are analogous to the state departments of health in the way that they link the national headquarters with local offices. The primary work at this level is to coordinate local efforts and to ensure that policies developed at the national headquarters are carried out. The state-level office may also provide training services for employees and volunteers of local-level offices and are usually available as consultants and problem solvers. In recent years, some voluntary agencies have been merging several state offices into one to help reduce overhead expenses.

The local-level office of each voluntary agency is usually managed by a paid staff worker who has been hired either by the state-level office or by a local board of directors. Members of the local board of directors usually serve in that capacity on a voluntary basis. Working under the manager of each agency are local volunteers, who are the backbone of voluntary agencies. It has been said that the local level is where the "rubber meets the road." In other words, this is where most of the money is raised, most of the education takes place, and most of the service is rendered. Volunteers are of two types, professional and lay. Professional volunteers have had training in a medical profession, while lay volunteers have had no medical training. The paid employees help facilitate the work of the volunteers with expertise, training, and other resources.

Purpose of Voluntary Health Agencies

Voluntary agencies share four basic objectives: (1) to raise money to fund their programs, with the majority of the money going to fund research, (2) to provide education both to professionals and to the public, (3) to provide service to those individuals and families that are afflicted with the disease or health problem, and (4) to advocate for beneficial policies, laws, and regulations that affect the work of the agency and in turn the people they are trying to help.

Fund-raising is a primary activity of many voluntary agencies. While in the past this was accomplished primarily by door-to-door solicitations, today mass-mailing and telephone solicitation are more common. In addition, most agencies sponsor special events like golf outings, dances, or dinners. One type of special event that is very popular today is the "a-thon" (see Figure 2.10). The term "a-thon" is derived from the name of the ancient Greek city Marathon, and usually signified some kind of "endurance" event. Examples include bike-a-thons, rock-a-thons, telethons, skate-a-thons, and dance-a-thons. These money-making "a-thons" seem to be

FIGURE 2.10
Most voluntary health agencies hold special events to raise money for their causes.

limited in scope only by the creativity of those planning them. In addition, some of these agencies have become United Way agencies and receive some funds derived from the annual United Way campaign, which conducts fund-raising efforts at worksites. The three largest voluntary agencies in the United States today (in terms of dollars raised) are the American Cancer Society (see Box 2.3), the American Heart Association, and the American Lung Association.

Over the years, the number of voluntary agencies formed to help meet special health needs has continually increased. Due to the growth in the number of new agencies, several consumer "watchdog" groups have taken a closer look into the practices of the agencies. A major concern of these consumer groups has been the amount of money that the voluntary agencies spend on the cause (e.g., cancer, heart disease, AIDS, etc.) and how much they spend on fund-raising and overhead (e.g., salaries, office furniture, leasing of office space). Well-run agencies will spend less than 15% of what they raise on fund-raising. Some of the not so well-run agencies spend as much as 80% to 90% on fund-raising. All consumers should ask agencies how they spend their money prior to contributing.

Professional Health Organizations/Associations

Professional health organizations and associations are made up of health professionals who have completed specialized education and training programs and have met the standards of registration, certification, and/or licensure for their respective fields. Their mission is to promote high standards of professional practice for their specific profession, thereby improving the health of society by improving the people in the profession. Professional organizations are funded primarily by membership dues. Examples of such organizations are the American Medical Association, the American Dental Association, the American Nursing Association, the American Public Health Association, the American Association for Health Education, and the Society for Public Health Education, Inc.

Although each professional organization is unique, most provide similar services to their members. These services include the certification of continuing-education programs for professional renewal, the hosting of annual conventions where members share research results and interact with colleagues, and the publication of professional journals and other reports. Some examples of journals published by professional health associations are the *Journal of the American Medical Association,* the *American Journal of Public Health,* and the *American Journal of Health Education.*

Like voluntary health agencies, another important activity of some professional organizations is advocating on issues important to their membership. The American Medical Association, for example, has a powerful lobby nationally and in some state legislatures. Their purpose is to affect legislation in such a way as to benefit their membership and their profession. Many professional health organizations provide the opportunity for benefits, including group insurance and discount travel rates. There are hundreds of professional health organizations in the United States, and it would be difficult to describe them all here.

philanthropic foundation an endowed institution that donates money for the good of humankind

Philanthropic Foundations

Philanthropic foundations have made and continue to make significant contributions to community health in the United States and throughout the world. These foundations sup-

**A CLOSER LOOK AT ONE VOLUNTARY HEALTH AGENCY:
THE AMERICAN CANCER SOCIETY**

The American Cancer Society (ACS) was founded in 1913 by 10 physicians and five laymen. At that time, it was known as the American Society for the Control of Cancer. Today, with offices throughout the country and approximately two million volunteers, ACS is one of our largest voluntary health organizations. In spite of its success, its mission has remained constant since its founding. It is "dedicated to eliminating cancer as a major health problem by preventing cancer, saving lives, and diminishing suffering from cancer, through research, education, advocacy and service."[29]

The mission of the ACS includes both short- and long-term goals. Its short-term goals are to save lives and diminish suffering. This is accomplished through education, advocacy, and service. Its long-term goal, the elimination of cancer, is being approached through the society's support of cancer research.

The American Cancer Society's educational programs are targeted at two different groups—the general public and the health professionals who treat cancer patients. The public education program promotes the following skills and concepts to people of all ages: (1) taking the necessary steps to prevent cancer, (2) knowing the seven warning signals, (3) understanding the value of regular checkups, and (4) coping with cancer. The society accomplishes this by offering free public education programs, supported by up-to-date literature and audiovisual materials, whenever and wherever they may be requested. These programs may be presented in homes, worksites, churches, clubs, organizations, and schools. A few of their better-known programs include I Can Cope, Reach to Recovery, and Man to Man.[29] From time to time, the society also prepares public service messages for broadcasting or televising.

The society's professional education program is aimed at the professionals who work with oncology patients. The objective of this program is to motivate "medical and allied health professionals to use the latest and best possible cancer detection, diagnostic, and patient management techniques."[30] Such education is provided through professional publications, up-to-date audiovisual materials, conferences, and grants that fund specialized education experiences.

The ACS offers patient service and rehabilitation programs that ease the impact of cancer on those affected. The services offered include information and referral to appropriate professionals, home care supplies and equipment for the comfort of patients, transportation of patients to maintain their medical and continuing care programs, and specialized education programs for cancer patients to help them cope and feel better about themselves. There are also rehabilitation programs that provide social support for all cancer patients and specific programs for those who have had a mastectomy, laryngectomy, or ostomy.

The ACS is the largest source of private, not-for-profit cancer research funds in the United States, second only to the federal government in total dollars spent. Since 1946, when the ACS first started awarding grants, it has invested about $3.1 billion in cancer research. The research program consists of three components: extramural grants, intramural epidemiology and surveillance research, and the intramural behavioral research center.[29] The most recent addition to the work of the ACS is in the area of advocacy. Specifically, the ACS works to (1) support cancer research and programs to prevent, detect, and treat cancer; (2) expand access to quality cancer care, prevention, and awareness; (3) reduce cancer disparities in minority and medically underserved populations; and (4) reduce and prevent suffering from tobacco-related illnesses.[29]

All ACS programs—education, service, research, and advocacy—are planned primarily by the society's volunteers. However, the society does employ staff members to carry out the day-to-day operations and to help advise and support the work of the volunteers. This arrangement of volunteers and staff working together has created a very strong voluntary health agency.

port community health by funding programs and research on the prevention, control, and treatment of many diseases. Foundation directors, sometimes in consultation with a review committee, determine the types of programs that will be funded. Some foundations fund an array of health projects, whereas others have a much narrower scope of interests. Some foundations, such as the Bill and Melinda Gates Foundation, fund international health projects, whereas others restrict their funding to domestic projects. The geographical scope of domestic foundations can be national, state, or local. Local foundations may restrict their funding to projects that only benefit local citizens.

The activities of these foundations differ from those of the voluntary health agencies in two important ways. First, foundations have money to give away, and therefore no effort is spent on fund-raising. Second, foundations can afford to fund long-term or innovative research projects, which might be too risky or expensive for voluntary or even government-funded agencies. The development of a vaccine for yellow fever by a scientist funded by the Rockefeller Foundation is an example of one such long-range project.

Some of the larger foundations, in addition to the Bill and Melinda Gates Foundation, that have made significant commitments to community health are the Commonwealth Fund, which has contributed to community health in rural communities, improved hospital facilities, and tried to strengthen mental health services; the Ford Foundation, which has contributed greatly to family-planning efforts throughout the world; the Robert Wood Johnson Foundation, which has worked to improve access to medical and dental care throughout the United States and lessen the impact of tobacco on health; the Henry J. Kaiser Family Foundation, which has supported the development of health maintenance organizations (HMOs) and community health promotion; the W. K. Kellogg Foundation, which has funded many diverse health programs that address human issues and provide a practical solution; and the Milbank Memorial Fund, which has primarily funded preventive-medicine projects.

Service, Social, and Religious Organizations

Service, social, and religious organizations have also played a part in community health over the years (see Figure 2.11). Examples of service and social groups involved in community health are the Jaycees, Kiwanis Club, Fraternal Order of Police, Rotary Club, Elks, Lions, Moose, Shriners, American Legion, and Veterans of Foreign Wars. Members of these groups enjoy social interactions with people of similar interests in addition to fulfilling the groups' primary reason for existence—service to others in their communities. Although health may not be the specific focus of their mission, several of these groups make important contributions in that direction by raising money and funding health-related programs. Sometimes, their contributions are substantial. Examples of such programs include the Shriners' children's hospitals and burn centers, the Lions' contributions to pilot (lead) dog programs and other services for those who are visually impaired, such as the provision of eyeglasses for school-aged children unable to afford them, and the Lions' contributions to school health programs via the educational program named "Lions Quest."

FIGURE 2.11

Community service groups contribute needed resources for the improvement of the health of the community.

The contributions of religious groups to community health have also been substantial. Such groups also have been effective avenues for promoting health programs because (1) they have had a history of volunteerism and pre-existing reinforcement contingencies for volunteerism, (2) they can influence entire families, and (3) they have accessible meeting-room facilities.[31] One way in which these groups contribute is through donations of money for missions for the less fortunate. Examples of religious organizations that solicit donations from their members include the Protestants' One Great Hour of Sharing, the Catholics' Relief Fund, and the United Jewish Appeal. Other types of involvement in community health by religious groups include (1) the donation of space for voluntary health programs such as blood donations, Alcoholics Anonymous, and other support groups, (2) the sponsorship of food banks and shelters for the hungry, poor, and homeless, (3) the sharing of the doctrine of good personal health behavior, and (4) allowing community health professionals to deliver their programs through the congregations. This latter contribution has been especially useful in black American communities because of the importance of churches in the culture of this group of people.

In addition, it should be noted that some religious groups have hindered the work of community health workers. Almost every community in the country can provide an example where a religious organization has protested the offering of a school district's sex education program, picketed a public health clinic for providing reproductive information or services to women, or has spoken out against homosexuality.

Corporate Involvement in Community Health

From the way it treats the environment by its use of natural resources and the discharge of wastes, to the safety of the work environment, to the products and services it produces and provides, to the provision of health care benefits for its employees, corporate America is very much involved in community health. Though each of these aspects of community health is important to the overall health of a community, because of the concern for the "bottom line" in corporate America, it is the provision of health care benefits that often receives the most attention. In fact, many corporations today find that their single largest annual expenditure behind salaries and wages is for employee health care benefits. Consider, for example, the cost of manufacturing a new car. The cost of health benefits for those who build the car now exceeds the cost of the raw materials for the car itself.

In an effort to keep a healthy workforce and reduce the amount paid for health care benefits, many companies support health-related programs both at and away from the worksite. Worksite programs aimed at trimming employee medical bills have been expanded beyond the traditional safety awareness programs and first aid services to include such programs as substance abuse counseling, nutrition education, smoking cessation, stress management, physical fitness, and disease management. Many companies also are implementing health promotion policies and enforcing state and local laws that prohibit (or severely restrict) smoking on company grounds or that mandate the use of safety belts at all times in all company-owned vehicles. (See Chapter 18 for more on safety and health in the workplace.)

CHAPTER SUMMARY

- Contemporary society is too complex to respond effectively to community health problems on either an emergency or a long-term basis. This fact necessitates organizations and planning for health in our communities.

- The different types of organizations that contribute to the promotion, protection, and maintenance of health in a community can be classified into three groups according to their sources of funding and organizational structure—governmental, quasi-governmental, and nongovernmental.

- Governmental health agencies exist at the local, state, federal, and international levels and are funded primarily by tax dollars.

- WHO is the largest and most visible governmental health agency on the international level.

- The Department of Health and Human Services (HHS) is the U.S. government's principal agency for the pro-

tection of the health of all Americans and for providing essential human services, especially for those who are least able to help themselves.

- The core functions of public health include the assessment of information on the health of the community, comprehensive public health policy development, and assurance that public health services are provided to the community.

- Quasi-governmental agencies, such as the American Red Cross, share attributes with both governmental and nongovernmental agencies.

- Nongovernmental organizations include voluntary and professional associations, philanthropic foundations, and service, social, and religious groups.

- Corporate America has also become more involved in community health, both at the worksite and within the community.

REVIEW QUESTIONS

1. What characteristics of modern society necessitate planning and organization for community health?

2. What is a governmental health agency?

3. What is the World Health Organization (WHO) and what does it do?

4. What federal department in the United States is the government's principal agency for protecting the health of all Americans and for providing essential human services, especially to those who are least able to help themselves? What major services does this department provide?

5. What are the three core functions of public health?

6. What are the 10 essential public health services?

7. How do state and local health departments interface?

8. What is meant by the term *coordinated school health program?* What are the major components of it?

9. What is meant by the term *quasi-governmental agency?* Name one such agency.

10. Describe the characteristics of a nongovernmental health agency.

11. What are the major differences between a governmental health organization and a voluntary health agency?

12. What does a health professional gain from being a member of a professional health organization?

13. How do philanthropic foundations contribute to community health? List three well-known foundations.

14. How do service, social, and religious groups contribute to the health of the community?

15. Why has corporate America become involved in community health?

ACTIVITIES

1. Using a local telephone book, list all the health-related organizations that service your community. Divide your list by the three major types of health organizations noted in this chapter.

2. Make an appointment to interview someone at one of the organizations identified in Activity 1. During your visit, find answers to the following questions:

   a. How did the organization begin?

   b. What is its mission?

   c. How is it funded?

   d. How many people (employees and volunteers) work for the organization, and what type of education/training do they have?

   e. What types of programs/services does the organization provide?

3. Obtain organizational charts from the U.S. Department of Health and Human Services (a copy is in this chapter), your state department of health, and your local health department. Compare and contrast these charts and describe their similarities and differences.

4. Call a local voluntary health organization in your community and ask if you could volunteer to work 10 to 15 hours during this academic term. Then volunteer those hours and keep a journal of your experience.

5. Carefully review your community newspaper each day for an entire week. Keep track of all articles or advertisements that make reference to local health organizations. Summarize your findings in a one-page paper. (If you do not subscribe to your local paper, copies are available in libraries.)

SCENARIO: ANALYSIS AND RESPONSE

After having read this chapter, please respond to the following questions in reference to the scenario at the beginning of the chapter.

1. What type of health agency do you think will be of most help to Mary?

2. If this scenario were to happen to someone in your community, what recommendations would you give to him or her on seeking help from health agencies?

3. The Internet has many sources of information that could help Mary. Use a search engine (e.g., Google) and enter the word "cancer." Find the Web site of one governmental health agency at the national level and one voluntary health agency that might be able to help her. Explain how these agencies could be of help.

4. If Mary did not have Internet access, how would you suggest she find out about local health agencies in her area that could help her?

COMMUNITY HEALTH ON THE WEB

The Internet contains a wealth of information about community and public health. Increase your knowledge of some of the topics presented in this chapter by accessing the Jones and Bartlett Publishers Web site at **http://health.jbpub.com/book/communityhealth/6e** and follow the links to complete the following Web activities.

- World Health Organization
- Department of Health and Human Services
- Association of State and Territorial Health Officials

REFERENCES

1. Green, L. W. (1990). "The Revival of Community and the Public Obligation of Academic Health Center." In R. E. Bulger and S. J. Reiser, eds. *Integrity in Institutions: Humane Environments for Teaching, Inquiry and Health.* Iowa City: University of Iowa Press, 163-180.

2. World Health Organization (2006). "World Health Organization." Available at http://www.who.int/about/en/.

3. United Nations (2000). *United Nations Millennium Declaration.* New York: Author.

4. United Nations (2002). *Road Map Towards the Implementation of the United Nations Millennium Declaration.* New York: Author.

5. World Health Organization (2003). *World Health Report 2003: Shaping the Future.* Geneva, Switzerland: Author.

6. Dodd, R., and A. Cassels (2006). "Health, Development and the Millennium Development Goals." *Annals of Tropical Medicine and Parasitology,* 100(5/6): 379-387.

7. World Health Organization (2005). *Health and the Millennium Development Goals.* Geneva, Switzerland: Author.

8. U.S. Department of Health and Human Services (2006). "United States Department of Health and Human Services." Available at http://www.hhs.gov/about/whatwedo.html.

9. Government Printing Office Access (2006). *Budget of the United States Government: Browse Fiscal Year 2007.* Available at http://origin.www.gpoaccess.gov/usbudget/fy07/browse.html.

10. Agency for Healthcare Research and Quality (2004). "What Is AHRQ?" Available at http://www.ahrq.gov/about/Whatis.htm.

11. Agency for Toxic Substances and Disease Registry (2006). "About the Agency for Toxic Substances and Disease Registry." Available at http://www.atsdr.cdc.gov/about.html.

12. Falk, H. (2003) "A Message from Dr. Henry Falk, ATSDR Assistant Administrator." *Public Health and the Environment,* 2(1/2): 1.

13. Centers for Disease Control and Prevention (2006). "Centers for Disease Control and Prevention." Available at http://www.cdc.gov/.

14. U.S. Food and Drug Administration (2006). "FDA's Mission Statement." Available at http://fda.gov/opacom/morechoices/mission.html.

15. Health Resources and Services Administration (2006). "About HRSA." Available at http://www.hrsa.gov/about/default.htm.

16. Indian Health Service (2006). "Indian Health Service Fact Sheet." Available at http:www.ihs.gov/PublicInfo/PublicAffairs/Welcome_Info/ThisFacts.asp.

17. National Institutes for Health (2006). "Questions and Answers about NIH." Available at http://www.nih.gov/about/Faqs.thm#NIH.

18. Substance Abuse and Mental Health Services Administration (2006). "SAMSHA: Who Are We?" Available at http://www.samhsa.gov/about/background.aspx.

19. National Academy of Sciences, Institute of Medicine (1988). *The Future of Public Health.* Washington, DC: National Academy Press.

20. Office of Disease Prevention and Health Promotion (2004). "Public Health in America." Available at http://web.health.gov/phfunctions/public.htm.

21. Jeep, C. J. (2005). *National Profile of Local Health Departments.* Washington, DC: National Association of County and City Health Officials.

22. Allensworth, D. D., and L. J. Kolbe (1987). "The Comprehensive School Health Program: Exploring an Expanded Concept." *Journal of School Health,* 57(10): 409-412.

23. Butler, S. C. (1993). "Chief State School Officers Rank Barriers to Implementing Comprehensive School Health Education." *Journal of School Health,* 63(3): 130-132.

24. Clark, N. M. (2002). *A Letter from the Dean.* Ann Arbor, MI: University of Michigan, School of Public Health.

25. Institute of Medicine (2003). *The Future of the Public's Health.* Washington, DC: The National Academies Press.

26. Joint Committee on Health Education and Promotion Terminology (2001). "Report of the 2000 Joint Committee on Health Education and Promotion Terminology." *American Journal of Health Education,* 32(2): 89-103.

27. American Red Cross (2006). "Frequently Asked Questions." Available at http://www.redcross.org/faq.

28. International Committee of the Red Cross (2006). "About the Red Cross/Red Crescent Emblem: Questions and Answers." Available at http://www.icrc.org.

29. American Cancer Society (2006). "About the American Cancer Society." Available at http://www.cancer.org/docroot/AA/AA_0.asp.

30. American Cancer Society (2006). "Continuing Medical Education." Available at http://www.cancer.org/docroot/PRO/content/PRO_2_Continuing_Medical_Education.asp.

31. Lasater, T. M., B. L. Wells, R. A. Carleton, and J. P. Elder (1986). "The Role of Churches in Disease Prevention Research Studies." *Public Health Report,* 101(2) 123-131.

Chapter 3

Epidemiology: The Study of Disease, Injury, and Death in the Community

Chapter Objectives

After studying this chapter you will be able to:

1 Define the terms *epidemic, epidemiology,* and *epidemiologist,* and explain their importance in community health.

2 List some diseases that caused epidemics in the past and some that are causing epidemics today.

3 Discuss how the practice of epidemiology has changed since the days of Benjamin Rush and John Snow.

4 Explain why rates are important in epidemiology and list some of the commonly used rates.

5 Define incidence and prevalence rates and provide examples of each.

6 Calculate a variety of rates from the appropriate data.

7 Discuss the importance of disease reporting to a community's health and describe the reporting process.

8 Define the following standardized measurements of health status—life expectancy, years of potential life lost (YPLL), disability-adjusted life years (DALYs), and health-adjusted life expectancy (HALE).

9 Identify sources of standardized data used by epidemiologists, community health workers, and health officials and list the types of data available from each source.

10 List and describe the various types of epidemiological studies and explain the purpose of each.

SCENARIO

John thought about this afternoon's picnic. Everyone had a blast. For a while it had seemed almost too warm, but plenty of cold drinks were available, and by late afternoon it had become quite pleasant. The games were fun too . . . frisbee, soccer, softball, and volleyball. Then there was the picnic itself—turkey, potato salad, bread and butter, milk, and dessert—served about noon.

It was now 8 P.M. that same night, and instead of studying as he had planned, John was lying on his bed with a bad stomachache. He was experiencing severe diarrhea and had made several hurried trips to the bathroom in the last half-hour.

The telephone rang, and it was Michael, John's roommate. He had gone to his girlfriend's house after the picnic to work on a class project with her. He and Caroline were both sick with stomach cramps and diarrhea, and Michael was calling to ask whether John was sick too. As John was answering, he realized that he needed to run to the bathroom again. He quickly hung up, promising to call back soon. Moments later as he returned to his bedroom, John began to think about what a coincidence it was that all three of them were sick with the same symptoms at about the same time. Could they have become ill from food they ate at the picnic? There were about 50 people at the picnic; How many others might also be sick? Was it the heat? Was it the food? Was this an epidemic? A half-hour later, John

called Michael back to tell him that he had decided to go to the campus health center.

Elsewhere . . .

This had turned out to be an interesting volunteer experience. As a requirement for her community health class, Kim had agreed to volunteer at the local health department. The spring semester was almost over now, and she was writing a final report of her activities. During the term, she had spent her Friday afternoons accompanying a sanitarian on his inspections of restaurants and retail food stores. She also had helped him complete his reports on substandard housing and malfunctioning septic tanks.

Dr. Turner, the health officer, had given Kim permission to use one of the department's personal computers for preparing her final report. Because it was Sunday evening, she was alone in the health department office when the telephone rang. She briefly considered not answering it but finally picked up the receiver. It was Dr. Lee from the University Health Center. He said he was calling in the hope that someone might be there because he needed to reach Dr. Turner immediately. He said that he had admitted six students to the infirmary with severe stomach cramps, vomiting, and diarrhea. The students had been at a picnic earlier, and he thought they could have food poisoning. He called to ask Dr. Turner to investigate this outbreak and asked Kim to try to reach him as soon as possible.

INTRODUCTION

When you become ill and visit a doctor, the first thing the physician does is take measurements and collect information. The measurements include your temperature, heart rate, and blood pressure. The information includes time of onset of your illness, where you have traveled, and what you might have eaten. Next, you may be given a physical examination and asked to provide a specimen such as urine or blood for laboratory examination. The information gathered helps the physician understand the nature of your illness and prescribe an appropriate treatment.

While a primary care physician is concerned with the course of disease in an individual patient, an epidemiologist is concerned with the course of disease in a population. When illness, injury, or death occur at unexpected or unacceptable levels in a community or population, epidemiologists seek to collect information about the disease status of the community. First, epidemiologists want to know *how many* people are sick. Second, they want to know *who* is sick—the old? the young? males? females? rich? poor? They also want to know *when* the people became sick, and finally, *where* the sick people live or have traveled. In summary, epidemiologists want to know what it is that the sick people have in common. For this reason, epidemiology is sometimes referred to as *population medicine*.

epidemiology
the study of the distribution and determinants of health-related states or events in specified populations

Epidemiology is one of the community health activities "aimed at protecting or improving the health of a population or community" discussed in Chapter 1. Information gathered from epidemiological studies assists community decision makers to make the best use of the community's human and financial health resources. Data gathered at local, state, and national levels can be used not only to prevent disease outbreaks or control those that are in progress, but also to assess whether an ongoing disease prevention program is effective.

Definition of Epidemiology

epidemic
an unexpectedly large number of cases of an illness, specific health-related behavior, or other health-related event in a particular population

Before we discuss the types of questions an epidemiologist asks, we need to define the term *epidemiology*. **Epidemiology** is "the study of the distribution and determinants of health-related states or events in specified populations, and the application of this study to control health problems."[1] The term *epidemiology* is derived from Greek words that can be translated into the phrase "the study of that which is upon the people." The goal of epidemiology is to limit disease, injury, and death in a community by intervening to prevent or limit outbreaks or epidemics of disease and injury. This is accomplished by describing outbreaks and designing studies to analyze them and to validate new approaches to prevention, control, and treatment. Through these practices, epidemiologists contribute to our knowledge of how diseases begin and spread through populations, and how they can be prevented, controlled, and treated.

endemic disease
a disease that occurs regularly in a population as a matter of course

The question might be asked, how many cases are required before a disease outbreak is considered an epidemic—10 cases? 100 cases? 1,000 cases? The answer is that it depends upon the disease and the population, *but any unexpectedly large number of cases of an illness, specific health-related behavior, or other health-related event* in a particular population at a particular time and place can be considered an **epidemic.** Some recent epidemics in the United States are presented in Table 3.1.

The question might be asked, what are diseases called that occur regularly in a population but are not epidemic? These diseases are referred to as **endemic diseases.** Whether a disease is epidemic or endemic depends on the disease and the population. Heart disease is endemic in America, while in many regions of equatorial Africa, malaria is endemic.

epidemiologist
one who practices epidemiology

An **epidemiologist** is "an investigator who studies the occurrence of disease or other health-related conditions or events in defined populations."[1] Some epidemics begin as outbreaks of disease in animals, known as *epizootics*, and then spread to human populations. Examples are bubonic plague that first affects rodents, and West Nile fever virus that first affects birds. Occasionally, an epidemic will spread over a wide area, perhaps even across an entire continent or around the world. Such a widespread epidemic is termed a **pandemic.**

pandemic
an outbreak of disease over a wide geographical area such as a continent

The influenza pandemic of 1918 is an example (see Figure 3.1). This disease spread in Europe, Asia, and North America simultaneously.[2] An estimated 25 million people died over several years as a result of this pandemic. Could another influenza pandemic occur (see Box 3.1)? The

Table 3.1
Recent Epidemics in the United States

Disease	Cases in Previous Years	Epidemic Period	Number of Cases
St. Louis encephalitis	5–72	1975	1,815 [4]
Legionnaires' disease	Unknown	1976	235 [5]
Toxic shock syndrome	11–272	1980	877 [6]
HIV/AIDS	Unknown	1981–2004	944,305 [7]
Lyme disease	Unknown	1990–2004	222,350 [8-10]
Plague	13–19	1983	40 [5]
West Nile virus	Unknown	1999–2005	18,756 [11]
Mumps	231–314	2006	5,423 [12]

FIGURE 3.1
More than 25 million people died during the influenza pandemic of 1918–1919.

| BOX 3.1 | INFLUENZA: THE NEXT PANDEMIC? |

In 1997, in Hong Kong, the first documented cases occurred in which avian influenza virus infected humans directly from birds. Previous human influenza virus infections had been traced to pig intermediaries. Because pigs can also be infected with human influenza virus, they are a host in which the two influenza virus strains can mix. A possible outcome of such mixing can be a strain that can be transmitted from human to human. In fact, this happens regularly, and new vaccines are introduced annually to combat the latest new strain or strains of influenza virus emanating from Asia.

The avian flu virus strain that infected people directly has been identified as the virulent H5N1 strain. Avian and human immunity to this strain is very low, so that most birds and people who become infected become very ill and many die. In December 2003, 19,000 of 25,000 chickens died on a farm in the Republic of Korea, and over the next several weeks more than a million chickens and ducks died. The virus next turned up in Vietnam and then Thailand, where human cases were reported. In these two countries there were 19 deaths among the 25 human cases in 2004. Since 2003, human H5N1 cases have been reported in Azerbaijan, Cambodia, China, Djibouti, Egypt, Indonesia, Iraq, and Turkey, according to the Centers for Disease Control and

Prevention (CDC). Since the first human case in 2003 through the middle of September 2006, 246 cases have been reported, with 144 deaths.

Health officials are concerned that the H5N1 strain could become pandemic because

- It is especially virulent.
- It is being spread by migratory birds.
- It can be transmitted from birds to mammals and in some limited circumstances to humans.
- Like other influenza viruses, it continues to evolve.

The best source of information about avian influenza is the CDC Web site (http://pandemicflu.gov/). It provides scientific information about the flu virus, documents aimed at helping individuals and communities prepare for a possible flu pandemic, and links to state and local planning documents.

Another useful site is the World Health Organization's Web site (www.who.int/csr/disease/avian_influenza/en/), where you can read a history of the avian flu epidemic and get the latest information on the avian flu situation.

Sources: Centers for Disease Control and Prevention. "PandemicFlu.gov." Available at http://pandemicflu.gov/; and World Health Organization. "Avian Influenza." Available at http://www.who.int/csr/disease/avian_influenza/en/.

current outbreak of acquired immunodeficiency syndrome (AIDS) is another example of a pandemic. During 2005, an estimated 2.8 million people died of AIDS worldwide and 38,600,000 people were living with HIV (human immunodeficiency virus).[3]

History of Epidemiology

If one searches diligently, it is possible to trace the roots of epidemiological thinking back to the "Father of Medicine," Hippocrates, who as early as 300 B.C. suggested a relationship between the occurrence of disease and the physical environment.[13] For example, cases of a disease fitting the description of malaria were found to occur in the vicinity of marshes and swamps.

With the fall of the classical civilizations of Greece and Rome and the return in Europe to a belief in spiritual causes of disease, few advances were made in the field of epidemiology. As a result, epidemics continued to occur. There were three waves of plague—one in 542-543, one in 1348-1349, and another in 1664-1665.[14] There were also epidemics of leprosy, smallpox, malaria, and, later, syphilis and yellow fever.

Epidemics occurred in the New World as well. One such epidemic of yellow fever struck Philadelphia in 1793, causing the death of 4,044 people. Yellow fever was epidemic again in Philadelphia in 1797, 1798, and in 1803.[15] Dr. Benjamin Rush, a prominent Philadelphia physician and signatory of the Declaration of Independence, was able to trace the cases of yellow fever to the docks where ships arrived from tropical ports. However, his conclusion that the disease was caused by vapors arising from decaying coffee beans in port warehouses was incorrect. He could not have known that yellow fever is caused by a virus and is carried by the yellow fever mosquito, *Aedes aegypti*. These facts were discovered by Major Walter Reed of the U.S. Army and his associates a century later.

In 1849, some 50 years after the yellow fever outbreaks in Philadelphia, cholera became epidemic in London. A prominent physician, John Snow, investigated the outbreak by interviewing numerous victims and their families. He concluded that the source of the epidemic was probably water drawn from a particular communal well located on Broad Street. Snow extinguished the epidemic in 1854 when he removed the pump handle from the Broad Street pump, thus forcing people to obtain their water elsewhere.[16]

John Snow's quashing of the London cholera epidemic in 1854 is a classic example of how epidemiological methods can be used to limit disease and deaths. His achievement was even more remarkable because it occurred 30 years before Louis Pasteur proposed his "germ theory of disease." It was not until 1883 that Robert Koch discovered the organism that causes cholera, *Vibrio cholerae*.

From its early use for the description and investigation of communicable diseases, epidemiology has developed into a sophisticated field of science. Epidemiological methods are used to evaluate everything from the effectiveness of vaccines to the possible causes of occupational illnesses and unintentional injury deaths.

Knowledge of epidemiology is important to the community health worker who wishes to establish the presence of a set of needs or conditions for a particular health service or program or to justify a request for funding. Likewise, epidemiological methods are used to evaluate the effectiveness of programs already in existence and to plan to meet anticipated needs for facilities and personnel.

THE IMPORTANCE OF RATES

Epidemiologists are concerned with numbers. Of prime importance is the number of health-related events, the number of **cases** (people who are sick), and, of course, the number of deaths. These numbers alone, however, are not enough to provide a description of the extent of the dis-

cases
people afflicted with a disease

rate
the number of events that occur in a given population in a given period of time

natality (birth) rate
the number of live births divided by the total population

morbidity rate
the rate of illness in a population

ease in a community. Epidemiologists must also know the total number in the susceptible population so that rates can be calculated. A **rate** is the number of events (births, cases of disease, or deaths) in a given population over a given period or at a given point in time. Three general categories of rates are **natality (birth) rates, morbidity** (sickness) **rates,** and **mortality or fatality (death) rates.**

Why are rates important? Why not simply enumerate the sick or dead? The answer is that rates enable one to compare outbreaks that occur at different times or in different places. For example, by using rates it is possible to determine whether there are more cases of gonorrhea per capita this year than there were last year or whether there are more homicides per capita in City A than in City B.

For example, suppose you wish to compare transportation deaths associated with travel by autos and airplanes. To examine this hypothetical situation, consider that for a given time period, 1,000 people died in auto crashes while 50 people died in airplane crashes. Without calculating rates, one might assume that auto travel is more dangerous than air travel. However, if you knew the population exposed (100,000 people for auto travel versus 1,000 people for air travel), you could calculate fatality rates, the number of deaths divided by the population, for each mode of travel.[17] (See Table 3.2.) These rates have greater meaning because they are based upon the **population at risk,** those who are susceptible to disease or death from a particular cause. In this case, the fatality rates are 1/100 for autos and 5/100 for airplanes, thus indicating that in this hypothetical example air travel is five times more dangerous than auto travel.

Incidence, Prevalence, and Attack Rates

Three important types of morbidity rates are incidence rates, prevalence rates, and attack rates. An **incidence rate** is defined as the number of new health-related events or cases of a disease in a population exposed to that risk in a given time period—the number of *new* cases of influenza in a community over a week's time, for example. Those who became ill with influenza during the previous week and remain ill during the week in question are not counted in an incidence rate. Incidence rates are important in the study of **acute diseases,** diseases in which the peak severity of symptoms occurs and subsides within days or weeks. These diseases usually move quickly through a population. Examples of acute diseases are the common cold, influenza, chickenpox, measles, and mumps.

Prevalence rates are calculated by dividing *all* current cases of a disease (*old and new*) by the total population. Prevalence rates are useful for the study of **chronic disease,** diseases that usually last three months or longer. In these cases, it is more important to know how many people are currently suffering from a chronic disease—such as arthritis, heart disease, cancer, or diabetes—than it is to know when they became afflicted. Furthermore, with many chronic diseases, it is difficult or impossible to determine the date of onset of disease. Because a preponderance of health services and facilities are used for the treatment of persons with chronic diseases and conditions, prevalence rates are more useful than incidence rates for the planning of public health programs, personnel needs, and facilities.

mortality (fatality) rate the number of deaths in a population divided by the total population

population at risk those in the population who are susceptible to a particular disease or condition

incidence rate the number of new health-related events or cases of a disease in a population exposed to that risk during a particular period of time, divided by the total number in that same population

acute disease a disease that lasts three months or less

prevalence rate the number of new and old cases of a disease in a population in a given period of time, divided by the total number in that population

chronic disease a disease or health condition that lasts longer than three months

Table 3.2
Hypothetical Number of Deaths and Death Rates for Two Modes of Travel

	Source of Fatalities	
	Auto	**Airplane**
Number of fatalities per year	1,000	50
Number exposed to risk	100,000	1,000
Rate of fatality	0.01 (1/100)	0.05 (5/100)

Table 3.3
Incidence Rates, Prevalence Rates, and Attack Rates

Name of Rate		Definition of Rate	
Incidence rate	=	$\dfrac{\text{Number of new health-related events or cases of a disease}}{\text{Number of people exposed to risk during this period}}$	
Prevalence rate	=	$\dfrac{\text{Total number of all individuals who have an attribute or disease at a time}}{\text{Population at risk of having the attribute or disease at this point or period of time}}$	
Attack rate*	=	$\dfrac{\text{The cumulative incidence of infection in a group observed during an epidemic}}{\text{Number of people exposed}}$	× 100

*Attack rates are usually given as a percentage.

attack rate
an incidence rate calculated for a particular population for a single disease outbreak and expressed as a percentage

An **attack rate** is a special incidence rate calculated for a particular population for a single disease outbreak and expressed as a percentage (see Table 3.3). For example, suppose a number of people who traveled on the same airline flight developed a similar illness, and epidemiologists suspected that the cause of this illness was associated with the flight itself. An attack rate could be calculated for the passengers on that flight to express the percentage who became ill. Furthermore, attack rates could be calculated for various subpopulations, such as those seated at various locations in the plane, those who selected specific entrees from the menu, those of particular age groups, or those who boarded the flight at specific stops. Differences in attack rates for different subpopulations might indicate to the epidemiologists the source or cause of the illness.

Crude and Age-Adjusted Rates

crude rate
a rate in which the denominator includes the total population

crude birth rate
the number of live births per 1,000 in a population in a given period of time

Incidence and prevalence rates can be expressed in two forms—crude and specific. **Crude rates** are those in which the denominator includes the total population. The most important of these are the crude birth rate and the crude death rate. The **crude birth rate** is the number of live births in a given year, divided by the midyear population. The **crude death rate (CDR)** is the total number of deaths in a given year from all causes, divided by the midyear population (see Table 3.4). Crude rates are relatively easy to obtain and are useful when comparing similar populations. But they can be misleading when populations differ by age structure or by some other attribute. For example, crude birth rates are normally higher in younger populations, which have a higher proportion of people of reproductive age, than in populations with more elderly people. Conversely, CDRs are normally higher in older populations. This makes it difficult to use crude rates to compare the risk of death in different populations, such as those of the states of Florida and Alaska. To show what the level of mortality would be if the age composition of different populations were the same, epidemiologists use **age-adjusted rates.** For example, because of its larger senior population, Florida has a higher crude death rate (991.0 per 100,000) compared with Alaska's (490.1 per 100,000), where the population is younger.

crude death rate (CDR)
the number of deaths (from all causes) per 1,000 in a population in a given period of time

age-adjusted rate
rate used to make comparisons of relative risks across groups and over time when groups differ in age structure

Table 3.4
Crude Rates

Name of Rate		Definition of Rate		Multiplier
Crude birth rate	=	$\dfrac{\text{Number of live births}}{\text{Estimated midyear population}}$	×	1,000
Crude death rate	=	$\dfrac{\text{Number of deaths (all causes)}}{\text{Estimated midyear population}}$	×	1,000

Table 3.5
Crude and Age-Adjusted Mortality Rates for Alaska and Florida, 2003

State	Number of Deaths	Crude Death Rate*	Age-Adjusted Death Rate*
Alaska	3,180	490.1	829.8
Florida	168,657	991.0	776.0

*Deaths per 100,000 population.

Source: Hoyert, D. L., M. P. Heron, S. L. Murphy, and H. C. Kung (2006). "Deaths: Final Data for 2003." *National Vital Statistics Report,* 54(13): 1–120.

However, when these death rates are adjusted for differences in the age structures of the populations of these two states, one can see that the death rate in Florida (776.0 per 100,000) compares favorably with the death rate in Alaska (829.8 per 100,000). See Table 3.5.[18] Methods for calculating age-adjusted rates can be found in standard epidemiology textbooks.

Specific Rates

Specific rates measure morbidity and mortality for particular populations or for particular diseases. One could, for example, calculate the age-specific mortality rate for a population of 35- to 44-year-olds by dividing the number of deaths in that age group by the midyear population of 35- to 44-year-olds. Similarly, one could calculate race- and sex-specific mortality rates.

A very important specific rate is the **cause-specific mortality rate (CSMR),** which measures the death rate for a specific disease. This rate can be calculated by dividing the number of deaths due to a particular disease by the total population. One could also calculate an age–specific, cause-specific mortality rate. Because fewer people can be expected to die from each cause than to die from all causes, CSMRs are usually reported per 100,000 population. Table 3.6 lists some important rates used in epidemiology, defines them, and gives an example of each.

specific rate
a rate that measures morbidity or mortality for particular populations or diseases

cause-specific mortality rate (CSMR)
the death rate due to a particular disease

Table 3.6
Important Rates in Epidemiology

Rate		Definition		Multiplier	Examples (U.S. 2004)[20,21]
Crude birth rate	=	$\dfrac{\text{Number of live births}}{\text{Estimated midyear population}}$	×	1,000	14.0/1000
Crude death rate	=	$\dfrac{\text{Number of deaths (all causes)}}{\text{Estimated midyear population}}$	×	1,000	8.0/1000
Age-specific death rate	=	$\dfrac{\text{Number of deaths, 15–24}}{\text{Estimated midyear population, 15–24}}$	×	100,000	79.2/100,000
Infant mortality rate	=	$\dfrac{\text{Number of deaths under 1 year of age}}{\text{Number of live births}}$	×	100,000	6.76/1000
Neonatal mortality rate	=	$\dfrac{\text{Number of deaths under 28 days of age}}{\text{Number of live births}}$	×	100,000	4.5/1000
Cause-specific death rate	=	$\dfrac{\text{Number of deaths (diabetes mellitus)}}{\text{Estimated midyear population}}$	×	100,000	24.8/100,000
Age-specific, cause-specific death rate	=	$\dfrac{\text{Number of deaths, 15–24 (motor vehicles)}}{\text{Estimated midyear population}}$	×	100,000	26.1/100,000

case fatality rate (CFR)
the percentage of cases of a particular disease that result in death

proportionate mortality ratio (PMR)
the percentage of overall mortality in a population that is attributable to a particular cause

notifiable diseases
infectious diseases for which health officials request or require reporting for public health reasons

Two other important measures of disease are the **case fatality rate (CFR)** and the **proportionate mortality ratio (PMR).** The CFR is simply the percentage of cases that result in death. It is a measure of the severity of a disease and is directly related to the virulence of the disease agent. It is calculated by dividing the number of deaths from a particular disease in a specified period of time by the number of cases of that same disease in the same time period. The resulting fraction is multiplied by 100 and is reported as a percentage. For example, if there were 200 cases of a severe illness and 10 of them resulted in death, the CFR would be $10 \div 200 \times 100 = 5\%$.

The PMR describes the relationship between the number of deaths from a specific cause to the total number of deaths attributable to all causes. It is calculated by dividing the number of deaths attributed to a particular disease by the total number of deaths from all causes in the same population during the same period of time. This rate is also reported as a percentage. For example, in the United States, there were 652,486 deaths due to diseases of the heart in 2004, and 2,397,615 total deaths reported that same year.[19] Thus, the PMR for cardiovascular disease can be calculated as follows: $652,486 \div 2,397,615 \times 100 = 27\%$. In other words, in the United States, heart disease was responsible for 27% of all deaths in 2004.

REPORTING OF BIRTHS, DEATHS, AND DISEASES

It is important to epidemiologists that births, deaths, and cases of diseases be recorded promptly and accurately. Physicians, clinics, and hospitals are required by law to report all births and deaths as well as all cases of certain **notifiable diseases** to their local health departments. Notifiable diseases are infectious diseases that can become epidemic and for which health officials maintain weekly records. The Centers for Disease Control and Prevention (CDC) issues a list of notifiable diseases for which it requests reports from each state health department. This list is revised periodically. In 2004, the CDC designated more than 60 diseases as notifiable at the national level (see Table 3.7). Several diseases caused by possible

Table 3.7
Reported Cases of Notifiable Diseases, United States, 2004

Disease*	No. of Cases	Rank†	Rate§
AIDS¶	44,108	3	15.2
Botulism			
Foodborne	16	55	0
Infant	87	47	0
Other (includes wound and unspecified)	30	51	0
Brucellosis	114	43	0
Chancroid**	30	51	0
Chlamydia**††	929,462	1	319.6
Cholera	5	62	0
Coccidioidomycosis§§	6,449	13	4.1
Cryptosporidiosis	3,557	18	1.2
Cyclosporiasis	171	39	0.1
Ehrlichiosis			
Human granulocytic	537	30	0.2
Human monocytic	338	32	0.1
Encephalitis/meningitis, arboviral			
California serogroup	112	44	0
Eastern equine	6	61	0
Powassan	1	65	S¶¶
St. Louis	12	56	0
West Nile	1,142	27	0.4

Disease*	No. of Cases	Rank†	Rate§
Enterohemorrhagic *Escherichia coli* (EHEC)			
EHEC O157:H7	2,544	20	0.9
EHEC non-O157	308	35	0.1
EHEC, not serogrouped	316	34	0.1
Giardiasis	20,636	8	8.3
Gonorrhea**	330,132	2	113.5
Haemophilus influenzae, invasive, all ages/serotypes	2,085	22	0.7
Age < 5 yr, serotype b	19	54	0
Age < 5 yr, nonserotype b	135	40	0
Age < 5 yr, unknown	177	38	0.9
Hansen disease (leprosy)	105	45	0
Hantavirus pulmonary syndrome	24	53	0
Hemolytic uremic syndrome, postdiarrheal	200	37	0.1
Hepatitis A, acute	5,683	16	1.9
Hepatitis B, acute	6,212	15	2.1
Hepatitis C, acute	720	29	0.3
Legionellosis	2,093	21	0.7
Listeriosis	753	28	0.3
Lyme disease	19,804	9	6.8
Malaria	1,458	24	0.5
Measles	37	49	0
Meningococcal disease	1,361	25	0.5
Mumps	258	36	0.1
Pertussis	25,827	7	8.9
Plague	3	64	S
Psittacosis	12	56	0
Q fever	70	48	0
Rabies			
Animal	6,345	14	2.2
Human	7	60	0
Rocky Mountain spotted fever	1,713	23	0.6
Rubella	10	58	0
Salmonellosis	42,197	4	14.5
Shigellosis	14,627	10	5.0
Streptococcal disease, invasive, group A	4,395	17	1.8
Streptococcal toxic-shock syndrome	132	42	0.1
Streptococcus pneumoniae, invasive			
Drug-resistant§§	2,590	19	1.5
Age, < 5 yr§§	1,162	26	0.6
Syphilis, total, all stages	33,041	5	11.5
Congenital (age < 1 yr)**	353	31	0.1
Primary and secondary**	7,980	12	2.7
Tetanus	34	50	0
Toxic-shock syndrome	95	46	0
Trichinellosis	5	62	0
Tuberculosis***	14,517	11	5.0
Tularemia	134	41	0
Typhoid fever	322	33	0.1
Vancomycin-resistant *Staphylococcus aureus*	1	65	S
Varicella (chickenpox)§§	32,931	6	18.4
Varicella deaths†††	9	59	0

*No cases of anthrax; diphtheria; influenza-associated pediatric mortality; paralytic poliomyelitis; rubella, congenital syndrome; severe acute respiratory syndrome–associated coronavirus; smallpox; vancomycin-intermediate *Staphylococcus aureus*; western equine encephalitis; or yellow fever were reported in 2004.

†Diseases are ranked in order of the total number of incident cases reported. The disease with the highest number of cases is assigned a rank of 1. Diseases with equal case counts are assigned the same rank, and the disease with the next rank is augmented to reflect the number of diseases with an equal ranking immediately preceding it.

(*continues*)

Table 3.7 (continued)

---

§Per 100,000 population.

¶Total number of acquired immunodeficiency syndrome (AIDS) cases reported to the Division of HIV/AIDS Prevention—Surveillance and Epidemiology, National Center for HIV, STD, and TB Prevention (NCHSTP), through December 31, 2005.

**Totals reported to the Division of Sexually Transmitted Diseases Prevention, NCHSTP, as of May 20, 2005.

††Chlamydia refers to genital infections caused by *Chlamydia trachomatis*.

§§Notifiable in < 40 states.

¶¶Rates are suppressed if fewer than five incident cases were reported.

***Totals reported to the Division of TB Elimination, NCHSTP, as of April 15, 2005.

†††Death counts provided by Epidemiology and Surveillance Division, National Immunization Program.

Source: Centers for Disease Control and Prevention (2006). "Summary of Notifiable Diseases—United States, 2004." *MMWR,* 53(53): 18-19.

National Electronic Telecommunications System (NETS) the electronic reporting system used by state health departments and the CDC

bioterrorism agents, such as anthrax and Q fever, were added. Individual states may require the reporting of additional diseases that are of local public health concern. Local health departments are required by their respective state health departments to summarize all records of births (see Figure 3.2), deaths, and notifiable diseases, and to report them. State health departments summarize these reports and relay them to the CDC through the **National Electronic Telecommunications System (NETS).** The reporting scheme for notifiable disease is shown in Figure 3.3.

The CDC summarizes state and territorial data and uses it to plan epidemiological research, conduct investigations, and issue reports. One series of reports, published weekly by the CDC, is called the *Morbidity and Mortality Weekly Report (MMWR). MMWRs* are available to the public at the CDC Web site, www.cdc.gov/mmwr. Paper copies can usually be found in the government documents areas of certain larger libraries.

Unfortunately, the information reported is not always as good as it should be. One study estimated that local health departments may receive notification of only 35% of the cases of some communicable diseases and that many physicians are not familiar with the requirement of reporting. Clinics may not report each and every case of measles or gonorrhea. Doctors' offices and clinics may be understaffed or simply too busy to keep up with reporting. In other cases, patients recover—with or without treatment—before a diagnosis is confirmed. Also, changes in local and state government administration or other key personnel often interfere with the timely reporting of disease data. The accuracy of disease reporting also depends on the type of disease. In this regard, serious diseases are more likely to be reported than milder ones. Rabies cases, for example, are almost 100% reported, whereas German measles cases may be only 80% to 90% reported. Therefore, morbidity data—while useful for reflecting disease trends—cannot always be considered to be precise counts of the actual number of cases of diseases.

STANDARDIZED MEASUREMENTS OF HEALTH STATUS OF POPULATIONS

It is often difficult to precisely measure the level of wellness or, for that matter, ill health. On the other hand, death can be clearly defined. For this reason, mortality statistics continue to be the single most reliable indicator of a population's health status. While mortality statistics do not completely describe the health status of a population, they can be used to calculate other useful measurements; two of these are life expectancy and years of potential life lost. Finally, there are measurements of ill health that, while less precise than mortality, can

FIGURE 3.2

Birth certificates are issued by local health departments that have jurisdiction where the birth occurred.

• 73 •

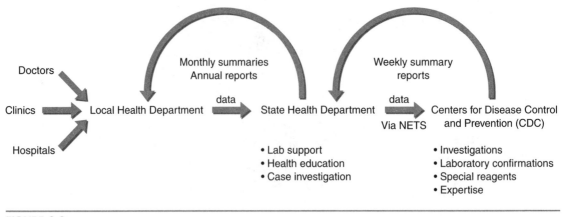

FIGURE 3.3
Scheme for the reporting of notifiable diseases.

nonetheless be meaningful. Such measurements are disability-adjusted life years and health-adjusted life expectancy.

Mortality Statistics

In 2004, 2,397,615 deaths were registered in the United States. The crude mortality rate was 816.5 per 100,000. The age-adjusted death rate, which eliminates the effects of the aging population, was 854.5 deaths per 100,000 U.S. standard population. This was a record low.[19,20] Age-adjusted death rates show what the level of mortality would be if no changes occurred in the age make-up of the population from year to year. Thus, they are a better indicator than unadjusted (crude) death rates for examining changes in the risk of death over a period of time when the age distribution of the population is changing. Death rates and age-adjusted death rates for the 15 leading causes of death for the entire population in the United States in 2004 are presented in Table 3.8.

Naturally, morbidity and mortality rates vary greatly depending on age, sex, race, and ethnicity. For example, while heart disease is the leading cause of death for the general population and especially for seniors (those who have reached 65 years of age), cancer is the leading cause of death for the 45- to 64-years age group, and unintentional injuries are the leading cause of death for all age groups between 1 and 44. (In Chapters 7–10, we will discuss the differences in the health statistics of people in different age, sex, and minority groups.)

A study of the mortality statistics for the twentieth century reveals a shift in the leading causes of death. When the century began, communicable diseases such as pneumonia, tuberculosis, and gastrointestinal infections were the leading causes of death. However, a century of progress in public health practice and in biomedical research has resulted in a significant reduction in the proportion of deaths from communicable diseases, so that the four leading causes of death today are noncommunicable diseases (see Table 3.9). At the beginning of the twenty-first century, the five leading causes of death in the United States—heart disease, cancer, stroke, chronic obstructive pulmonary disease, and unintentional injuries (accidents and adverse effects)—account for about 68% of all deaths (see Table 3.9).[19]

This domination of annual mortality statistics by noncommunicable diseases masks the importance of communicable diseases as causes of deaths in certain age groups. For example,

Table 3.8

Percentage of Total Deaths, Death Rates, and Age-Adjusted Death Rates for 2004, the Percent Change in Age-Adjusted Death Rates from 2003 to 2004, and the Ratio of Age-Adjusted Death Rates by Race and Sex for the 15 Leading Causes of Death for the Total U.S. Population in 2004

Rank*	Cause of Death (Based on the International Classification of Diseases, Tenth Revision, 1992)	Number	Percentage of Total Deaths	2004 Crude Death Rate	Age-Adjusted Death Rate 2004	Percent Change from 2003 to 2004	Ratio Male to Female	Ratio Black to White	Ratio Hispanic† to non-Hispanic White
...	All causes	2,397,615	100.0	816.5	800.8	-3.8	1.4	1.3	0.7
1	Diseases of heart	652,486	27.2	222.2	217.0	-6.6	1.5	1.3	0.7
2	Malignant neoplasms	553,888	23.1	188.6	185.8	-2.3	1.4	1.2	0.6
3	Cerebrovascular diseases	150,074	6.3	51.1	50.0	-6.5	1.0	1.5	0.8
4	Chronic lower respiratory diseases	121,987	5.1	41.5	41.1	-5.1	1.4	0.7	0.4
5	Accidents (unintentional injuries)	112,012	4.7	38.1	37.7	1.1	2.1	0.9	0.8
6	Diabetes mellitus	73,138	3.1	24.9	24.5	-3.2	1.3	2.2	1.5
7	Alzheimer's disease	65,965	2.8	22.5	21.8	1.9	0.7	0.8	0.6
8	Influenza and pneumonia	59,664	2.5	20.3	19.8	-10.0	1.4	1.1	0.9
9	Nephritis, nephrotic syndrome, and nephrosis	42,480	1.8	14.5	14.2	-1.4	1.4	2.3	0.9
10	Septicemia	33,373	1.4	11.4	11.2	-3.4	1.2	2.2	0.8
11	Intentional self-harm (suicide)	32,439	1.4	11.0	10.9	0.9	4.0	0.4	0.5
12	Chronic liver disease and cirrhosis	27,013	1.1	9.2	9.0	-3.2	2.2	0.9	1.6
13	Essential (primary) hypertension and hypertensive renal disease	23,076	1.0	7.9	7.7	4.1	1.0	2.8	1.0
14	Parkinson's disease	17,989	0.8	6.1	6.1	-1.6	2.3	0.4	0.6
15	Assault (homicide)	17,357	0.7	5.9	5.9	-1.7	3.7	5.6	2.7
...	All other causes (residual)	414,674	17.3	141.2	...	...	...	...	...

Note: Death rates are on an annual basis per 100,000 population; age-adjusted rates are per 100,000 U.S. standard population.

. . . Category not applicable.

*Rank is based on number of deaths.

†Data for Hispanic origin should be interpreted with caution because of inconsistencies between reporting Hispanic origin on death certificates and on censuses and surveys.

Source: Miniño, A. M., M. Heron, S. L. Murphy, and K. D. Kochanek (2006). "Deaths: Final Data for 2004." NCHS Health E-Stats. Available at http://www.cdc.gov/nchs/products/pubs/pubd/hestats/finaldeaths04/finaldeaths04.htm.

Table 3.9
Leading Causes of Death in the United States: 1900, 1940, 2004

1900

1.	Pneumonia, influenza
2.	Tuberculosis
3.	Diarrhea
4.	Diseases of the heart
5.	Cerebrovascular diseases (stroke)
6.	Nephritis
7.	Unintentional injuries (accidents)
8.	Malignant neoplasms (cancers)
9.	Senility
10.	Diphtheria

1940

1.	Diseases of the heart
2.	Malignant neoplasms (cancers)
3.	Cerebrovascular diseases (stroke)
4.	Nephritis
5.	Pneumonia, influenza
6.	Unintentional injuries (non-motor vehicle)
7.	Tuberculosis
8.	Diabetes mellitus
9.	Unintentional injuries (motor vehicle)
10.	Premature birth

2004

1.	Diseases of the heart
2.	Malignant neoplasms (cancers)
3.	Cerebrovascular diseases (stroke)
4.	Chronic obstructive pulmonary diseases
5.	Unintentional injuries (all)
6.	Diabetes mellitus
7.	Alzheimer's disease
8.	Influenza and pneumonia
9.	Nephritis (kidney diseases)
10.	Septicemia

pneumonia and influenza still kill many seniors in this country each year. Also, HIV/AIDS, listed as the eighth overall leading cause of death for Americans as recently as 1996, kills more males than females. Thus, it is important to remember that viewing the leading causes of death for the entire population does not provide a clear picture of the health for any one segment of the population.

Life Expectancy

life expectancy
the average number of years a person from a specific cohort is projected to live from a given point in time

Life expectancy is another standard measurement used to compare the health status of various populations. Also based on mortality, **life expectancy** is defined as the average number of years a person from a specific cohort is projected to live from a given point in time. While life insurance companies are interested in life expectancy at every age, health statisticians are usually concerned with life expectancy at birth, at the age of 65 years, and, more recently, at age 75. It must be remembered that life expectancy is an average for an entire cohort (usually of a single birth year) and is not necessarily a useful prediction for any one individual. Moreover, it certainly cannot describe the quality of one's life. However, the ever-increasing life expectancy for Americans suggests that, as a country, we have managed to control some of those factors that contribute to early deaths.

Table 3.10
Life Expectancy at Birth, at 65 Years of Age, and at 75 Years of Age According to Sex:
In the United States, During the Selected Years 1900–2003

Year	At Birth Both Sexes	Male	Female	At 65 Years Both Sexes	Male	Female	At 75 Years Both Sexes	Male	Female
1900	47.3	46.3	48.3	11.9	11.5	12.2	*	*	*
1950	68.2	65.6	71.1	13.9	12.8	15.0	*	*	*
1960	69.7	66.6	73.1	14.3	12.8	15.8	*	*	*
1970	70.8	67.1	74.7	15.2	13.1	17.0	*	*	*
1980	73.7	70.7	77.4	16.4	14.1	18.3	10.4	8.8	11.5
1990	75.4	71.8	78.8	17.2	15.1	18.9	10.9	9.4	12.0
2003	77.5	74.8	80.1	18.4	16.8	19.8	11.8	10.5	12.6

*Data not available.

Source: Adapted from the National Center for Health Statistics (2006). *Health, United States, 2006 with Chartbook on Trends in the Health of Americans.* (DHHS pub. no. 2006-1232). Hyattsville, MD: Public Health Service.

Table 3.10 provides a summary of life expectancy figures for the United States from 1900 to 2003. The data presented indicate that the overall life expectancy at birth, at 65 years, and at 75 years has generally increased since 1900. Life expectancies at birth for both sexes rose from 47.3 years in 1900 to 77.5 years in 2003, when the life expectancy of a newborn baby girl was 80.1 years compared with a newborn baby boy—74.8 years.[22]

When compared with the life expectancy figures of other countries (see Table 3.11), the United States figures roughly correspond with those of other countries with well-developed economies. The highest life expectancy figures are reported in Japan (86 years for females); while the lowest are reported from countries in Africa.[23] In three African countries—Congo, Malawi, and South Africa—life expectancy has declined since 1980, in part because of HIV/AIDS.

Table 3.11
Life Expectancy at Birth for Selected Countries by Sex in 2005

	Male	Female
Ethiopia	50	53
Malawi	47	46
India	62	64
Nicaragua	68	73
Ecuador	70	75
Congo	54	55
Thailand	67	73
Malaysia	69	74
South Africa	50	52
Brazil	68	75
Latvia	65	76
Republic of Korea	75	82
Greece	77	82
New Zealand	77	82
United Kingdom	77	81
United States	75	80
Sweden	79	83
Japan	79	86

Source: World Bank (2007). http://www.who.int/whosis/whostat2007/en/index.html. Reprinted wth permission.

Years of Potential Life Lost

While standard mortality statistics, such as leading causes of death, provide one measure of the importance of various diseases, **years of potential life lost (YPLL)** provides another, different measure. YPLL is calculated by subtracting a person's age at death from his or her life expectancy. Such calculations are difficult because each person may have a different life expectancy at any given time. Thus, the ages 65 years or 75 years are often used in these calculations. For a person who dies at age 59, the YPLL-75 is 16. For many years in the United States, a death prior to 65 years was considered a premature death, perhaps because 65 was the standard age of retirement and when full Social Security payments could begin. Now, however, 75 years of age is increasingly being used to calculate YPLL because the life expectancy for a child born today is closer to 75 years (see Table 3.10). People are living longer, and many of us know people who continue to work beyond the age of 65; examples include former President Ronald Reagan, his successor, George H. W. Bush, and the late South Carolina Senator Strom Thurmond, who served as a U.S. senator into his 90s.

YPLL weights deaths such that the death of a very young person counts more than the death of a very old person. Table 3.12 provides a summary of the age-adjusted YPLL before 75 (YPLL-75) for the 10 leading causes of death in the United States for 1990 and 2003.[22] In examining this table, note that the number of YPLL-75 per 100,000 population was higher for malignant neoplasms (cancer) than for heart disease. Also, YPLL resulting from unintentional injuries was third highest. This is because unintentional injuries and malignant neoplasms (cancer) often kill people when they are young. These differences can also be seen in the two pie charts shown in Figure 3.4. Also, notice that the YPLL-75 per 100,000 population declined for most of the leading causes of death between 1990 and 2003. An important exception is for diabetes mellitus, a disease that is becoming epidemic in the United States.

YPLL from specific causes varies depending upon the gender and face of the subpopulation under consideration. For example, the YPLL-75 per 100,000 population due to unintentional injuries is nearly three times as high for men as it is for women. The YPLL-75 per 100,000 for diseases of the heart for blacks is nearly twice that for whites, and for homicide, it is nearly six times greater.[22]

Table 3.12
Age-Adjusted Years of Potential Life Lost Before 75 (YPLL-75) for the 10 Leading Causes of Death, United States, 1990 and 2003

	YPLL per 100,000 Population	
Cause	1990	2003
Diseases of the heart	1,617.7	1,187.9
Malignant neoplasms (cancer)	2,003.8	1,586.9
Cerebrovascular diseases (stroke)	259.6	203.6
Chronic lower respiratory diseases	187.4	183.9
Unintentional injuries	1,162.1	1,084.6
Influenza and pneumonia	141.5	90.8
Diabetes mellitus	155.9	159.6
Human immunodeficiency virus infection (HIV/AIDS)	383.8	153.3
Suicide	393.1	343.3
Homicide and legal intervention	417.4	274.3

Source: Adapted from National Center for Health Statistics (2003). *Health, United States, 2006 with Chartbook on Trends in the Health of Americans* (HHS pub. no. 2006-1232). Hyattsville, MD: Author.

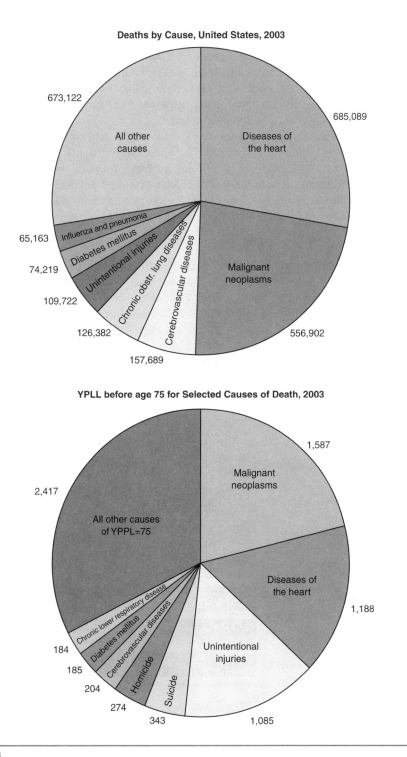

FIGURE 3.4

Deaths by cause in the United States, 2003, and the years of potential life lost before age 75 (YPLL-75) per 100,000 population for selected causes of death within the United States, 2003.

Source: National Center for Health Statistics (2006). *Health, United States, 2006 with Chartbook on Trends in the Health of Americans* (HHS pub. no. 2006-1232). Hyattsville, MD: Author.

Disability-Adjusted Life Years

disability-adjusted life years (DALYs)
a measure for the burden of disease that takes into account premature death and loss of healthy life resulting from disability

Mortality does not entirely express the burden of disease. For example, chronic depression and paralysis caused by polio are responsible for great loss of healthy life but are not reflected in mortality tables. Because of this, the World Health Organization (WHO) and the World Bank have developed a measure called the **disability-adjusted life years (DALYs).**[23]

One DALY is one lost year of healthy life. Total DALYs for a given condition for a particular population can be calculated by estimating the total YPLL and the total years of life lived with disability, and then by summing these totals. As an example, the DALYs incurred through firearm injuries in the United States could be calculated by adding the total of YPLL incurred from fatal firearm injuries to the total years of life lived with disabilities by survivors of firearm injuries. Figure 3.5 illustrates the number of DALYs lost per 1,000 in 2001 from seven demographic regions of the world.[23,24]

Health-Adjusted Life Expectancy

Health-adjusted life expectancy (HALE)
the number of years of healthy life expected, on average in a given population

Health-adjusted life expectancy (HALE), sometimes referred to as *healthy life expectancy*, is the number of years of healthy life expected, on average, in a given population or region of the world. The HALE indicator used by the WHO is similar to the disability-adjusted life expectancy (DALE) first reported in the original Global Burden of Disease study.[23] The methods used to calculate HALE are beyond the scope of this textbook, but have been described elsewhere.[25] Worldwide, HALE at birth in 2001 was 57.4 years, 7.5 years lower than overall life expectancy at birth. As with life expectancy, HALE in sub-Saharan Africa is very low—less than 40 years for males, compared with about 70 years for females in high-income countries (Figure 3.6).[24]

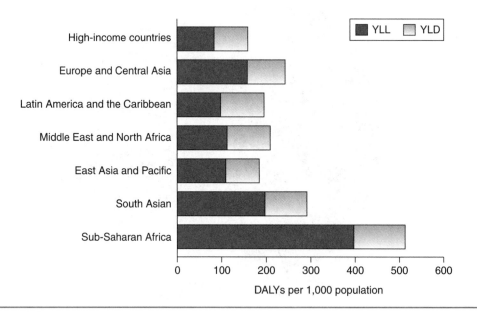

FIGURE 3.5

Burden of disease: years of life lost due to premature mortality (YLL) and years of life lived with a disability (YLD) per thousand by region, 2001. DALYs, disability-adjusted life years.

Source: Lopez, A. S., C. D. Mathers, M. Ezzati, D. T. Jamison, and C. J. L. Murray, eds. (2006). *Global Burden of Disease and Risk Factors*. Washington, DC: The World Bank and Oxford University Press. Used with permission of the International Bank for Reconstruction and Development/The World Bank.

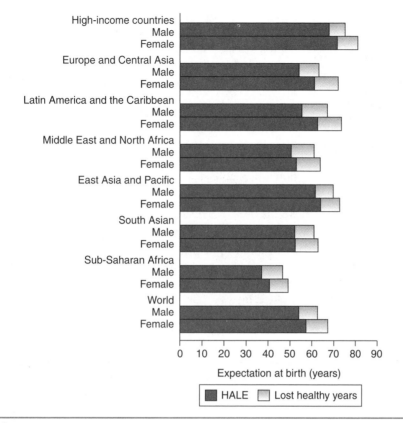

FIGURE 3.6

Life expectancy, health-adjusted life expectancy (HALE), and lost healthy years by region and sex, 2001.

Source: Lopez, A. S., C. D. Mathers, M. Ezzati, D. T. Jamison, and C. J. L. Murray, eds. (2006). *Global Burden of Disease and Risk Factors*. Washington, DC: The World Bank and Oxford University Press. Used with permission of the International Bank for Reconstruction and Development/The World Bank.

SOURCES OF STANDARDIZED DATA

Because demographic and epidemiological data are used in the planning of public health programs and facilities, students of community health should be aware of the sources of these standardized data. Students can obtain standardized data for use in community health work from the following sources: The U.S. Census, the *Statistical Abstract of the United States,* the *Monthly Vital Statistics Report, Morbidity and Mortality Weekly Report,* the National Health Interview Survey, the National Health and Nutrition Examination Survey, the Behavioral Risk Factor Surveillance System, the Youth Risk Behavior Surveillance System, the National Hospital Discharge Survey, and the National Hospital Ambulatory Medical Care Survey.

Each of these sources of national data has a specific value and usefulness to those in the public health field. Students interested in studying local health problems can obtain data from state and local health departments, hospitals, volunteer agencies, and disease registries. The study and analysis of these data provide a basis for planning appropriate health programs and facilities in your communities.

The U.S. Census

The **U.S. Census,** taken every 10 years, is an enumeration of the population living in the United States. George Washington ordered the first census in 1790 for the purpose of

U.S. Census
the enumeration of
the population of the
United States that is
conducted every
10 years

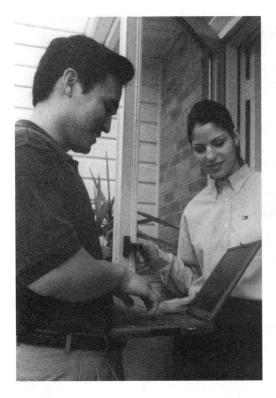

FIGURE 3.7
A census worker collects data used to calculate disease rates.

apportioning representation to the House of Representatives. Through the years, the census form has become much more complex than the one filled out over 200 years earlier. Data are gathered about income, employment, family size, education, dwelling type, and many other social indicators (see Figure 3.7). Copies of the U.S. Census results are available in most libraries.

Census data are important to health workers because they are used for calculating disease and death rates and for program planning. The U.S. Census is carried out by the Bureau of the Census, located in the U.S. Department of Commerce. Information is available at www.census.gov.

Statistical Abstract of the United States

Another Bureau of the Census publication is the *Statistical Abstract of the United States* (SA). This book, published annually, is the standard summary of statistics on the social, political, and economic organization of the United States. Information is divided into sections under headings such as Population, Vital Statistics, Health and Nutrition, Education, Law Enforcement, Courts and Prisons, and many more. Data contained in the SA are extremely useful and are reasonably up-to-date. (A new edition is published every January and includes data from two years before the publication date.) The SA can be purchased from the Government Printing Office for about $50 and is available in most libraries. Information is also available at www.census .gov/statab/www/.

Monthly Vital Statistics Report

The National Center for Health Statistics (NCHS), one of the Centers for Disease Control and Prevention, provides the most up-to-date national vital statistics available. These statistics appear in the *Monthly Vital Statistics Report,* published by the NCHS in Hyattsville, Maryland. **Vital statistics** are statistical summaries of vital records, that is, records of major life events. Listed are live births, deaths, marriages, divorces, and infant deaths. Death rates are also calculated by race and age, and in some issues, by cause. Selected issues also provide mortality data for specific causes (for example, diabetes, drug overdoses, and heart disease). Copies of this publication are available in government document areas of university and large public libraries, on the Web at www.cdc.gov/nchs/, or by writing directly to the NCHS (6525 Belcrest Rd., Hyattsville, MD 20782).

vital statistics statistical summaries of records of major life events such as births, deaths, marriages, divorces, and infant deaths

Morbidity and Mortality Weekly Report

Reported cases of specified notifiable diseases are reported weekly in the *Morbidity and Mortality Weekly Report* (*MMWR*), which lists morbidity and mortality data by state and region of the country. The report is prepared by the CDC based upon reports from state health departments. This report is printed and distributed through an agreement with the Massachusetts Medical Society, publishers of the *New England Journal of Medicine.* Each weekly issue also contains several reports of outbreaks of disease, environmental hazards, unusual cases, or other public health problems. The *MMWR* and its annual summary reports are available in larger libraries, on the Web at www.cdc.gov/mmwr, and by subscription from the Massachusetts Medical Society (P.O. Box 9120, Waltham, MA 02254-9120).

National Health Surveys

Another source of standardized data is the National Health Surveys. These surveys are a result of the National Health Survey Act of 1956. This act authorized a continuing survey of the amount, distribution, and effects of illness and disability in the United States. The intent of this act is currently being fulfilled by three types of surveys: (1) health interviews of people; (2) clinical tests, measurements, and physical examinations of people; and (3) surveys of places where people receive medical care, such as hospitals, clinics, and doctors' offices. The following paragraphs describe these surveys. More information about these surveys and results is available at the National Center for Health Statistics Web site, www.cdc.gov/nchs.

National Health Interview Survey

In the *National Health Interview Survey* (NHIS), conducted by the National Center for Health Statistics (NCHS), people are asked numerous questions about their health. One of the questions asks respondents to describe their health status using one of five categories—excellent, very good, good, fair, or poor. Fewer than 1 in 10 of the respondents in 2004 described their health status as either fair or poor, while nearly 7 in 10 Americans believe they are in very good or excellent health. College graduates (40%) were about three times as likely as persons who had not graduated from high school (15%) to be in excellent health.

Persons with family incomes of $75,000 or more were almost twice as likely as those with incomes of less than $20,000 to be in excellent health (51% vs. 26%).[26]

It is important to remember that these data were generated by self-reported responses to NHIS questions and not by actual examinations objectively generated in a clinic. As such, respondents may overreport good health habits or underreport bad ones. Such reporting is often dependent on the respondent's perceived social stigma or support for a response and the degree to which people's responses are confidential or anonymous. Furthermore, people have widely divergent views on what constitutes poor or good health. For example, many sedentary, cigarette-smoking, high-stress people see themselves as being in good health, while "health nuts" feel their health is deteriorating when they miss a day of exercise. In general, the young assess their health better than the old do, males better than females, whites better than blacks, and those with large family incomes better than those with smaller ones.

National Health and Nutrition Examination Survey

Another of the National Health Surveys is the *National Health and Nutrition Examination Survey* (NHANES). The purpose of the NHANES is to assess the health and nutritional status of the general U.S. population. Using a mobile examination center (see Figure 3.8), the data are collected through direct physical examinations, clinical and laboratory testing, and related procedures on a representative group of Americans. These examinations result in the most authoritative source of standardized clinical, physical, and physiological data on the American people. Included in the data are the prevalence of specific conditions and diseases and data on blood pressure, serum cholesterol, body measurements, nutritional status and deficiencies, and exposure to environmental toxins.

The first series of these surveys, known as *National Health Examination Surveys* (NHES), were carried out during the 1960s. Beginning in the 1970s, nutrition was added as a new focus, and the surveys became known as the *National Health and Nutrition Examination Survey* (NHANES). Three cycles of the NHANES have been conducted by the National Center for Health Statistics. The third (and most recent) cycle (NHANES III) began in 1988 and ended in 1994. During that six-year period, approximately 40,000 persons were examined (see Figure 3.8). A special version of this survey, the *Hispanic Health and Nutrition Examination Survey,* was conducted in 1982 to 1984. This survey provided data on a 12,000-person sample of three subgroups of the Hispanic population: Mexican Americans in the Southwest; Cubans in Miami (Dade County), Florida; and Puerto Ricans in the New York City area.

FIGURE 3.8
A National Health and Nutrition Examination Survey (NHANES) mobile examination center.

Behavioral Risk Factor Surveillance System

The *Behavioral Risk Factor Surveillance System* (BRFSS) is a state-based telephone survey of the civilian, noninstitutional, adult population conducted by the Behavioral Surveillance Branch, a division of Adult and Community Health, National Center for Chronic Disease Prevention and Health Promotion at the CDC. This survey seeks to ascertain the prevalence of such high-risk behaviors as cigarette smoking, excessive alcohol consumption, and physical inactivity, and the lack of preventive health care such as screening for cancer. These results are published periodically as part of *MMWR*'s *CDC Surveillance Summaries* and are available wherever copies of the CDC *MMWR* are found. Information is also available at www.cdc.gov/brfss.

Youth Risk Behavior Surveillance System

"The Youth Risk Behavior Surveillance System (YRBSS) monitors six categories of priority health-risk behaviors among youth and young adults, including behaviors that contribute to unintentional injuries and violence; tobacco use; alcohol and other drug use; sexual behaviors that contribute to unintended pregnancy and sexually transmitted diseases (STDs), including human immunodeficiency virus (HIV) infections; unhealthy dietary behaviors; and physical inactivity."[27]

YRBSS includes a national school-based survey conducted by the CDC, and state and local school-based surveys conducted by state and local education and health agencies. The YRBSS is conducted by the CDC's National Center for Chronic Disease Prevention and Health Promotion. More information about YRBSS is available at www.cdc.gov/healthyyouth/yrbs/index.htm.

National Health Care Survey

The *National Health Care Survey* (NHCS) includes about eight different national surveys that gather information on the nation's health care system. Two of the best known health care surveys are the *National Hospital Discharge Survey* (NHDS) and the *National Hospital Ambulatory Medical Care Survey* (NHAMCS). The NHDS provides data on the characteristics of patients discharged from nonfederal, short-stay hospitals. These data can be used to examine a variety of

important public health issues such as hospitalization rates for selected inpatient surgical procedures, infectious diseases, injuries, substance abuse, and other health problems. It can also be used
to estimate costs for public health problems. The NHAMCS gathers and disseminates information
about the health care provided by hospital outpatient departments and emergency departments.
Summaries of the results of these surveys are published by the National Center for Health Statistics and are available at www.cdc.gov/nchs/nhcs.

EPIDEMIOLOGICAL STUDIES

When disease and/or death occurs in unexpected or unacceptable numbers, epidemiologists
may carry out investigations. These investigations may be descriptive or analytic (observational or experimental/interventional) in nature, depending upon the objectives of the specific
study.

Descriptive Studies

Descriptive studies seek to describe the extent of disease in regard to person, time, and
place. These studies are designed to answer the questions *who, when,* and *where.* To answer
the first question, epidemiologists first take a "head count" to determine how many cases of a
disease have occurred. At this time, they also try to determine who is ill—children, elders,
men, women, or both. The data they gather should permit them to develop a summary of
cases by age, sex, race, marital status, occupation, and employer.

To answer the second question (*when*), epidemiologists must determine the time of the
onset of illness for each case. The resulting data can be used to prepare an **epidemic curve,** a
graphic display of the cases of disease by the time or date of the onset of their symptoms. Three
types of epidemic curves are commonly used in descriptive studies—secular, seasonal, and single
epidemic curves. The secular display of a disease shows the distribution of cases over many years
(e.g., cases of paralytic poliomyelitis for the period 1972 to 2002; see Figure 3.9). Secular graphs
illustrate the long-term trend of a disease. A graph of the case data by season or month is usually
prepared to show cyclical changes in the numbers of cases of a disease. Cases of arthropodborne
viral infections, for example, peak in the late summer months, following the seasonal rise in populations of the mosquitoes that transmit them (see Figure 3.10).

Epidemic curves for single epidemics vary in appearance with each disease outbreak; however, two classic types exist. The first is the **point source epidemic curve** (see Figure 3.11). In
a point source epidemic, each case can be traced to an exposure to the same source—spoiled
food, for example. Because an epidemic curve shows cases of a disease by time or date of the
onset of their symptoms, the epidemic curve for a single epidemic can be used to calculate the
incubation period, the period of time between exposure to an infectious agent and the onset
of symptoms. The incubation period, together with the symptoms, can often help epidemiologists determine the cause of the disease.

The second type of epidemic curve for a solitary outbreak is a **propagated epidemic
curve.** In this type of epidemic, primary cases appear first at the end of the incubation period
following exposure to an infected source. *Secondary cases* arise after a second incubation
period, and they represent exposure to the primary cases; *tertiary cases* appear even later due
to exposure to secondary cases, and so on. Because new cases give rise to more new cases, this
type of epidemic is termed a *propagated epidemic.* Epidemics of communicable diseases such
as chickenpox follow this pattern (see Figure 3.12).

Finally, epidemiologists must determine *where* the outbreak occurred. To determine
where the illnesses may have originated, the residential address and travel history, including
restaurants, schools, shopping trips, and vacations, of each case are recorded. This information
provides a geographic distribution of cases and helps to delineate the extent of the outbreak.

descriptive study
an epidemiological
study that describes
an epidemic with
respect to person,
place, and time

epidemic curve
a graphic display of
the cases of disease
according to the time
or date of onset of
symptoms

**point source
epidemic curve**
an epidemic curve
depicting a
distribution of cases
which all can be
traced to a single
source of exposure

incubation period
the period between
exposure to a disease
and the onset of
symptoms

**propagated
epidemic curve**
an epidemic curve
depicting a
distribution of cases
traceable to multiple
sources of exposure

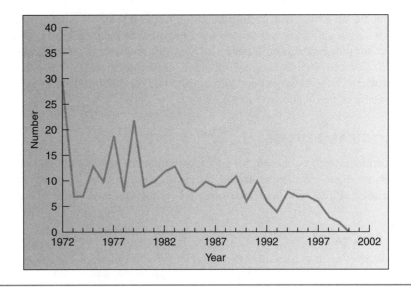

FIGURE 3.9

Vaccine-associated paralytic poliomyelitis: reported cases by year, United States, 1972–2002.

Note: An inactivated poliomyelitis vaccine (IPV) was first licensed in 1955. An oral vaccine was licensed in 1961. No cases of vaccine-associated paralytic poliomyelitis have been reported since the all-IPV schedule was implemented in 2000.

Source: Centers for Disease Control and Prevention (2004). "Summary of Notifiable Diseases—United States, 2002." *MMWR*, 51(53): 1–88.

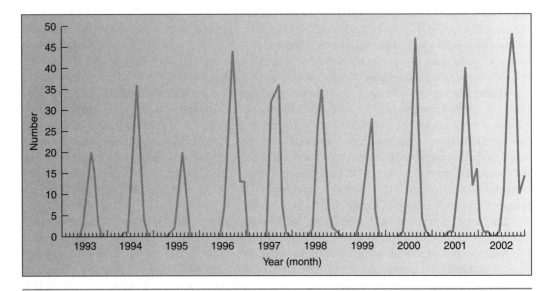

FIGURE 3.10

Encephalitis/meningitis: reported cases of California serogroup viruses by month of onset, United States, 1993–2002.

Source: Centers for Disease Control and Prevention (2004). "Summary of Notifiable Diseases—United States, 2002." *MMWR*, 51(53): 1–88.

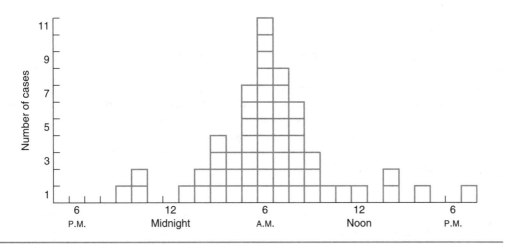

FIGURE 3.11

Point source epidemic curve: Cases of gastroenteritis following ingestion of a common food source.

Source: Centers for Disease Control and Prevention.

FIGURE 3.12

Propagated epidemic curve: Cases of chickenpox during April through June.

Source: Centers for Disease Control and Prevention.

By plotting cases on a map, along with natural features such as streams and humanmade structures such as factories, it is sometimes possible to learn something about the source of the disease.

A descriptive study is usually the first epidemiological study carried out on a disease. Descriptive data provide valuable information to health care providers and administrators, enabling them to allocate resources efficiently and to plan effective prevention and education programs. Also, detectable patterns of cases may provide investigators with ideas that can lead to a hypothesis about the cause or source of the disease outbreak. This hypothesis can subsequently be tested in an analytic study.

As important and useful as they are, descriptive studies have some limitations. Results from descriptive studies are usually not applicable to outbreaks elsewhere. Also, the investigation of a single epidemic cannot provide information about disease trends. Lastly, with few exceptions, descriptive studies by themselves rarely identify with certainty the cause of an outbreak.

Analytic Studies

A second type of epidemiological study is the **analytic study.** The purpose of analytic studies is to test hypotheses about relationships between health problems and possible **risk factors,** factors that increase the probability of disease. While front-line community health workers usually do not conduct analytic studies, it is important that students of community health understand how they are carried out and what kinds of data they generate. Only through such an understanding can those who work in community health interpret the findings of these studies to others in the community, who may then apply the knowledge to improve their own health and that of the community.

An example of an analytic study might be one designed to discover whether diabetes (health problem) is associated with obesity (possible risk factor), or whether lung cancer (health problem) is associated with cigarette smoking (possible risk factor). It is important to remember that the associations discovered through analytic epidemiological studies are not always cause-and-effect associations.

There are two types of analytic studies—observational and experimental (interventional). These differ in the role played by the investigator. In **observational studies** the investigator simply observes the natural course of events, taking note of who is exposed or unexposed and who has or has not developed the disease of interest. In experimental studies, the investigator actually allocates the exposure and subsequently follows the subjects for the development of disease.

Observational studies can be further divided into either case/control or cohort studies. The choice of which study to use when studying a particular disease-exposure relationship depends on the nature of the disease (rare or common) and the time and resources available. **Case/control studies** are analytic studies that compare people with disease (cases) to healthy people of similar age, sex, and background (controls) with respect to proportion of prior exposure to possible risk factors. These case/control studies are aimed at identifying familial, environmental, or behavioral factors that are more common or more pronounced in the case group than in the control group. Such factors could be associated with the disease under study. For example, epidemiologists might wish to study the factors associated with cervical cancer in women.

To carry out this study, epidemiologists would identify a number of women with cervical cancer (cases) and an equal or larger number of healthy women (controls). Medical histories for each group would be obtained and compared. In this hypothetical example, an examination of the histories suggests that cigarette smoking is more prevalent in the case group. If exposure to the possible risk factor (smoking) is significantly greater in the cases (of cervical cancer) than in the controls, an association is said to exist. Note that this association may or may not be one of cause and effect. Further studies are usually necessary to confirm initial findings. Case/control studies almost never prove causation by themselves. Instead, they usually indicate the direction for future studies.

Cohort studies are epidemiological studies in which the researcher selects a **cohort,** a large number of healthy subjects that share a similar experience, such as year of birth or high school graduation. Subjects in this cohort are then classified on the basis of their exposure to one or more possible causative factors, such as cigarette smoking, dietary habits, or other factors. The entire cohort is then observed for a number of years to determine the rate at which disease develops in each subgroup that was classified by exposure factor.

It is important to note the difference in the type of results obtained from case/control and cohort studies and the advantages and disadvantages of each type of study. In case/control studies, results obtained are not true incidence rates because disease was already present at the beginning of the study; that is, there were cases and controls to begin with, rather than a pop-

analytic study
an epidemiological study aimed at testing hypotheses

risk factors
factors that increase the probability of disease, injury, or death

observational study
an analytic, epidemiological study in which the investigator observes the natural course of events, noting exposed and unexposed subjects and disease development

case/control study
a study that seeks to compare those diagnosed with a disease with those who do not have the disease for prior exposure to specific risk factors

cohort study
an epidemiological study in which a cohort is classified by exposure to one or more specific risk factors and observed to determine the rates at which disease develops in each class

cohort
a group of people who share some important demographic characteristic (year of birth, for example)

ulation at risk. For this reason, case/control studies cannot calculate the incidence rate of development of disease. They can only provide a probability statement about the association between factor and disease. This probability statement can be stated mathematically as an odds ratio. The following is a hypothetical example of such a probability statement: Lung cancer patients have a probability of having smoked cigarettes that is 11 times greater than that of the control group. The **odds ratio** in this case is 11:1. (For a more detailed description of how to calculate an odds ratio and relative risk, see Appendix 1.)

In cohort studies, one begins with a population at risk, and therefore is able to calculate the incidence rate for developing disease associated with each exposure factor. This **relative risk** states the relationship between the rate of acquiring the disease in the presence of the risk factor to the rate of acquiring the disease in the absence of the risk factor. An example of a relative risk statement is as follows: Smokers are 11 times more likely to develop lung cancer than are nonsmokers.

Although cohort studies yield a relative risk, they have three distinct disadvantages: (1) they are expensive, (2) they usually take many years to complete, and (3) they are not very useful for studying rare diseases because the disease may not develop in the cohort. Case/control studies, on the other hand, are less expensive to carry out, can be completed more quickly, and are useful for studying rare diseases because one can select the cases. Unfortunately, they cannot yield a true risk for acquiring a disease.

Experimental studies are carried out in order to identify the cause of a disease or to determine the effectiveness of a vaccine, therapeutic drug, or surgical procedure. The central feature of experimental (interventional) studies is that the investigator can control the intervention or variable of interest. The subjects may be humans but more often are animals such as laboratory mice, rats, or monkeys. The use of research animals in experimental studies is necessary to determine the safety and effectiveness of new therapeutic agents or medical procedures with minimum risk to human health.

Whether animals or humans are used, every effort is made to reduce unwanted variability of factors other than the risk factors under study among the experimental subjects. In the case of animal studies, the variables over which the experimenter may wish to exert control include age, sex, diet, and environmental conditions. In addition to controlling variables, three other principles are essential to properly designed experimental studies—*control groups, randomization*, and *blinding*.

The use of *control groups* means that the experimental treatment (intervention) such as a drug, vaccine, smoke-free environment, or special diet, is withheld from a portion of the subjects. These subjects belong to the control group, which receives blank doses or treatments, called **placebos.** In order for a treatment regimen to be considered effective or for a factor to be considered causally related, it must significantly affect the *treatment group* differently (usually determined using a statistical test) from the control group.

Randomization refers to the practice of assigning subjects to treatments or control groups in a completely random manner. This can be accomplished by assigning numbers to subjects and then having numbers selected randomly. Numbers can be selected randomly from a table of random numbers, by drawing lots, or by using a computer-generated list of random numbers. Thus, each research subject, human or animal, has an equal chance of being placed in the treatment group.

Blinding refers to the practice in which the investigator(s) and/or subjects remain uninformed and unaware of the groups to which subjects are assigned throughout the period of experimentation and data gathering. This prevents the investigator(s) from looking favorably or unfavorably on the responses of any particular subject or group while gathering data during the experiment. Thus, the researcher can remain unbiased. When both the observer and subjects are kept ignorant, the study is referred to as a *double-blind trial*.

odds ratio
a probability statement about the association between a particular disease and a specific risk factor, resulting from a case/control study

relative risk
a statement of the relationship between the risk of acquiring a disease when a specific risk factor is present and the risk of acquiring that same disease when the risk factor is absent

experimental (interventional) studies
analytic studies in which the investigator allocates exposure or intervention and follows development of disease

placebo
a blank treatment

Table 3.13
Percentage of Subjects Abstaining from Smoking 6, 12, 26, and 52 Weeks after the Start of the Program

Week Number	Percentage of People Remaining Abstinent	
	Nicotine Patch	Placebo Patch
6	53	17
12	41	10
26	24	5
52	17	4

Source: Tonnesen, P., J. Norregaard, K. Simonsen, and U. Sawe (1991). "A Double-Blind Trial of a 16-Hour Transdermal Nicotine Patch in Smoking Cessation." *New England Journal of Medicine,* 325(5): 311–315.

When studies involve human subjects, they often involve the use of a placebo, such as a saline (saltwater) injection or sugar pill. The use of a placebo prevents subjects from determining by observation whether or not they are receiving treatment. This is important because human thought processes are such that some people begin to feel better if they believe they have received a treatment. In order for a vaccine or therapeutic drug to be labeled as effective, it must consistently perform better than a placebo.

An example of just such an experiment was performed by Tonnesen and his colleagues, who studied the effectiveness of a 16-hour nicotine patch on smoking cessation.[28] They used a double-blind randomized design to compare the effects of a nicotine skin patch with those of a placebo skin patch. Subjects were assigned to the active treatment or the placebo according to computer-generated random numbers. There were 145 subjects who received a nicotine patch and 144 who received the placebo. Subjects were scheduled for visits 1, 3, 6, 12, 26, and 52 weeks after the first visit—the day smoking cessation was to begin. Table 3.13 presents the results of cessation for each group 6, 12, 26, and 52 weeks after the study began. The results of this study indicated that there was a significant difference between the effectiveness of the nicotine patch and the placebo patch with regard to smoking cessation.

Controlling variables, the use of treatment and control groups, randomization, and blinding are techniques aimed at ensuring objectivity and avoiding bias in experimental studies. Through strict adherence to these principles, investigators hope to achieve experimental results that accurately reflect what occurs in a natural setting.

By carrying out carefully planned descriptive studies, epidemiologists define outbreaks of disease, injury, and death in specific populations and develop hypotheses about the causes of these outbreaks. By designing and carrying out analytic and experimental studies, epidemiologists test these hypotheses. In the next chapter, we will examine how this knowledge is used to prevent and control diseases in the community.

CHAPTER SUMMARY

- Epidemiology is the study of the distribution and determinants of health-related states or events in specified populations, and the application of this study to control health problems.

- Rates of birth, death, injury, and disease are essential tools for epidemiologists.

- Incidence rates are a measurement of the number of new cases of disease, injury, or death in a population over a given period of time. Prevalence rates measure all cases. An attack rate is a special kind of incidence rate used for a single outbreak.

- Cases of certain diseases, called notifiable or reportable diseases, are reported by doctors, clinics, medical laboratories, and hospitals to local health agencies.

These agencies then report them to state health agencies, who then forward the data to the CDC. These reports assist epidemiologists who study disease trends.

- The health status of a population or community can be measured in a number of different ways, including mortality statistics, life expectancy, years of potential life lost (YPLL), disability-adjusted life years (DALYs), and health-adjusted life expectancy (HALE).

- Epidemiologists also consult the data available from the U.S. Census, the *Statistical Abstract of the United States,* the *Monthly Vital Statistics Report,* the *Morbidity and Mortality Weekly Report,* and a variety of national health surveys.

- Epidemiologists conduct three general types of studies to learn about disease and injury in populations—descriptive studies, analytic studies, and experimental studies.

- Descriptive studies describe the extent of outbreaks in regard to person, place, and time.

- Analytic studies test hypotheses regarding associations between diseases and risk factors.

- Analytic studies can be either observational or experimental.

- Observational studies can be either case/control or cohort in design.

- Experimental studies examine the effects of specific factors under carefully controlled conditions.

- The purpose of each of these studies is to help determine the cause of disease, injury, and death in the community and to provide information that will assist in controlling current outbreaks and preventing future ones.

REVIEW QUESTIONS

1. What is an epidemic? A pandemic? Name some diseases that caused epidemics in the past. Name some diseases that are epidemic today.

2. Why are epidemiologists sometimes interested in epizootics?

3. What does the term *endemic disease* mean? Give examples of such diseases.

4. What is the difference between natality, morbidity, and mortality?

5. Why are rates important in community health?

6. What is the difference between crude and specific rates?

7. Why are prevalence rates more useful than incidence rates for measuring chronic diseases?

8. What is an infant mortality rate? Why is it such an important rate in community health?

9. What are notifiable diseases? Give some examples.

10. In general, contrast the leading causes of death in the United States in 1900 with those in 2000. Comment on the differences.

11. At what ages is life expectancy calculated? What does it tell us about a population? Which country has the longest life expectancy?

12. What are years of potential life lost (YPLL)? How does calculating YPLL change the way we think about the leading causes of death?

13. How would you define disability-adjusted life years (DALYs)? How would you define health-adjusted life expectancy (HALE)?

14. What is the U.S. Census? How often is it conducted? What types of data does it gather?

15. What types of information can you find in the *Statistical Abstract of the United States?*

16. What kinds of data would you expect to find in the Centers for Disease Control and Prevention's *Morbidity and Mortality Weekly Report?*

17. List five important national health surveys that are valuable sources of data about the health and health care of our population.

18. What can be said about the reliability of self-reported health data?

19. What is the National Health Care Survey? Why is it carried out?

20. In a descriptive epidemiological study, what types of information does the epidemiologist gather?

21. What is the purpose of an analytic study? Contrast observational and experimental studies in regard to methodology and usefulness.

22. With regard to observational studies, how do case/control studies and cohort studies differ in design and in the kinds of results obtainable?

23. How do experimental studies differ from observational studies? What value do they have in epidemiology? To what principles must investigators adhere in order to properly carry out an experimental study?

SCENARIO: ANALYSIS AND RESPONSE

Assume that you were Kim and you were able to reach Dr. Turner, the local health officer. He then asked whether you would like to help in the investigation of the foodborne outbreak mentioned in the scenario. You agreed to help. So far, you have learned that on Sunday, May 28, 49 people were at a picnic where they had eaten, beginning about noon. People began to report their illnesses later that night. Dr. Turner developed a foodborne outbreak investigation worksheet, which you helped to complete by making numerous phone calls and house visits with the public health nurse. The histories of people attending the picnic appear in Table 3.14.

Using Table 3.15, the Epidemic Curve Tally Sheet, you tally the cases by hour of onset of illness. Using the results of the tally, you establish the incubation period—the range of hours (after the meal) over which symptoms started. Next, you prepare a graph to illustrate the epidemic curve of the outbreak. Try to answer the following questions:

1. What is the incubation period?
2. Does the curve you prepared suggest a single- or multiple-exposure epidemic?
3. Based solely on the incubation period, can you make a guess as to the cause of the outbreak?

Table 3.14
Histories Obtained from Persons Eating Picnic Lunch

Person No.	Bread	Butter	Turkey	Potato Salad	Milk	Jell-O	Ill*	Not Ill
1			X	X	X		7:30	
2	X	X		X	X			X
3	X	X	X	X	X	X	8:00	
4			X		X	X		X
5			X	X	X		9:15	
6			X	X	X		7:40	
7	X	X		X	X			X
8	X	X	X	X	X	X	8:10	
9			X		X	X		X
10			X	X	X	X	10:15	
11	X			X		X		X
12	X	X	X	X	X	X	8:30	
13			X		X			X
14	X	X	X	X	X	X	9:30	
15	X	X		X	X	X		X
16	X			X		X		X
17	X	X	X	X	X	X	8:35	
18			X		X			X
19	X	X	X	X	X	X	10:05	
20	X	X		X	X	X		X
21			X		X	X	9:15	
22	X	X		X	X	X		X
23	X	X			X	X	8:30	
24	X	X			X	X		X
25	X	X	X	X	X	X	12:30 A.M.	
26			X		X	X	9:20	
27	X	X		X	X	X		X
28	X	X	X		X	X	8:40	
29	X	X			X	X		X
30	X	X	X	X	X		12:15 A.M.	
31			X	X	X		7:30	
32	X	X		X	X			X
33	X	X	X	X	X	X	8:00	
34			X		X	X		X
35			X	X	X		10:30	

(continues)

Table 3.14 (continued)

Person No.	Bread	Butter	Turkey	Potato Salad	Milk	Jell-O	Ill*	Not Ill
36			x	x	x		7:30	
37	x	x		x	x			x
38	x	x	x	x	x	x	8:05	
39			x		x	x		x
40			x	x	x	x	9:45	
41	x			x		x		x
42	x	x	x	x	x	x	8:30	
43			x		x			x
44	x	x	x	x	x	x	9:30	
45	x	x		x	x	x		x
46	x			x		x		x
47	x	x	x	x	x	x	8:30	
48			x		x	x		x
49	x	x	x	x	x	x	10:10	

*All time is p.m. unless otherwise indicated.

Table 3.15
Epidemic Curve Tally Sheet

Time of Onset	Tally	Number	Incubation Period
7:00–7:59			
8:00–8:59			
9:00–9:59			
10:00–10:59			
11:00–11:59			
12:00–12:59			

Unfortunately, by the time the investigation began, all the picnic food had been discarded, and no samples were available for laboratory testing. In order to determine which food at the picnic might have caused the outbreak, you need to calculate attack rates for people eating each food as well as for people not eating each food. Using Table 3.16, the Attack Rate Worksheet, calculate the attack rates for those who ate and did not eat each food served.

1. Which food would you most suspect of causing the illness?
2. Based on this information, what might the causative agent have been?
3. How could the Internet be of assistance to health department officials in this situation?

Table 3.16
Attack Rate Worksheet

Food	Persons Eating Food				Persons Not Eating Food			
	Total	Ill	Well	Attack Rate	Total	Ill	Well	Attack Rate
Bread								
Butter								
Turkey								
Potato salad								
Milk								
Jell-O								

Activities

1. When you hear the word *epidemic*, what disease comes to your mind first? Ask this question of 10 people you know, allowing them time to think and give you an answer. Try to find people of different ages as you complete your informal poll. List their answers on paper. Are there any answers that surprise you? Does your list include both classic and contemporary epidemic diseases?

2. Look at the data in Table 3.17. What conclusion can you draw about the risk for acquiring tuberculosis for populations in each age group? Write down your answer. Now examine Table 3.18. Which age groups exhibit the highest disease rates? Explain why it is important to calculate rates to report disease outbreaks accurately.

3. There are 346 students at Hillside School. During March and April, 56 pupils were absent with chickenpox. What is the attack rate for chickenpox at Hillside School? The 56 pupils who were absent had 88 brothers and sisters at home. Of the 88 siblings, 19 developed chickenpox. What was the attack rate among these children? Of the 75 total cases of chickenpox, one child died. Calculate the case fatality rate for chickenpox in this epidemic.

4. In an epidemic in Sample City (population 100,000— 60,000 males and 40,000 females), there were 600 cases (350 males, 250 females) of a severe disease. There were 70 deaths (all males) due to this disease and 880 deaths due to causes other than the specific disease. Calculate the following—crude death rate, cause-specific mortality rate, case fatality rate, cause-specific morbidity rate for females, and case fatality rate for males.

5. Visit, call, or write your state or local health department. Ask for the total number of birth and death certificates issued for the latest year for which complete data are available. Assuming no migration into or out of your state or county occurred, what is the natural rate of population increase (number of births minus number of deaths)? Try to obtain an estimate of the total population of the state or county for that same year. Calculate a crude birth rate and a crude death rate (number of births and deaths) per 1,000 population.

6. Using the data presented in Table 3.10, estimate (as best you can) the life expectancy of your siblings, parents, and grandparents at birth. If your grandparents are older than 65, determine what their life expectancies were when they turned 65. If you were to fulfill your life expectancy exactly, in what year can you expect to die?

7. Visit your campus library and locate the *American Journal of Epidemiology*. Examine several recent issues, taking note of the different types of articles as they appear in the Table of Contents. Select six articles and read the abstracts. On a piece of paper, list the titles of these articles. Were these descriptive, analytic, or experimental studies? After each title that you have listed, put either the letter D (descriptive), A (analytic), or E (experimental) to denote the type of study that you examined.

Community Health on the Web

The Internet contains a wealth of information about community and public health. Increase your knowledge of some of the topics presented in this chapter by accessing the Jones and Bartlett Publishers Web site at **http://health.jbpub.com/book/communityhealth/6e** and follow the links to complete the following activities.

- Epidemiology Program Office
- Morbidity and Mortality Weekly Report
- National Center for Health Statistics

Table 3.18
Reported Tuberculosis Cases and Incidence Rates per 100,000, Low Socioeconomic Area, City of Dixon, 1960

Age Group in Years	Number of Cases	Population of Age Group	Rate*
0–4	7	8,638	81.0
5–14	7	13,098	53.4
15–24	6	10,247	58.5
25–34	10	8,680	115.2
35–44	6	7,528	79.7
45–54	9	6,736	133.6
55–64	8	4,534	176.4
65+	7	4,075	171.8
Total	60	63,536	94.4

*Example: 7 cases ÷ 8,638 population × 100,000 = 81.0.

Table 3.17
Reported Tuberculosis Cases, by Age Group, Low Socioeconomic Area, City of Dixon, 1960

Age Group in Years	Number of Cases	Age Group in Years	Number of Cases
0–4	7	35–44	6
5–14	7	45–54	9
15–24	6	55–64	8
25–34	10	65+	7

REFERENCES

1. Last, J. M., ed. (2001). *A Dictionary of Epidemiology*. New York: Oxford University Press.

2. Taubenberer, J. K., and D. M. Morens (2006). "1918 Influenza: The Mother of All Pandemics." *Emerging Infectious Diseases,* 12(1): 15-22.

3. Joint United Nations Programme on HIV/AIDS (2006). *2006 Report on the Global AIDS Epidemic*. Geneva, Switzerland: Author. Available at http://www.unaids.org/en/HIV_data/2006GlobalReport/default.asp.

4. Monath, T. P. (1980). *St. Louis Encephalitis*. Washington, DC: American Public Health Association.

5. Centers for Disease Control and Prevention (2003). "Summary of Notifiable Diseases—United States, 2001." *Morbidity and Mortality Weekly Report*, 50(53): 1-108.

6. Centers for Disease Control and Prevention (1981). "Toxic Shock Syndrome—United States, 1970-1980." *Morbidity and Mortality Weekly Report*, 30(3): 25-33.

7. Centers for Disease Control and Prevention (2005). *HIV/AIDS Surveillance Report for 2004*, vol. 16. Atlanta, GA: Author. Available at http://www.cdc.gov/hiv/topics/surveillance/resources/reports/2004report/default.htm.

8. Centers for Disease Control and Prevention (2005). "Lyme Disease Statistics." Available at http://www.cdc.gov/ncidod/dvbid/lyme/ld_statistics.htm.

9. Centers for Disease Control and Prevention (2005). "Summary of Notifiable Diseases-United States, 2003." *Morbidity and Mortality Weekly Report*, 52(53): 1-86.

10. Centers for Disease Control and Prevention (2006). "Summary of Notifiable Diseases- United States, 2004." *Morbidity and Mortality Weekly Report*, 53(53): 1-82.

11. Centers for Disease Control and Prevention (2004). "West Nile Virus." Available at http://www.cdc.gov/ncidod/dvbid/westnile/index.htm.

12. Centers for Disease Control and Prevention (2006). "Summary of Provisional Cases of Selected Notifiable Diseases, United States, Cumulative, Week Ending July 29, 2006 (30th Week)." Available at http://www.cdc.gov/mmwr/index.html.

13. Markellis, V. C. (December 1985-January 1986). "Epidemiology: Cornerstone for Health Education." *Health Education*, 15-17.

14. Gale, A. H. (1959). *Epidemiologic Disease*. London: Pelican Books, 25.

15. Woodruff, A. W. (1977). "Benjamin Rush, His Work on Yellow Fever and His British Connections." *American Journal of Tropical Medicine and Hygiene*, 26(5): 1055-1059.

16. Snow, J. (1963). "The Broad Street Pump." In B. Rouche, ed., *Curiosities of Medicine*. Boston: Little, Brown.

17. Mausner, J. S., and S. Kramer (1985). *Epidemiology: An Introductory Text*. Philadelphia: WB Saunders, 5.

18. Hoyert, D. L., M. P. Heron, S. L. Murphy, and H. C. Kung (2006). "Deaths: Final Data for 2003." *National Vital Statistics Report*, 54(13): 1-120.

19. Miniño, A. M., M. Heron, S. L. Murphy, and K. D. Kochanek (2006). "Deaths: Final Data for 2004." NCHS Health E-Stats. Available at http://www.cdc.gov/nchs/products/pubs/pubd/hestats/finaldeaths04/finaldeaths04.htm.

20. Miniño, A. M., M. Heron, and B L. Smith (2006). "Deaths: Preliminary Data for 2004." *National Vital Statistics Report*, 54(19): 1-52.

21. Hamilton, B. E., S. J. Ventura, J. A. Martin, and P. D. Sutton (2005). "Preliminary Births for 2004." NCHS Health E-Stats. Available at http://www.cdc.gov/nchs/products/pubs/pubd/hestats/prelim_births/prelim_births04.htm.

22. National Center for Health Statistics (2006). *Health, United States, 2006 with Chartbook on Trends in the Health of Americans* (DHHS pub. no. 2006-1232). Hyattsville, MD: Author. Available at www.cdc.gov/nchs/hus.htm.

23. Murray, D. J. L., and A. D. Lopez, eds. (1996). *The Global Burden of Disease and Injury. Vol. 1: A Comprehensive Assessment of Mortality and Disability from Diseases, Injuries and Risk Factors in 1990 and Projected to 2020*. Cambridge, MA: Harvard School of Public Health on behalf of the World Health Organization.

24. Lopez, A. S., C. D. Mathers, M. Ezzati, D. T. Jamison, and C. J. L. Murray, eds. (2006). *Global Burden of Disease and Risk Factors*. Washington, DC: The World Bank and Oxford University Press.

25. Mathers, C. D., R. Sadana, J. A. Salomon, C. J. L. Murray, and A. D. Lopez (2001). Healthy life expectancies in 191 countries, 1999. *Lancet*, 357:1685-1691.

26. Adams, P. F., and P. M. Barnes. (2006). *Summary Health Statistics for the U.S. Population: National Health Interview Survey, 2004* (Vital and Health Statistics no. 10). Hyattsville, MD: National Center for Health Statistics.

27. Centers for Disease Control and Prevention (28 June 2002). "Youth Risk Behavior Surveillance—United States, 2001." *MMWR Surveillance Summaries*, 51(SS-4): 1-64.

28. Tonnesen, P., J. Norregaard, K. Simonsen, and U. Sawe (1991). "A Double-Blind Trial of a 16-Hour Transdermal Nicotine Patch in Smoking Cessation." *New England Journal of Medicine*, 325(5): 311-315.

Chapter 4

Epidemiology: Prevention and Control of Diseases and Health Conditions

Chapter Outline

Chapter Objectives

After studying this chapter you will be able to:

1 Explain the differences between communicable (infectious) and noncommunicable (noninfectious) diseases and between acute and chronic diseases and provide examples of each.

2 Describe and explain communicable and multicausation disease models.

3 Explain how communicable diseases are transmitted in a community using the "chain of infection" model and use a specific communicable disease to illustrate your explanation.

4 Explain why noncommunicable diseases are a community health concern and provide some examples of important noncommunicable diseases.

5 Explain the difference between primary, secondary, and tertiary prevention of disease and provide examples of each.

6 List and explain the various criteria that communities might use in order to prioritize their health problems in preparation for the allocation of prevention and control resources.

7 List and discuss important measures for preventing and controlling the spread of communicable diseases in a community.

8 List and discuss approaches to noncommunicable disease control in the community.

9 Define and explain the purpose and importance of *health screenings*.

10 Outline a chronic, noncommunicable disease control program that includes primary, secondary, and tertiary disease prevention components.

SCENARIO

Bob had always been an active and athletic person. He lettered in three sports in high school and played varsity tennis in college. Following graduation last May, he was lucky enough to land a job with one of the Fortune 500 companies in nearby Indianapolis. He shares an apartment with Chuck, a business colleague, and both work long hours in the hope that hard work will mean success and advancement. Neither seems to find time to exercise regularly, and both rely increasingly on fast-food restaurants. Bob's weight is now 12 pounds above his weight at graduation.

Bob is beginning to wonder whether he is compromising his health for financial success. When he first came to the company, he took the stairs between floors two at a time and was never winded, even after climbing several flights. Now he becomes tired after two flights. Also, Bob recently participated in a free serum cholesterol screening. Bob's cholesterol level was 259 mg/dL. Bob decided it was time to have a complete physical examination.

INTRODUCTION

In Chapter 3 we discussed the measurement and reporting of disease and the use of rates and ratios to describe disease incidence and prevalence. We then explained how epidemiologists describe disease outbreaks by person, place, and time, and how they search for causal associations through analytic and experimental studies.

In this chapter, we extend our discussion of epidemiology. We begin by describing the different ways to classify diseases and other health conditions. Then, we explain models of communicable and noncommunicable diseases, conceptual frameworks used by epidemiologists to develop prevention and control strategies. We also discuss criteria used by communities to prioritize their health problems and allocate health resources. Finally, we discuss some approaches to disease prevention and control; introduce the concepts of primary, secondary, and tertiary prevention; and provide examples of their application to a communicable and noncommunicable disease.

CLASSIFICATION OF DISEASES AND HEALTH PROBLEMS

Diseases and health problems can be classified in several meaningful ways. The public often classifies diseases by organ or organ system, such as kidney disease, heart disease, respiratory infection, and so on. Another method of classification is by causative agent—viral disease, chemical poisoning, physical injury, and so forth. In this scheme, causative agents may be biological, chemical, or physical. Biological agents include viruses, rickettsiae, bacteria, protozoa, fungi, and metazoa (multicellular organisms). Chemical agents include drugs, pesticides, industrial chemicals, food additives, air pollutants, and cigarette smoke. Physical agents that can cause injury or disease include various forms of energy such as heat, ultraviolet light, radiation, noise vibrations, and speeding or falling objects (see Table 4.1). In community health, diseases are usually classified as acute or chronic, or as communicable (infectious) or noncommunicable (noninfectious).

communicable (infectious) disease an illness caused by some specific biological agent or its toxic products that can be transmitted from an infected person, animal, or inanimate reservoir to a susceptible host

Communicable versus Noncommunicable Diseases

Another classification system divides diseases into communicable and noncommunicable diseases. **Communicable (infectious) diseases** are those diseases for which biological agents or their products are the cause and that are transmissible from one individual to another. The

Table 4.1
Causative Agents for Diseases and Injuries

Biological Agents	Chemical Agents	Physical Agents
Viruses	Pesticides	Heat
Rickettsiae	Food additives	Light
Bacteria	Pharmacologics	Radiation
Fungi	Industrial chemicals	Noise
Protozoa	Air pollutants	Vibration
Metazoa	Cigarette smoke	Speeding objects

disease process begins when the agent is able to enter and grow or reproduce within the body of the host. The entrance and growth of a microorganism or virus in the host is called *infection*.

Noncommunicable (noninfectious) diseases or illnesses are those that cannot be transmitted from one person to another. Delineating the causes of noncommunicable diseases is often more difficult because several, or even many, factors may contribute to the development of a given noncommunicable health condition. These contributing factors may be genetic, environmental, or behavioral in nature. For this reason, many noncommunicable health conditions are called multicausation diseases; an example of such is heart disease. Genetics, environmental factors such as stress, and behavioral choices such as poor diet and lack of exercise can all contribute to heart disease.

noncommunicable disease (noninfectious disease) a disease that cannot be transmitted from infected host to susceptible host

Acute versus Chronic Diseases and Illnesses

In the acute/chronic classification scheme, diseases are classified by their duration of symptoms. Acute diseases, as defined in Chapter 3, are diseases in which the peak severity of symptoms occurs and subsides within three months (usually sooner) and the recovery of those who survive is usually complete. Examples of acute communicable diseases include the common cold, influenza (flu), chickenpox, measles, mumps, Rocky Mountain spotted fever, and plague. Examples of acute noncommunicable illnesses are appendicitis, injuries from motor vehicle crashes, acute alcohol intoxication or drug overdose, and sprained ankles (see Table 4.2).

Chronic diseases or conditions are those in which symptoms continue longer than three months, and in some cases, for the remainder of one's life (see Figure 4.1). Recovery is slow and sometimes incomplete. These diseases can be either communicable or noncommunicable. Examples of chronic communicable diseases are AIDS, tuberculosis, herpes virus infections, syphilis, and Lyme disease. Chronic noncommunicable illnesses include hypertension, hypercholesterolemia, coronary heart disease, diabetes, and many types of arthritis and cancer.

Table 4.2
Classification of Diseases

Types of Diseases	Examples
Acute diseases	
Communicable	Common cold, pneumonia, mumps, measles, pertussis, typhoid fever, cholera
Noncommunicable	Appendicitis, poisoning, injury (due to motor vehicle crash, fire, gunshot, etc.)
Chronic diseases	
Communicable	AIDS, Lyme disease, tuberculosis, syphilis, rheumatic fever following streptococcal infections, hepatitis B
Noncommunicable	Diabetes, coronary heart disease, osteoarthritis, cirrhosis of the liver due to alcoholism

FIGURE 4.1
Arthritis is a noninfectious chronic condition that can persist for one's entire life.

infectivity
the ability of a biological agent to enter and grow in the host

pathogenicity
the capability of a communicable disease agent to cause disease in a susceptible host

COMMUNICABLE DISEASES

While **infectivity** refers to the ability of a biological agent to enter and grow in a host, the term **pathogenicity** refers to an infectious disease agent's ability to produce disease. Selected pathogenic agents and the diseases they cause are listed in Table 4.3. Under certain conditions, pathogenic, biological agents can be transmitted from an infected individual in the community to an uninfected, susceptible one. Communicable disease agents may be further classified according to the manner in which they are transmitted.

The elements of a simplified **communicable disease model**—agent, host, and environment—are presented in Figure 4.2. These three factors are the minimal requirements for the occurrence and spread of communicable diseases in a population. In this model, the

communicable disease model
a visual representation of the interrelationships between causative agent, host, and environment

Table 4.3
Biological Agents of Disease

Types of Agent	Name of Agent	Disease
Viruses	Varicella virus	Chickenpox
	Human immunodeficiency virus (HIV)	Acquired immunodeficiency syndrome (AIDS)
	Rubella virus	German measles
Rickettsiae	*Rickettsia rickettsii*	Rocky Mountain spotted fever
Bacteria	*Vibrio cholerae*	Cholera
	Clostridium tetani	Tetanus
	Yersinia pestis	Plague
	Borrelia burgdorferi	Lyme disease
Protozoa	*Entamoeba histolytica*	Amebic dysentery
	Plasmodium falciparum	Malaria
	Trypanosoma gambiense	African sleeping sickness
Fungi and yeasts	*Tinea cruris*	Jock itch
	Tinea pedis	Athlete's foot
Nematoda (worms)	*Wuchereria bancrofti*	Filariasis (elephantiasis)
	Onchocerca volvulus	Onchocerciasis (river blindness)

agent is the element that must be present in order for disease to occur. For example, the influenza virus must be present for a person to become ill with flu. The **host** is any susceptible organism—a single-celled organism, a plant, an animal, or a human—invaded by an infectious agent. The *environment* includes all other factors—physical, biological, or social—that inhibit or promote disease transmission. Communicable disease transmission occurs when a susceptible host and a pathogenic agent exist in an environment conducive to disease transmission.

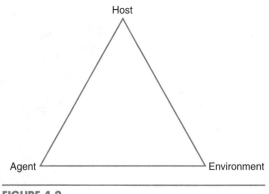

FIGURE 4.2
Communicable disease model.

Chain of Infection

Communicable disease transmission is a complicated but well-studied process that is best understood through a conceptual model known as the **chain of infection** (see Figure 4.3). Using the chain of infection model, one can visualize the step-by-step process by which communicable diseases spread from an infected person to an uninfected person in the community. The *pathogenic* (disease-producing) agent leaves its *reservoir* (infected host) via a *portal of exit*. *Transmission* occurs in either a direct or indirect manner, and the pathogenic agent enters a susceptible host through a *portal of entry* in order to establish infection. For example, let us follow the common cold through the chain of infection. The agent (the cold virus) leaves its reservoir (the throat of an infected person), perhaps when the host sneezes. The portals of exit are the nose and mouth. Transmission may be direct if saliva droplets enter the respiratory tract of a susceptible host at close range, or it may be indirect if droplets dry and become airborne. The portal of entry could be the nose or mouth of a susceptible host. The agent enters, and a new infection is established.

There are many variations in the chain of infection, depending upon the disease agent, environmental conditions, infectivity, and host susceptibility. For example, the reservoir for a disease may be a **case**—a person who has the disease—or a **carrier**—one who is well but infected and is capable of serving as a source of infection. A (disease) carrier could be one who is incubating the disease, such as a person who is HIV positive but has no signs of AIDS, or one who has recovered from the disease (is asymptomatic), as is sometimes the case in typhoid fever. For some diseases, the reservoir is not humans but animals. Diseases for which the reservoir resides in animal populations are called **zoonoses.** Plague, rabies, Rocky Mountain spotted fever, and Lyme disease are zoonoses. Diseases for which humans are

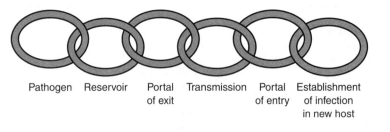

Pathogen   Reservoir   Portal of exit   Transmission   Portal of entry   Establishment of infection in new host

FIGURE 4.3
Chain of infection.

FIGURE 4.4
Portal of exit: The causative agents for many respiratory diseases leave their host via the mouth and nose.

the only known reservoir, like measles, are known as **anthroponoses.**

Portals of exit (see Figure 4.4) and entry vary from disease to disease. Natural portals of exit and examples of diseases that use them are the respiratory tract (cold, influenza, measles, tuberculosis, and whooping cough), urogenital tract (gonorrhea, syphilis, herpes, and AIDS), digestive tract (amebic dysentery, shigellosis, polio, typhoid fever, and cholera), and skin (ringworm and jock itch). The skin is actually a good barrier to infection, but it can be bypassed by a hypodermic needle or when there is an open wound. Blood-sucking insects and ticks make their own portals of entry with mouth parts that penetrate the skin. Finally, many pathogenic agents can cross the placenta from mother to fetus (for example, rubella virus, syphilis spirochetes, and hepatitis B virus).

anthroponosis
a disease that infects only humans

direct transmission
the immediate transfer of an infectious agent by direct contact between infected and susceptible individuals

Modes of Transmission

As noted in the previous paragraphs, communicable disease transmission may be direct or indirect. **Direct transmission** implies the immediate transfer of the disease agent between the infected and the susceptible individuals by direct contact "such as touching, biting, kissing, sexual intercourse, or by direct projection (droplet spread) of droplet spray onto the conjunctiva or onto the mucous membranes of the eye, nose or mouth during sneezing, coughing, spitting, singing or talking (usually limited to a distance of one meter or less)."[1] Examples of diseases for which transmission is usually direct are AIDS, syphilis, gonorrhea, rabies, and the common cold.

Indirect transmission may be one of three types—airborne, vehicleborne, or vectorborne. *Airborne transmission* is the dissemination of microbial aerosols to a suitable portal of entry, usually the respiratory tract. Microbial aerosols are suspensions of dust or droplet nuclei made up wholly or in part of microorganisms. These particles may remain suspended and infective for long periods of time. Tuberculosis, influenza, histoplasmosis, and legionellosis are examples of airborne diseases.

In *vehicleborne transmission,* contaminated materials or objects (fomites) serve as **vehicles**—nonliving objects by which communicable agents are transferred to a susceptible host. The agent may or may not have multiplied or developed on the vehicle. Examples of vehicles include toys, handkerchiefs, soiled clothes, bedding, food service utensils, and surgical instruments. Also considered vehicles are water, milk, food, or biological products such as blood, serum, plasma, organs, and tissues. Almost any disease can be transmitted by vehicles, including those for which the primary mode of transmission is direct, such as dysentery and hepatitis.

Vectorborne transmission is the transfer of disease by a living organism such as a mosquito, fly, or tick. Transmission may be mechanical, via the contaminated mouth parts or feet of the **vector,** or biological, which involves multiplication or developmental changes of the agent in the vector before transmission occurs. In *mechanical transmission,* multiplication and development of the disease organism usually do not occur. For example, organisms that cause

indirect transmission
communicable disease transmission involving an intermediate step

vehicle
inanimate materials or objects that can serve as a source of infection

vector
a living organism, usually an arthropod (e.g., mosquito, tick, louse, or flea), that can transmit a communicable agent to susceptible hosts

FIGURE 4.5
A blacklegged tick, *Ixodes scapularis* (nymph).
The nymph is the stage that is responsible for
transmitting most of the cases of Lyme disease.

dysentery, polio, cholera, and typhoid fever have been isolated from insects such as cockroaches and houseflies and could presumably be deposited on food prepared for human consumption.

In *biological transmission,* multiplication and/or developmental changes of the disease agent occur in the vector before transmission occurs. Biological transmission is much more important than mechanical transmission in terms of its impact on community health. Examples of biological vectors include mosquitoes, fleas, lice, ticks, flies, and other insects. Mosquitoes are by far the most important vectors of human disease. They transmit the viruses that cause yellow fever and dengue fever as well as more than 200 other viruses, including West Nile fever virus. They also transmit malaria, which infects 100 million people in the world each year (mostly in tropical areas), killing at least 1 million of them. Ticks, another important vector, transmit Rocky Mountain spotted fever, relapsing fever, and Lyme disease (see Figure 4.5). Other insect vectors (and the diseases they transmit) are flies (African sleeping sickness, onchocerciasis, loiasis, and leishmaniasis), fleas (plague and murine typhus), lice (epidemic typhus and trench fever), and kissing bugs (Chagas' disease).

NONCOMMUNICABLE DISEASES

etiology
the cause of a disease

Although communicable diseases remain an important concern for communities, certain noncommunicable diseases, such as heart disease, stroke, and cancer, now rank high among the nation's leading causes of death. While these diseases are not infectious, they nonetheless can occur in epidemic proportions. Furthermore, the chronic nature of many of these diseases means that they can deplete a community's resources quite rapidly.

The complex **etiologies** (causes) of many of the noncommunicable diseases, such as coronary heart disease, are best illustrated by the **multicausation disease model** (see Figure 4.6). In this model, the human host is pictured in the center of the environment in which he or she lives. Within the host, there exists a unique genetic endowment that is inalterable. The host exists in a complex environment that includes exposures to a multitude of *risk factors* that can contribute to the disease process. These environmental risk factors may be physical, chemical, biological, or social in nature.

multicausation disease model
a visual representation of the host together with various internal and external factors that promote and protect against disease

Physical factors include the latitude, climate, and physical geography of where one lives. The major health risks in the tropics—communicable and parasitic diseases—are different from those in temperate regions with cold winters—difficulty in finding food and remaining warm. Chemical factors include not only natural chemical hazards of polluted water and air but also the added pollutants of our modern, industrial society. Biological hazards include communicable disease agents such as pathogenic viruses, bacteria, and fungi. Social factors include one's occupation, recreational activities, and living arrangements. Poor choices in life can increase the number and severity of one's risk factors and be detrimental to one's health.

Diseases of the Heart and Blood Vessels

coronary heart disease (CHD)
a chronic disease characterized by damage to the coronary arteries in the heart

Diseases of the heart and blood vessels, cardiovascular diseases (CVDs), are a leading cause of death in the United States. **Coronary heart disease (CHD)** is the Number 1 killer of Americans. In 2004 alone, more than 652,000 people died of heart disease in the United States[2] and it was estimated that more than 71 million Americans have one or more types of CVD.[3]

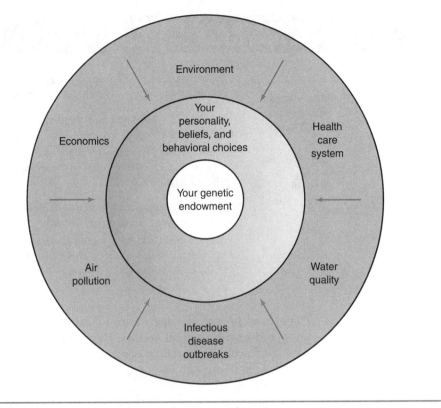

FIGURE 4.6
Multicausation disease model.

The American Heart Association lists nine types of CVDs: CHD, stroke, high blood pressure, arrhythmias, diseases of the arteries, congestive heart failure, valvular heart disease, rheumatic fever/rheumatic heart disease, and congenital heart defects.[3] CHD causes more than half of all cardiovascular disease deaths. Sometimes called *coronary artery disease,* CHD is characterized by damage to the coronary arteries, the blood vessels that carry oxygen-rich blood to the heart muscle. Damage to the coronary arteries usually evolves from the condition known as *atherosclerosis,* a narrowing of the blood vessels. This narrowing usually results from the buildup of fatty deposits on the inner walls of arteries. When blood flow to the heart muscle is severely reduced or interrupted, a heart attack can occur. If heart damage is severe, the heart may stop beating—a condition known as cardiac arrest.

Over the past 50 years, a more complete understanding of the processes involved in CVDs has resulted in a 56% decline in deaths from heart disease and stroke (see Box 4.1). Numerous risk factors for coronary artery disease have been identified. While some of these risk factors cannot be altered by changes in lifestyle or behavior, others can. Factors that cannot be altered include one's age, sex, race, and the genetic tendency toward developing the disease. Factors that can be modified include cigarette smoking, high blood pressure, high blood cholesterol, physical inactivity, obesity, diabetes, and stress.

Cerebrovascular disease (stroke) is the third leading cause of death in the United States. Strokes killed more than 150,000 people in 2004.[2] During a stroke, or cerebrovascular accident, the blood supply to the brain is interrupted.

cerebrovascular disease (stroke) a chronic disease characterized by damage to blood vessels of the brain resulting in disruption of circulation to the brain

You Gotta Have Heart

Since 1921, heart disease has been the leading cause of death, and since 1938, stroke has been the third leading cause of death. However, since 1950, age-adjusted death rates from cardiovascular disease (CVD) have declined 60%, representing one of the most important public health achievements in the twentieth century. This decline was made possible through a better under-standing of disease epidemiology and advances in pre-vention techniques, diagnoses, and treatment.

Disease Epidemiology

The risk-factor concept—the idea that particular biologic, lifestyle, and social conditions were associated with an increased risk for specific disease—developed as a result of population-based research into the causes of CVD.

Advances in Prevention, Diagnoses, and Treatment

Prevention efforts and improvements in early detection, treatment, and care have resulted in several beneficial trends that have likely contributed to declines in CVD.

Trends That Have Likely Contributed to Declines in Cardiovascular Disease

- A decline in cigarette smoking among adults
- A decrease in mean blood pressure levels
- A decrease in mean blood cholesterol levels

---

malignant neoplasm uncontrolled new tissue growth resulting from cells that have lost control over their growth and division

The risk factors for developing cerebrovascular disease are similar to those for CHD and include hereditary, behavioral, and environmental factors. Hypertension and cigarette smoking are especially important risk factors for cerebrovascular disease.

Malignant Neoplasms (Cancer)

Nearly 554,000 people died from malignant neoplasms (cancer) in 2004 making it the second leading cause of death in the United States.[2] **Malignant neoplasms** occur when cells lose control over their growth and division. Normal cells are inhibited from continual growth and division by virtue of their contact with adjacent cells. Malignant (cancerous) cells are not so inhibited; they continue to grow and divide, eventually piling up in a "new growth," a neo-plasm or tumor. Early-stage tumors, sometimes called *in situ cancers,* are more treatable than later-stage cancers. As tumor growth continues, parts of the neoplasm can break off and be carried to distant parts of the body, where they can lodge and continue to grow. When this occurs, the cancer is said to have **metastasized.** When malignant neoplasms have spread beyond the orginal cell layer where they developed, the cancer is said to be *invasive.*[4] The more the malignancy spreads, the more difficult it is to treat and the lower the survival rates. For more information on the staging of cancer, see Box 4.2.

metastasis the spread of cancer cells to distant parts of the body by the circulatory or lymphatic system

---

According to the American Cancer Society, "staging is the process of describing the extent or spread of the dis-ease at the time of diagnosis." A number of different staging systems exist. One of the most popular is the TNM staging system, which assesses tumors in three ways:

> The extent of the primary tumor (T), absence or presence of regional lymph node involvement (N), and absence or presence of distant metastases (M). Once the T, N, and M are determined, a stage of I,

II, III, or IV is assigned, with stage I being early stage and stage IV being advanced.

A different system of summary staging (in situ, local, regional, and distant) is used for descriptive and statistical analysis of tumor registry data. If cancer cells are present only in the layer of cells where they developed and have not spread, the stage is in situ. If the cancer has spread beyond the original layer of tissue, the cancer is invasive.

Source: American Cancer Society (2006). *Cancer Facts and Figures 2006.* Atlanta, GA: Author. Reprinted with permission.

Estimated New Cases*

Male	Female
Prostate 234,460 (33%)	Breast 212,920 (31%)
Lung & bronchus 92,700 (13%)	Lung & bronchus 81,770 (12%)
Colon & rectum 72,800 (10%)	Colon & rectum 75,810 (11%)
Urinary bladder 44,690 (6%)	Uterine corpus 41,200 (6%)
Melanoma of the skin 34,260 (5%)	Non-Hodgkin lymphoma 28,190 (4%)
Non-Hodgkin lymphoma 30,680 (4%)	Melanoma of the skin 27,930 (4%)
Kidney & renal pelvis 24,650 (3%)	Thyroid 22,590 (3%)
Oral cavity & pharynx 20,180 (3%)	Ovary 20,180 (3%)
Leukemia 20,000 (3%)	Urinary bladder 16,730 (2%)
Pancreas 17,150 (2%)	Pancreas 16,580 (2%)
All sites 720,280 (100%)	All sites 679,510 (100%)

Estimated Deaths

Male	Female
Lung & bronchus 90,330 (31%)	Lung & bronchus 72,130 (26%)
Colon & rectum 27,870 (10%)	Breast 40,970 (15%)
Prostate 27,350 (9%)	Colon & rectum 27,300 (10%)
Pancreas 16,090 (6%)	Pancreas 16,210 (6%)
Leukemia 12,470 (4%)	Ovary 15,310 (6%)
Liver & intrahepatic bile duct 10,840 (4%)	Leukemia 9,810 (4%)
Esophagus 10,730 (4%)	Non-Hodgkin lymphoma 8,840 (3%)
Non-Hodgkin lymphoma 10,000 (3%)	Uterine corpus 7,350 (3%)
Urinary bladder 8,990 (3%)	Multiple myeloma 5,630 (2%)
Kidney & renal pelvis 8,130 (3%)	Brain & other nervous system 5,560 (2%)
All sites 291,270 (100%)	All sites 273,560 (100%)

FIGURE 4.7

Leading sites of new cancer cases* and deaths—2006 estimates (percentages may not total 100% due to rounding.)

*Excludes basal and squamous cell skin cancer and in situ carcinomas except urinary bladder.

Source: American Cancer Society (2006). *Cancer Facts and Figures* 2006. Atlanta, GA: American Cancer Society. Used with permission from the American Cancer Society. All rights reserved.

Common cancer sites in order of frequency of reported cases and deaths for both men and women are shown in Figure 4.7. Cancer sites with the highest number of reported cases are the prostate gland (men) and breast (women), but cancer frequently occurs in other sites, including the lung, colon and rectum, pancreas, uterus, ovaries, mouth, bladder, and skin. Lung cancer is the leading cause of cancer deaths in both sexes. There were an estimated 174,470 new cases of lung cancer and an estimated 162,460 lung cancer deaths in 2006 alone. It has been estimated that 87% of these deaths can be attributed to smoking. Alcohol and smokeless tobacco contribute to cancers of the mouth, throat, larynx, esophagus, and liver.[4]

Approximately one million new cases of basal cell or squamous cell skin cancer are detected each year in the United States. Almost all of these cases are attributable to exposure to the sun, and yet many people continue to sunbathe or use tanning salons, believing that a tanned body is a healthy one. The number of cases of nonmelanoma skin cancer is expected to rise as long as the ozone layer in the atmosphere continues to be eroded (see Chapter 16). This is an example of how environmental policy affects public health.

Table 4.4
Some Noncommunicable Health Conditions That Affect Americans

Allergic disorders	Epilepsy	Osteoporosis
Arthritis	Fibrocystic breast condition	Premenstrual syndrome
Cerebral palsy	Lower back pain	Sickle cell trait and sickle cell disease
Endogenous depression	Multiple sclerosis	

Other Noncommunicable Disease Problems

Other noncommunicable diseases of major concern are (1) chronic obstructive pulmonary disease and allied conditions (the fourth leading cause of death), (2) diabetes mellitus (the seventh leading cause of death), and (3) chronic liver disease and cirrhosis (the tenth leading cause of death). Each of these chronic noncommunicable diseases and those listed in Table 4.4 places a burden not only on the afflicted individuals and their families but on the community's health resources as well.

PRIORITIZING PREVENTION AND CONTROL EFFORTS

Communities are confronted with a multitude of health problems—communicable and noncommunicable diseases, unintentional injuries, violence, substance abuse problems, and so on. How can health officials make logical and responsible choices about the allocation of community resources to prevent or control these problems? Which problems are indeed the most urgent? Which problems will benefit the most from a timely intervention? Several criteria are used to judge the importance of a particular disease to a community. Among these are (1) the number of people who die from a disease, (2) the number of years of potential life lost attributable to a particular cause, and (3) the economic costs associated with a particular disease or health condition.

Leading Causes of Death

The National Center for Health Statistics (NCHS) regularly publishes a list of the leading causes of death. For more than 80 years, the leading cause of death in America has been heart disease. Nearly one in every three deaths can be attributed to diseases of the heart. Cancers (malignant neoplasms) represent the second leading killer; nearly one in four deaths is the result of cancer. Cerebrovascular disease (stroke) ranks third, chronic lower pulmonary diseases rank fourth, and unintentional injuries rank fifth (see Table 3.8).[2]

One might prioritize expenditures of health care resources solely on the basis of the number of deaths, but in doing so one would spend about two-thirds of the entire health budget on the four leading health problems alone. Very little or perhaps none of the resources would be available for infant and childhood nutrition programs, for example, which have been shown to prevent more serious health care problems in later life. Nor would there be any funds available for the treatment of those with debilitating, but usually nonfatal, diseases such as chronic arthritis or mental illness.

Years of Potential Life Lost

Another approach to prioritizing a community's health care problems is by using the *years of potential life lost (YPLL)* statistic described in Chapter 3. Using this approach, diseases that kill people of all ages become as important as those that kill primarily the elderly. Recall, for example, that malignant neoplasms (cancers) are the leading cause of YPLL-75 in the United States and account for 21.3% of all YPLL-75 compared with CVD, which accounts for only about 15.9%. Unintentional injuries are the third leading cause of YPLL-75, accounting for 14.5% of the total YPLL (refer to Table 3.12 and Figure 3.4).[5]

Economic Cost to Society

Still another way to evaluate the impact of a particular disease or health problem is to estimate the economic cost to the country or community. Economic cost data are hard to come by, and sometimes even experts cannot agree on the estimates obtained. An example of such an estimate is the cost to society resulting from the use and abuse of alcohol and other drugs, a whopping $487 billion annually, more than $1 billion per day.[6] This figure includes not only the cost of treatment and the loss of productivity but also the cost of law enforcement, courts, jails, and social work (see Chapter 12).

PREVENTION, INTERVENTION, CONTROL, AND ERADICATION OF DISEASES

The goals of epidemiology are to prevent, control, and in rare cases, to eradicate diseases and injuries. **Prevention** implies the planning for and taking of action to prevent or forestall the occurrence of an undesirable event, and is therefore more desirable than **intervention,** the taking of action during an event. For example, immunizing to prevent a disease is preferable to taking an antibiotic to cure one.

Control is a general term for the containment of a disease and can include both prevention and intervention measures. The term *control* is often used to mean the limiting of transmission of a communicable disease in a population. **Eradication** is the uprooting or total elimination of a disease from the human population. It is an elusive goal, one that is only rarely achieved in public health. Smallpox is the only communicable disease that has been eradicated (see Box 4.3) This was possible only because humans are the only reservoir.

LEVELS OF PREVENTION

There are three levels of application of preventive measures in disease control—primary, secondary, and tertiary. The purpose of **primary prevention** is to forestall the onset of illness or injury during the prepathogenesis period (before the disease process begins). Examples of primary prevention include health education and health promotion programs, safe-housing projects, and character-building and personality development programs. Other examples are the use of immunizations against specific diseases, the practice of personal hygiene such as hand washing, the use of rubber gloves, and the chlorination of the community's water supply. These are illustrated in Figure 4.8.

Unfortunately, disease or injury cannot always be avoided. Chronic diseases in particular sometimes cause considerable disability before they are detected and treated. In these cases,

prevention
the planning for and taking of action to forestall the onset of a disease or other health problem

intervention
efforts to control a disease in progress

eradication
the complete elimination or uprooting of a disease (e.g., smallpox eradication)

primary prevention
preventive measures that forestall the onset of illness or injury during the prepathogenesis period

---

BOX 4.3	COMMUNITY HEALTH IN YOUR WORLD: SMALLPOX ERADICATION

December 2007 marked 30 years since the last naturally acquired case of smallpox in the world. This last case occurred in Somalia in October 1977.[1] Although two cases of smallpox were reported in the United Kingdom in 1978, these were associated with a research laboratory and did not represent a natural recurrence.

Smallpox is caused by the variola virus. In its severest form, it is a disfiguring and deadly disease. Manifestations of the disease include fever, headache, malaise, and prostration. A rash appears and covers the body, and there is bleeding into the skin, mucous linings, and genital tract. The circulatory system is also severely affected. Between 15% and 40% of cases die, usually within two weeks. Survivors are terribly scarred for life and are sometimes blinded.

Mass vaccinations and case-finding measures by the World Health Organization (WHO), with financial support from the United States, led to the eradication of smallpox from the world. Why was it possible to eradicate smallpox? Why have we been unable to eradicate any other diseases since 1977? Do you think we will ever be able to do so? If so, what disease will be eliminated next?

The Natural History of Any Disease of Humans

FIGURE 4.8
Applications of levels of prevention.

prompt *intervention* can prevent death or limit disability. **Secondary prevention** is the early diagnosis and prompt treatment of diseases before the disease becomes advanced and disability becomes severe.

One of the most important secondary prevention measures is *health screenings*. The goal of these screenings is not to prevent the onset of disease but rather to detect its presence during early pathogenesis, thus permitting early intervention (treatment) and limiting disability. It is important to note that the purpose of a health screening is not to diagnose disease. Instead, the purpose is to economically and efficiently sort those who are probably healthy from those who could possibly be positive for a disease (see Figure 4.9). Those who screen positively can then be referred for more specific diagnostic procedures. Screenings for diabetes and high blood pressure are popular examples of health screenings, as are breast self-examination and testicular self-examination.

The goal of **tertiary prevention** is to retrain, re-educate, and rehabilitate the patient who has already incurred a disability. Tertiary preventive measures include those that are applied after significant pathogenesis has occurred. Therapy for a heart patient is an example of tertiary prevention.

Prevention of Communicable Diseases

Prevention and control efforts for communicable diseases include primary, secondary, and tertiary approaches. Successful application of these approaches, particularly primary prevention, resulting in unprecedented declines in morbidity and mortality from communicable

secondary prevention preventive measures that lead to an early diagnosis and prompt treatment of a disease or injury to limit disability and prevent more severe pathogenesis

tertiary prevention measures aimed at rehabilitation following significant pathogenesis

FIGURE 4.9

Flow diagram for a mass screening test.

Source: Mausner, J. S., and S. Kramer (1985). *Epidemiology—An Introductory Text.* Philadelphia: W.B. Saunders Company. Reprinted with permission of Elsevier.

BOX
4.4 TEN GREAT PUBLIC HEALTH ACHIEVEMENTS, 1900–1999: CONTROL OF INFECTIOUS DISEASES

An Ounce of Prevention Is Worth a Century of Cure

Public health action to control infectious diseases in the twentieth century was founded on the late nineteenth century's discovery of microorganisms as causes of many diseases. Further scientific findings documented the interactions among humans, the environment, and microbes. Improvements in sanitation, hygiene, and food safety; the discovery of antibiotics; and the implementation of universal childhood vaccination programs resulted in the control of many fatal infectious diseases and the global eradication of one disease—smallpox. Scientific and technologic advances played a substantial role in these efforts. Today, those advances are the foundation for the disease surveillance and control systems that are used to combat all infectious diseases.

Sanitation and Hygiene

Early in the twentieth century, infections associated with overcrowding, poor housing, and contaminated water resulted in the transmission of tuberculosis, diphtheria, typhoid fever, and dysentery. Improvements in housing and public water supplies—including chlorination and filtration—and waste-disposal systems have resulted in swift progress in disease control.

Antibiotics and Other Antimicrobial Medicines

Antibiotics have been in common use since the 1940s and have saved the lives and health of persons with streptococcal and staphylococcal infections, gonorrhea, syphilis, and other infections. Penicillin was the first of many antibiotics that became widely available to cure previously untreatable bacterial diseases. Drugs also have been developed to treat viral, fungal, and parasitic diseases, but resistance to these miracle drugs is an ever increasing challenge.

Emerging Diseases

For continued success in controlling infectious disease, the U.S. public health system must address such diverse challenges as the emergence of new infectious disease—for example, HIV and hantavirus—and the re-emergence of old diseases, sometimes in drug-resistant forms—for example, tuberculosis and malaria. Bioterrorism and pandemic influenza are also potential public health crises requiring advance preparedness.

Marvel of Medical Science, Miracle for Mankind

Sometimes a miracle happens and a disease is eradicated. Biomedical science and public health create this miracle when medicines and vaccines are developed that enable disease control and prevention. At the beginning of the twentieth century, few effective treatments and preventitive measures existed to prevent infectious diseases. However, vaccines have been developed and are used to prevent many of the infectious diseases that threatened our parents, grandparents, and great-grandparents during the twentieth century.

Overall, U.S. vaccination coverage is at record high levels. Up-to-date training for the shot-givers and shot-callers is also at record high levels. Vaccines have the remarkable power to eradicate diseases. However, the combined effort of many partners is needed to achieve the full potential of these miraculous medicines.

diseases, has been one of the outstanding achievements in public health in this century (see Box 4.4).

Primary Prevention of Communicable Diseases

The primary prevention measures for communicable diseases can best be visualized using the chain of infection (see Figure 4.10). In this model, prevention strategies are evident at each link in the chain. Successful application of each strategy can be seen as weakening a link, with the ultimate goal of breaking the chain of infection, or interrupting the disease transmission cycle. Examples of community measures include chlorination of the water supply, the inspection of restaurants and retail food markets, immunization programs that reach all citizens, the maintenance of a well-functioning sewer system, the proper disposal of solid waste, and the control of vectors and rodents. To these can be added personal efforts at primary prevention, including hand washing, the proper cooking of food, adequate clothing and housing, the use of condoms, and obtaining all the available immunizations against specific diseases.

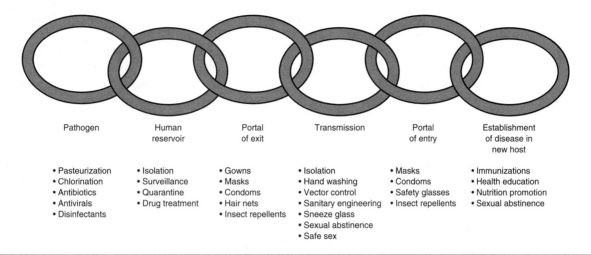

Pathogen	Human reservoir	Portal of exit	Transmission	Portal of entry	Establishment of disease in new host
• Pasteurization • Chlorination • Antibiotics • Antivirals • Disinfectants	• Isolation • Surveillance • Quarantine • Drug treatment	• Gowns • Masks • Condoms • Hair nets • Insect repellents	• Isolation • Hand washing • Vector control • Sanitary engineering • Sneeze glass • Sexual abstinence • Safe sex	• Masks • Condoms • Safety glasses • Insect repellents	• Immunizations • Health education • Nutrition promotion • Sexual abstinence

FIGURE 4.10

Chain of infection model showing disease prevention and control strategies.

Secondary Prevention of Communicable Diseases

Secondary preventive measures against communicable diseases for the individual involve either (1) self-diagnosis and self-treatment with nonprescription medications or home remedies, or (2) diagnosis and treatment with an antibiotic prescribed by a physician. Secondary preventive measures undertaken by the community against infectious diseases are usually aimed at controlling or limiting the extent of an epidemic. Examples include carefully maintaining records of cases and complying with the regulations requiring the reporting of notifiable diseases (see Chapter 3) and investigating cases and contacts—those who may have become infected through close contact with known cases.

Occasionally, secondary disease control measures may include isolation and quarantine. These two practices are quite different from one another and are often confused. **Isolation** is the separation, for the period of communicability, of infected persons or animals from others so as to prevent the direct or indirect transmission of the communicable agent to a susceptible person. **Quarantine** is the limitation of the freedom of movement of well persons or animals that have been exposed to a communicable disease until the incubation period has passed. Further control measures may include **disinfection,** the killing of communicable agents outside of the host, and mass treatment with antibiotics. Finally, public health education and health promotion should be used as both primary and secondary preventive measures.

Tertiary Prevention of Communicable Diseases

Tertiary preventive measures for the control of communicable diseases for the individual include convalescence from infection, recovery to full health, and return to normal activity. In some cases, such as paralytic poliomyelitis, return to normal activity may not be possible even after extensive physical therapy. At the community level, tertiary preventive measures are aimed at preventing the recurrence of an epidemic. The proper removal, embalming, and burial of the dead is an example. Tertiary prevention may involve the reapplication of primary and secondary measures in such a way as to prevent further cases. For example, in some countries, such as the Republic of Korea, people with colds or flu wear gauze masks in public to reduce the spread of disease.

isolation
the separation of infected persons from those who are susceptible

quarantine
limitation of freedom of movement of those who have been exposed to a disease and may be incubating it

disinfection
the killing of communicable disease agents outside the host, on counter tops, for example

Application of Preventive Measures in the Control of a Communicable Disease: AIDS

Acquired immunodeficiency syndrome (AIDS) is a progressive disease that is caused by human immunodeficiency virus (HIV) infection. Individuals can become infected when they come in contact with the virus through sexual activity, intravenous drug use, or blood exposure. It usually takes between two and six months for antibodies to appear in the blood of an infected person. When this happens, these people are referred to as being *HIV positive* or *seropositive.* Epidemiologically, these symptomless, HIV-positive people are an important virus reservoir and can serve as a source of infection for other community members. At some time later (six months to 10 or more years later), as the HIV infection weakens their immune system, they will usually develop signs and symptoms of illnesses caused by opportunistic infections or AIDS indicator infections. Once they do, they are referred to as *HIV positive with symptoms,* and may be diagnosed as having AIDS. It may take as long as 15 years for an infected person, without prophylactic drug treatment, to develop AIDS.[7] Their diagnosis is then referred to as *HIV positive with AIDS.*

HIV is responsible for a pandemic of unprecedented size. The WHO estimates that 39 million people are living with HIV/AIDS worldwide. During 2005, 4.1 million people were newly infected with HIV and 2.8 million people died of AIDS.[8] In the United States, through December 2004, a cumulative total of 944,305 persons with AIDS were reported to the CDC by state and territorial health departments.[9] The reservoir for HIV virus is the infected human population; there are no known animal or insect reservoirs. Referring to the chain of infection, HIV normally leaves its infected host (reservoir) during sexual activity. The portal of exit is the urogenital tract. Transmission is direct and occurs when reproductive fluids or blood are exchanged with the susceptible host. In the case of injection drug users, however, transmission is indirect, by contaminated needles (vehicle). The portal of entry is usually either genital, oral, or anal in direct (sexual) transmission or transdermal in the case of injection drug users or blood transfusion recipients. Transmission can also occur during medical procedures if there is an accidental needlestick or some other type of contamination with blood or other potentially infectious material.

A closer examination of the chain of infection reveals that prevention or control measures can be identified for each link. The pathogen in the diseased host can be held in check by the appropriate drug. Outside the host, measures such as sterilizing needles and other possible vehicles and disinfecting surfaces readily kill the virus and reduce the likelihood of transmission by contamination. The infected host (reservoir) can be identified through blood tests and educated to take precautions against the careless transmission of live virus through unsafe sex and needle sharing. Portals of exit (and entry) can be protected by the use of condoms. Transmission can be stopped by the practice of abstinence or reduced by limiting the number of sexual partners. Urogenital portals of entry can be protected through sexual abstinence and the use of condoms. One of the stated objectives of *Healthy People 2010* is to increase condom use (see Box 4.5). In the case of injection drug users, abstinence from such drug use would preclude transmission by needles and syringes. A more realistic approach to reducing the spread of HIV/AIDS in the injection-drug-using population might be a more reasonable syringe sale and possession policy (see Box 4.6).[10]

For those working in the health professions, the risk of acquiring an HIV infection in the workplace is of particular concern. The Occupational Safety and Health Administration (OSHA) estimates that 5.6 million workers in the health care industry and related occupations are at risk of occupational exposure to **bloodborne pathogens,** including HIV, hepatitis B virus (HBV), hepatitis C virus (HCV), and others.[10] In 1991 OSHA, recognizing that workers in the health care industry were at risk of occupational exposure to bloodborne pathogens, issued the **Bloodborne Pathogens Standard.**

bloodborne pathogens disease agents, such as HIV, that are transmissible in blood and other body fluids

Bloodborne Pathogens Standard a set of regulations promulgated by OSHA that sets forth the responsibilities of employers and employees with regard to precautions to be taken concerning bloodborne pathogens in the workplace

BOX
4.5
HEALTHY PEOPLE 2010: OBJECTIVES

Goal: Prevent HIV infection and its related illness and death.

Objective 13-6a: Increase the proportion of condom use by partners of sexually active unmarried females (aged 18 to 44 years).

	Baseline Year	Baseline	2002	Target 2010
Race and ethnicity				
American Indian or Alaska Native	1995	DSU	DSU	50%
Asian or Pacific Islander	1995	DSU	DSU	50%
Asian	1995	DNC	DSU	50%
Native Hawaiian and other Pacific Islander	1995	DNC	DSU	50%
Black or African American	1995	22%	33%	50%
White	1995	23%	30%	50%
Hispanic or Latino	1995	17%	25%	50%
Persons aged 18 to 19 years	1995	16%	DSU	NA
Persons aged 20 to 24 years	1995	18%	35%	NA
Persons aged 25 to 29 years	1995	19%	30%	NA
Persons aged 30 to 34 years	1995	22%	18%	NA
Persons aged 35 to 44 years	1995	9%	13%	NA
Not Hispanic or Latino	1995	24%	33%	NA
Black or African American, not Hispanic/Latino	1995	22%	33%	50%
Persons aged 18 to 19 years	1995	31%	DSU	NA
Persons aged 20 to 24 years	1995	35%	37%	NA
Persons aged 25 to 29 years	1995	23%	30%	NA
Persons aged 30 to 34 years	1995	17%	31%	NA
Persons aged 35 to 44 years	1995	12%	29%	NA
White, not Hispanic or Latino	1995	24%	32%	50%
Persons aged 18 to 19 years	1995	39%	60%	NA
Persons aged 20 to 24 years	1995	29%	39%	NA
Persons aged 25 to 29 years	1995	24%	29%	NA
Persons aged 30 to 34 years	1995	14%	21%	NA
Persons aged 35 to 44 years	1995	18%	18%	NA
Family income level				
Poor	1995	16%	25%	50%
Near poor	1995	21%	26%	50%
Middle/high income	1995	27%	32%	50%
Education level (aged 25 to 44 years)				
Less than high school	1995	7%	20%	50%
High school graduate	1995	15%	25%	50%
At least some college	1995	25%	34%	50%
Geographic location				
Urban (metropolitan statistical area)	1995	24%	32%	50%
Rural (nonmetropolitan statistical area)	1995	18%	29%	50%
Disability status				
Persons with disabilities	1995	DNA	30%	50%
Persons without disabilities	1995	DNA	32%	50%
Sexual orientation	1995	DNC	DNC	50%

Note: Data may include revisions and may differ from those shown previously. Any displayed age-adjusted data are adjusted to the 2000 standard population.

DNA = Data have not been analyzed. DNC = Data for specific population are not collected. DSU = Data do not meet the criteria for statistical reliability, data quality, or confidentiality. NA = Not applicable.

Source: CDC (2007). *DATA2010 . . . The Healthy People 2010 Database—January, 2007 Edition.* Available at http://wonder.cdc.gov.

For Further Thought

Unprotected sexual contact, whether homosexual or heterosexual, with a person infected with HIV is one of the most important ways HIV infections are transmitted. An important way to slow the rate of new AIDS cases is to increase the proportion of sexually active females whose partners use condoms. Can you think of other ways to increase the rate of condom use in sexually active persons?

BOX
4.6
INJECTION DRUG USE, HIV/AIDS, AND PUBLIC HEALTH: PROMOTING HEALTH AND SAFETY IN AMERICA THROUGH A REASONABLE SYRINGE SALE AND POSSESSION POLICY

Injection drug use is the second most frequently reported risk factor for AIDS, accounting for 193,527 cases through December 1995. In 2000, 35% of all AIDS cases occurred among injection drug users (IDUs), their heterosexual sex partners, and children whose mothers were IDUs or sex partners of IDUs. Transmission of HIV infection by IDUs occurs primarily through multiperson use of syringes— needle sharing. (In this discussion, the term *syringe* includes both syringes and needles.) When an IDU injects drugs, the syringe becomes contaminated with that person's blood and bloodborne pathogens that can then be transmitted to another IDU who uses the same syringe.

In an effort to control the widespread use of opium, morphine, cocaine, and heroin in the late nineteenth and early twentieth centuries, states passed laws restricting the freedom of physicians to dispense the drugs. These laws also regulated the sale and distribution of syringes. In 1979, the Drug Enforcement Administration wrote the Model Drug Paraphernalia Act (MDPA), versions of which were adopted by many states. These laws were adopted in response to the proliferation of drug paraphernalia industry and the numerous "head shops" operated nationwide. Included as drug paraphernalia are "hypodermic syringes, needles, and other objects used, intended for use, and designed for use in parenterally injecting controlled substances into the human body."

A survey reveals that 47 states and the District of Columbia have passed drug paraphernalia statutes. Ten states have laws, regulations, or ordinances that require a prescription for the purchase of syringes, and 16 additional states have laws or regulations that can otherwise limit the sale and purchase of syringes. To the extent that these laws, regulations, and ordinances restrict access to sterile syringes, they contribute to the spread of bloodborne diseases among IDUs, their sexual contacts, and their children. Some, but not all, of these states have carved out some provisions to exempt operators and participants of syringe exchange programs (SEPs) from prosecution under these laws.

Pharmacists face substantial legal and professional hurdles if they sell syringes to IDUs. Physicians and other health professionals face potentially dire legal consequences when they prescribe syringes or otherwise directly assist IDUs in obtaining sterile syringes. Criminal and professional sanctions prevent these professionals from providing important HIV prevention services to persons who continue to inject drugs. Most of the laws that restrict the sale, possession, or distribution of syringes were promulgated before the HIV/AIDS epidemic.

The dual epidemics of drug use and the human immunodeficiency virus and acquired immunodeficiency syndrome (HIV/AIDS) are significant burdens on the health and safety of Americans. There are between 1 and 2 million IDUs in the United States who are at risk for acquiring a variety of bloodborne pathogens such as hepatitis B and C, HIV/AIDS, endocarditis, and malaria. Futhermore, illicit drug use results in destruction of families, domestic abuse and neglect, and a variety of social and economic problems. Drug abuse is also associated with higher rates of crime against people and property. The annual cost to society of drug abuse has been estimated at nearly $60 billion.

Many public health, medical, and legal organizations have supported the deregulation of syringes as a strategy to prevent HIV/AIDS and other bloodborne diseases among IDUs. What do you think?

1. What are the legitimate medical (public health) purposes of sterile syringes?
2. Should drug paraphernalia laws be modified?
3. Should syringe prescription laws be changed to exempt authorized use of syringes to prevent multiperson use of syringes in syringe exchange programs, for example?
4. Should pharmacy regulations that prevent pharmacists from dispensing sterile needles to IDUs be repealed?
5. Should there be in-service training for pharmacists and other health professionals and criminal justice personnel so they can advance public health goals?
6. Should states allow local discretion in establishing syringe exchange programs?
7. What kinds of programs should be developed to reduce the number of contaminated syringes in circulation and reduce health risks to the public?

Source: Gostin, L. O., Z. Lazzarini, T. S. Jones, and K. Flaherty (1997). "Prevention of HIV/AIDS and Other Blood-borne Diseases among Injection Drug Users: A National Survey on the Regulation of Syringes and Needles." *JAMA,* 277(1): 53–62.

In November 2000, Congress, acknowledging the estimates of 600,000 to 800,000 needlestick and other percutaneous injuries occurring among health care workers annually, passed the Needlestick Safety and Prevention Act.[11] In 2001, in response to the Needlestick Safety and Prevention Act, OSHA revised its Bloodborne Pathogens Standard. This revised standard, currently in effect, "clarifies the need for employers to select safer needle devices and to involve employees in identifying and choosing these devices" and to maintain a log of injuries from contaminated sharps.[12] The goal of all of these regulations and standards is to reduce the number of HIV/AIDS cases, as well as cases of other bloodborne diseases, resulting from workplace exposure.

Prevention of Noncommunicable Diseases

Both the individual and the community can contribute substantially to the prevention and control of multicausation diseases. The community can provide a pro-health environment—physical, economic, and social—in which it becomes easier for individuals to achieve a high level of health.

Primary Prevention of Noncommunicable Diseases

Primary preventive measures for noncommunicable diseases include adequate food and energy supplies, good opportunities for education, employment, and housing, and efficient community services. Beyond this foundation, a community should provide health promotion and health education programs, health and medical services, and protection from environmental and occupational hazards.

Individuals can practice primary prevention by obtaining a high level of education that includes a knowledge about health and disease and the history of disease of others in one's family. In particular, the individual should take responsibility for eating properly, exercising adequately, maintaining appropriate weight, and avoiding the overuse of alcohol and other drugs. Individuals can also protect themselves from injury by wearing safety belts, safety goggles, and sunscreen lotions.

Secondary Prevention of Noncommunicable Diseases

Secondary preventive measures the community can take include the provision of mass screenings for chronic diseases (see Figure 4.11), case-finding measures, and the provision of adequate health personnel, equipment, and facilities for the community. Secondary prevention responsibilities of individual citizens include personal screenings such as self-examination of breasts or testes (for cancer of these organs), the hemocult test (for colorectal cancer), and medical screenings such as the Pap test (for cervical cancer), the PSA test for cancer of the prostate, mammography, and screenings for diabetes, glaucoma, or hypertension. Participating in such health screenings and having regular medical and dental checkups represent only the first step in the secondary prevention of noncommunicable diseases. This must be followed by the pursuit of definitive diagnosis and prompt treatment of any diseases detected.

FIGURE 4.11

Mammography, used for screening and early detection of breast cancer, is an example of secondary prevention.

Tertiary Prevention of Noncommunicable Diseases

Tertiary preventive measures for a community include adequate emergency medical personnel, services, and facilities to meet the needs of those citizens for whom primary and secondary preventive measures were unsuccessful. Examples include ambulance services, hospitals, physicians and surgeons, nurses, and other allied health professionals. Interestingly, most communities are doing a more-than-adequate job in tertiary prevention. Many experts feel that most communities in America need to reallocate resources from tertiary prevention to primary and secondary preventive measures.

Tertiary prevention for the individual often requires significant behavioral or lifestyle changes. Examples include strict adherence to prescribed medications, exercise programs, and diet. For example, a heart attack patient could receive nutrition education and counseling and be encouraged to participate in a supervised exercise program, thus maximizing the use of remaining capabilities. This could lead to a resumption of employment and the prevention of a second heart attack. For certain types of noncommunicable health problems, such as those involving substance abuse, regular attendance at support group meetings or counseling sessions may constitute an important part of a tertiary prevention program.

Application of Preventive Measures in the Control of a Noncommunicable Disease: CHD

Despite considerable progress, CHD remains America's Number 1 killer. Reducing CHD deaths is one of the *Healthy People 2010* objectives (see Box 4.7). Many factors contribute to one's risk of developing this disease. Both the community and the individual can contribute to the prevention of CHD.

The Community's Role

The community must recognize the importance of preventing chronic disease; intervention following a crisis, such as a heart attack, is the least effective and most expensive way to provide help to a CHD patient. While individual behavioral changes hold the best prospects for reducing the prevalence of heart disease in this country, communities can provide a supporting environment for these behavioral changes. For example, the community can support restricting smoking areas and can provide a clear message to youth that smoking is damaging to health. Communities also can provide adequate opportunity for health screening for risk factors such as hypertension and serum cholesterol levels. In particular, schools can permit the administration of Youth Risk Behavior Surveillance System surveys (see Chapter 3) and utilize these occasions as opportunities to teach students about the importance of healthy behavioral choices. Communities also can promote and assist in the development of areas for recreation and exercise, such as safe paths for jogging or cycling and lighted sidewalks for walking. Exercise reduces obesity and increases the high-density lipoproteins (HDLs) in the blood, thereby lowering risk for a heart attack. Finally, communities should promote sound nutrition throughout the life span, but particularly in schools.

unmodifiable risk factors factors contributing to the development of a noncommunicable disease that cannot be altered by modifying one's behavior or environment

The Individual's Role

The risk factors for CHD are multiple. Some of these risk factors are unmodifiable, whereas other risk factors can be modified (reduced) to improve one's health. Each person can increase his or her resistance to CHD by knowing the difference between the types of risk factors and by adopting behaviors that prevent or postpone the onset of CHD.

Each person is endowed with a unique genetic code. An individual's innate resistance or susceptibility to heart disease is encoded in the genes. **Unmodifiable risk factors** for CHD include one's race, gender, personality type, age, and basic metabolic rate. Also inherited is

HEALTHY PEOPLE 2010: OBJECTIVES

Objective 12.1:   Reduce coronary heart disease deaths to 166 deaths per 100,000 population.

	Baseline Year	Baseline	2004	Target 2010
Race and ethnicity				
American Indian or Alaska Native	1999	a\148	112	b\162
Asian or Pacific Islander	1999	a\124	90	b\162
Asian	1999	a\DNC	DNA	b\162
Native Hawaiian and other Pacific Islander	1999	a\DNC	DNA	b\162
Black or African American	1999	a\248	204	b\162
White	1999	a\200	157	b\162
Hispanic or Latino	1999	a\169	127	b\162
Not Hispanic or Latino	1999	a\204	161	b\162
Black or African American, not Hispanic/Latino	1999	a\250	207	b\162
White, not Hispanic or Latino	1999	a\201	159	b\162
Gender				
Female	1999	a\161	125	b\162
Male	1999	a\260	204	b\162
Education level (persons aged 25 to 64 years)				
Less than high school	1999	a,1\97	2\101	NA
High school graduate	1999	a,1\80	2\73	NA
At least some college	1999	a,1\36	2\30	NA
Disability status				
Persons with disabilities	1999	a\DNC	DNC	b\162
Persons without disabilities	1999	a\DNC	DNC	b\162

Note: Data may include revisions and may differ from those shown previously. Any displayed age-adjusted data are adjusted to the 2000 standard population.

DNA = Data have not been analyzed. DNC = Data for specific population are not collected. NA = Not applicable.

a\Baseline has been revised.

b\Target has been revised.

1\Total of 46 reporting states and the District of Columbia.

2\Total of 36 reporting states and the District of Columbia. Data are not directly comparable to those of previous year.

Source: CDC (2007). *DATA2010 . . . The Healthy People 2010 Database—January, 2007 Edition.* Available at http://wonder.cdc.gov.

For Further Thought

Important contributing factors to CHD are high blood cholesterol, high blood pressure, and obesity. What is the prevalence of high blood pressure in your community? What is the prevalence of obesity in your state? Do you know your serum cholesterol level?

one's baseline serum cholesterol level. That is, children whose parents had high serum cholesterol levels are at risk for those same higher levels, independent of their diet.

Modifiable risk factors for CHD include environmental and behavioral factors over which an individual has some control. Modifiable risk factors that would increase the likelihood of CHD include smoking, a diet too rich in fats, lack of exercise, obesity, uncontrolled hypertension, and too much stress. Although none of these factors alone is likely to cause a premature heart attack, each can contribute to the likelihood of CHD.

modifiable risk factors
factors contributing to the development of a noncommunicable disease that can be altered by modifying one's behavior or environment

CHAPTER SUMMARY

- Diseases can be classified as communicable (infectious) or noncommunicable (noninfectious), and acute or chronic.

- Acute diseases last for less than three months, whereas chronic diseases continue longer than three months.

- Communicable diseases are caused by biological agents and are transmissible from a source of infection to a susceptible host.

- The process of communicable disease transmission is best understood by the chain of infection model, in which the interruption of disease transmission can be visualized as the breaking of one or more links in the chain.

- Noncommunicable diseases are often the result of multiple risk factors that can be genetic, behavioral, and environmental in origin.

- Several of the noncommunicable diseases rank among the leading causes of death in America.

- There are three levels of disease prevention—primary, secondary, and tertiary.

- Primary prevention includes measures that forestall the onset of disease or injury, while secondary prevention encompasses efforts aimed at early detection and intervention to limit disease and disability. Tertiary prevention includes measures aimed at re-education and rehabilitation after significant pathogenesis has occurred.

- Both the spread of communicable diseases and the prevalence of noncommunicable diseases can best be reduced by the appropriate application of primary, secondary, and tertiary preventive measures by the community and the individual.

- The prevention and control of noncommunicable diseases require both individual and community efforts.

REVIEW QUESTIONS

1. What are some of the ways in which diseases and health problems are classified in community health?
2. Contrast the terms *acute disease* and *chronic disease*. Provide three examples of each type of disease.
3. Contrast the terms *communicable disease* and *noncommunicable disease*. Provide three examples of each type of disease.
4. What is the difference between a communicable agent and a pathogenic agent?
5. What are the components of a simplified communicable disease model?
6. List some examples of environmental factors that can influence the occurrence and spread of disease.
7. Draw and explain the model for multicausation diseases.
8. What is the difference between prevention and intervention?
9. Explain the difference between primary, secondary, and tertiary prevention and provide an example of each.
10. What is the chain of infection model of disease transmission? Draw the model and label its parts.
11. Again referring to the chain of infection, indicate how prevention and control strategies could be implemented to interrupt the transmission of gonorrhea. Are most of these strategies primary, secondary, or tertiary prevention measures?
12. Define the following terms—*case, carrier, vector, vehicle.*
13. List five examples each of vectorborne diseases and nonvectorborne diseases.
14. Explain the difference between the public health practices of isolation and quarantine.

SCENARIO: ANALYSIS AND RESPONSE

1. If Bob's roommate, Chuck, were to begin to show signs of the flu, what could Bob do to lessen his chances of becoming infected himself? (*Hint:* Think about the chain of infection.)
2. As an accountant, Bob spends most of his day behind a desk. To identify primary, secondary, and tertiary preventive measures Bob should take to reduce his risk for heart disease, visit one governmental and one nongovernmental Web site and find some information about prevention of heart disease. For each preventive measure you list, indicate whether it is primary, secondary, or tertiary prevention.
3. In what other health screenings should Bob and Chuck participate? Are there any health screenings available on the Internet?
4. What kinds of thoughts, behaviors, and conditions prevent people from participating in health screenings?

15. Apply the principles of prevention and the examples given in this chapter to outline a prevention strategy for breast cancer that includes primary, secondary, and tertiary prevention components.

ACTIVITIES

1. Call your state health department and find out which are the top communicable (infectious) disease problems reported in your state. Which are the rarest? Is Lyme disease reportable?

2. List some of the infections you have had. How were these infections transmitted to you—directly, by vehicle, or by vector? Talk to someone who is very old about diseases they can recall from their youth and how these diseases affected them and their families. Take notes on the response and hand them in or share them orally in class.

3. Look up the disease bubonic plague in an encyclopedia or on the Internet. After reading about the disease, see if you can complete a chain of infection model for plague. Identify the causative agent, the vector, the reservoir, and the mode of transmission. What types of prevention and control strategies were used in the past to stop the spread of this disease? What can be done differently today if there is an epidemic of plague?

4. Think about motor vehicle crashes. List some primary, secondary, and tertiary preventive measures that the community and you can take to reduce the number and seriousness of injuries caused by auto accidents.

COMMUNITY HEALTH ON THE WEB

The Internet contains a wealth of information about community and public health. Increase your knowledge of some of the topics presented in this chapter by accessing the Jones and Bartlett Publishers Web site at **http://health.jbpub.com/book/communityhealth/6e** and follow the links to complete the following Web activities.

- National Center for Infectious Diseases
- National Center for Chronic Disease Prevention and Health Promotion
- Epidemic Intelligence Service

REFERENCES

1. Heymann, D. L., ed. (2004). *Control of Communicable Diseases Manual*, 18th ed. Washington, DC: American Public Health Association.

2. Hoyert, D. L., M. P. Heron, S. L. Murphy, and H. C. Kung. 2006. "Deaths: Final Data for 2003." *National Vital Statistics Report*, 54(13): 1–120.

3. American Heart Association (2006). *Heart Disease and Stroke Statistics—2006 Update*. Dallas, TX: Author. Available at http://www.americanheart.org.

4. American Cancer Society (2006). *Cancer Facts and Figures—2006*. Atlanta, GA: Author. Available at http://www.cancer.org.

5. National Center for Health Statistics (2006). *Health, United States, 2006 with Chartbook on Trends in the Health of Americans* (DHHS pub. no. 2006-1232). Hyattsville, MD: Author. Available at: http://www.cdc.gov/nchs/hus.htm.

6. Horgan, C., K. C. Skwara, and G. Strickler (2001). *Substance Abuse: The Nation's Number One Health Problem*. Princeton, NJ: Robert Wood Johnson Foundation.

7. Payne, W. A., D. B. Hahn, and E. B. Lucas (2006). *Understanding Your Health*, 9th ed. New York: McGraw-Hill Higher Education.

8. Joint United Nations Programme on HIV/AIDS (2006). *2006 Report on the Global AIDS Epidemic*. Geneva, Switzerland: Author. Available at http://www.who.int/hiv/epiupdates/en/index.html.

9. Centers for Disease Control and Prevention (2005). *HIV/AIDS Surveillance Report, 2004. Vol. 16: Basic Statistics*, 1–46. Available at http://www.cdc.gov/hiv/stats/hasrlink.htm.

10. Occupational Safety and Health Administration (2004). "Bloodborne Pathogens and Needlestick Prevention: Hazard Recognition." Available at http://www.osha.gov/SLTC/bloodbornepathogens/recognition.html.

11. U.S. Congress (2000). "An Act to Require Changes in the Bloodborne Pathogens Standard in Effect under the Occupational Safety and Health Act of 1970." *Congressional Record*, 146(2000): October 3.

12. Occupational Safety and Health Administration (2004). "Safety and Health Topics: Bloodborne Pathogens and Needlestick Prevention." Available at http://www.osha.gov/SLTC/bloodbornepathogens/index.html.

Chapter 5

Community Organizing/ Building and Health Promotion Programming

Chapter Outline

Chapter Objectives

After studying this chapter you will be able to:

1 Define *community organizing, community capacity, community participation,* and *empowered community.*

2 Identify the assumptions that underlie the process of community organization.

3 Briefly explain the difference between locality development, social planning, and social action approaches to community organization.

4 Explain the difference between needs-based and strength-based community organizing models.

5 List the steps for a generalized model for community organizing/building.

6 Explain what is meant by community building.

7 Explain the difference between health education and health promotion.

8 Briefly explain Healthy Cities/Health Communities, PATCH, and MAPP.

9 State and summarize the steps involved in creating a health promotion program.

10 Define the term *needs assessment.*

11 Briefly explain the six steps used in assessing needs.

12 Explain the difference between goals and objectives.

13 List the different types of intervention strategies.

14 Explain the purposes of pilot testing in program development.

15 State the difference between formative and summative evaluation.

SCENARIO

It was becoming obvious to many that the suburb of Kenzington now had a drug problem, but few wanted to admit it. The community's residents liked their quiet neighborhoods, and most never thought that drugs would be a problem. In fact, the problem really sneaked up on everyone. The town only had one bar, and while occasionally someone drank too much, the bar's patrons usually controlled their drinking and didn't bother anyone. Occasionally, two or three high school seniors would be caught drinking beer purchased at a store in a nearby town. Yet these isolated incidents gave no indication of Kenzington's impending drug problem.

Within the past year, the climate of the town had changed considerably. Incidents of teenagers being arrested for possession of alcohol or even other drugs, such as marijuana, were being reported more regularly in the newspaper. There seemed to be more reports of burglaries, too. There had even been a robbery and two assaults reported within the last month. The population of young adults in the community seemed to be increasing, and many of these seemed to be driving impressive cars and wearing the latest clothes. All of these signs were obvious to a group of concerned citizens in Kenzington and suggested the possibility of a drug problem. So the concerned citizens decided to take their concern to the city council.

INTRODUCTION

In order to deal with the health issues that face many communities, community health professionals must possess specific knowledge and skills. They need to be able to identify problems, develop a plan to attack each problem, gather the resources necessary to carry out that plan, implement that plan, and then evaluate the results to determine the degree of progress that has been achieved. In the previous two chapters, we described epidemiological methods as essential tools of the community health professional. In this chapter, we present two other important capabilities that each successful community health worker must master: the skills to organize a community and to plan a health promotion program.

COMMUNITY ORGANIZING/BUILDING

Community health problems can range from small and simple to large and complex. Small, simple problems that are local and involve few people can be solved with the effort of a small group of people and a minimal amount of organization. Large, complex problems that involve whole communities require significant skills and resources for their solution. For these larger problems, a considerable effort must be expended to organize the citizens of the community to work together to implement a lasting solution to their problem. For example, a trained smoking cessation facilitator could help a single person or a small group of people to stop smoking. But to reduce the smoking rates community-wide, community collaboration is needed. The same smoking cessation facilitators are needed to work with individuals, but others are also needed. Schools are needed to provide appropriate tobacco education programs to youth, organizations (e.g., worksites) and institutions (e.g., religious communities) are needed to create smoking policies, government agencies are needed to enforce the laws associated with the sale of tobacco, and cities, counties, and states are needed to create clean indoor air ordinances or laws. This more comprehensive approach to reducing smoking rates needs to bring together, in an organized and coordinated effort, the people and groups interested in the issue and the resources necessary for change. In other words, a community organization effort is needed.

Table 5.1
Terms Associated with Community Organizing/Building

Community capacity	"The characteristics of communities that affect their ability to identify, mobilize, and address social and public health problems"[3]
Empowered community	"One in which individuals and organizations apply their skills and resources in collective efforts to meet their respective needs"[4]
Participation and relevance	"Community organizing that starts where the people are and engages community members as equals"[1]
Social capital	"Relationships and structures within a community that promote cooperation for mutual benefit"[1]

community organizing process through which communities are helped to identify common problems or goals, mobilize resources, and in other ways develop and implement strategies for reaching their goals they have collectively set

"The term *community organization* was coined by American social workers in the late 1880s to describe their efforts to coordinate services for newly arrived immigrants and the poor."[1] More recently, *community organization* has been used by a variety of professionals, including community health workers, and refers to various methods of interventions to deal with social problems. More formally, **community organizing** has been defined as a "process through which communities are helped to identify common problems or goals, mobilize resources, and in other ways develop and implement strategies for reaching their goals they have collectively set."[1] Community organizing is not a science but an art of consensus building within a democratic process[2] (see Table 5.1).

Need for Organizing Communities

In recent years, the need to organize communities seems to have increased. Advances in electronics (e.g., digital and satellite television) and communications (e.g., multifunction cell phones, fax machines, and the Internet), household upgrades (e.g., energy efficiency), and increased mobility (i.e., frequency of moving and ease of worldwide travel) have resulted in a loss of a sense of community. Individuals are much more independent than ever before. The days when people knew everyone on their block are past. Today, it is not uncommon for people to never meet their neighbors (see Figure 5.1). In other cases, people see or talk to their neighbors only once or twice each year. Because of these changes in community social structure, it now takes specific skills to organize a community to act together for the collective good. Note that the usefulness of community organizing skills extends beyond community health.

FIGURE 5.1
In today's complex communities, it is not uncommon for people never to meet their neighbors.

Assumptions of Community Organizing

According to Ross,[2] those who organize communities do so while making certain assumptions. The assumptions Ross outlines can be summarized as follows:

1. Communities of people can develop the capacity to deal with their own problems.
2. People want to change and can change.
3. People should participate in making, adjusting, or controlling the major changes taking place within their communities.
4. Changes in community living that are self-imposed or self-developed have a meaning and permanence that imposed changes do not have.
5. A "holistic approach" can successfully address problems with which a "fragmented approach" cannot cope.
6. Democracy requires cooperative participation and action in the affairs of the community, and people must learn the skills that make this possible.

7. Frequently, communities of people need help in organizing to deal with their needs, just as many individuals require help in coping with their individual problems.

Community Organizing Methods

There is no single, preferred method for organizing a community. In fact, a careful review reveals that several different approaches have been successful, which led Rothman and Tropman to state, "We would speak of community organization methods rather than the community organization method."[5]

The early approaches to community organization used by social workers emphasized the use of consensus and cooperation to deal with community problems.[6] However, in recent years, three primary methods of community organization have developed—locality development, social planning, and social action.[5] *Locality development* is based on the concept of broad self-help participation from the local community. It is "heavily process oriented, stressing consensus and cooperation aimed at building group identity and a sense of community."[1]

Social planning is heavily task oriented, stressing rational-empirical problem solving and involves various levels of participation from many people and outside planners.[1]

The third method, *social action,* is "both task and process oriented"[1] and has been useful in helping to organize disadvantaged segments of the population. It often involves trying to redistribute power or resources, which enables institutional or community change. This method is not used as much as it once was, but it was useful during the civil rights and gay rights movements and in other settings where people have been oppressed.

Though locality development, social planning, and social action methods have been the primary means by which communities have organized over the years, they do have their limitations. Maybe the greatest limitation is that they are primarily "problem-based and organizer-centered, rather than strength-based and community-centered."[7] Thus, some of the newer models are based more on collaborative empowerment and community building. However, all models—old or new—revolve around a common theme: The work and resources of many have a much better chance of solving a problem than the work and resources of a few.

Minkler and Wallerstein have done a nice job of summarizing the models, old and new, by presenting a typology that incorporates both needs- and strength-based approaches (see Figure 5.2).[1] Their typology is divided into four quadrants, with strength-based and needs-based on the vertical axis and consensus and conflict on the horizontal axis. Though this typology separates and categorizes the various methods of community organizing and building, Minkler and Wallerstein point out that

> Community organizing and community building are fluid endeavors. While some organizing efforts primarily have focused in one quadrant, most incorporate multiple tendencies, possibly starting from a specific need or crisis and moving to a strength-based community capacity approach. Different organizing models, such as coalitions, lay health worker programs, political action groups, leadership development or grassroots organizing may incorporate needs- or strength-based approaches at different times, depending on the starting place and the ever changing social dynamic. It is important, however, that organizing efforts clarify their assumptions and make decisions about primary strategies based on skills of group members, history of the group, willingness to take risks, or comfort level with different approaches.[1]

No matter what community organizing/community building approach is used, they all incorporate some fundamental principles. These include "the principle of relevance, or starting where the people are; the principle of participation; and the importance of creating environments in which individuals and communities can become empowered as they increase their community problem-solving ability."[1]

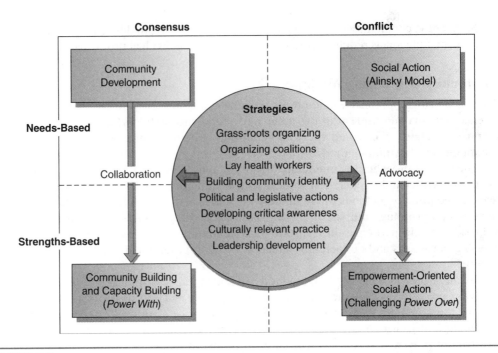

FIGURE 5.2
Community organization and community building typology.

Source: Minkler, M., and N. Wallerstein (2005). "Improving Health through Community Organization and Community Building." In M. Minkler, ed., *Community Organizing and Community Building for Health,* 2nd ed. New Brunswick, NJ: Rutgers University Press, 32.

THE PROCESS OF COMMUNITY ORGANIZING/BUILDING

It is beyond the scope of this textbook to explain all the approaches to community organizing and building in detail. Instead, we will present a generic approach (see Figure 5.3) created by McKenzie, Neiger, and Thackeray that draws upon many of these other approaches.[8] The 10 steps of this generic approach are briefly reviewed in the sections that follow.

Recognizing the Issue

The process of community organizing/building begins when someone recognizes that a problem exists in a community and decides to do something about it. This person (or persons) is referred to as the initial organizer. This individual may not be the primary organizer throughout the community organizing/building process. He or she is the one who gets things started. For the purposes of this discussion, let us assume the problem is violence. People in most communities would like to have a violence-free community, but it would be most unusual to live in a community that was without at least some level of violence. How much violence is too much? At what point is a community willing to organize to deal with the problem? In a small-town community, an acceptable level of violence would be very low, while in a large city, an acceptable level would be much higher.

The people, or organizers, who first recognize a problem in the community and decide to act can be members of the community or individuals from outside the community. If those who initiate community organization are members of the community, then the movement is referred to as being **grass-roots,** *citizen initiated,* or organized from the *bottom up*. Community members who might recognize that violence is a problem could include teachers, police officers, or other concerned citizens. When community organization is initiated by

grass-roots
a process that begins with those who are affected by the problem/concern

individuals from outside of the community, the problem is said to be organized from the *top down* or *outside in.* Individuals from outside the community who might initiate organization could include a judge who presides over cases involving violence, a state social worker who handles cases of family violence, or a politically active group that is against violent behavior wherever it happens. In cases where the person who recognizes the community problem is not a community member, great care must be taken when notifying those in the community that a problem exists. "It is difficult for someone from the outside coming in and telling community members that they have problems or issues that have to be dealt with and they need to organize to take care of them."[8]

Gaining Entry into the Community

This second step in the community organizing process may or may not be needed, depending on whether the issue in step 1 was identified by someone from within the community or outside. If the issue is identified by someone outside the community, this step becomes a critical step in the process.[8] Gaining entry may seem like a relatively easy matter, but an error by organizers at this step could ruin the chances of successfully organizing the community. This may be the most crucial step in the whole process.

Braithwaite and colleagues have stressed the importance of tactfully negotiating entry into a community with the individuals who control, both formally and informally, the "political climate" of the community.[9] These people are referred to as the **gatekeepers.** Thus the term indicates that you must pass through this "gate" to get to your priority population.[10] These "power brokers" know their community, how it functions, and how to accomplish tasks within it. Long-time residents are usually able to identify the gatekeepers of their community. A gatekeeper can be a representative of an intermediary organization—such as a church or school—that has direct contact with your priority audience.[10] Examples include politicians, leaders of activist groups, business and education leaders, and clergy, to name a few.

Organizers must approach such figures on the gatekeepers' own terms and play the gatekeepers' ball game. However, before approaching these important individuals, organizers must study the community well. They must be *culturally sensitive* and work toward *cultural competence.* That is, they must be aware of the cultural differences within a community and effectively work with the cultural context of the community. They need to know where the power lies, the community power dynamics, what type of politics must be used to solve a problem, and

FIGURE 5.3

A summary of steps in community organizing and building.

Source: McKenzie, J. F., B. L. Neiger, and R. Thackeray (2009). *Planning, Implementing, and Evaluating Health Promotion Programs: A Primer,* 5th ed. San Francisco, CA: Benjamin Cummings. Reprinted with permission from Pearson Education, Inc.

gatekeepers
those who control, both formally and informally, the political climate of the community

whether the particular problem they wish to solve has ever been dealt with before in the community.[11] In the violence example, organizers need to know (1) who is causing the violence and why, (2) how the problem has been addressed in the past, (3) who supports and who opposes the idea of addressing the problem, and (4) who could provide more insight into the problem. This is a critical step in the community organization process because failure to study the community carefully in the beginning may lead to a delay in organizing it later and a subsequent waste of time and resources.

Once the organizers have a good understanding of the community, they are then ready to approach the gatekeepers. In keeping with the violence example, the gatekeepers would probably include the police department, elected officials, school board members, social service personnel, members of the judicial system, and possibly some of those who are creating the violence.

When the top-down approach is being used, organizers might find it advantageous to enter the community through a well-respected organization or institution that is already established in the community, such as a church, a service group, or another successful local group. If those who make up such an organization/institution can be convinced that the problem exists and needs to be solved, it can help smooth the way for gaining entry and achieving the remaining steps in the process.

Organizing the People

Obtaining the support of community members to deal with the problem is the next step in the process. It is best to begin by organizing those who are already interested in seeing that the problem is solved. This core group of community members, sometimes referred to as "executive participants,"[12] will become the backbone of the workforce and will end up doing the majority of the work. For our example of community violence, the core group could include law enforcement personnel, former victims of violence and their families (or victims' support groups), parent-teacher organizations, and public health officials. It is also important to recruit people from the subpopulation that is most directly affected by the problem. For example, if most of the violence in a community is directed toward teenagers, teenagers need to be included in the core group. If elderly persons are affected, they need to be included.

"From among the core group, a leader or coordinator must be identified. If at all possible, the leader should be someone with leadership skills, good knowledge of the concern and the community, and most of all, someone from within the community. One of the early tasks of the leader will be to help build group cohesion."[8]

Although the formation of the core group is essential, this group is usually not large enough to do all the work itself. Therefore, one of the core group's tasks is to recruit more members of the community to the cause. This step can take place via a *networking process,* which is when organizers make personal contacts with others who might be interested. Or, the organizers can call an organizing meeting at a local school, community center, or church. By broadening the constituency, the core group can spread out the workload and generate additional resources to deal with the problem. However, recruiting additional workers can often be difficult. Over the last 30 years, the number of people in many communities interested in volunteering their time has decreased. Today, if you ask someone to volunteer, you may hear the reply, "I'm already too busy." There are two primary reasons for this response. First, there are many families in which both husband and wife work outside the home. And second, there are more single-parent households.

Therefore, when organizers are expanding their constituencies, they should be sure to (1) identify people who are affected by the problem that they are trying to solve, (2) provide "perks" for or otherwise reward volunteers, (3) keep volunteer time short, (4) match volunteer assignments with the abilities and expertise of the volunteers, and (5) consider providing appropriate training to make sure volunteers are comfort-able with their tasks. For example, if the organizers need someone to talk with law enforcement groups, it would probably be a good idea to solicit the help of someone who feels comfortable around such groups and who is respected by them, such as another law enforcement person.

When the core group has been expanded to include these other volunteers, the larger group is sometimes referred to as an *association* or a *task force.* There may even be an occasion where a coalition is formed. A **coalition** is "a formal, long-term alliance among a group of individuals representing diverse organizations, factors or constituencies within the community who agree to work together to achieve a common goal"[13]—often, to compensate for deficits in power, resources, and expertise. A larger group with more resources, people, and energy has a greater chance of solving a community problem than a smaller, less powerful group (see Figure 5.4). "Building and maintaining effective coalitions have increasingly been recognized as vital components of much effective community organizing and community building."[14]

FIGURE 5.4
Coalition building is often an important step in successful community organization.

coalition
formal, long-term alliance among a group of individuals representing others within the community who agree to work together to achieve a common goal

Assessing the Community

Earlier in this chapter we referred to Rothman and Tropman's typology for organizing a community—locality development, social planning, and social action.[5] Each of these community organizing strategies operates "from the assumption that problems in society can be addressed by the community becoming better or differently 'organized,' with each strategy perceiving the problems and how or whom to organize in order to address them somewhat differently."[15] In contrast to these strategies is community building. **Community building** "is an orientation to community that is strength-based rather than need-based and stresses the identification, nurturing, and celebration of community assets."[14] Thus, one of the major differences between community organizing and community building is the type of assessment that is used to determine where to focus the community's efforts. In the community organizing approach, the assessment is focused on the needs of the community, while in community building, the assessment focuses on the assets and capabilities of the community. It is assumed that a clearer picture of the community will be revealed and a stronger base will be developed for change if the assessment includes the identification of both needs and assets/capacities and involves those who live in the community. It is from these capacities and assets that communities are built.[16]

community building
an orientation to community that is strength-based rather than need-based and stresses the identification, nurturing, and celebration of community assets

In order to determine the needs and assets/capacities of a community, an assessment must be completed. There are two reasons for completing an effective and comprehensive assessment: "Information is needed for change, and it is also needed for empowerment."[17] This could include a traditional *needs assessment* and/or a newer technique called *mapping community capacity*. A needs assessment is a process by which data about the issues of concern are collected and analyzed. From the analyzed data, concerns or problems emerge and are prioritized so that strategies can be created to tackle them. (*Note:* Needs assessment is discussed in greater length in the second half of this chapter, with regard to program planning.)

Mapping community capacity, on the other hand, is a process of identifying community assets, not concerns or problems. It is a process by which organizers literally use a map to identify the different assets of a community. McKnight and Kretzmann[16] have categorized assets into three different groups based on their availability to the community and refer to them as building blocks. *Primary building blocks* are the most accessible assets. They are located in the neighborhood and are controlled by those who live in the neighborhood. Primary building blocks can be organized into the assets of individuals (e.g., skills and talents) and those of organizations or associations (e.g., religious and citizen organizations). The next most accessible building blocks are secondary building blocks. *Secondary building blocks* are assets located in the neighborhood but largely controlled by people outside (e.g., social service agencies, schools, hospitals, and housing structures). The least accessible assets are referred to as potential building blocks. *Potential building blocks* are resources originating outside the neighborhood and controlled by people outside (e.g., welfare expenditures and public information). By knowing both the needs and assets of the community, organizers can work to identify the true concerns or problems of the community and use the assets of the community as a foundation for dealing with the concerns or problems.

Determining the Priorities and Setting Goals

An analysis of the community assessment data should result in the identification of the problems to be addressed. However, more often than not, the resources needed to solve all identified problems are not available. Therefore, the problems that have been identified must be prioritized. This prioritization is best achieved through general agreement or consensus of those who have been organized so that "ownership" can take hold. It is critical that all those working with the process feel that they "own" the problem and want to see it solved. Without this sense of ownership, they will be unwilling to give of their time and energy to solve it. For example, if a few highly vocal participants intimidate people into voting for certain activities to be the top priorities before a consensus is actually reached, it is unlikely that those who disagreed on this assignment of priorities will work enthusiastically to help solve the problem. They may even drop out of the process because they feel they have no ownership in the decision-making process.

Miller (as cited in Minkler and Wallenstein[1]) has identified five criteria that community organizers need to consider when selecting a priority issue or problem. The issue or problem (1) must be winnable, ensuring that working on it does not simply reinforce fatalistic attitudes and beliefs that things cannot be improved; (2) must be simple and specific, so that any member of the organizing group can explain it clearly in a sentence or two; (3) must unite members of the organizing group and must involve them in a meaningful way in achieving resolution of the issue or problem; (4) should affect many people and build up the community; and (5) should be a part of a larger plan or strategy to enhance the community.[18]

Once the problems have been prioritized, goals need to be identified and written that will serve as guides for problem solving. The practice of consensus building should again be employed during the setting of goals. These goals, which will become the foundation for all the work that follows, can be thought of as the "hoped-for end result." In other words, once community action has occurred, what will have changed? In the community where violence is a problem, the goal may be to reduce the number of violent crimes or eliminate them altogether. Sometimes at this point in the process, some members of the larger group drop out because they do not see their priorities or goals included on consensus lists. Unable to feel ownership, they are unwilling to expend their resources on this process. Because there is strength in numbers, efforts should be made to keep them in. One strategy for doing so is to keep the goal list as long as possible.

Arriving at a Solution and Selecting Intervention Strategies

There are alternative solutions for every community problem. The group should examine the alternatives in terms of probable outcomes, acceptability to the community, probable long- and short-term effects on the community, and the cost of resources to solve the problem.[19] A

Table 5.2
Intervention Strategies and Example Activities

---

1. *Health communication strategies:* Mass media, billboards, booklets, bulletin boards, flyers, direct mail, newsletters, pamphlets, posters, and video and audio materials
2. *Health education strategies:* Educational methods (such as lecture, discussion, and group work) as well as audiovisual materials, computerized instruction, laboratory exercises, and written materials (books and periodicals)
3. *Health policy/enforcement strategies:* Executive orders, laws, ordinances, policies, position statements, regulations, and formal and informal rules
4. *Environmental change strategies:* Those that are designed to change the structure of services or systems of care to improve health promotion services, such as safety belts and air bags in cars, speed bumps in parking lots, or environmental cues such as No Smoking signs
5. *Health-related community services:* The use of health risk appraisals (HRAs), community screening for health problems, and immunization clinics
6. Other strategies
    a. *Behavior modification activities:* Modifying behavior to stop smoking, start to exercise, manage stress, and regulate diet
    b. *Community advocacy activities:* Mass mobilization, social action, community planning, community service development, community education, and community advocacy (such as a letter-writing campaign)
    c. *Organizational culture activities:* Activities that work to change norms and traditions
    d. *Incentives and disincentives:* Items that can either encourage or discourage people to behave a certain way, which may include money and other material items or fines
    e. *Social intervention activities:* Support groups, social activities, and social networks
    f. *Technology-delivered activities:* Educating or informing people by using technology (e.g., computers and telephones)

Source: McKenzie, J. F., B. L. Neiger, and R. Thackeray (2009). *Planning, Implementing, and Evaluating Health Promotion Programs: A Primer,* 5th ed. San Francisco, CA: Benjamin Cummings.

---

solution involves selecting one or more intervention strategies (see Table 5.2). Each type of intervention strategy has advantages and disadvantages. The group must try to agree upon the best strategy and then select the most advantageous intervention activity or activities. Again, the group must work toward consensus through compromise. If the educators in the group were asked to provide a recommended strategy, they might suggest offering more preventive-education programs; law enforcement personnel might recommend more enforceable laws; judges might want more space in the jails and prisons. The protectionism of the subgroups within the larger group is often referred to as *turfism.* It is not uncommon to have turf struggles when trying to build consensus.

The Final Steps in the Community Organizing/Building Process: Implementing, Evaluating, Maintaining, and Looping Back

The last four steps in this generalized approach to organizing/building a community include implementing the intervention strategy and activities that were selected in the previous step, evaluating the outcomes of the plans of action, maintaining the outcomes over time, and if necessary, going back to a previous step in the process—"looping back"—to modify or restructure the work plan to organize the community.

Implementation of the intervention strategy includes identifying and collecting the necessary resources for implementation and creating the appropriate time line for implementation. Often the resources can be found within a community, and thus horizontal relationships, the interaction of local units with one another, are needed.[20] Other times the resources must be obtained from units located outside the community; in this case, vertical relationships, those where local units interact with extracommunity systems, are needed.[20] An example of this latter relationship is the interaction "between a local nonprofit organization and a state agency with which it has contact."[15]

Evaluation of the process involves comparing the outcomes of the process to the goals that were set in an earlier step. Maintaining or sustaining the outcomes may be one of the most difficult steps in the entire process. It is at this point that organizers need to seriously consider the need for a long-term capacity for problem solving. Finally, through the steps of implementation, evaluation, and maintenance of the outcomes, organizers may see the need to "loop back" to a previous step in the process to rethink or rework before proceeding onward in their plan.

Other Models Used for Community Organizing/Building

So far, this chapter has presented background information on community organizing/building and a generic step-by-step approach that could be used for community health efforts. However, it should be noted that there are some models for community organizing/building that have been created by governmental agencies and professional associations for specific projects or programs. Some of the better-known models include Healthy Cities/Healthy Communities, Planned Approach to Community Health (PATCH), and Mobilizing for Action through Planning and Partnerships (MAPP). Each is briefly discussed here.

Healthy Cities/Healthy Communities

Healthy Cities/Healthy Communities is an initiative of the World Health Organization (WHO). This model has been implemented widely throughout the world and is characterized by community ownership and empowerment and driven by the values, needs, and participation of community members with consultation from health professionals.

Although various models are used in Healthy Cities/Healthy Communities, the U.S. Department of Health and Human Services has produced a guide entitled *Healthy People in Healthy Communities* that provides a five-step framework for the Healthy Communities process.[21] Step 1, Mobilize Key Individuals and Organizations, identifies and organizes people who care about the health of their community. This step also involves creating a vision for a healthy community among this core group of individuals that reflects their values and personalities. Eventually, this small core group expands into a larger coalition of individuals and organizations who share in the established vision.

Step 2, Assessing Community Needs, Strengths, and Resources, involves gathering and evaluating a wide range of data about the community and setting priorities. Step 3, Plan for Action, requires the coalition to plan an approach to address the priorities that were analyzed earlier. As with other models, this involves creating objectives, identifying appropriate interventions, assigning specific responsibilities to individuals or organizations, and developing time lines. Coalition members must understand their roles and responsibilities, communicate effectively, follow up meticulously, and track and measure the success of all program components. Step 4, Implement the Action Plan, and step 5, Track Progress and Outcomes, follow patterns much like those presented in the generic approach discussed earlier in this chapter.

Planned Approach to Community Health (PATCH)

PATCH was created in the mid-1980s by the Centers for Disease Control and Prevention (CDC) to "strengthen state and local health departments' capacities to plan, implement, and evaluate community-based health promotion activities targeted toward priority health problems."[22] PATCH is a team approach in which the people of the community make the decisions (via a consensus process) and do the work, with technical assistance from the state and local health departments and the CDC. These team members not only facilitate the necessary work but also provide financial support for the project. Since its development, PATCH has proved to be a useful process with a "good track record for facilitating collaborative, community-based programs."[23] The essential elements of PATCH (see Figure 5.5) include organizing the community with local support, participation, and leadership; choosing health priorities via community

FIGURE 5.5

The five phases of PATCH.

Source: Centers for Disease Control and Prevention. *Planned Approach to Community Health: Guide for the Local Coordinator.* Available at http://www.cdc.gov/nccdphp/publications/PATCH/pdf/00patch.pdf.

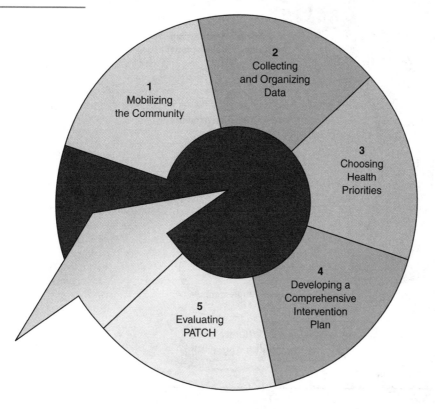

members using local health data; developing and carrying out a comprehensive intervention plan; and evaluating the results.[23]

Mobilizing for Action through Planning and Partnerships (MAPP)

The National Association of County and City Health Officials (NACCHO) developed MAPP. Thus, it represents a planning approach common to local health departments. The vision of the MAPP approach is to improve health and quality of life through mobilized partnerships and taking strategic action.[24]

MAPP is composed of multiple steps in six general phases (see Figure 5.6). In the first phase of MAPP, Organizing for Success and Partnership Development, core planners assess whether the MAPP process is timely, appropriate, and even possible. If the decision is made to undertake a MAPP process, the following work groups are created: (1) a core support team, which prepares most, if not all, of the material needed for the process; (2) the MAPP committee, composed of key sponsors and *stakeholders* (those who have a stake in the outcome of the process) who guide and oversee the process; and (3) the community itself, which provides input, representation, and decision making.

Phase 2 of the MAPP process, Visioning, guides the community through a process that results in a shared vision (what the ideal future looks like) and common values (principles and beliefs that will guide the remainder of the planning process).[24]

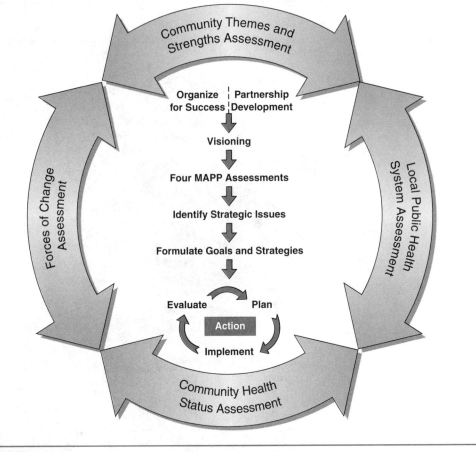

FIGURE 5.6

Mobilizing for Action through Planning and Partnerships (MAPP).

Source: National Association of County and City Health Officials. *Mobilizing for Action through Planning and Partnerships.* Available at http://mapp.naccho.org/MappModel.asp. Used with permission.

Phase 3, the Four MAPP Assessments, is the strength and defining characteristic of the MAPP model. The four assessments are (1) the community themes and strengths assessment (community or consumer opinion), (2) the local public health assessment (general capacity of the local health department), (3) the community health status assessment (measurement of the health of the community), and (4) the forces of change assessment (forces such as legislation, technology, and other environmental or social phenomena that do or will affect the community). This phase provides insight into the gaps that exist between the current status in the community and what was learned in the visioning phase as well as strategic direction for goals and strategies.[24]

In phase 4 of MAPP, Identify Strategic Issues, a prioritized list of the most important issues facing the health of the community is developed. Only issues that jeopardize the vision and values of the community are considered.

Phase 5, Formulate Goals and Strategies, creates goals related to the vision and priority strategic issues. It also selects and adopts strategies. Finally, phase 6, the Action Cycle, is similar to implementation and evaluation phases in other planning models. In this phase, implementation details are considered, evaluation plans (gathering credible evidence) are developed, and plans for disseminating results are made.[24]

A Special Note about Community Organizing/Building

Before we leave the processes of community organizing/building, it should be noted that no matter what approach is used in organizing/building a community—locality development, social planning, social action, or the generalized approach outlined here—not all problems can be solved. In other cases, repeated attempts may be necessary before a solution is reached. In addition, it is important to remember that if a problem exists in a community, there are probably some people who benefit from its existence and who may work toward preventing a successful solution to the problem. Whether or not the problem is solved, the final decision facing the organized group is whether to disband the group or to reorganize in order to take on a new problem or attack the first problem from a different direction.

HEALTH PROMOTION PROGRAMMING

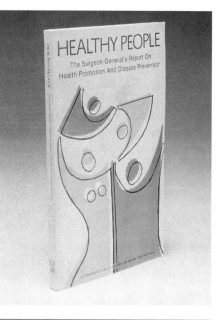

FIGURE 5.7

Healthy People, the 1979 Surgeon General's report on health promotion and disease prevention, charted a new course for community health.

In Chapters 2 through 4, we discuss how communities describe, analyze, and intervene to solve existing health problems such as disease outbreaks or other community problems. However, the 1979 Surgeon General's report on health promotion and disease prevention, *Healthy People* (see Figure 5.7), charted a new course for community health—away from curing diseases and toward preventing diseases and promoting health. Health promotion programming has now become an important tool of community health professionals. The second half of this chapter presents the process of health promotion programming.

Basic Understanding of Program Planning

Prior to discussing the process of program planning, two relationships must be presented. These are the relationships between health education and health promotion, and program planning and community organizing/building.

Health education and *health promotion* are terms that are sometimes used interchangeably. This is incorrect because health education is only a part of health promotion. The Joint Committee on Health Education and Promotion Terminology defined the process of **health education** as "any combination of planned learning experiences based on sound theories that provide individuals, groups, and communities the opportunity to acquire information and the skills to make quality health decisions."[25] The committee defined **health promotion** as "any planned combination of educational, political, environmental, regulatory, or organizational mechanisms that support actions and conditions of living conducive to the health of individuals, groups, and communities."[25] From these definitions, it is obvious that the terms are not the same and that *health promotion* is a much more encompassing term than *health education.* Figure 5.8 provides a graphic representation of the relationship between the terms.

The first half of this chapter described the process of community organizing/building—the process by which individuals, groups, and organizations engage in planned action to influence social problems. Program planning may or may not be associated with community

health education
any combination of planned learning experiences based on sound theories that provide individuals, groups, and communities the opportunity to acquire information and the skills to make quality health decisions

health promotion
any planned combination of educational, political, environmental, regulatory, or organizational mechanisms that support actions and conditions of living conducive to the health of individuals, groups, and communities

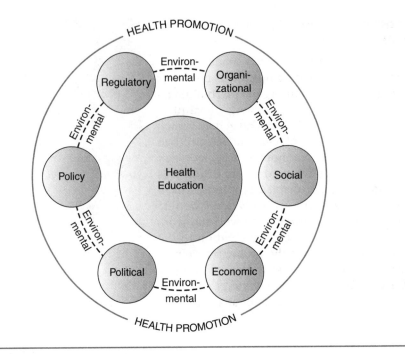

FIGURE 5.8

The relationship of health education and health promotion.

Source: McKenzie, J. F., B. L. Neiger, and R. Thackeray (2009). *Planning, Implementing, and Evaluating Health Promotion Programs: A Primer,* 5th ed. San Francisco, CA: Benjamin Cummings. Reprinted with permission from Pearson Education, Inc.

program planning
a process by which an intervention is planned to help meet the needs of a priority population

organizing/building. **Program planning** is a process in which an intervention is planned to help meet the needs of a specific group of people. It may take a community organizing/building effort to be able to plan such an intervention. The antiviolence campaign used earlier in the chapter is such an example, where many resources of the community were brought together in order to create interventions (programs) to deal with the violence problem. However, program planning need not be connected to community organizing/building. For example, a community organizing/building effort is not needed before a company offers a smoking cessation program for its employees or a religious organization offers a stress management class for its members. In such cases, only the steps of the program planning process need to be carried out. These steps are described in the following section.

CREATING A HEALTH PROMOTION PROGRAM

The process of developing a health promotion program, like the process of community organizing/building, involves a series of steps. Success depends upon many factors, including the assistance of a professional experienced in program planning.

Experienced program planners use models to guide their work. Planning models are the means by which structure and organization are given to the planning process. Many different planning models exist, some of which are used more often than others. Some of the more frequently used models include the PRECEDE/PROCEED model,[26] probably the best known and most often used; the Multilevel Approach to Community Health (MATCH);[27] Intervention Mapping,[28] and the more recently developed consumer-based planning models that are based upon health communication and social marketing such as CDCynergy[29] and Social Marketing Assessment and Response Tool (SMART).[30] Each of these planning models has its strengths

FIGURE 5.9

A generalized model for program planning.

Source: McKenzie, J. F., B. L. Neiger, and R. Thackeray (2009). *Planning, Implementing, and Evaluating Health Promotion Programs: A Primer,* 5th ed. San Francisco, CA: Benjamin Cummings. Reprinted with permission from Pearson Education, Inc.

and weaknesses, and each has distinctive components that make it unique. In addition, each of the models has been used to plan health promotion programs in a variety of settings, with many successes.

It is not absolutely necessary that the student studying community health for the first time have a thorough understanding of the models mentioned here, but it is important to know the basic steps in the planning process. Therefore, we are presenting a generalized program development model[8] that draws on the major components of these other models. The steps of this generalized model are presented in Figure 5.9 and explained in the following paragraphs.

Prior to undertaking the first step in the generalized model it is important to understand the community and engage the **priority population (audience),** those whom the health promotion program is intended to serve. Understanding the community means finding out as much as possible about the priority population and the environment in which it exists. Engaging the priority population means getting those in the population involved in the early stages of the health promotion program planning process. If the priority population was composed of the employees of a corporation, the planners would want to read all the material they could find about the company, spend time talking with various individuals and subgroups in the company (e.g., new employees, employees who had been with the company for a long time, management, clerical staff, labor representatives, etc.) to find out what they wanted from a health promotion program, and review old documents of the company (e.g., health insurance records, labor agreements, written history of the company, etc.). Also, the planners should consider forming a program planning committee with representation from the various subgroups of the workforce (i.e., management, labor, and clerical staff). The planning committee can help ensure all segments of the priority population will be engaged in the planning process.

priority population (audience) those whom a program is intended to serve

needs assessment the process of collecting and analyzing information, to develop an understanding of the issues, resources, and constraints of the priority population, as related to the development of the health promotion program

Assessing the Needs of the Priority Population

In order to create a useful and effective program for the priority population, planners, with the assistance of the planning committee, must determine the needs and wants of the priority population. This procedural step is referred to as a *needs assessment.* A **needs assessment** is the process of collecting and analyzing information to develop an understanding of the issues, resources, and constraints of the priority population, as related to the development of the health promotion program.[31] The assessment's purpose is to determine whether the needs of the people are being met (see Figure 5.10).

FIGURE 5.10

A telephone survey is a common form of data collection for a health needs assessment.

For those interested in a detailed explanation of the process of conducting a needs assessment, extensive accounts are available.[32,33] The following is a simplified six-step approach.[8]

Step 1: Determining the Purpose and Scope of the Needs Assessment
The first step in the needs assessment process is to determine the purpose and the scope of the needs assessment. That is, what is the goal of the needs assessment? What does the planning committee hope to gain from the needs assessment? How extensive will the assessment be? What kind of resources will be available to conduct the needs assessment? Once these questions are answered, the planners are ready to begin gathering data.

Step 2: Gathering Data
The second step in the process is gathering the data that will help to identify the true needs of the priority population. Such data are categorized into two groups—primary and secondary. Primary data are those that are collected specifically for use in this process. An example is having those in the priority population complete a needs assessment questionnaire about their health behavior. Secondary data are data that have already been collected for some other purpose, such as health insurance claims records or BRFSS data. Using both primary and secondary data usually presents the clearest picture of the priority population's needs.

Step 3: Analyzing the Data
Collected data can be analyzed in one of two ways—formally or informally. Formal analysis consists of some type of statistical analysis, assuming that the appropriate statistical criteria have been met. However, a more common means of analysis is an informal technique referred to as "eyeballing the data." With this technique, program developers look for the obvious differences between the health status or conditions of the priority population and the programs and services available to close the gap between what is and what ought to be. Regardless of the method used, data analysis should yield a list of the problems that exist, with a description of the nature and extent of each.

The final part of this step is prioritizing the list of problems. Prioritization must take place because though all needs are important, seldom are there enough resources (money and time) available to deal with all the problems identified. When prioritizing, planners should consider (1) the importance of the need, (2) how changeable the need is, and (3) whether adequate resources are available to deal with the problem.

Step 4: Identifying the Factors Linked to the Health Problem
In this step of the process, planners need to identify and prioritize the risk factors that are associated with the health problem. Thus, if the prioritized health problem identified in step 3 is heart disease, planners must analyze the health behaviors and environment of the priority population for known risk factors of heart disease. For example, higher than expected smoking behavior may be present in the priority population in addition to a community that lacks recreational areas for exercise. Once these risk factors are identified, they also need to be prioritized.

Step 5: Identifying the Program Focus
With risk factors identified and prioritized, planners need to identify those predisposing, enabling, and reinforcing factors that seem to have a direct impact on the targeted risk factors. In the heart disease example, those in the priority population may not (1) have the skills to begin an exercise program (predisposing factor), (2) have access to recreational facilities (enabling factor), or (3) have people around them who value the benefits of exercise (reinforcing factor). Once the predisposing, enabling, and reinforcing factors have been identified, they too need to be prioritized. As in step 2 earlier, planners can prioritize these factors

according to their importance and changeability.[26] The resulting prioritized list provides the program focus.

Step 6: Validating the Prioritized Need

The final step in this process is to double-check or to confirm that the identified need and resulting program focus indeed need to be addressed in the priority population. For example, a limited amount of data may indicate the primary need of the priority group to be one thing—heart disease, for example. However, more extensive data or more comprehensive networking may identify another problem, such as diabetes or malnutrition. Before step 6 is completed, planners must make sure they have indeed identified a true need. In short, all work should be double-checked.

At the conclusion of a needs assessment, planners should be able to answer the following questions:[33]

1. Who is the priority population?
2. What are the needs of the priority population?
3. Which subgroups within the priority population have the greatest need?
4. Where are the subgroups located geographically?
5. What is currently being done to resolve identified needs?
6. How well have the identified needs been addressed in the past?

Setting Appropriate Goals and Objectives

Once the problem has been well defined and the needs prioritized, the planners can set goals and develop objectives for the program. The goals and objectives should be thought of as the foundation of the program. The remaining portions of the programming process—intervention development, implementation, and evaluation—will be designed to achieve the goals by meeting the objectives.

The words *goals* and *objectives* are often used interchangeably, but there is really a significant difference between the two. "A goal is a future event toward which a committed endeavor is directed; objectives are the steps taken in pursuit of a goal."[34] To further distinguish between goals and objectives, McKenzie and colleagues[8] have stated that goals (1) are much more encompassing and global than objectives, (2) are written to cover all aspects of a program, (3) provide overall program direction, (4) are more general in nature, (5) usually take longer to complete, (6) are usually not observed but inferred,[35] and (7) often are not easily measured. Goals are easy to write and include two basic components—who will be affected and what will change because of the program. Here are some examples of program goals:

1. To help employees learn how to manage their stress
2. To reduce the number of teenage pregnancies in the community
3. To help cardiac patients and their families deal with the lifestyle changes that occur after a heart attack

Objectives are more precise and can be considered the steps to achieve the program goals. Because some program goals are more complex than others, the number and type of objectives will vary from program to program. For example, the process of getting a group of people to exercise is a more complex activity than trying to get a group to learn the four food groups. The more complex a program, the greater the number of objectives needed. To deal with these different types of programs, McKenzie and colleagues[8] adapted a hierarchy of program objectives first developed by Deeds[36] and later updated by Cleary and Neiger.[37] Table 5.3 presents the hierarchy and an example of an objective at each of the levels within the hierarchy.

Table 5.3
Hierarchy of Objectives and Examples of Each

Type of Objective	Program Outcomes	Possible Evaluation Measures	Type of Evaluation	Example Objective
Process/administrative objectives	Activities presented and tasks completed	Number of sessions held, exposure, attendance, participation, staff performance, appropriate materials, adequacy of resources, tasks on schedule	Process (form of formative)	On June 12, 2008, a breast cancer brochure will be distributed to all female customers over the age of 18 at the Ross grocery store.
Learning objectives	Change in awareness, knowledge, attitudes, and skills	Increase in awareness, knowledge, attitudes, and skill development/acquisition	Impact (form of summative)	When asked in class, 50% of the students will be able to list the four principles of cardiovascular conditioning.
Action/behavioral objectives	Change in behavior	Current behavior modified or discontinued, or new behavior adopted	Impact (form of summative)	During a telephone interview, 35% of the residents will report having had their blood cholesterol checked in the last six months.
Environmental objectives	Change in the environment	Protection added to, or hazards or barriers removed from, the environment	Impact (form of summative)	By the end of the year, all senior citizens who requested transportation to the congregate meals will have received it.
Program objectives	Change in quality of life (QOL), health status, or risk, and social benefits	QOL measures, morbidity data, mortality data, measures of risk (e.g., HRA)	Outcome (form of summative)	By the year 2008, infant mortality rates will be reduced to no more than 7 per 1,000 in Franklin County.

Source: Adapted from Deeds, S. G. (1992). *The Health Education Specialist: Self-Study for Professional Competence.* Los Alamitos, CA: Loose Canon; Cleary, M. J., and B. L. Neiger (1998). *The Certified Health Education Specialist: A Self-Study Guide for Professional Competence,* 3rd ed. Allentown, PA: National Commission for Health Education Credentialing; and McKenzie, J. F., B. L. Neiger, and R. Thackeray (2009). *Planning, Implementing, and Evaluating Health Promotion Programs: A Primer* (5th ed.). San Francisco, CA: Benjamin Cummings.

From the examples presented in Table 5.3, it should be obvious that the hierarchy goes from less complex to more complex levels. Thus, it takes less energy and fewer resources to increase awareness in the priority population than to improve its health status. Close examination of the example objectives reveals that the objectives are written in specific terms. They are composed of four parts (who, what, when, and how much) and outline changes that should result from the implementation of the program.[38] As such, the objectives are written so that the level of their attainment is observable and measurable.

One final note about objectives: In Chapter 1, *Healthy People 2010,* the national health goals and objectives of the nation, was discussed. Selected objectives from this publication are presented in boxes throughout this text (see Box 5.1). These goals and objectives provide a good model for developing goals and objectives for a new program. In fact, these goals and objectives can be adapted for use in most community health promotion programs.

Creating an Intervention That Considers the Peculiarities of the Setting

The next step in the program planning process is to design activities that will help the priority population meet the objectives and, in the process, achieve the program goals. These activities are collectively referred to as an **intervention,** or treatment. This intervention or treatment constitutes the program that the priority population will experience.

The number of activities in an intervention may be many or only a few. Although no minimum number has been established, it has been shown that multiple activities are often more

intervention an activity or activities designed to create change in people

BOX
5.1

HEALTHY PEOPLE 2010: OBJECTIVES

Educational and Community-Based Programs

7-5. Increase the proportion of worksites that offer a comprehensive employee health promotion program to their employees.

Objective	Increase in Worksites Offering a Comprehensive Employer-Sponsored Health Promotion Program	1999* Baseline	2010 Target
		Percent	
7-5a.	Worksites with <50 employees	Developmental	
7-5b.	Worksites with 50 or more employees	34%	75%
7-5c.	Worksites with 50 to 99 employees	33%	75%
7-5d.	Worksites with 100 to 249 employees	33%	75%
7-5e.	Worksites with 250 to 749 employees	38%	75%
7-5f.	Worksites with 750 or more employees	50%	75%

*No measurement since baseline.

7-6. Increase the proportion of employees who participate in employer-sponsored health promotion activities.

Target: 75 percent.

Baseline: 61 percent of employees aged 18 years and older participated in employer-sponsored health promotion activities in 1994; 1998 status 59%.

7-10. (Developmental) Increase the proportion of tribal and local health service areas or jurisdictions that have established a community health promotion program that addresses multiple *Healthy People 2010* focus areas.

7-12. Increase the proportion of older adults who have participated during the preceding year in at least one organized health promotion activity.

Target: 90 percent.

Baseline: 12 percent of adults aged 65 years and older participated during the preceding year in at least one organized health promotion activity in 1998 (age adjusted to the year 2000 standard population).

Note: Objectives 7-7, 7-8, 7-9, and 7-11 were deleted at the midcourse review.

For Further Thought

If you had the opportunity to write one more objective dealing with the implementation of health promotion pro-grams for use in *Healthy People 2010,* what would it be? What is your rationale for selecting such an objective?

effective than a single activity. For example, if the planners wanted to change the attitudes of community members toward a new landfill, they would have a greater chance of doing so by distributing pamphlets door to door, writing articles for the local newspaper, and speaking to local service groups, than by performing any one of these activities by itself. In other words, the size and amount of intervention are of the 'dose' is important in health promotion programming. Few people change their behavior based on a single exposure; instead, multiple exposures are generally needed to change most behaviors. It stands to reason that 'hitting' the priority population from several angles or through multiple channels should increase the chances of making an impact.[8]

The choice of strategies for an intervention depends on a number of variables. McLeroy and colleagues have indicated that the levels of influence need to be considered when developing interventions.[39] These levels of influence are included in the ecological perspective, which "recognizes that health behaviors are part of the larger social system (or ecology) of behaviors and social influences, much like a river, forest or desert is part of a larger biological system (ecosystem), and that lasting changes in health behaviors require supportive changes in the whole system, just as the addition of a power plant, the flooding of a reservoir, or the growth of a city in a desert produce changes in the whole ecosystem."[40] This perspective includes five levels of influence on health-related behaviors and conditions:

1. Intrapersonal or individual factors
2. Interpersonal factors
3. Institutional or organizational factors
4. Community factors
5. Public policy factors

Thus, interventions can be developed to "attack" a health concern of a priority population at any or all of these levels. The intervention strategies designed to solve problems associated with community organizing/building, as presented in Table 5.2, are the same strategies being discussed here.

Implementing the Intervention

The moment of truth is when the intervention is implemented. **Implementation** is the actual carrying out or putting into practice the activity or activities that make up the intervention. More formally, implementation has been defined as "the act of converting planning, goals, and objectives into action through administrative structure, management activities, policies, procedures, regulations, and organizational actions of new programs."[41] It is at this point that the planners will learn whether the product (intervention) they developed will be useful in producing the measurable changes as outlined in the objectives.

To ensure a smooth-flowing implementation of the intervention, it is wise to pilot test it at least once and sometimes more. A **pilot test** is a trial run. It is when the intervention is presented to just a few individuals who are either from the intended priority population or from a very similar population. For example, if the intervention is being developed for fifth graders in a particular school, it might be pilot tested on fifth graders with similar educational backgrounds and demographic characteristics but from a different school.

The purpose of pilot testing an intervention is to determine whether there are any problems with it. Some of the more common problems that pop up are those dealing with the design or delivery of the intervention; however, any part of it could be flawed. For example, it could be determined during pilot testing that there is a lack of resources to carry out the intervention as planned or that those implementing the intervention need more training. When minor flaws are detected and corrected easily, the intervention is then ready for full implementation. However, if a major problem surfaces—one that requires much time and many resources to correct—it is recommended that the intervention be pilot tested again with the improvements in place before implementation.

An integral part of the piloting process is collecting feedback from those in the pilot group. By surveying the pilot group, planners can identify popular and unpopular aspects of the intervention, how the intervention might be changed or improved, and whether the program activities were effective. This information can be useful in fine-tuning this intervention or in developing future programs.

Once the intervention has been pilot tested and corrected as necessary, it is ready to be disseminated and implemented. If the program that has been planned is being implemented with a large priority population and there is a lot at stake with the implementation, it is advisable that the intervention be implemented gradually rather than all at once. One way of doing so is by phasing in the intervention. **Phasing in** refers to a step-by-step implementation in which the intervention is introduced first to smaller groups instead of the entire priority

implementation
putting a planned program into action

pilot test
a trial run of an intervention

phasing in
implementation of an intervention with a series of small groups instead of the entire population

population. Common criteria used for selecting participating groups for phasing in include participant ability, number of participants, program offerings, and program location.[10]

The following is an example of phasing in by location. Assume that a local health department wants to provide smoking cessation programs for all the smokers in the community (priority population). Instead of initiating one big intervention for all, planners could divide the priority population by residence location. Facilitators would begin implementation by offering the smoking cessation classes on the south side of town during the first month. During the second month, they would continue the classes on the south side and begin implementation on the west side of town. They would continue to implement this intervention until all sections of the town were included.

Evaluating the Results

The final step in the generalized planning model is the evaluation. Although evaluation is the last step in this model, it really takes place in all steps of program planning. It is very important that planning for evaluation occur during the first stages of program development, not just at the end.

Evaluation is the process in which planners determine the value or worth of the object of interest by comparing it against a **standard of acceptability**.[42] Common standards of acceptability include, but are not limited to, mandates (policies, statues, and laws), values, norms, and comparison/control groups.

Evaluation can be categorized further into summative and formative evaluation. **Formative evaluation** is done during the planning and implementing processes to improve or refine the program. For example, validating the needs assessment and pilot testing are both forms of formative evaluation. **Summative evaluation** begins with the development of goals and objectives and is conducted after implementation to determine the program's impact on the priority population.

Like other steps in the planning model, this step can be broken down into smaller steps. The mini-steps of evaluation include planning the evaluation, collecting the necessary evaluative data, analyzing the data, and reporting and applying the results.

Planning the Evaluation

As noted earlier, planning for summative evaluation begins with the development of the goals and objectives of the program. These statements put into writing what should happen as a result of the program. Also in this planning mini-step, it should be determined who will evaluate the program—an *internal evaluator* (one who already is involved in the program) or an *external evaluator* (one from outside the program). In addition, this portion of the evaluation process should identify an evaluation design and a time line for carrying out the evaluation.

Collecting the Data

Data collection includes deciding how to collect the data (e.g., with a survey instrument, from existing records, by observation, etc.), determining who will collect them, pilot testing the procedures, and performing the actual data collection.

Analyzing the Data

Once the data are in hand, they must be analyzed and interpreted. Also, it must be decided who will analyze the data and when the analysis is to be completed.

Reporting the Results

Next the evaluation report should be written. Decisions must be made (if they have not been made already) regarding who should write the report, who should receive the report, in what form, and when.

evaluation
determining the value or worth of an object of interest

standard of acceptability
a comparative mandate, value, norm, or group

formative evaluation
the evaluation that is conducted during the planning and implementing processes to improve or refine the program

summative evaluation
the evaluation that determines the impact of a program on the priority population

Applying the Results

With the findings in hand, it then must be decided how they will be used. When time, resources, and effort are spent on an evaluation, it is important that the results be useful for reaching a constructive end and for deciding whether to continue or discontinue the program or to alter it in some way.

CHAPTER SUMMARY

- A knowledge of community organizing and program planning is essential for community health workers whose job it is to promote and protect the health of the community.

- Community organizing is a process through which communities are helped to identify common problems or goals, mobilize resources, and in other ways develop and implement strategies for reaching their goals that they have collectively set.

- Community building is an orientation to community that is strength-based rather than need-based and stresses the identification, nurturing, and celebration of community assets.

- The steps of the general model for community organizing/building include recognizing the issue, gaining entry into the community, organizing the people, assessing the community, determining the priorities and setting goals, arriving at a solution and selecting the intervention strategies, implementing the plan, evaluating the outcomes of the plan of action, maintaining the outcomes in the community, and, if necessary, looping back.

- Community organizing/building models available from others include Healthy Cities/Healthy Communities, PATCH, and MAPP.

- Program planning is a process in which an intervention is planned to help meet the needs of a priority population (audience).

- The steps in the program planning process include assessing the needs of the priority population, setting appropriate goals and objectives, creating an intervention that considers the peculiarities of the setting, implementing the intervention, and evaluating the results.

REVIEW QUESTIONS

1. What is community organizing?
2. What are the assumptions (identified by Ross) under which organizers work when bringing a community together to solve a problem?
3. What is the difference between top-down and grass-roots community organizing?
4. What is meant by the term *gatekeepers*? Who would they be in your hometown?

SCENARIO: ANALYSIS AND RESPONSE

The town of Kenzington sounds like a good candidate for a community organizing/building effort. Assume that Kenzington is the town in which you now live and you belong to the group that has taken the issue to the city council. Based upon what you know about the problem in the scenario and what you know about your town, answer the following questions.

1. What is the real problem?
2. Who do you think the gatekeepers are in the community?
3. What groups of people in the community might be most interested in solving this problem?
4. What groups might have a vested interest in seeing the problem remain unsolved?
5. What interventions would be useful in dealing with the problem?
6. How would you evaluate your efforts to solve the problem?
7. What strategies might you recommend to make the solution lasting?
8. If you were to look for help on the Internet to deal with this problem, what key words would you use to search the Web for help?

5. Identify the steps in the generalized approach to community organizing/building presented in this chapter.

6. What is meant by community building?

7. Healthy Cities/Healthy Communities, PATCH, and MAPP are models developed by whom for what purposes?

8. What is a needs assessment? Why is it important in the health promotion programming process?

9. What are the five major steps in program development?

10. What are the differences between goals and objectives?

11. What are intervention strategies? Provide five examples.

12. What is meant by the term *pilot testing*? How is it useful when developing an intervention?

13. What is the difference between formative and summative evaluation?

14. Name and briefly describe the five major components of program evaluation.

ACTIVITIES

1. From your knowledge of the community in which you live (or from the yellow pages of the telephone book), generate a list of 7 to 10 agencies that might be interested in creating a coalition to deal with community drug problems. Provide a one-sentence rationale for each why it might want to be involved.

2. Ask your instructor if he or she is aware of any community organizing/building efforts in a local community. If you are able to identify such an effort, make an appointment—either by yourself or with some of your classmates—to meet with the person who is leading the effort and ask the following questions:

   What is the problem that faces the community?

   What is the goal of the group?

   What steps have been taken so far to organize/build the community, and what steps are yet to be taken?

   Who is active in the core group?

   Did the group conduct a community assessment?

   What intervention will be/has been used?

   Is it anticipated that the problem will be solved?

3. Using a smoking cessation program, write one program goal and an objective for each of the levels presented in Table 5.3.

4. Visit a voluntary health agency in your community, either by yourself or with classmates. Ask employees if you may review any of the standard health promotion programs the agency offers to the community. Examine the program materials, locating the five major components of a program development discussed in this chapter. Then, in a two-page paper, summarize your findings.

COMMUNITY HEALTH ON THE WEB

The Internet contains a wealth of information about community and public health. Increase your knowledge of some of the topics presented in this chapter by accessing the Jones and Bartlett Publishers Web site at **http://health.jbpub.com/book/communityhealth/6e** and follow the links to complete the following Web activities.

- MAPP
- Community Health Status Indicators
- Public Health Functions Project

REFERENCES

1. Minkler, M., and N. Wallerstein (2005). "Improving Health through Community Organization and Community Building: A Health Education Perspective." In M. Minkler, ed., *Community Organizing and Community Building for Health*, 2nd ed. New Brunswick, NJ: Rutgers University Press, 26–50.

2. Ross, M. G. (1967). *Community Organization: Theory, Principles, and Practice*. New York: Harper and Row, 86–92.

3. Goodman, R. M., M. A. Speers, K. McLeroy, S. Fawcett, M. Kegler, E. Parker, S. R. Smith, T. D. Sterling, and N. Wallerstein (1999). "Identifying and Defining the Dimensions of Community Capacity to Provide a Basis for Measurement." *Health Education and Behavior*, 25(3), 258–278.

4. Israel, B. A., B. Checkoway, A. Schultz, and M. Zimmerman (1994). "Health Education and Community Empowerment: Conceptualizing and Measuring Perceptions of Individual, Organizational, and Community Control." *Health Education Quarterly*, 21(2): 149–170.

5. Rothman, J., and J. E. Tropman (1987). "Models of Community Organization and Macro Practice Perspectives: Their Mixing and Phasing." In F. M. Cox, J. L. Erlich, J. Rothman, and J. E. Tropman, eds., *Strategies of Community Organization: Macro Practice*. Itasca, IL: F. E. Peacock, 3–26.

6. Garvin, C. D., and F. M. Cox (2001). "A History of Community Organizing Since the Civil War with Special Reference to Oppressed Communities." In J. Rothman, J. L. Erlich, and J. E. Tropman, eds., *Strategies of Community Intervention*, 5th ed. Itasca, IL: Peacock, 65–100.

7. Checkoway, B. (1989). "Community Participation for Health Promotion: Prescription for Public Policy." *Wellness Perspectives: Research, Theory, and Practice*, 6(1): 18–26.

8. McKenzie, J. F., B. L. Neiger, and R. Thackeray (2009). *Planning, Implementing, and Evaluating Health Promotion Programs: A Primer*, 5th ed. San Francisco: Benjamin Cummings.

9. Braithwaite, R. L., F. Murphy, N. Lythcott, and D. S. Blumenthal (1989). "Community Organization and Development for Health Promotion within an Urban Black Community: A Conceptual Model." *Health Education*, 20(5): 56–60.

10. Wright, P. A. (1994). *A Key Step in Developing Prevention Materials Is to Obtain Expert and Gatekeepers' Reviews* (Technical Assistance Bulletin). Bethesda, MD: Center for Substance Abuse Prevention (CASP) Communications Team, 1–6.

11. Perlman, J. (1978). "Grassroots Participation from Neighborhood to Nation." In S. Langton, ed., *Citizen Participation in America*. Lexington, MA: Lexington Books, 65–79.

12. Brager, G., H. Specht, and J. L. Torczyner (1987). *Community Organizing*. New York: Columbia University Press, 55.

13. Butterfoss, F. D., and M. D. Whitt (2003). "Building and Sustaining Coalitions." In R. J. Bensley and J. Brookins-Fisher, eds., *Community Health Education Methods*, 2nd ed. Boston: Jones and Bartlett, 325–356.

14. Minkler, M. (2005). "Introduction to Community Organizing and Community Building." In M. Minkler, ed., *Community Organizing and Community Building for Health*, 2nd ed. New Brunswick, NJ: Rutgers University Press, 1–21.

15. Walter, C. L. (2005). "Community Building Practice: A Conceptual Framework." In M. Minkler, ed., *Community Organizing and Community Building for Health*, 2nd ed. New Brunswick, NJ: Rutgers University Press, 66–78.

16. McKnight, J. L., and J. P. Kretzmann (2005). "Mapping Community Capacity." In M. Minkler, ed., *Community Organizing and Community Building for Health*, 2nd ed. New Brunswick, NJ: Rutgers University Press, 158–172.

17. Hancock, T., and M. Minkler (2005). "Community Health Assessment or Healthy Community Assessment." In M. Minkler, ed., *Community Organizing and Community Building for Health*, 2nd ed. New Brunswick, NJ: Rutgers University Press, 138–157.

18. Miller, M. (1986). "Turning Problems into Actionable Issues." Unpublished paper. San Francisco: Organize Training Center.

19. Archer, S. E., and R. P. Fleshman (1985). *Community Health Nursing*. Monterey, CA: Wadsworth Health Sciences.

20. Warren, R. L. (1963). *The Community in America*. Chicago: Rand-McNally.

21. U.S. Department of Health and Human Services (2001). *Healthy People in Healthy Communities: A Community Planning Guide Using Healthy People 2010*. Washington, DC: Author.

22. Kreuter, M. W. (1992). "PATCH: Its Origin, Basic Concepts, and Links to Contemporary Public Health Policy." *Journal of Health Education*, 23(3), 135–139.

23. Speers, M. (1992). "Preface." *Journal of Health Education*, 23(3), 132–133.

24. National Association of County and City Health Officials. *Mobilizing for Action through Planning and Partnerships*. Available from http://mapp.naccho.org/MappModel.asp.

25. Joint Committee on Health Education and Promotion Terminology (2001). "Report of the 2000 Joint Committee on Health Education and Promotion Terminology." *American Journal of Health Education*, 32(2): 89–103.

26. Green, L. W., and M. W. Kreuter (2005). *Health Program Planning: An Educational and Ecological Approach*, 4th ed. Boston: McGraw-Hill.

27. Simons-Morton, D. G., W. H. Greene, and N. H. Gottlieb (1995). *Introduction to Health Education and Health Promotion*, 2nd ed. Prospect Heights, IL: Waveland Press.

28. Bartholomew, L. K., G. S. Parcel, G. Kok, and N. H. Gottlieb (2006). *Planning Health Promotion Programs: An Intervention Mapping Approach*, 2nd ed. San Francisco: Jossey-Bass.

29. Centers for Disease Control and Prevention, U.S. Department of Health and Human Services (2003). *CDCynergy 3.0: Your Guide to Effective Health Communication* [CD-ROM Version 3.0]. Atlanta, GA: Author.

30. Neiger, B. L., and R. Thackeray (1998). "Social Marketing: Making Public Health Sense." Paper presented at the annual meeting of the Utah Public Health Association, Provo, UT.

31. Anspaugh, D. J., M. B. Dignan, and S. L. Anspaugh (2000). *Developing Health Promotion Programs*. Boston: McGraw-Hill Higher Education.

32. Gilmore, G. D., and M. D. Campbell (2005). *Needs and Capacity Assessment Strategies for Health Education and Health Promotion*, 3rd ed. Sudbury, MA: Jones and Bartlett.

33. Peterson, D. J., and G. R. Alexander (2001). *Needs Assessment in Public Health: A Practical Guide for Students and Professionals*. New York: Kluwer Academic/Plenum Publishers.

34. Ross, H. S., and P. R. Mico (1980). *Theory and Practice in Health Education*. Palo Alto, CA: Mayfield, 219.

35. Jacobsen, D., P. Eggen, and D. Kauchak (1989). *Methods for Teaching: A Skills Approach*, 3rd ed. Columbus, OH: Merrill.

36. Deeds, S. G. (1992). *The Health Education Specialist: Self-Study for Professional Competence*. Los Alamitos, CA: Loose Canon Publications.

37. Cleary, M. J., and B. L. Neiger (1998). *The Certified Health Education Specialist: A Self-Study Guide for Professional Competence*, 3rd ed. Allentown, PA: National Commission for Health Education Credentialing.

38. McKenzie, J. F. (2005). "Planning and Evaluating Interventions." In J. Kerr, R. Weitkunat, and M. Moretti, eds., *ABC of Behavior Change: A Guide to Successful Disease Prevention and Health Promotion*. Oxford, England: Elsevier, 41–54.

39. McLeroy, K. R., D. Bibeau, A. Steckler, and K. Glanz (1988). "An Ecological Perspective for Health Promotion Programs." *Health Education Quarterly*, 15(4): 351–378.

40. O'Donnell, M. P. (1996). "Editor's Notes." *American Journal of Health Promotion*, 10(4): 244.

41. Timmreck, T. C. (1997). *Health Services Cyclopedic Dictionary*, 3rd ed. Boston: Jones and Bartlett.

42. Green, L. W., and F. M. Lewis (1986). *Measurement and Evaluation in Health Education and Health Promotion*. Palo Alto, CA: Mayfield.

Chapter 6

The School Health Program: A Component of Community Health

Chapter Outline

Chapter Objectives

After studying this chapter you will be able to:

1 Define *coordinated school health program*.

2 List the ideal members of a school health council.

3 Explain why a school health program is important.

4 Identify the major foundations of a coordinated school health program.

5 Define written *school health policies* and explain their importance to the school health program.

6 Explain processes for developing and implementing school health policies.

7 List the eight components of a coordinated school health program.

8 Describe the role of the school health coordinator.

9 Identify those services offered as part of school health services and explain why schools are logical places to offer such services.

10 Explain what is meant by a *healthy school environment* and discuss the two major environments.

11 Define *school health education*.

12 Identify the eight National Health Education Standards.

13 Explain how a health educator could locate credible health education curricula.

14 Identify and briefly explain four issues that are faced by school health advocates.

SCENARIO

Seldom does an elementary school teacher have a typical day. Each day seems to bring a variety of new experiences. Take, for example, the day Ms. Graff experienced last Wednesday. Even before the first bell at 8:30 A.M. she was summoned to the hallway, where one of her second-graders became ill and threw up. Remembering her teachers' in-service workshop on HIV and AIDS, Ms. Graff put into action her new knowledge of universal precautions for handling blood and body fluids.

After that incident, her day seemed to be going along well until two of Ms. Graff's students began fighting in the lunch room. They were arguing over who had the healthier lunch. It seemed that Billy thought his peanut butter and jelly sandwich was healthier than Tommy's cheese sandwich and bag of potato chips. Ms. Graff was skillful in helping to settle the dispute.

After lunch, Ms. Graff began her lesson on drug education. She wasn't 10 minutes into her lesson when the school nurse stuck her head in the door and asked if Ms. Graff could send five students for their annual vision screening. Reluctantly, Ms. Graff excused five of her students.

During the last half-hour of the school day, Ms. Graff provided the children with quiet time so that they could read or work on some of their homework. Just before the last bell was to ring, Annie came up to Ms. Graff's desk and told her that the girl sitting in front of her kept rubbing her eye and it seemed really red. Annie said, "I think she has pinkeye."

Just another "typical day" for Ms. Graff.

INTRODUCTION

The school health program is an important component of community health. Though the primary responsibility for the health of school-aged children lies with their parents/guardians, the schools have immeasurable potential for affecting the health of children, their families, and the health of the community. Full-service community schools provide a good example of the link between school health and community health. These schools, using an integrated approach, offer a variety of educational, counseling, social, and health services to families in one location. Such schools focus on the well-being of the child and family, and some of their services are available on a 24-hour basis. These school buildings serve as neighborhood hubs and institutions that are safe, attentive, and comfortable.[1,2]

In this chapter, we define *coordinated school health program*, explain who is involved in school health programs, explore the reasons why school health is important, discuss the components of school health, and present some of the issues facing school health programs today.

Coordinated School Health Program Defined

A **coordinated school health program (CSHP)** has been defined as "an organized set of policies, procedures, and activities designed to protect, promote, and improve the health and well-being of students and staff, thus improving a student's ability to learn. It includes, but is not limited to comprehensive school health education; school health services; a healthy school environment; school counseling; psychological and social services; physical education; school nutrition services; family and community involvement in school health; and school-site health promotion for staff."[3] This definition is based on the work of Allensworth and Kolbe[4] and is represented in Figure 6.1.

The school health program has great potential for affecting the health of many. There are over 55 million school-aged children attending over 120,000 schools and over 6 million instructional and noninstructional employees in the United States.[5] This represents about one-

coordinated school health program (CSHP) an organized set of policies, procedures, and activities designed to protect, promote, and improve the health and well-being of students and staff, thus improving a student's ability to learn. It includes, but is not limited to, comprehensive school health education; school health services; a healthy school environment; school counseling; psychological and social services; physical education; school nutrition services; family and community involvement in school health; and school-site health promotion for staff

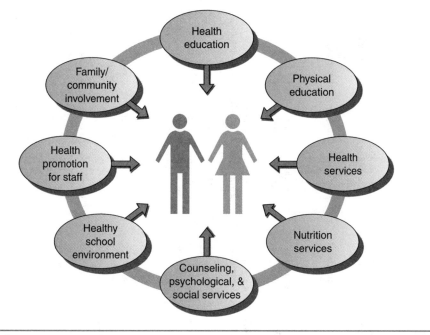

FIGURE 6.1

The coordinated school health program.

Source: Division of Adolescent and School Health, Centers for Disease Control and Prevention (2005). *Coordinated School Health Program.* Available at http://www.cdc.gov/healthyyouth/CSHP/.

fifth of the entire U.S. population. "The knowledge, attitudes, behavior, and skills developed as a result of effective school health programs enable individuals to make informed choices about behavior that will affect their own health throughout their lives, as well as the health of the families for which they are responsible, and the health of the communities in which they live."[6] However, in practice the quality and quantity of CSHPs, in school districts throughout the United States vary greatly. In the majority of school districts, school health programs are not well defined or coordinated; "most schools have some elements of a coordinated school health program, few have a health program that includes all components at a full functioning level, and fewer still effectively coordinate all."[7] For example, it is not unusual for a health teacher to be talking about the importance of aerobic exercise but never tell the physical education teacher. Similarly, a science teacher may be teaching about pathogens and the prevention of communicable diseases, but yet the restrooms in a school are not properly equipped for adequate hand washing. Additionally, there is little coordination between school districts and community health agencies to improve the health of the school-aged child. Table 6.1 provides some possibilities for such interaction.

The School Health Council

In order for CSHPs to fulfill their potential, a great deal of time and effort must be expended by those involved in the program's various components. When these individuals work together to plan and implement a school health program, they are referred to as the **school health council.** The primary role of this council is to provide coordination of the various components of CSHP to help students reach and maintain high-quality health. An ideal council would include representation from administrators, food service workers, counseling personnel, maintenance workers, medical personnel (especially a school nurse and school physician), social workers, parents and other caregivers, students, teachers (especially those who teach health,

school health council individuals from a school or school district and its community who work together to provide advice on aspects of the school health program

Table 6.1
Selected Examples of the Interactions of School and Community Programs

Institutionalized Mechanisms for Interaction	Dynamics of Exchange		
	One-Way	Two-Way	Three-Way
Information	Distribution of materials produced by voluntary health agencies	Delivery of workshops/seminars on parenting health issues by school and agency experts	Distribution to multiple agencies of newsletters, calendars of events, and/or directory of services
Service	Screening for health problems by volunteer community lay and/or health professionals	Cooperative venture utilizing school setting for training of medical students, nursing students, etc.	Collaborative venture by school and community agencies to provide school clinics
Advising and decision making	Formation of school health advisory council	Collaboration by physician/teacher to improve health status and educational attainment	Formation of an interagency management system
Planning and development	Utilization of school recreational facilities for fitness programs by community residents	Utilization of parents as partners in specific instructional strategies	Development of a consortium to implement a validated curriculum
Research and evaluation	Providing access for researchers from higher educational institutions	Cooperative submission of a grant proposal by schools and community agency	Utilization of multiagency task force to gather specific health, epidemiological, social, and economic data on adolescent health problems
Monitoring and reporting	School counselor monitoring at-risk students	Monitoring referrals of students between health and social service agencies to ensure continued treatment	Development of Adolescent Services Network to monitor health/educational needs and referral from one agency to another
Training	Utilization of community professionals as consultants for in-service or instructional programs	Utilization of community agencies as learning laboratories for students who serve as volunteers in service/instructional capacities	Utilization of personnel in Adolescent Health Service Network to provide in-service programs for respective members
Advocacy	Utilization of parents as fund raisers	Initiation and development of a regional school health education coalition by a state health education advocacy network	Formation of a coalition to publicize the benefits of comprehensive school health
Electoral/legislative	Citizen campaigning for individuals running for school board	Campaigning for individual whose platform is supportive of school health	Formation of a coalition to promote legislative mandate

Source: Adapted from Killip, D. C., S. R. Lovick, L. Goldman, and D. D. Allensworth (1987). "Integrated School and Community Programs." *Journal of School Health,* 57(10): 437–444.

physical education, and family and consumer science classes), and personnel from appropriate community health agencies. From this group must come a leader or coordinator. This coordinator should have an educational background that includes training and certification in school health. In addition, the coordinator should "be able to plan, implement, and evaluate a coordinated school health program; be familiar with existing community resources; and have connections to local, state, and national health and education organizations."[8] Most often the coordinator of the school health council is a health educator or school nurse.

The School Nurse

As previously noted, the school nurse is one of several people who is positioned to provide leadership for a CSHP (Figure 6.2). The nurse not only has medical knowledge, but should also have formal training in health education and an understanding of the health needs of all children in kindergarten through the twelfth grade. Some of the key responsibilities of the school nurse as a member of the school health team include the following:[9]

1. Providing direct health care to students and staff
2. Providing leadership for the provision of health services
3. Providing screening and referral for health conditions
4. Promoting a healthy school environment
5. Promoting health
6. Serving in a leadership role for health policies and programs
7. Serving as a liaison between school personnel, family, community, and health care providers

FIGURE 6.2

The school nurse is in a good position to guide the school health program.

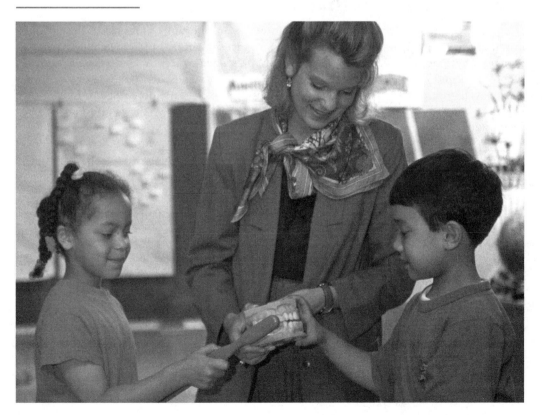

It should be noted that even though school nurses are in a good position to provide leadership to the school health council, there are many school districts that do not have the resources to hire a full-time school nurse. It is not uncommon for a school district to contract with an outside health agency such as a local health department for nursing services. When this scenario occurs, it is normal for the contracted nurse to complete only the nursing tasks required by state law and not to take on the leadership responsibilities for the school health council. This task may then be fulfilled by a school health educator. In fact, the health educator may even be responsible when a full-time nurse is present.

The Teacher's Role

Though the school nurse might provide the leadership for a CSHP, the classroom teachers carry a heavy responsibility in seeing that the program works (see Figure 6.3). On the average school day, teachers spend more waking hours with school-aged children than the parents of the children. A teacher may spend six to eight hours a day with any given child, while the parents spend an hour with that child before school and maybe four to five hours with the child after school and before bedtime. Teachers are also in a position to make observations on the "normal and abnormal" behaviors and conditions of children because they are able to compare the students in their classroom each day. Furthermore, many health teachers are receiving leadership training regarding CSHPs in their undergraduate or postgraduate coursework, thus making them ideal individuals to lead the coordination. Table 6.2 presents a suggested list of competencies for teachers who expect to be involved in school health education and leadership of a CSHP.

THE NEED FOR SCHOOL HEALTH

The primary role of schools is to educate. However, an unhealthy child has a difficult time learning. Consider, for example, a student who arrives at school without having breakfast, with poor hygiene, and without adequate sleep. This student will be unable to concentrate on school work and may distract others. As a reader, you know how difficult it is to study for a test or even to read this textbook when you do not feel well or are depressed or hungry (see Box 6.1). See Chapters 7 and 8 for specific information related to the health behaviors of school-aged children and adolescents.

"Health of children and their learning are reciprocally related."[10] One cannot exist without the other. That is to say, "education and health for children are inextricably intertwined. A student who is not healthy, who suffers from an undetected vision or hearing defect, or who is hungry, or who is impaired by drugs or alcohol, is not a student who will profit from the educational process. Likewise, an individual who has not been provided assistance in the shaping of healthy attitudes, beliefs, and habits early in life, will be more likely to suffer the consequences of reduced productivity in later years."[11] A CSHP provides the integration of education and health.

The importance of the school health program is also evident by its inclusion in the national health objectives for the year 2010. Of all the objectives listed in the publication *Healthy People 2010: Understanding and Improving Health,* a significant

FIGURE 6.3

The classroom teacher's participation is essential for a successful school health program.

Table 6.2
Health Education Standards for School Health Educators

Standard I: Assess individual and community needs for health education.
A. Obtain health-related data about social and cultural environments, growth and development factors, needs, and interests of students.
B. Distinguish between behaviors that foster and those that hinder well-being.
C. Determine health education needs based on observed and obtained data.

Standard II: Plan effective health education programs.
A. Recruit school and community representatives to support and assist in program planning.
B. Develop a logical scope and sequence plan for a health education program.
C. Formulate appropriate and measurable learner objectives.
D. Design educational strategies consistent with specified learner objectives.

Standard III: Implement health education programs.
A. Analyze factors affecting the successful implementation of health education and coordinated school health programs.
B. Select resources and media best suited to implement program plans for diverse learners.
C. Exhibit competence in carrying out planned programs.
D. Monitor educational programs, adjusting objectives and instructional strategies as necessary.

Standard IV: Evaluate the effectiveness of coordinated school health programs.
A. Develop plans to assess student achievement of program objectives.
B. Carry out evaluation plans.
C. Interpret results of program evaluation.
D. Infer implications of evaluation findings for future program planning.

Standard V: Coordinate provision of health education programs and services.
A. Develop a plan for coordinating health education with other components of a school health program.
B. Demonstrate the dispositions and skills to facilitate cooperation among health educators, other teachers, and the appropriate school staff.
C. Formulate practical modes of collaboration among health educators in all settings and other school and community health professionals.
D. Organize professional development programs for teachers, other school personnel, community members, and other interested individuals.

Standard VI: Act as a resource person in health education.
A. Utilize computerized health information retrieval systems effectively.
B. Establish effective consultative relationships with those requesting assistance in solving health-related problems.
C. Interpret and respond to requests for health information.
D. Select effective educational resource materials for dissemination.

Standard VII: Communicate health and health education needs, concerns, and resources.
A. Interpret concepts, purposes, and theories of health education.
B. Predict the impact of societal value systems on health education programs.
C. Select a variety of communication methods and techniques in providing health information.
D. Foster communication between health care providers and consumers.

Source: American Association for Health Education (2003). "AAHE/NCATE Health Education Standards and Key Elements." Available at http://www.aahperd.org/aahe/template.cfm?Template=ncate_elements.html.

number can either be directly attained by schools or their attainment can be influenced in important ways by schools (see Box 6.2).

Nevertheless, a CSHP is not a cure-all. There are no quick and easy solutions to improving the overall health of a community. However, a CSHP provides a strong base upon which to build.

BOX
6.1

IT IS HARDER TO LEARN IF YOU ARE NOT HEALTHY!

It stands to reason that if children are not healthy it is harder for them to concentrate and in turn to have a meaningful learning experience. One such example that is significantly affecting students and schools is the obesity epidemic. Experts have determined that body mass index (BMI) is the most practical tool available to define obesity and screen for it.

Childhood obesity, often referred to as *overweight* when talking about children, is often accompanied by numerous other health conditions, such as increased rates of type 2 diabetes, cardiovascular problems, sleep apnea, and asthma. The reasons for the obesity epidemic are varied, but are slowly becoming understood. Increased soft drink consumption is one such reason, as consumption of soft drinks increased 41% in the first five years of the 1990s. The impact of soft drink consumption is not just felt by those who consume the drinks, but also by those who benefit from the consumption—schools. In 2000, the School Health Policies and Programs Study (SHPPS) found that one-half of all school districts had a soft drink contract, and nearly 80% received a percentage of the sales receipts. Couple this with schools failing to provide the recommended daily physical education and providing poor nutritional offerings, and it is no wonder that the obesity problem is affecting schools.

Researchers are beginning to determine some of the social, psychological, and educational consequences of obesity. A review of the literature determined that over-weight and obese children are more likely to have low self-esteem, higher rates of anxiety disorders, and depression. Severely obese kids report many more missed days of school than the general student population. What is yet to be understood is why these kids miss more school—are they embarrassed to participate in physical activity? Are health conditions (e.g., asthma) keeping them from school? Are they experiencing bullying or teasing? Although there is no known reason, the consequences are significant.

One way schools are addressing concerns about overweight children is by establishing policies related to improved nutritional offerings in the cafeteria, school parties and events, and vending machines, as well as increasing nutrition education and physical activity. The Child Nutrition and WIC Reauthorization Act of 2004 (Public Law 108-265) required all schools participating in the federally funded school feeding programs to establish a local wellness policy by the first day of the 2006–2007 school year. This law helped many districts begin the process of improving the school environment, not just to improve the obesity problem, but to make school a healthier place for all.

Sources: Division of Adolescent and School Health, Centers for Disease Control and Prevention (2006). *School Health Policies and Programs Study*. Available at http://www.cdc.gov/healthyyouth/shpps/index.htm; and Taras, H., and W. Potts-Datema (2005). "Obesity and Student Performance at School." *Journal of School Health,* 75(8): 291–295.

FOUNDATIONS OF THE SCHOOL HEALTH PROGRAM

The true foundations of any school health program are (1) a school administration that supports such an effort, (2) a well-organized school health council that is genuinely interested in providing a coordinated program for the students, and (3) written school health policies. A highly supportive administration is a must for a quality CSHP. In almost all organizations—and schools are no different—the administration controls resources. Without leadership and support from top school administrators, it will be an ongoing struggle to provide a quality program. Furthermore, every effort should be made to employ personnel who are appropriately trained to carry out their responsibilities as members of the school health council. For example, the American Association for Health Education has recommended that the "minimal requirements for school nurses should be state licensure as a registered professional nurse and a baccalaureate degree with study in school health,"[12] yet many school nurses without college degrees and training in health education are asked to teach. Conversely, certified teachers who lack preparation in school health are required to teach health in order to secure a job. Qualified personnel are a must.

HEALTHY PEOPLE 2010: OBJECTIVES

Objective 7-2: Increase the proportion of middle, junior high, and senior high schools that provide school health education to prevent health problems in the following areas: unintentional injury; violence; suicide; tobacco use and addiction; alcohol and other drug use; unintended pregnancy, HIV/AIDS, and STD infection; unhealthy dietary patterns; inadequate physical activity; and environmental health.

Target, 2000 status, and baseline:

Objective	Schools Providing School Health Education in Priority Areas	1994 Baseline	2000 Status**	2010 Target
			Percent	
7-2a.	All components	28	25	70
7-2b.	Unintentional injury	66	68	90
7-2c.	Violence	58	73	80
7-2d.	Suicide	58	59	80
7-2e.	Tobacco use and addiction	86	88	95
7-2f.	Alcohol and other drug use	90	89	95
7-2g.	Unintended pregnancy, HIV/AIDS, and STD infection	65	62	90
7-2h.	Unhealthy dietary patterns	84	84	95
7-2i.	Inadequate physical activity	78	76	90
7-2j.	Environmental health	60	60	80

Objective 7-4: Increase the proportion of the nation's elementary, middle, junior high, and senior high schools that have a nurse-to-student ratio of at least 1:750.

Target, 2000 status, and baseline:

Objective	Increase in Schools with Nurse-to-Student Ratio of at Least 1:750	1994 Baseline	2000 Status	2010 Target
			Percent	
7-4a.	All middle, junior high, and senior high schools	28	53	50
7-4b.	Senior high schools	28	26	50
7-4c.	Middle and junior high schools	32	*	50
7-4d.	Elementary schools	Developmental		

* = Data not available.
** = No new data available at midcourse review.

For Further Thought
Assuming money is available, why doesn't every school district in the nation have a coordinated school health program?

SCHOOL HEALTH POLICIES

School health policies are written statements that provide a framework[13] to guide all those who work within the program.[14] The written policy also describes the nature of the program and the procedure for its implementation to those outside the program.[15] Well-written school health policies provide a sense of direction and a means of accountability and credibility, and strengthen the possibility that a school health program will become "an institutionalized part of the school culture."[13] Steps for creating local health-related policies include the following:[16,17]

1. Identify the policy development team.
2. Assess the district's needs.

school health policies
written statements that describe the nature and procedures of a school health program

3. Prioritize needs and develop an action plan.
4. Draft a policy.
5. Build awareness and support.
6. Adopt and implement the policy.
7. Maintain, measure, and evaluate.

Policy Development

The development of a set of written policies is not an easy task. This challenging and time-consuming task should be executed by the school health council, because the council includes those most knowledgeable about the school health program in addition to representing many different constituencies in the school community.

The policies should cover all facets of the school health program. Table 6.3 provides a checklist that can be used for developing policies. Also, several professional associations that have an interest in school health programs have written a number of policy statements relating to school health issues. A few such associations are the American Academy of Pediatrics (information available at www.aap.org/), the American School Health Association (information available at www.ashaweb.org), the American Association for Health Education (information available at www.aahperd.org/aahe/), and the Association for Supervision and Curriculum Development (information available at www.ascd.org).

Once the policies have been written, it is important that they receive approval at three levels. Approval should come from (1) the school district's medical advisor, (2) the school administration, and (3) the board of education. The approval process provides credibility to the policies as well as legal protection for those who must implement the policies.[15]

Policy Implementation

The development of written policies is an important step in building a solid base for a CSHP. However, if the policies are never implemented, the school district will be no better off than before their development.

Implementation begins with the distribution of the policies to those who will be affected by them—faculty, staff, students, and parents. Some ideas for carrying out this process include (1) distributing the policies with a memorandum of explanation, (2) placing the policies in both faculty/staff and student handbooks, (3) presenting them at a gathering of the different groups (e.g., at staff or PTO meetings, or an open house), (4) holding a special meeting for the specific purpose of explaining the policies, and (5) placing them in the school district newsletter. News releases might even be considered if the policies include major changes. Each school district must decide the best way to disseminate its school health policies.

Policy Development Resources

Because of the Child Nutrition and WIC Reauthorization Act of 2004's requirements to implement a school wellness policy by districts,[18] numerous resources have become available to help schools develop policies. *Action for Healthy Kids* (AFHK) is one such organization that is advocating and providing support for making changes in schools that will address the epidemic of overweight, undernourished, and sedentary youth. AFHK has created a public-private partnership of more than 50 national organizations and government agencies representing health, education, fitness, and nutrition to support state, district, and school action toward developing healthier youth.[19] Sample wellness policies and a clearinghouse of related resources, including policy development guides, are available at the AFHK Web site (www.actionforhealthykids.org). Tools to assist schools in conducting needs assessments

Table 6.3
A Checklist for Developing Written Policies

	PIP	PN	NA
I. Administration and Organization			
A. Duties and Responsibilities of the Coordinator of the School Health Program			
B. Duties and Responsibilities of the School Health Team			
C. Responsibilities of School Health Personnel			
D. School Health Records			
E. General School Health Policies			
1. Use of prescribed medication in the school			
2. Report of child abuse and neglect			
3. Substance use/abuse			
4. Student health insurance			
5. Home health visits			
6. Health policies for after-school activities (including emergency care)			
7. Sending ill/injured students home			
8. Relationships with community health agencies/organizations			
9. In-service health programs for teachers			
II. School Health Services			
A. Emergency Care for Illness/Injury			
B. Students with Special Needs			
C. Health Appraisal			
1. Medical examinations			
2. Screening programs			
3. Dental examinations			
4. Social and psychological evaluations			
5. Policy for health referrals to parents			
D. Communicable Disease Control			
E. Health Advising			
III. Healthy School Environment			
A. Safety Program			
B. Safety Patrol and Bus Safety			
C. Emergency Drills (fire, tornado, etc.)			
D. Drug-Free Schools			
E. Safe/Violence-Free Schools			
F. Student Discipline			
G. Universal Precautions			
H. Hazardous Materials			
IV. Health Instruction			
A. Procedures for Curriculum Development and Revision			
B. Individual Education Programs for Special Needs Students			
V. School Food Service			
VI. School Counseling			
VII. School Physical Education			
VIII. School-Site Health Promotion for Faculty and Staff			
IX. Integrated School and Community Health Promotion Efforts			

Code: PIP = Policy in place. PN = Policy needed. NA = Not applicable to our district.

Source: Adapted from McKenzie, J. F. (1983). "Written Policies: Developing a Solid Foundation for a Comprehensive School Health Program." *Future Focus: Ohio Journal of Health, Physical Education, Recreation and Dance,* 4(3): 9–11.

related to the CSHP include the *School Health Index,* available free from the CDC (http://apps.nccd.cdc.gov/shi/default.aspx) and *Creating a Healthy School Using the Healthy School Report Card: An ASCD Action Tool,* available for purchase from the Association for Supervision and Curriculum Development (ASCD) (http://shop.ascd.org).

Monitoring the Status of School Health Policy in the United States

Because school health policy is an important foundation for CSHPs, the Division of Adolescent Health at the Centers for Disease Control and Prevention (CDC) conducts a national survey to assess school health policies and programs at the state, district, school, and classroom levels. The survey, which is titled the School Health Policies and Programs Study (SHPPS), has been conducted every six years since 1994. Specifically, SHPPS is used to:[20]

- Monitor the status of the nation's school health policies and programs.
- Describe the professional background of the personnel who deliver each component of the school health program.
- Describe coordination among components of school health programs.
- Describe relationships between state and district policies and school health programs and practices.
- Identify factors that facilitate or impede delivery of effective school health programs.

Results of these national surveys are available at the Division of Adolescent and School Health's Web site.

COMPONENTS OF A COORDINATED SCHOOL HEALTH PROGRAM

If implemented appropriately, a coordinated approach to school health can have a significant positive impact on the overall health status of students, staff, and the community, which, in turn, can be linked to higher academic achievement for students. In order to do so, all eight components illustrated in Figure 6.1 need to be provided. Because of the limitation of space, we will discuss the importance of the administration and organization of the eight components, provide an overview of the three traditional components of the school health program—(1) school health services, (2) healthy school environment, and (3) health education—and provide a brief explanation of the five additional components. Examples of successful implementation of CSHPs can be found in the document *Stories from the Field: Lessons Learned about Building Coordinated School Health Programs*.[21]

Administration and Organization

school health coordinator
a professional at the district (or school) level responsible for management and coordination of all school health policies, activities, and resources

Effective administration and organization of the school health program ensures that the people and activities that constitute the program work in a coordinated manner to meet the program's goals. As previously noted, the responsibility for coordinating the program in each school district should be delegated to a properly trained and knowledgeable individual. Logical choices for this position of **school health coordinator** would be a trained school nurse or a health educator.[22] While approximately one-half of the states and territories in the United States have school districts who employ school health coordinators, there are only a few states that require such a person.[23,24]

The American Cancer Society has taken a leadership role in training leaders for school health programs. In 1999 the American Cancer Society conducted the first National School Health Coordinator Leadership Institute, the beginning of a three-year training program for school health coordinators around the United States. As a result of the success of the Institute, a number of replications have been implemented around the country, some as state replication programs and others with specific school districts, such as urban school districts.[25] The American Cancer Society recommends that school health coordinators have the following responsibilities, regardless of the coordinator's professional preparation or training:[22]

- Assessing the local need for and status of health education
- Articulating the importance of and gaining support for school health programs within the school and community
- Providing leadership for the school health program team to ensure a coordinated approach and for the community-represented school health council
- Planning effective school health instruction based on a K–12 sequential framework
- Identifying current school health-related funding streams and coordinating with the school health program council to maximize usage
- Planning for and providing access to school health professional preparation opportunities
- Assisting with the identification, evaluation, and selection of resources
- Providing assistance in designing and evaluating the different components of the school health program

School Health Services

School health services are those health "services provided for students to appraise, protect, and promote health."[26] Specifically, those services offered by schools include health appraisals (screenings and examinations), emergency care for injury and sudden illness, management of chronic disease, prevention and control of communicable disease, provisions for special needs students, health advising, and remediation of detected health problems within the limits of state laws through referral and follow-up by the school nurse and teachers (see Figure 6.4). Originally the intent of school health services was to supplement rather than to supplant the family's responsibility for meeting the health care needs of its children. However, due to the poorer health status of youth, the involvement of youth in high-risk behaviors (such as smoking, drinking, substance abuse, and unprotected sexual intercourse), and such barriers to health care as inadequate health insurance and lack of providers, there has been a broadening of the role of schools in providing health care.

school health services
health services provided by school health workers to appraise, protect, and promote the health of students

Because school attendance is required throughout the United States, schools represent our best opportunity to reach many of those children in need of proper health care. More than 95% of all youths aged 5 to 17 years are enrolled in schools.[27] "The school's ability to reach children and youth slipping through the cracks of the health care system and at highest risk for poor health and potentially health-threatening behaviors is unmatched."[28] The advantages of having school health services include the following:[29]

1. Equitability: School health services provide a point of entry into the health care system for all children in school.
2. Breadth of coverage: Many preventive services are provided that are not covered in a majority of health insurance policies.
3. Confidentiality.
4. User friendliness: The school is an environment with which students are familiar and in which they feel comfortable.
5. Convenience: Services are accessible to all students.

Each school district is unique, from the demographics of its students to the availability of its health resources. As such, three

FIGURE 6.4
Health screenings are important components of school health services.

models have been developed that describe the delivery of school health services: (1) core health services, (2) core plus expanded school health services model, and (3) services through school-based or school-linked health centers.[29] The core health services model views the school district in the role of health screener. In this model, emphasis is placed on the detection of health problems and the referral to providers in the community for treatment. This is the model most commonly found in schools today.

The core plus expanded school health model builds upon the core health services model and extends it by providing additional services when students are unable to access community-based services or when the communities lack health care providers.[30] The most common services added for students include assistance with behavioral, mental health, and substance abuse treatment.[30]

The third model for offering school health services is through either school-based or school-linked health centers. Such centers are the most comprehensive means for offering school health services. Though the services offered by the centers differ by location, many operate like many primary care clinics. School-based health centers (SBHCs) have been defined as "a health center located in a school or on school grounds that provides, at a minimum, on-site primary and preventive health care, mental health counseling, health promotion, referral and follow-up services for young people enrolled."[31] School-linked health centers (SLHCs) have been defined as health centers "located beyond school property that serve one or more schools."[31] SLHCs usually have formal or informal agreements with schools and may serve more than just young people enrolled in school.[31] Both SBHCs and SLHCs employ a number of health care professionals on a full-time basis. The idea of school-based/linked clinics is gaining momentum throughout the country and will be discussed in greater detail later in this chapter.

> **healthy school environment** the promotion, maintenance, and utilization of safe and wholesome surroundings in a school

Healthy School Environment

The term *healthy school environment* designates the part of a CSHP that provides for a safe—both physically and emotionally—learning environment (see Figure 6.5). If children are not placed in a safe environment, learning becomes difficult at best. The most recent comprehensive definition of healthy environment was provided by the 1972–1973 Joint Committee on Health Education Terminology. They stated that providing a **healthy school environment** includes "the promotion, maintenance, and utilization of safe and wholesome surroundings, organization of day-by-day experiences and planned learning procedures to influence favorable emotional, physical and social health."[32]

By law, school districts are required to provide a safe school environment. However, the responsibility for maintaining this safe environment should rest with all who use it. Everyone, including those on the board of education, administrators, teachers, custodial staff, and students, must contribute to make a school a safer place through their daily actions. An unsafe school environment can exist only if those responsible for it and those who use it allow it to exist.

The Physical Environment

The physical environment of a school can be divided into two major categories. The first is the actual physical plant—the buildings and surrounding areas and all that come with them. The second is the behaviors of those using the buildings. The factors that must be considered when looking at the physical plant include (1) where the school is located, (2) the age of the buildings, (3) the traffic patterns in and around the school, (4) temperature control, (5) lighting, (6) acoustics, (7) water

FIGURE 6.5

The school should be a safe and healthy place to learn.

supply, (8) sanitation, (9) food service, (10) playgrounds, (11) school bus safety, and other items. Each school district should have an appropriate protocol for dealing with and maintaining these aspects of the physical environment.

The behavior of both the school personnel and students in the school environment also has an impact on the safety of the environment. Each year a significant number of students throughout the country are injured on their way to, at, or on their way home from school. Some of these injuries occur from an unsafe physical plant that is in need of repair, but many occur from inappropriate behavior. Unsafe behavior that is observed too frequently in schools includes acts of violence between students and lack of proper supervision by school employees. However, most do not worry about a safe environment until they are faced with a problem. Every school building in the United States could become a safer environment if greater attention were given to prevention than to a cure.

The Psychosocial Environment

Although a safe physical environment is important, a safe psychosocial environment is equally important. This portion of the school environment "encompasses the attitudes, feelings, and values of students and staff."[33] Students who are fearful of responding to a teacher's question because the teacher might make fun of them if they answer incorrectly or students who are afraid to say hello to the school principal because he is never nice to anyone are not learning in a healthy psychosocial environment. For many, learning does not come easily, and anxiety-producing factors like these can only make it more difficult.

The ways in which school personnel and students treat each other can also add much to the teaching/learning process (see Figure 6.6). All individuals within the school should

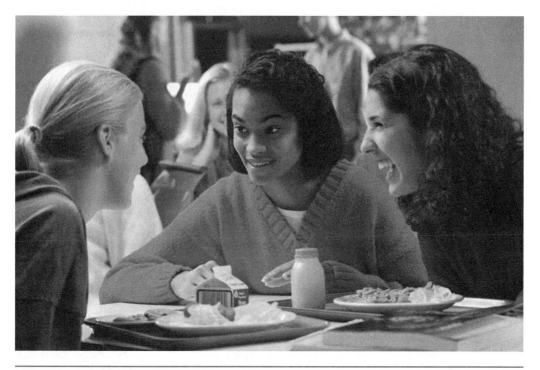

FIGURE 6.6
A healthy social environment, conducive to learning, is an important component of good school health.

be treated with respect. People should be polite and courteous to each other. This does not mean that high academic standards should be abandoned and that everyone should agree with all that others do, but students and teachers should not be afraid to express themselves in a cooperative, respectful way. For example, think back to your middle school and high school days. Think about the teachers you liked best. Did you like them because they were great teachers and knew their subject well? Or, did you like them because of the way they treated and respected you? The psychosocial environment can have a significant impact on the school environment!

School Health Education

school health education
the development, delivery, and evaluation of a planned curriculum, kindergarten through grade 12

School health education (e.g., classroom instruction)[34] has been defined as the "planned, sequential, K–12 curriculum that addresses the physical, mental, emotional and social dimensions of health. The curriculum is designed to motivate and assist students to maintain and improve their health, prevent disease, and reduce health-related risk behaviors."[26] If designed properly, school health education could be one of the most effective means to reduce serious health problems in the United States, including cardiovascular disease, cancer, motor vehicle crashes, homicide, and suicide.[35] Such a curriculum should focus on promoting the following priority health content:[36]

- An alcohol- and drug-free lifestyle
- Healthy eating
- Mental and emotional health
- Personal health and wellness
- Physical activity
- Safety/unintentional injury prevention
- Sexual health (abstinence and risk avoidance)
- Tobacco-free lifestyle
- Violence prevention

curriculum
a written plan for instruction

School health education includes all health education in the school. It includes health education that takes place in the classroom as well as any other activities designed to positively influence the health knowledge and skills of students, parents, and school staff. For example, health education can take place when the school nurse gives a vision screening test to a student or when coaches talk with their teams about the abuse of drugs.

scope
part of the curriculum that outlines what will be taught

For health education to be effective, it should be well conceived and carefully planned. The written plan for school health education is referred to as the health **curriculum.** The curriculum not only outlines the **scope** (what will be taught), and the **sequence** (when it will be taught), but also provides (1) learning objectives, (2) standards (see Box 6.3), (3) learning activities, (4) possible instructional resources, and (5) methods for assessment to determine the extent to which the objectives and standards are met. If health instruction is to be effective, the health curriculum should include lessons of appropriate scope and sequence for all grades from kindergarten through the twelfth grade.

sequence
part of the curriculum that states in what order the content will be taught

As with the CSHP, results from CDC's School Health Policies and Program Study (SHPPS) show that good school health instruction is not widespread. To enhance the state of health instruction in schools, the Joint Committee for National Health Education Standards was developed in 1993 by five health organizations—the American Association for Health Education, the American School Health Association, the American Public Health Association, the American Cancer Society, and the Society of State Directors of Health, Physical Education, and Recre-

BOX
6.3

NATIONAL HEALTH EDUCATION STANDARDS

1. Students will comprehend concepts related to health promotion and disease prevention to enhance health.
2. Students will analyze the influence of family, peers, culture, media, technology, and other factors on health behaviors.
3. Students will demonstrate the ability to access valid information and products and services to enhance health.
4. Students will demonstrate the ability to use interpersonal communication skills to enhance health and avoid or reduce health risks.
5. Students will demonstrate the ability to use decision-making skills to enhance health.
6. Students will demonstrate the ability to use goal setting to enhance health.
7. Students will demonstrate the ability to practice health-enhancing behaviors to avoid or reduce health risks.
8. Students will demonstrate the ability to advocate for personal, family, and community health.

Source: Joint Committee on National Health Standards (2007). *National Health Standards*, 2nd ed. Atlanta, GA: Author.

ation. The Joint Committee developed a set of standards that "describe the knowledge and skills essential to the development of health literacy.[37] The standards were developed "to serve as a framework for organizing health knowledge and skills into curricula at the state and local levels,"[39] and were not intended to define a national curriculum or to be a federal mandate. The original National Health Education Standards were reviewed and revised in 2006.[38]

There are eight standards (see Box 6.3), and each standard has grade-level performance indicators set for grades preK–2, 3–5, 6–8, and 9–12. "The standards evolved from the health education profession's current thinking about what constitutes grade-appropriate and challenging content and performance expectations for students."[37] Currently, over 75% of states mandating standards-based health education have used the National Health Education Standards as their basis for requirements and recommendations.[20]

Development of and Sources of Health Education Curricula

Each year, many school districts throughout the United States are faced with the task of developing a curriculum to guide health education. Such a task can be completed in one of several ways. First, a school district could obtain a prepackaged curriculum that has been developed by nationally recognized specialists. Some of these are prepared and sold by for-profit organizations and others are available free of charge from nonprofit agencies (i.e., voluntary health agencies). A second means would be to use the approved curriculum of either the state departments of education or health. A third method would be to adopt a new health textbook series and consider the series as a district's curricular guide. And fourth, some districts may even develop their own in-house curriculum. Each of these approaches has its strengths and weaknesses, and school districts have to decide which approach best suits their particular situation.

Determining what is and what is not a good curriculum can be a difficult process. Some very poor curricula, packaged in a slick way, can convince administrators that they have purchased a very fine product. Conversely, some educationally sound programs may not be well packaged. Fortunately, resources are available to help reduce the guesswork for those who must select curricula. See Box 6.4 for a summary of characteristics of effective health education curricula, which can serve as a guide when evaluating and selecting materials.

A number of federal agencies have created processes for reviewing, approving, and rating health education programs that are effective. The CDC maintains a list of registries sponsored by federal agencies that include programs effective in reducing youth risk behaviors.[39] Most of these registries allow curriculum developers to nominate their curricula for review. The review process typically involves peer review by three or more professionals with expertise

---

BOX 6.4

CHARACTERISTICS OF EFFECTIVE HEALTH EDUCATION CURRICULA

- Focuses on specific behavioral outcomes
- Is research-based and theory-driven
- Addresses individual values and group norms that support health-enhancing behaviors
- Focuses on increasing perceptions of risk and harmfulness of engaging in specific health-risk behaviors as well as reinforcing protective factors
- Addresses social pressures and influences
- Builds personal and social competence
- Provides functional health knowledge that is basic and accurate, and directly contributes to health-promoting decisions and behaviors
- Uses strategies designed to personalize information and engage students
- Provides age-appropriate and developmentally appropriate information, learning strategies, teaching methods, and materials

- Incorporates learning strategies, teaching methods, and materials that are culturally inclusive
- Provides adequate time for instruction and learning
- Provides opportunities to reinforce skills and positive health behaviors
- Provides opportunities to make connections with influential others (e.g., parents or other caregivers, teachers, youth leaders, clergy)
- Includes teacher information and professional development and training that enhances the effectiveness of instruction and student learning

Source: Centers for Disease Control and Prevention (pending). *Health Education Curriculum Assessment Tool.* Atlanta, GA: Author, 8-10.

---

in the specific area. Following the review, programs receive a rating, such as "promising," "exemplary," "effective," or "model" programs. Model programs, according to the National Registry of Effective Programs and Practices, which facilitates the review processes for the Substance Abuse and Mental Health Services Administration (SAMHSA) and CDC, are well-implemented, well-evaluated programs whose developers have agreed to participate in SAMHSA dissemination efforts and provide training and technical assistance to practitioners who wish to adopt their programs.[40]

In addition to the curricula that appear on the CDC's *Registries of Programs Effective in Reducing Youth Risk Behaviors,*[39] there are a number of other sources for obtaining health curricula. As a matter of fact, if we tried to create a list, it would consume many pages of this book and probably still would not be entirely inclusive. The following is a list of places where you may be able to find other health curricula. Some of them may be comprehensive (include a variety of topics and for every grade level, K–12), and others may be topic and/or grade-level specific. These other sources include the following:

1. The Centers for Disease Control and Prevention: Over the past several years the CDC has developed guidelines to assist schools and others in developing programs for healthy lifestyles. Examples include (a) Guidelines for School Health Programs to Prevent Tobacco Use and Addiction,[41] (b) Guidelines for School Health Programs to Promote Lifelong Healthy Eating,[42] and (c) Guidelines for School and Community Health Programs to Promote Physical Activity Among Young People.[43] and (d) Guidelines for School Programs to Prevent Skin Cancer.[44] These and others are available from CDC, Division of Adolescent and School Health (DASH).[45]

2. State departments of education or health: A number of states have either recommended or required a particular curriculum. Some states do not have comprehensive curricula but require instruction in some of the more controversial health topics, such as substance use and abuse and sexuality education.

3. Health agencies and associations: Many of the voluntary health agencies (e.g., American Cancer Society, American Heart Association, and American Lung Association) and other

health-related associations (e.g., National Dairy Council, American Health Foundation, and United Way) have developed curricula for grades K–12. Most of these are not comprehensive, but they are usually well done, supported by audiovisuals and handouts, and available either at very low or no cost.

4. Commercially produced curricula: These curricula have been developed by private corporations for schools.

Counseling, Psychological, and Social Services

Counseling, psychological, and social services are services provided to improve students' mental, emotional, and social health. These services can include individual and group assessments, interventions, and referrals. Professionals such as certified school counselors, psychologists, and social workers provide these services.[26]

Physical Education

Physical education is defined as a "planned, sequential K–12 curriculum that provides cognitive content and learning experiences in a variety of activity areas."[26] Emphasis is placed on physical fitness and skill development that lead to lifelong physical activity. Physical education should be taught by qualified teachers.[26]

School Nutrition Services

School nutrition services should provide access to a variety of nutritious and appealing meals that accommodate the health and nutrition needs of all students in a school district. Additionally, the school nutrition services program should offer students a learning laboratory for classroom nutrition and health education. The program should also serve as a resource for links with nutrition-related community services.[26]

Family/Community Involvement for School Health

Family/community involvement allows for an "integrated school, parent, and community approach for enhancing the health and well-being of students."[26] The school is an agency within a community that cannot function in isolation. Schools that actively engage parents and community resources in their school health councils, curriculum committees, and other health-related programming respond more effectively to the health-related needs of students.[26]

School-Site Health Promotion for Staff

School-site health promotion for staff includes "opportunities for school staff to improve their health status" through health-related assessments and activities.[26] These opportunities encourage staff to engage in healthy behaviors, resulting in improved health status, improved morale, positive health role modeling, reduced health insurance costs, and decreased absenteeism.[26]

ISSUES AND CONCERNS FACING THE SCHOOL HEALTH PROGRAM

Like most other community health programs, the school health program is not without its issues and concerns. "In the 1940's, the three leading school discipline problems were talking, chewing gum, and making noise."[46] Today, many of the leading school discipline problems are related to health, such as the distribution of prescription medications, violence, obesity, and the consequences of low self-esteem. In the remainder of this chapter, we will summarize a few of the challenges that still lie ahead of those who work in school health.

Lack of Support for Coordinated School Health Programs

"Schools offer the most systematic and efficient means available to improve the health of youth and enable young people to avoid health risks,"[47] yet, ironically, school health advocates have been unsuccessful in getting a CSHP implemented in even a majority of the school districts in the country. We have already pointed out that healthy children are better learners and that a CSHP can contribute to the health of children. More globally, a CSHP "facilitates the attainment of the goal of schooling; an educated populace whose health permits continued productivity through the lifespan."[48]

While many Americans support the idea that everyone is entitled to good health, we have not supported through legislation the notion that everyone is entitled to a CSHP. Obviously, getting legislation passed is a complicated process and is dependent on a number of different circumstances, including, but not limited to, economics, social action, and politics. This difficult task should not deter those who feel coordinated school health is vital (see Box 6.5). It is becoming clearer that many of the answers to current and future health problems lie with the resources found in the school—the one institution of society through which all of us must pass. The following are a few examples of the impact school health can have:

1. At the present time, the key to dealing with the AIDS problem is education.
2. The biggest stride in improving the health of the country will not come from new technology but from the health behavior in which we engage.
3. Many of the primary health care services needed by the children of this country are not available because of the barriers of the health care system.
4. "Every dollar invested in effective tobacco education saves society an estimated $18.80 in health care and other costs caused by smoking. Each dollar invested in alcohol and other drug prevention saves an estimated $5.69. And each education dollar spent to prevent too-early and unprotected sexual behaviors saves $5.10."[49]

BOX
6.5

BARRIERS TO COMPREHENSIVE SCHOOL HEALTH EDUCATION

Although the importance of comprehensive school health education is being recognized more and more, there are several barriers to its implementation. Research by various authors has informed health educators of barriers to establishing effective comprehensive health instruction. Those barriers include the following:

1. Lack of local administrative commitment
2. Lack of adequately prepared teachers
3. Lack of time in the school day/year
4. Lack of money/funds
5. Health education's lack of credibility as an academic subject
6. Lack of community/parental support for controversial topics
7. Policy constraints
8. Teacher priorities
9. Pressure to focus on subjects included in high-stakes tests

10. General lack of reinforcement by state and local education policy makers.

The top three barriers tend to be seen as the most significant. Recommendations to address them include

1. Inviting administrators to workshops and conferences dealing with current health issues
2. Conducting quality in-service programs
3. Advocacy to school administrators and professors of education

Sources: Bender, S. J., J. J. Neutens, S. Skonie-Hardin, and W. D. Sorochan (1997). *Teaching Health Science: Elementary and Middle School*, 4th ed. Boston: Jones and Bartlett, 32; Butler, S. C. (1993). "Chief State School Officers Rank Barriers to Implementing Comprehensive School Health Education." *Journal of School Health*, 63(3): 130–132; Telljohann, S. K., C. W. Symons, and B. Pateman (2007). *Health Education: Elementary and Middle School Applications*, 5th ed. New York: McGraw-Hill, 50; and Thackeray, R., B. L. Neiger, H. Bartle, S. C. Hill, and M. D. Barnes (2002). "Elementary School Teachers' Perspectives on Health Instruction: Implications for Health Education." *American Journal of Health Education*, 33(2): 77–82.

The need for coordinated school health should be obvious to all. We have taken the liberty to rephrase a quote from a group of school health experts who say it best: Society should not be as concerned with what happens when we implement a CSHP as about what is likely to happen if we do not.[50] Although garnering support for CSHPs has been an uphill battle, we are moving in the right direction. As mentioned earlier in the chapter, with the passing of the Child Nutrition and WIC Reauthorization Act of 2004,[18] school districts are required to institute local wellness policies promoting better nutrition, physical activity, and wellness. Some states have taken this one step further by passing state legislation requiring districts to institute coordinated school health advisory councils.[51] The inclusion of "coordinated school health" in the title of these councils encourages many districts to begin talking about, developing, and/or implementing a CSHP.

Controversy Regarding the School Health Curriculum

The words *sexual intercourse, suicide, substance use and abuse, sexually transmitted diseases, abortion, contraception,* and *death and dying* get attention. The very nature of the topics covered in a school health education curriculum today create controversy. Yet, controversy is not new to school health education; it has followed health education ever since it first attempted to deal with the many issues that face youth (see Figure 6.7).

Controversy is a part of health education for a number of reasons. Part of it deals with the pressure applied to schools by present-day conservative groups. These groups are interested in discouraging health instruction that includes values-clarification activities and open-ended decision-making processes.[52] Others believe that controversy exists due to the differences in family value systems and religious beliefs. Bensley and Harmon[53] have suggested that controversies fall into two major categories: issues that center around the values and beliefs of the content taught and issues that arise from improper implementation of the curriculum. The former category deals with questions such as (1) Do students really need to learn in school how to use a condom? (2) Doesn't talk of suicide lead some students to think that it might be the best alternative for them? (3) Aren't chiropractors just health quacks? and (4) Why do students need to know about funeral preplanning in high school? These are legitimate concerns, but they are also issues that today's adolescents face. Lack of awareness, knowledge, and skills are not excuses for undesirable health behavior. If the students do not get this information at school, where will they get it? Studies have shown that the institutions of church and family have taught little about the controversial topics included in health curricula.

Improper implementation of the curriculum is indeed a concern. Because health is not considered a "core" subject in most school districts, it has received little attention and support. In many school districts throughout the United States, the low priority given to health has meant that much of the health education is provided by individuals other than health education specialists. These people are not incapable of teaching health, but they have not been educated to do so. Therefore, the health curriculum is sometimes improperly implemented, and controversy arises.

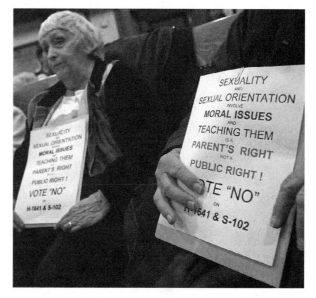

FIGURE 6.7

There are still many controversial issues that surround health coordinated school health programs.

School districts can help reduce controversy by (1) implementing age-appropriate curricula, (2) using acceptable teaching methods, (3) gaining parent/guardian approval of curricula and teaching methods, (4) developing a school policy that enables parents/guardians to review the curricula and to withdraw their children from lessons that go against family or religious beliefs, (5) implementing a school policy that provides for the handling of concern by parents/guardians,[49] and (6) making sure qualified and interested teachers teach health.

School-Based Health Centers or School-Linked Health Centers

Earlier in the chapter we mentioned that a number of school districts across the country are opening school-based or school-linked health centers to help meet the health needs of their students. Yet, the concept of offering comprehensive health care services through school-based or school-linked health centers is a relatively new one. In 1970, only one U.S. school had a SBHC/SLHC.[54] By 1984, that number had jumped to 31; by 1989 it had increased to 150.[55] In 2004, there were more than 1,350 SBHCs in 45 states.[56] Most (63%) of the SBHCs operating today are found in urban areas. Of these 1,350 SBHCs, 39% are found in high schools, 18% in middle schools, and 23% in elementary schools. The other 20% are located in alternative, K–8, 6–12, or K–12 schools.[56]

Although there is no single model for SBHCs, they share some common features:[57]

- They are located in schools.
- Parents sign written consents for their children to enroll in the health center.
- An advisory board of community representatives, parents, youth, and family organizations participate in planning and oversight of the health center.
- The health center works cooperatively with school nurses, coaches, counselors, classroom teachers, and school principals and their staff to assure that the health center is an integral part of the life of the school.
- Clinical services are the responsibility of a qualified health provider (hospital, health center, health department, group medical practice, etc.).
- A multidisciplinary team of nurse practitioners, clinical social workers, physicians, and other health professionals care for students.
- The health center provides a comprehensive range of services that specifically meets the serious health problems of young people in the community as well as provides general medical care.

As mentioned earlier in the chapter, there are a number of sound reasons why health centers should be based in schools—the primary reason being the ability to reach, in a cost-effective manner, a large segment of the population that is otherwise without primary health care. Yet, SBHCs have been the frequent targets of intense criticism at the local and national levels by political and religious groups.[58-60] Much of the controversy surrounding SBHCs has centered on three issues: (1) cultural wars, (2) funding, and (3) partisan politics.[61] The issue of cultural wars revolves around the views of conservatives versus liberals, and how and where people should receive their health care. While some people who support SBHCs would want their child treated as quickly and effectively as possible for a health problem, others who oppose the centers can see nothing but the "image of a condom on a cafeteria tray."[61] The key to working through the "cultural wars" problem is compromise. That is, each area of the country is different and what would be reasonable health services provided in an SBHC in one area would be unacceptable in another. Thus, advocates of the centers would say that the services provided by SBHCs are so badly needed that a single issue such as reproductive health care should not keep an SBHC from existing.[61]

Since their inception, funding for SBHCs has always been an issue. They do not have the sophisticated computers to bill for services, and they are typically not open 24 hours a day to qualify, at least in the eyes of insurance companies, as primary care health centers.[59] Also, the SBHCs' means of operation really do not match well with the concept of managed care (see Chapter 14). Therefore, most of the funding for SBHCs comes from state appropriations (61%), maternal and child health block grants (19%), and Medicaid (19%). Only 1% comes from private insurance.[62]

Violence in Schools

Over the years, schools have been viewed as safe and nurturing environments.[63] But more recently, there have been a number of high-profile incidents of violence in schools (e.g., Paducah, KY; Pearl, MS; Moses Lake, WA; Springfield, OR; Littleton, CO; and San Diego, CA) that have made the general public more aware of the violence in schools. "Violence in schools is certainly not new; almost every adult remembers the school bully."[64] The difference between violence in the schools today and years past is the means by which disagreements are settled. "Today the possibility that a disagreement among students will be settled with some type of weapon rather than an old-fashioned fist fight has significantly increased."[65] (See Chapter 8 for data on students carrying weapons.) CDC Youth Risk Behavior data indicate that 6% of U.S. high school students had missed at least one day of school in the preceding month because they felt unsafe either being at school or going to and from school; one of 13 students had been threatened or injured with a weapon on school property during the preceeding year; one of seven had been in a physical fight on school property; and approximately one in three had his or her property stolen or deliberately damaged on school grounds.[66]

We know that males are involved in more violent acts than females.[66] We also know that certain racial and ethnic groups participate and are victims of violence at school more often than other students.[66] Yet, it is close to impossible to predict who will be next to commit a violent act in a school. (See Chapter 8 for a more detailed description of adolescent risk behaviors.)

Another form of violence that has received significant attention recently is bullying. Bullying can be defined as "aggressive behavior that is intentional and that involves an imbalance of power or strength."[67] Bullying can take many forms, such as physical (hitting); verbal (teasing or name calling); emotional (gestures or social exclusion); and cyber (sending insulting messages by e-mail). Research indicates that between 15% and 25% of students are bullied with some frequency, and 15% to 20% report that they engage in bullying behavior. Being bullied can affect academic achievement and self-esteem. Bullying can also affect bystanders by creating a climate of fear and disrespect in schools. Furthermore, bullying behavior can be a sign of other serious antisocial or violent behavior by those who bully their peers.[67]

Like most other health problems, risk factors need to be identified and steps taken to reduce the risk of violent acts occurring in the schools. Many schools have taken steps to try to reduce the chances for violence, yet many more have stated that violence is not a problem at "our school." These are the schools that are most vulnerable to such a problem. The CDC makes the following recommendations, and outlines specific strategies, to guide schools in their efforts toward preventing unintentional injuries, violence, and suicide:[68]

- Social environment: Establish a social environment that promotes safety and prevents unintentional injuries, violence, and suicide.
- Physical environment: Provide a physical environment, inside and outside school buildings, that promotes safety and prevents unintentional injuries.
- Health education: Implement health and safety education curricula and instruction that help students develop knowledge, attitudes, behavioral skills, and confidence needed to adopt and maintain safe lifestyles and to advocate for health and safety.

- Physical education and physical activity programs: Provide safe physical education and extracurricular physical activity programs.
- Health services: Provide health, counseling, psychological, and social services to meet the physical, mental, emotional, and social health needs of students.
- Crisis response: Establish mechanisms for short- and long-term responses to crisis, disasters, and injuries that affect the school community.
- Family and community: Integrate school, family, and community efforts to prevent unintentional injuries, violence, and suicide.
- Staff members: For all school personnel, provide staff development services that impart the knowledge, skills, and confidence to effectively promote safety and prevent unintentional injuries, violence, and suicide and support students in their efforts to do the same.

Violence is not a problem that will be going away soon. Many school personnel do not believe it is something that can happen in their schools. As life has shown us, it can happen anywhere. Violence is an issue that all schools need to face and something for which they need to plan to reduce the risks to school children and personnel.

CHAPTER SUMMARY

- The potential impact of a coordinated school health program on the health of children, their families, and the community is great, because the school is the one institution through which we all must pass.
- To date, the full potential of school health has not been reached, due to lack of support and interest.
- If implemented properly, coordinated school health programs can improve access to health services, educate students about pressing health issues, and provide a safe and healthy environment in which students can learn and grow.
- The foundations of the school health program include (1) a school administration that supports such an effort, (2) a well-organized school health council that is genuinely interested in providing a coordinated program for the students, and (3) written school health policies.
- School health policies are critical for ensuring accountability, credibility, and the institutionalization of programs and efforts to make schools a healthy learning environment.
- The components of a coordinated school health program include (1) school health services, (2) a healthy school environment, (3) school health education, (4) counseling, psychological, and social services, (5) physical education, (6) school nutrition services, (7) family/community involvement for school health, and (8) school-site health promotion for staff.
- The eight National Health Education Standards emphasize a skills-based curriculum focusing on the following: (1) core concepts; (2) analyzing influences;

(3) accessing valid health information, products, and services; (4) demonstrating interpersonal communication skills; (5) utilizing decision-making skills; (6) utilizing goal-setting skills; (7) practicing health-enhancing behaviors; and (8) advocating for personal, family, and community health.

- A number of registries of effective health education programs are maintained to assist health educators locate and assess available curricula.
- There are a number of issues that face school health advocates, including a lack of support for coordinated school health, dealing with controversy in the health curriculum, the implementation of school-based health centers, and violence in schools.

REVIEW QUESTIONS

1. What is meant by the term *coordinated school health program*?
2. What individuals (name by position) should be considered for inclusion on the school health council?
3. What foundations are needed to ensure a coordinated school health program? Why?
4. Why are written school health policies needed?
5. Who should approve written school health policies?
6. What are the eight components of a coordinated school health program as noted by Allensworth and Kolbe?
7. What are the differences among (a) core health services, (b) core plus expanded school health services, and (c) services through school-based or school-linked health centers?

8. Explain the importance of using a standards-based health curriculum.

9. How would a health educator go about locating credible health education curricula?

10. State four issues facing school health advocates and explain why they are issues.

ACTIVITIES

1. Make arrangements to observe an elementary classroom in your town for a half-day. While observing, keep a chart of all the activities that take place in the classroom that relate to a coordinated school health program. Select one activity from your list and write a one-page paper describing the activity, why it was health related, how the teacher handled it, and what could have been done differently to improve the situation.

2. Visit a voluntary health agency in your community and ask the employees to describe the organization's philosophy on health education and inquire if their health education materials are available for use in a school health program. Summarize your visit with a one-page reaction paper.

3. Make an appointment to interview either a school nurse or a school health coordinator. During your interview, ask the person to provide an overview of what his or her school offers in the way of a coordinated school health program. Ask specifically about the eight components of the school health program and the issues of controversy presented in this chapter. Summarize your visit with a two-page written paper.

4. Make arrangements to interview a school administrator or school board member in a district where a school-based or school-linked center exists. Ask the person to describe the process that the school district went through to start the center, what resistance the district met in doing so, and what the district would do differently if it had to implement it again or start another center.

COMMUNITY HEALTH ON THE WEB

The Internet contains a wealth of information about community and public health. Increase your knowledge of some of the topics presented in this chapter by accessing the Jones and Bartlett Publishers Web site at **http://health.jbpub.com/book/communityhealth/6e** and follow the links to complete the following Web activities.

- American School Health Association
- Action for Healthy Kids
- Division of Adolescent and School Health

REFERENCES

1. U.S. Department of Health and Human Services, Public Health Service (1996). *Progress Review: Educational and Community-Based Programs*. Washington, DC: U.S. Government Printing Office.

2. Dryfoos, J. (2000). "The Mind-Body-Building Equation." *Educational Leadership*, 57(6): 14–17.

3. Joint Committee on Health Education and Promotion Terminology (2001). "Report of the 2000 Joint Committee on Health Education and Promotion Terminology." *American Journal of Health Education*, 32(2): 89–103.

SCENARIO: ANALYSIS AND RESPONSE

It was obvious that Ms. Graff had a very full day, which included several issues related to a coordinated school health program. Based upon what you read in this chapter and other knowledge you have about school health, respond to the following questions:

1. Identify five school health concerns with which Ms. Graff had to deal.

2. For each of the concerns you identified in Question 1, state how written policies may have helped or hindered Ms. Graff with her responsibilities.

3. How important do you feel is the role of the classroom teacher in making a coordinated school health program work? Why do you feel this way?

4. Say the school district in which Ms. Graff works was interested in opening up a school-based health center, but the superintendent needed more data to help "sell" the idea to the school board. Using a search engine on the Internet (e.g., Google), enter "school-based health centers." Could you recommend some Web sites to the superintendent that would be useful?

4. Allensworth, D. D., and L. J. Kolbe (1987). "The Comprehensive School Health Program: Exploring an Expanded Concept." *Journal of School Health*, 57(10): 409–412.

5. U.S. Census Bureau (2006). "Back to School: 2006-2007." In *U.S. Census Bureau News: Facts for Features*. Washington, DC: U.S. Department of Commerce.

6. McGinnis, J. M., and C. DeGraw (1991). "Healthy Schools 2000: Creating Partnerships for the Decade." *Journal of School Health*, 61(7): 292-296.

7. American Cancer Society (1999). *Improving School Health: A Guide to School Health Councils*. Atlanta, GA: American Cancer Society.

8. Fetro, J. V. (1998). "Implementing Coordinated School Health Programs in Local Schools." In E. Marx, S. F. Wooley, and D. Northrop, eds., *Health Is Academic: A Guide to Coordinated School Health Programs*. New York: Teachers College Press, 15-42.

9. National Association of School Nurses (2002). "Issue Brief: Role of the School Nurse." Available at http://www.nasn.org/briefs/briefs.htm.

10. Cornacchia, H. J., L. K. Olsen, and J. M. Ozias (1996). *Health in Elementary Schools*, 9th ed. St. Louis, MO: Mosby, 47-48.

11. McGinnis, J. M. (1981). "Health Problems of Children and Youth: A Challenge for Schools." *Health Education Quarterly*, 8(1): 11-14.

12. American Association for Health Education (2002). *The School Nurse in Education: A Position Statement*. Available at http://www.aahperd.org/aahe/template.cfm?template=publications-position.html.

13. Grebow, P. M., B. Z. Greene, J. Harvey, and C. J. Head (2000). "Shaping Health Policies." *Educational Leadership*, 57(6): 63-66.

14. Bruess, C. E., and J. E. Gay (1978). *Implementing Comprehensive School Health*. New York: Macmillan.

15. McKenzie, J. F. (1983). "Written Policies: Developing a Solid Foundation for a Comprehensive School Health Program." *Future Focus: Ohio Journal of Health, Physical Education, Recreation, and Dance*, 4(3): 9-11.

16. Bureau of Health and Nutrition Services and Child/Family/School Partnerships (2006). *Action Guide for School Nutrition and Physical Activity Policies*. Middletown, CT: Connecticut State Department of Education.

17. U.S. Department of Agriculture, Food and Nutrition Service (2007). "The Local Process: How to Create and Implement a Local Wellness Policy." Available at http://www.fns.usda.gov/tn/Healthy/wellnesspolicy_steps.html.

18. Child Nutrition and WIC Reauthorization Act of 2004, Pub. L. No. 108-265, § 204 (2004). Available at http://www.fns.usda.gov/TN/Healthy/108-265.pdf.

19. Action for Healthy Kids (2007). "About Us." Available at http://www.actionforhealthykids.org.

20. Division of Adolescent and School Health, Centers for Disease Control and Prevention (2004). *School Health Policies and Programs Study*. Available at http://www.cdc.gov/healthyyouth/shpps/index.htm.

21. Centers for Disease Control and Prevention (2003). *Stories from the Field: Lessons about Building Coordinated School Health Programs*. Available at http://www.cdc.gov/healthyyouth/publications/stories.htm.

22. American Cancer Society (1999). *Improving School Health: A Guide to the Role of the School Health Coordinator*. Atlanta, GA: Author.

23. Maylath, N. S. (1991). "Employment of School Health Coordinators." *Journal of School Health*, 61(2): 98-100.

24. National Association of State Boards of Education (2007). *State-by-State School Health Program Coordinators*. Available at http://www.nasbe.org/HealthySchools/States/Topics.asp?Category=F&Topic=2.

25. Winnail, S., S. Dorman, and B. Stevenson (2004). "Training Leaders for School Health Programs: The National School Coordinator Leadership Institute." *Journal of School Health*, 74(3): 79-84.

26. Division of Adolescent and School Health, Centers for Disease Control and Prevention (2005). *Coordinated School Health Program*. Available at http://www.cdc.gov/healthyyouth/CSHP/.

27. U.S. Department of Health and Human Services (2000). *Healthy People 2010: Understanding and Improving Health*. Washington, DC: U.S. Government Printing Office.

28. Schlitt, J. J. (June 1991). "Issue Brief—Bringing Health to School: Policy Implications for Southern States." Washington, DC: Southern Center on Adolescent Pregnancy Prevention and Southern Regional Project on Infant Mortality. Printed in *Journal of School Health*, 62(2): 60a-60h.

29. Klein, J. D., and L. S. Sadowski (1990). "Personal Health Services as a Component of Comprehensive Health Programs." *Journal of School Health*, 60(4): 164-169.

30. Duncan, P., and J. B. Igoe (1998). "School Health Services." In E. Marx, S. F. Wooley, and D. Northrop, eds., *Health Is Academic: A Guide to Coordinated School Health Programs*. New York: Teachers College Press, 169-194.

31. National Health and Education Consortium (1995). *Starting Young: School-Based Health Centers at the Elementary Level*. Washington, DC: Author.

32. Joint Committee on Health Education Terminology (1974). "New Definitions: Report of the 1972-73 Joint Committee on Health Education Terminology." *Journal of School Health*, 44(1): 33-37.

33. Henderson, A., and D. E. Rowe. (1998). "A Healthy School Environment." In E. Marx, S. F. Wooley, and D. Northrop, eds., *Health Is Academic: A Guide to Coordinated School Health Programs*. New York: Teachers College Press, 96-115.

34. Grunbaum, J. A., L. Kann, B. I. Williams, S. A. Kinchen, J. L. Collins, E. R. Baumler, and L. J. Kolbe (2000). "Surveillance for Characteristics of Health Education among Secondary Schools—School Health Education Profiles, 1998." *Morbidity and Mortality Weekly Report*, 49(SS-8): 1-41.

35. Institute of Medicine (1997). *Schools and Health: Our Nation's Investment*. Washington, DC: National Academies Press.

36. Centers for Disease Control and Prevention (pending). *Health Education Curriculum Assessment Tool*. Atlanta, GA: Author, 8-10.

37. Joint Committee on National Health Education Standards (1995). *National Health Education Standards*. Atlanta, GA: American Cancer Society.

38. Joint Committee on National Health Education Standards (2007). *National Health Education Standards* (2nd ed.). Atlanta, GA: Author.

39. Division of Adolescent and School Health, Centers for Disease Control and Prevention (2006). "Adolescent Health: Registries of Programs Effective in Reducing Youth Risk Behaviors." Available at http://www.cdc.gov/healthyyouth/AdolescentHealth/registries.htm.

40. Center for Substance Abuse Prevention, Substance Abuse and Mental Health Services Administration (2004). "SAMHSA Model Programs: Background Information." Available at http://modelprograms.samhsa.gov/template.cfm?page=background.

41. Centers for Disease Control and Prevention (1994). "Guidelines for School Health Programs to Prevent Tobacco Use and Addiction." *Morbidity and Mortality Weekly Report*, 43(RR-2): 1-18.

42. Centers for Disease Control and Prevention (1996). "Guidelines for School Health Programs to Promote Lifelong Healthy Eating." *Morbidity and Mortality Weekly Report*, 45(RR-9): 1-41.

43. Centers for Disease Control and Prevention (1997). "Guidelines for School and Community Health Programs to Promote Physical Activity among Young People." *Morbidity and Mortality Weekly Report*, 46(RR-6): 1-36.

44. Centers for Disease Control and Prevention (2002). "Guidelines for School Programs to Prevent Skin Cancer." *Morbidity and Mortality Weekly Report*, 54(RR-04): 1-16.

45. Division of Adolescent and School Health, Centers for Disease Control and Prevention (2004). "Healthy Youth! Publications and Links." Available at http://www.cdc.gov/healthyyouth/publications/index.htm.

46. U.S. Department of Health and Human Services, Office for Substance Abuse Prevention (1989). *Drug-Free Committees: Turning Awareness into Action* (DHHS pub. no. ADM 89-1562). Washington, DC: U.S. Government Printing Office.

47. "Healthy People 2000: National Health Promotion and Disease Prevention Objectives and Health Schools." (1991). *Journal of School Health*, 61(7): 298-299.

48. Association for the Advancement of Health Education (1991). *Position Statement: Comprehensive School Health*. Reston, VA: Author.

49. Centers for Disease Control and Prevention, Division of Adolescent and School Health (1997). "Is School Health Education Cost-Effective? An Exploratory Analysis of Selected Exemplary Components." As quoted in F. D. McKenzie and J. B. Richmond (1998). "Linking Health and Learning: An Overview of Coordinated School Health Programs." In E. Marx, S. F. Wooley, and D. Northrop, eds., *Health Is Academic: A Guide to Coordinated School Health Programs*. New York: Teachers College Press, 1-14.

50. Gold, R. S., G. S. Parcel, H. J. Walberg, R. V. Luepker, B. Portnoy, and E. J. Stone (1991). "Summary and Conclusions of the THTM Evaluation: The Expert Work Group Perspective." *Journal of School Health*, 61(1): 39-42.

51. Student Nutrition and Physical Activity. S. Enrolled Act No. 111, 114th Gen. Assem., 2d Reg. Sess. (Ind. 2006). Available at http://www.in.gov/legislative/bills/2006/SE/SE0111.1.html.

52. Cleary, M. J. (1991). "School Health Education and a National Curriculum: One Disconcerting Scenario." *Journal of School Health*, 61(8): 355-358.

53. Bensley, L. B., Jr., and E. O. Harmon (May/June 1992). "Addressing Controversy in Health Education." *Update*, 9-10.

54. Council on Scientific Affairs, American Medical Association (1990). "Providing Medical Services through School-Based Health Programs." *Journal of School Health*, 60(3): 87-91.

55. Lear, J. G., L. L. Montgomery, J. J. Schlitt, and K. D. Rickett (1996). "Key Issues Affecting School-Based Health Centers and Medicaid." *Journal of School Health*, 66(3): 83-88.

56. Geierstanger, S. P., and G. Amaral (2005). "School-Based Health Centers and Academic Performance: What Is the Intersection?" Available at http://www.nasbhc.org/nasbhc_resources.htm.

57. Making the Grade (2001). *School-Based Health Centers: Background*. Available at http://www.gwu.edu/~mtg/sbhcs/sbhc.htm.

58. Pacheco, M., W. Powell, C. Cole, N. Kalishman, R. Benon, and A. Kaufmann (1991). "School-Based Clinics: The Politics of Change." *Journal of School Health*, 61(2): 92-94.

59. Rienzo, B. A., and J. W. Button (1993). "The Politics of School-Based Clinics: A Community-Level Analysis." *Journal of School Health*, 63(6): 266-272.

60. The School-Based Adolescent Health Care Program (1993). *The Answer Is at School: Bringing Health Care to Our Students*. Washington, DC: Author.

61. Morone, J. A., E. H. Kilbreth, and K. M. Langwell (2001). "Back to School: A Health Care Strategy for Youth." *Health Affairs*, 20(1): 122-136.

62. Making the Grade (1999). *School-Based Health Centers: National Survey, 1997/1998 Report*. Washington, DC: Author.

63. Hill, S. C., and J. C. Drolet (1999). "School-Related Violence among High School Students in the United States, 1993-1995." *Journal of School Health*, 69(7): 264-272.

64. Prothrow-Smith, D., and S. Quanday (1996). "Communities, Schools, and Violence." In A. M. Hoffman, ed., *Schools, Violence, and Society*. Westport, CT: Praeger, 153-161.

65. Anspaugh, D. J., and G. Ezell (2001). *Teaching Today's Health*, 6th ed. Boston: Allyn and Bacon.

66. Centers for Disease Control and Prevention (2006). "Youth Risk Behavior Surveillance—United States, 2005." *MMWR Surveillance Summaries*, 55(SS-5).

67. Health Resources and Services Administration (2007). "What We Know about Bullying." Available at http://www.stopbullyingnow.hrsa.gov.

68. Centers for Disease Control and Prevention (2001). "School Health Guidelines to Prevent Unintentional Injuries and Violence." *Morbidity and Mortality Weekly Report*, 50(RR-22): 1-75.

UNIT TWO

THE NATION'S HEALTH

Chapter 7

Maternal, Infant, and Child Health

Chapter Outline

Chapter Objectives

After studying this chapter you will be able to:

1 Define *maternal, infant,* and *child health.*

2 Explain the importance of maternal, infant, and child health as indicators of a society's health.

3 Define *family planning* and explain why it is important.

4 Identify consequences of teenage pregnancies.

5 Define *legalized abortion* and discuss *Roe v. Wade* and the pro-life and pro-choice movements.

6 Define *maternal mortality rate.*

7 Define *prenatal care* and the influence this has on pregnancy outcome.

8 List the major factors that contribute to infant health and mortality.

9 Explain the differences among infant mortality, neonatal mortality, and postneonatal mortality.

10 Identify the leading causes of childhood morbidity and mortality.

11 List the immunizations required in order for a two-year-old child to be considered fully immunized.

12 Explain how health insurance and health care services affect childhood health.

13 Identify important governmental programs developed to improve maternal and child health.

14 Briefly explain what WIC programs are and who they serve.

15 Identify the major groups who are recognized as advocates for children.

SCENARIO

Joan is 18 years old and a recent high school graduate. She lives in a small town of about 2,700 people. Most of the town's residents rely on a larger city nearby for shopping, recreation, and health care. Joan had dated Dave the past two years, but there was never any talk of marriage. Just before graduation she learned that she was pregnant. At Thanksgiving, just as she was completing her seventh month of pregnancy, she went into premature labor. An ambulance rushed her to the emer-

gency room of the hospital in the nearby city for what became a premature birth of her baby. While Joan was in recovery, doctors determined that her baby was not only premature, it also appeared to have other "developmental abnormalities." When asked whether she had received any prenatal care, Joan replied, "No, I couldn't afford it; besides, I didn't know where to go to get help."

INTRODUCTION

Creating a health profile of Americans requires a clear understanding of the health-related problems and opportunities of all Americans. In Chapter 3 we dicussed the role of descriptive epidemiology in understanding the health of populations. In describing the personal characteristics of a population, age is the first and perhaps the most important population characteristic to consider when describing the occurrence of disease, injury, and/or death in a population. Almost every health-related event or state has greater differences with age than in any other population characteristic. For this reason, community health professionals use age-specific rates when comparing the amount of disease between populations. When they analyze data by age, they use groups that are narrow enough to detect any age-related patterns, which may be present as a result of either the natural life cycle or behavioral patterns. Viewing age-group profiles in this manner enables community health workers to identify risk factors for specific age groups within the population and to develop and propose interventions aimed at reducing these risk factors. Health promotion and disease prevention programs successful at reducing exposure of specific age groups to such risk factors can improve the health status of the entire population.

In this chapter, we present a health profile of mothers, infants (those younger than 1 year), and children (ages 1–14 years). In the following two chapters, the health profiles will be presented of adolescents and young adults (15–24), adults (25–64), and older adults or seniors (65 and older). These same age subgroupings are used by the *Healthy People 2010* report and many other documents produced by the National Center for Health Statistics (NCHS) to describe and measure the health status of Americans.

maternal, infant, and child health the health of women of childbearing age and that of the child through adolescence

Maternal, infant, and child health encompasses the health of women of childbearing age from pre-pregnancy, through pregnancy, labor, and delivery, and the postpartum period and the health of the child prior to birth through adolescence.[1] In this chapter, we define and discuss commonly used indicators for measuring maternal, infant, and child health; examine the risk factors associated with maternal, infant, and child morbidity and mortality; and review selected community programs aimed at improving the health of women of childbearing age, infants, and children in the United States.

Maternal, infant, and child health are important to a community for several reasons. First, maternal, infant, and child health statistics are regarded as important indicators of the effectiveness of the disease prevention and health promotion services in a community. It is known that unintended pregnancies, lack of prenatal care, poor maternal and child nutrition, maternal drug use, low immunization rates, poverty, limited education, and insufficient child care—

combined with a lack of access to health care services in a community—are precursors to high rates of maternal, infant, and childhood morbidity and mortality. Second, we now know that many of the risk factors specified can be reduced or prevented with the early intervention of educational programs and preventive medical services for women, infants, and children. These early community efforts provide a positive environment that supports the physical and emotional needs of the woman, infant, and family and reduce the need for more costly medical or social assistance to these same members of society later in their lives (see Figure 7.1).

During the past several decades the United States has made important progress in reducing infant and maternal mortality (see Figures 7.2 and 7.3). However, despite these declines in mortality rates, challenges remain. Possibly the most important concern is that infant and maternal mortality data for the United States are characterized by a continual and substantial disparity between mortality rates for whites and blacks. The mortality rate among black infants (14.1 per 1,000 live births) was about two and one-half times the rate among white infants (5.8 per 1,000 live births) in 2003 (see Figure 7.2). The mortality rate among black women (31.2 per 100,000 births) was about four times the rate among white women (8.1 per 100,000 live births) in 2000 (see Figure 7.3). These disparities are not directly attributable to race or ethnicity, although certain diseases occur more often in certain races or ethnicities. Rather, the

FIGURE 7.1
The health of a nation is often judged by the health of its mothers and children.

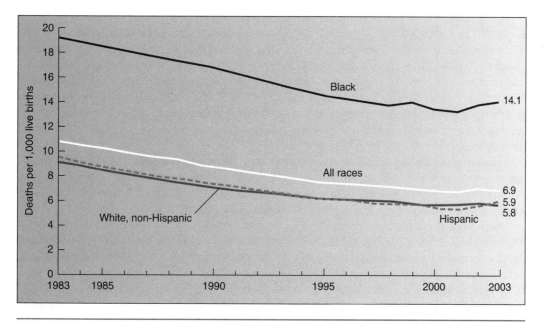

FIGURE 7.2
U.S. mortality rates among infants younger than 1 year, by maternal race/ethnicity, 1983–2003.
Source: Centers for Disease Control and Prevention, National Center for Health Statistics, National Vital Statistics System.

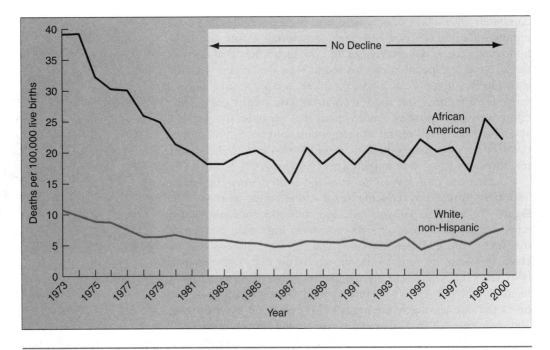

FIGURE 7.3

African American and white women who died of pregnancy-related complications: United States, 1973–2000 (annual number of deaths during pregnancy or within 42 days after delivery, per 100,000 live births).

*The apparent increase in the number of maternal deaths between 1998 and 1999 is the result of changes in how maternal deaths are classified and coded.

Source: Centers for Disease Control and Prevention, National Center for Health Statistics.

disparity can be traced to differences in the socioeconomic status between segments of the American population. For example, research indicates that low income and limited education correlate very highly with poor health status.[2] Second, the United States has higher infant and maternal mortality rates than other industrialized nations; it ranked 28th in infant mortality (see Figure 7.4) and 20th in maternal mortality in 2002.[2] These differences among industrialized nations mirror differences in the health status of women before and during pregnancy as well as the ease of access and quantity and quality of primary care for pregnant women and their infants.

Similar to the decline in infant and maternal mortality rates, the mortality rates of *children* (ages 1–14) have gone down significantly in the past couple of decades. The death rate declined by more than one-half in 1- to 4-year-old children (see Figure 7.5) and by nearly one-half in 5- to 14-year-old children from 1980 to 2002 (see Figure 7.6).[2]

Even with these improvements in child mortality rates, there is still much to be done to improve the health of American children. First, we must recognize that children today face other concerns that can significantly put them at risk for poor health. These concerns have been referred to as the "new morbidities" and include their family and social environments, behaviors, economic security, and education (see Box 7.1).[2] Second, we must be concerned about the difference in mortality rates between races. If the young are indeed the hope for the future, the United States must continue to work hard to ensure the health of each infant and child, regardless of race or socioeconomic status.

Whereas there are numerous factors that affect the health of both infant and child, many reflect or are related to the health status of the mother and her immediate environment. One of the first steps to ensure healthy children is to ensure that pregnant women have access to prenatal

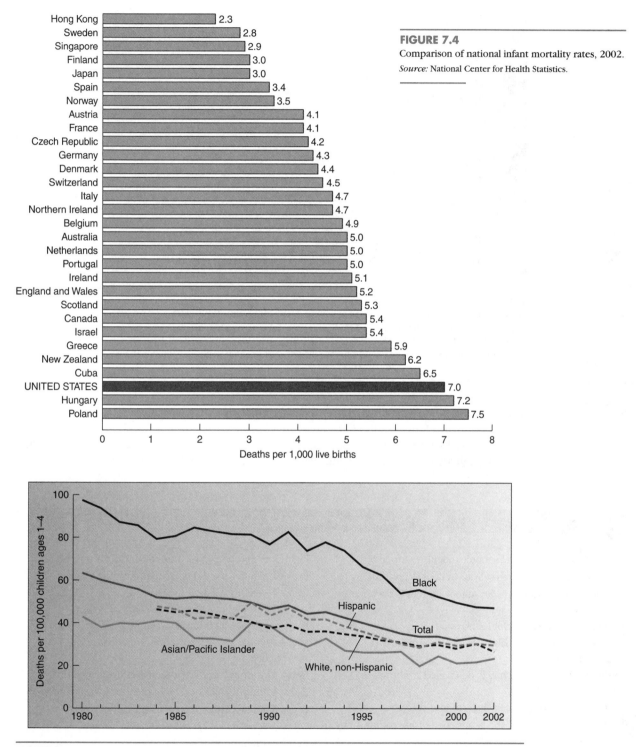

FIGURE 7.4

Comparison of national infant mortality rates, 2002.

Source: National Center for Health Statistics.

FIGURE 7.5

Death rates among children ages 1–4 by race and Hispanic origin, 1980–2002.

Note: Death rates for American Indians/Alaska Natives are included in the total but are not shown separately because the numbers of deaths were too small to calculate reliable rates.

Source: Centers for Disease Control and Prevention, National Center for Health Statistics, National Vital Statistics System.

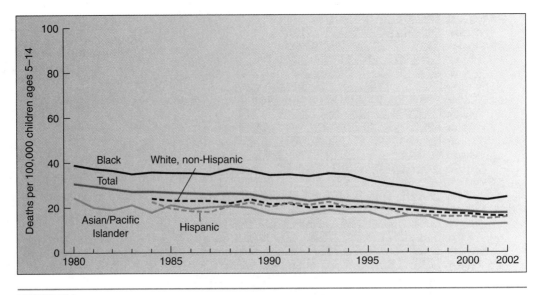

FIGURE 7.6

Death rates among children ages 5 to 14 by race and Hispanic origin, 1980–2002.

Note: Death rates for American Indians/Alaska Natives are included in the total but are not shown separately because the numbers of deaths were too small to calculate reliable rates.

Source: Centers for Disease Control and Prevention, National Center for Health Statistics, National Vital Statistics System.

care early in a pregnancy and that they receive proper care throughout it. There is nothing more dependent than a fetus in a mother's uterus relying on her to eat nutritiously and to avoid drugs or a newborn that is reliant upon an adult to survive and develop into a healthy child. Therefore, we will begin by looking at the health status of mothers and the family structure.

BOX **7.1**

KEY FACTS ABOUT AMERICAN CHILDREN

Every second a public school student is suspended.

Every 9 seconds a high school student drops out.

Every 13 seconds a public school student is corporally punished.

Every 20 seconds a child is arrested.

Every 22 seconds a baby is born to an unmarried mother.

Every 35 seconds a child is confirmed as abused or neglected.

Every 35 seconds a baby is born into poverty.

Every 38 seconds a baby is born to a mother who is not a high school graduate.

Every 51 seconds a baby is born without health insurance.

Every minute a baby is born to a teen mother.

Every 2 minutes a baby is born at low birth weight.

Every 4 minutes a child is arrested for drug abuse.

Every 4 minutes a baby is born to a mother who received late or no prenatal care.

Every 8 minutes a child is arrested for violent crimes.

Every 19 minutes a baby dies before his or her first birthday.

Every 41 minutes a child or teen dies in an accident.

Every 3 hours a child or teen is killed by a firearm.

Every 5 hours a child or teen commits suicide.

Every 6 hours a child is killed by abuse or neglect.

Every day a mother dies in childbirth.

Source: Children's Defense Fund (2007). Retrieved from www.childrensdefense.org. Reprinted with permission.

FAMILY AND REPRODUCTIVE HEALTH

The family is one of society's most treasured foundations. It represents a primary social group that influences and is influenced by other people and establishments. Moreover, families are the primary unit in which infants and children are nurtured and supported regarding their healthy development.[1] The U.S. Census Bureau defines a family as "a group of two people or more (one of whom is the householder) related by birth, marriage, or adoption and residing together; all such people (including related subfamily members) are considered as members of one family."[3] This definition does not include a variety of cultural styles and optional family structures that exist in our society today. Friedman broadens the definition of family to include "two or more persons who are joined together by bonds of sharing and emotional closeness and who identify themselves as being part of the family."[4] These definitions not only provide a basis for delineating a family, but are important to consider because most people, at some point in their life, will consider becoming a parent.

From a community health perspective, a marriage, or having two parents, serves as an important family characteristic in relation to a child's well-being. Research indicates there are increased health risks for infants and children who are raised in single-parent families, including adverse birth outcomes, low birth weight, and infant mortality, and that these children are more likely to live in poverty than children of married mothers.[5,6] Additionally, unmarried mothers generally have lower education, lower incomes, and greater dependence on welfare assistance than do married mothers. In 2004, the percentage of births to unmarried women was 35.8%, or nearly double that of the 18.4% of live births to unmarried women that occurred in 1980.[6] Younger women who give birth are substantially more likely than older women to have that birth outside of marriage. In 2003, 97.1% of teenagers under 15, 81.3% of 15- to 19-year-olds, and 53.2% of 20- to 24-year-olds who gave birth were unmarried, compared with 26.4% of 25- to 29-year-olds and approximately 15% of women in their thirties (see Figure 7.7).[7]

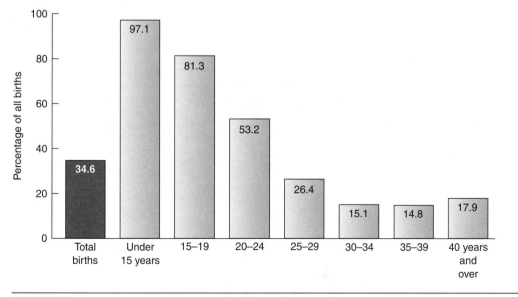

FIGURE 7.7

Percentage of all births that were to unmarried women, by age, 2003.

Source: Martin, J. A., B. E. Hamilton, P. D. Sutton, S. J. Ventura, F. Menacker, and M. Munson (2005). "Births: Final Data for 2003." *National Vital Statistics Reports*, 54(2): 1–30.

Teenage Births

Teenage childbearing represents a significant social and financial burden on both the family and the community. Teenagers who become pregnant and have a child are more likely than their peers who are not mothers to (1) drop out of school, (2) not get married or to have a marriage end in divorce, (3) rely on public assistance, and (4) live in poverty.[5,8] Teenage pregnancy and childbearing also have substantial economic consequences for society in the form of increased welfare costs. Each year teenage childbearing costs taxpayers at least $7 billion in direct costs associated with health care, foster care, criminal justice, and public assistance, as well as lost tax revenues.[9] Furthermore, teenage pregnancy and childbearing have considerable long-term consequences for teenage parents and their children. For instance, teenagers who give birth are less likely to graduate from high school and more likely to have a larger number of children in poverty than are nonparenting teenagers. Also, children born to teenage mothers may experience lower educational attainment and higher rates of teenage childbearing themselves when compared with children born to older mothers.

Teenage pregnancies also result in serious health consequences for these women and their babies. Teenage mothers are much less likely than women over the age of 20 to receive early prenatal care and are more likely to smoke during pregnancy and have a preterm birth and low-birth-weight baby (see Figure 7.8).[8] As a consequence of these and other factors, babies born to teenagers are more likely to die during the first year of life and more likely to suffer certain serious health problems than a baby born to a mother in her twenties and thirties. A teenage mother is at greater risk than a woman over the age of 20 for pregnancy complications (such as premature labor, anemia, and high blood pressure).[8] Therefore, teenage pregnancies are a significant community health concern in the United States.

Due in large part to effective community and public health campaigns aimed at reducing teenage pregnancies, teen pregnancy and birth rates have declined steadily in recent years. Between 1991 and 2004, the teenage birth rate in the United States declined 33% to a record low of 41.2 births per 1,000 teenage girls in 2004.[6] Despite the recently declining rates, 31%

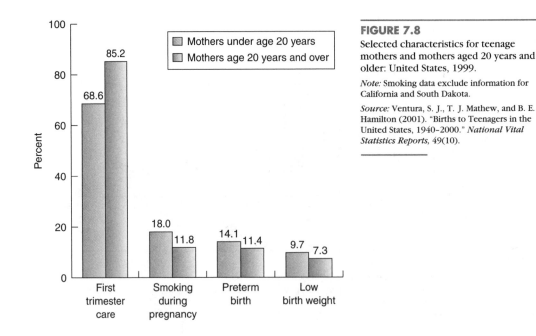

FIGURE 7.8

Selected characteristics for teenage mothers and mothers aged 20 years and older: United States, 1999.

Note: Smoking data exclude information for California and South Dakota.

Source: Ventura, S. J., T. J. Mathew, and B. E. Hamilton (2001). "Births to Teenagers in the United States, 1940–2000." *National Vital Statistics Reports,* 49(10).

of teenage girls get pregnant at least once before they reach age 20, resulting in approximately 750,000 teen pregnancies a year.[6] In fact, the United States still leads the industrialized world in teen pregnancy and birth rates by a large margin. U.S. rates are at least double those of other Western countries, which places the United States at a significant competitive disadvantage in the global economy.[10]

As stated in the introduction, the future of our nation depends on our children. The extent to which we actually believe this can be measured by the degree to which we plan, provide for, educate, and protect our children. Yet, every day in America, 3,879 babies are born to unmarried mothers; 2,482 children are confirmed abused or neglected; 2,447 babies are born into poverty; 2,252 babies are born to mothers who are not high school graduates; 1,701 babies are born without health insurance; 1,154 babies are born to teenage mothers; 888 babies are born at low birth weight; 367 babies are born to mothers who received late or no prenatal care; and 77 babies die before their first birthdays.[11] The need to plan a pregnancy and thereby place children first in families and in communities must be re-emphasized. Unwanted and unplanned childbearing has long been linked with adverse consequences for mothers, couples, and families, as well as for the children themselves.[12]

The choice to become a parent is a critical decision that affects the individual and the community. People who become parents acquire the major responsibility for another human being. They must provide an environment conducive to child development—one that protects and promotes health. However, the broader community also contributes to this growth and development.[12] This is best illustrated by an African proverb "it takes an entire village to educate and raise a child."[13] Therefore, the community must also make provisions for a child's care, nurture, and socialization.

Family Planning

Planning for the birth of a child can be one of life's splendid experiences. The first step is making a conscious decision on whether or not to become a parent. This determination will perhaps be one of the most important and consequential decisions couples will make during their lifetime. Parenthood requires enormous amounts of time, energy, and financial commitment, but most notably it requires the willingness to take full responsibility for a child's growth and development. In general, it is considered important that a pregnancy be planned to ensure the best health for the mother and fetus during the pregnancy. Unfortunately, approximately one-half of pregnancies in the United States are unintended, and half of those end in abortion.[14] The United States has set a national goal of decreasing unintended pregnancies to 30% by 2010.[12]

An unintended pregnancy is a pregnancy that is either mistimed (the woman did not want to be pregnant until later) or unwanted (the woman did not want to be pregnant at any time) at the time of conception. Unintended pregnancy is associated with a range of behaviors that can adversely affect the health of mothers and their babies. These risky behaviors include delayed entry into prenatal care, inadequate weight gain, cigarette smoking, and the use of alcohol and other drugs.[15] Women of all ages may have unintended pregnancies, but some groups are at a higher risk, including teenagers, those living in poverty, and those with limited education.[15,16]

The National Family Growth Study collects information to better understand unintended pregnancy. Using a 10-point scale, with 1 being "very unhappy to be pregnant" and 10 being "very happy to be pregnant," women were asked to report their feelings of pregnancy. The average mean rating was 9.2 for intended pregnancies and 4.2 for unintended pregnancies.[17] These indicators re-emphasize the importance of community health education programs regarding family planning.

family planning
determining the preferred number and spacing of children and choosing the appropriate means to accomplish it

Therefore, an important approach to reducing unwanted pregnancies and their adverse consequences is effective family planning by the community.[12] **Family planning** is defined as the process of determining the preferred number and spacing of children in one's family and choosing the appropriate means to achieve this preference. Although many maternal, infant, and child morbidity and mortality outcomes cannot be completely prevented by effective family planning, the frequency of occurrence can be reduced. Thus, preconception education and good gynecological, maternal, and child health care are required for effective family planning.[12]

Community involvement in family planning and care programs has historically included both governmental and nongovernmental health organizations in the United States (see Box 7.2). The federal and state governments provide funding assistance through a myriad of family planning services, including Title X of the Public Health Service Act, Medicaid, state funds, the Maternal and Child Health Bureau, and Social Service block grants. Of these, Title X, or the Family Planning Act, is the only federal program dedicated solely to funding family planning and related reproductive health care services through the National Family Planning Program (PL 91-572).[18] **Title X** of the Public Health Service Act was signed into law by President Nixon in 1970 to provide family planning services and help to all who wanted them but could not afford them. For more than three decades, Title X has been this nation's major program to reduce unintended pregnancy by providing contraceptive and other reproductive health care services to low-income women. Currently, it provides funding support to approximately 61% of the 4,000-plus family planning clinics nationwide. Every year more than 4.8 million women receive health care services at family planning clinics funded by Title X.[19,20] Those served are predominantly young, poor, uninsured, and have never had a child.[21]

Title X
a portion of the Public Health Service Act of 1970 that provides funds for family planning services for low-income people

---

BOX
7.2 **Ten Great Public Health Achievements, 1900–1999: Family Planning**

Changes in Family Planning

In 1900, the average life span was 47 years, and 10% of infants died during their first year of life. The average woman had 3.5 children, and 6 to 9 women per 1,000 died in childbirth. Distribution of information regarding contraception and contraceptive devices was generally illegal under federal and state Comstock laws, which had been enacted in the late 1800s. In 1900, the most common methods of contraception included withdrawal before ejaculation, rhythm, contraceptive douches, and vaginal pessaries (diaphragms, for example).

Milestones in Family Planning, United States, 1900–1999

1914	Margaret Sanger arrested for distributing information regarding birth control
1916	First birth control clinic, Brooklyn, New York; closed after 10 days by the New York City Vice Squad
1917	Federal registration of birth certificates
1928	Timing of ovulation during the menstrual cycle established
1955	First national fertility survey
1960	First licensure of birth control pills
1960	Modern intrauterine device licensed
1965	*Griswold v. Connecticut;* Supreme Court legalizes contraception
1970	Title X created
1972	Medicaid funding for family planning services authorized
1972	*Roe v. Wade;* Supreme Court legalizes abortion
1973	First National Survey of Family Growth taken
1990	Norplant licensed
1992	Depo-Provera licensed
1993	Female condom licensed

Source: Available at http://www.cdc.gov/phtn/tenachievements/family2/fp2.htm.

These family planning clinics are located in every state and in 85% of all counties. The administration of all Title X grants is through state health departments or regional agencies that subcontract with local agencies and clinics. Currently, slightly more than half of the grants are administered by state and local health departments, one-fifth by Planned Parenthood affiliates, and the remaining one-fourth by regional or local family planning councils located in community organizations and hospitals.[21]

For clinics to receive funding under the Title X program, they must offer a broad range of acceptable family planning methods (oral contraceptives, condoms, sterilization, and abstinence); they must encourage family participation; they must give priority to low-income families, and they must not use abortion as a method of family planning.[18] In addition to family planning methods, clinics also provide a comprehensive group of other health services critical to their clients' sexual and reproductive health (see Figure 7.9).

In 1981, family planning clinics that received federal funds were required to provide counseling on all options open to a pregnant woman, including abortion, as outlined in Title X. However, these facilities were not allowed to perform abortions. In 1988, the "**gag rule**" regulations were enacted. These regulations barred physicians and nurses in clinics receiving federal funds from counseling clients about abortions. Family planning providers challenged this legislation on the grounds that it denied women their rights to information that was needed to make an informed decision. Many health care providers felt that the gag rule restricted their rights to counsel a client even when childbirth could be detrimental to her health.[18] Supporters of the gag rule regulation felt that Title X was created to help prevent unwanted pregnancy by providing education and contraception services and was not intended to provide services related to pregnancy options.

In 1992, congressional action loosened the gag rule and allowed for abortion options to be discussed between a client and her physician at Title X facilities. While this may appear to be a reasonable compromise, in reality most women who visit family planning clinics are served by a nurse or nurse-practitioner and never see a physician; therefore this change in the gag rule still did not permit the free exchange of information between clients and all professionals in the clinic. In 1993, President William Clinton signed a presidential memorandum to reverse the

gag rule
regulations that barred physicians and nurses in clinics receiving federal funds from counseling clients about abortions

Family planning agencies offer a range of services beyond contraception.

FIGURE 7.9

A significant proportion of women rely on family planning clinics for their reproductive health care.

Source: Alan Guttmacher Institute (2000). *Fulfilling the Promise: Public Policy and U.S. Family Planning Clinics.* New York: Author, 18. Reprinted with permission.

gag rule regulations. This change enabled Title X facilities to discuss abortion as an option to pregnancy. In 2003, President George W. Bush reimposed the gag rule to cover State Department family-planning grants. This tug-of-war over the gag rule is expected to continue.

Controversy regarding acceptable family planning methods is not new in our country. In the early 1900s, a maternity nurse by the name of Margaret Sanger delivered babies in the homes of poor, mostly immigrant women. She described her experiences by writing: "Tales were poured into my ears, a baby born dead, great relief, the death of an older child, sorrow but again relief of a sort, . . . the story told a thousand times of death and abortion and children going into institutions. I shuddered with horror as I listened to the details and studied the reasons in back of them—destitution with excessive childbearing. The waste of life seemed utterly senseless."[22]

The women Sanger cared for knew nothing of how to prevent pregnancy and because of the "Comstock Laws" they could get no information from their doctors. Sanger further explained her experiences by writing "I came to a sudden realization that my work as a nurse and my activities in social service were entirely palliative and consequently futile and useless to relieve the misery I saw all about me."[22] So, disheartened by her ability to care for them, she decided to try to prevent these unwanted conditions in the first place.

In 1914, Margaret Sanger, with the help of funds from numerous supporters worldwide, founded the National Birth Control League. The establishment of this organization is credited with starting the birth control movement in the United States. The purpose of this organization was to win greater public support for birth control by demonstrating the association between a woman's ability to limit her fertility and the improvement of both her health and the health of children. In addition, Sanger also challenged the morality of the times by declaring that women had the right to experience sexual pleasure and that freeing them from the fear of pregnancy would assist women in achieving this. In 1942, the National Birth Control League joined with hundreds of family planning clinics nationwide and formed the Planned Parenthood Federation of America.

Today, Planned Parenthood Federation of America, Inc., has grown to be the largest voluntary reproductive health care organization in the world and is still dedicated to the principle that every woman has the fundamental right to choose when or whether to have children.[23] Currently, Planned Parenthood operates nearly 900 health centers, which are located in every state and the District of Columbia. This not-for-profit organization serves nearly 5 million women and men each year.[23]

Evaluating the Success of Community Health Family Planning Programs

The establishment of local family planning clinics, many of which receive funding through Title X, has resulted in an improvement in maternal and child health indicators for the communities served.[21] Many people in need of family planning services are uninsured, and private health insurance usually does not provide coverage for contraceptive services. Title X funding enables for the support network of over 4,000 clinics that provide comprehensive family planning services to nearly 5 million women each year, 85% of whom are low income and a third of whom are adolescents. By providing access to contraceptive materials and instructions on how to use these materials effectively and counseling about reproductive health matters, community family planning clinics are able to show large reductions in unintended pregnancies, abortions, and births. Each year, publicly subsidized family planning services help prevent 1.3 million unplanned pregnancies, which would otherwise result in 632,300 abortions, 533,800 unintended births, and 165,000 miscarriages.[21]

Publicly funded family planning services are vital to enabling low-income women to avoid unintended pregnancy. From an economic perspective, each public health dollar spent by federal and state governments to provide family planning services saves $3 in Medicaid costs for pregnancy-related and newborn care.[24] The total annual savings is estimated at nearly $2 billion, which represents money currently being spent on welfare, medical, and nutritional services as required by law. A 2006 report projected that by expanding Medicaid eligibility for family planning services and providing new participants with family planning services and supplies, the programs would prevent between 375,000 and 723,000 unintended pregnancies—reducing the current national incidence of unintended pregnancy by between 20% and 39%.[25]

Abortion

One of the most important outcomes of community family planning programs is preventing abortions. Abortion has been legal throughout the United States since 1973 when the Supreme Court ruled in the ***Roe v. Wade*** case that women, in consultation with their physician, have a constitutionally protected right to have an abortion in the early stages of pregnancy free from government interference.[26] Since the early 1970s, the Centers for Disease Control and Prevention (CDC) has been documenting the number and characteristics of women obtaining legal induced abortions to monitor unintended pregnancy and to assist with efforts to identify and reduce preventable causes of morbidity and mortality associated with abortions.[27] As a result of the *Roe v. Wade* decision, the number of women dying from illegal abortions has diminished sharply during the last three decades in the United States. However, doubters remain, largely among those whose main strategy for reducing abortion is to outlaw it. However, while it may seem paradoxical, the legal status of abortion appears to have relatively little connection to its overall pervasiveness.

Starting in 1973, the number, ratio, and rate of legal abortions in the United States increased steadily until 1979 and remained stable in the 1980s and early 1990s; it has declined in most years thereafter (see Figure 7.10). In 2002, 854,122 abortions were reported.[27] According to the CDC, the overwhelming majority of all abortions were performed on unmarried mothers (82%), of whom 55% were white and approximately half (51%) were under age 25 (see Figure 7.11).

Roe v. Wade
a 1973 Supreme Court decision that made it unconstitutional for state laws to prohibit abortions

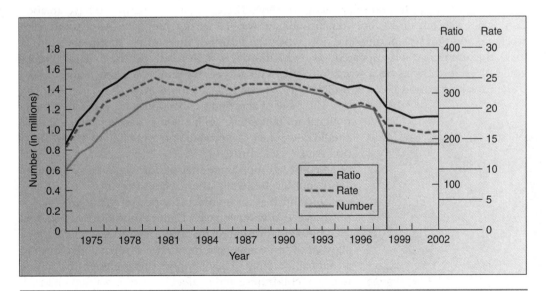

FIGURE 7.10

Number, ratio, and rate of legal abortions performed, by year: United States, 1973–2002.

Note: Ratio is calculated as number of abortions per 1,000 live births; rate is calculated as number of abortions per 1,000 women aged 15 to 44 years. For 1998-2002, data are from 48 reporting areas.

Source: Strauss, L.T., J. Herdon, J. Change, W. Parker, S. Bowens, and C. Berg (2005). "Abortion Surveillance—United States, 2002." *Morbidity and Mortality Weekly Report,* 54(SS 7): 1-15.

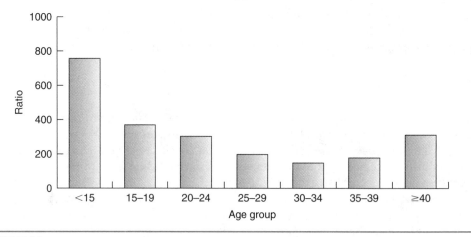

FIGURE 7.11

Abortion ratio, by age group of women who obtained a legal abortion in selected states: United States, 2002.

Note: Ratio is calculated as number of abortions per 1,000 live births. Data are from 46 states, the District of Columbia, and New York City.

Source: Strauss, L.T., J. Herdon, J. Change, W. Parker, S. Bowens, and C. Berg (2005). "Abortion Surveillance—United States, 2002." *Morbidity and Mortality Weekly Report*, 54(SS 7): 1–15.

pro-life
a medical/ethical position that holds that performing an abortion is an act of murder

pro-choice
a medical/ethical position that holds that women have a right to reproductive freedom

The fate of legalized abortion itself is as unclear as the right of a client to discuss abortion options in federally funded clinics. The Hyde Amendment of 1976 made it illegal to use federal funds to perform an abortion except in cases where the woman's life was in danger. In 1992, the Supreme Court was asked to rule on the constitutionality of the landmark court decision of *Roe v. Wade*. The *Roe v. Wade* Supreme Court ruling made it unconstitutional for state laws to prohibit abortions. In effect, this decision concluded that an unborn child is not a person and therefore has no rights under the law. The decision of whether to have an abortion or not was left up to the woman until she was 12 weeks' pregnant. After the twelfth week, an abortion was permissible only when the health of the mother was in question. In 1989, the Supreme Court appeared to reverse this decision. It ruled that the individual states could place restrictions on a woman's right to obtain an abortion. Some states now have a 24-hour waiting period after counseling before permitting an abortion.

The issue of abortion has become a hotly debated topic. Political appointments can be won or lost depending upon a candidate's stance as "pro-life" or "pro-choice" on the abortion issue (see Figure 7.12).

Pro-life groups argue that performing an abortion is an act of murder. Generally, they believe that life begins at conception and that an embryo is a person. The **pro-choice** position is that women have a right to reproductive freedom. Pro-choice advocates feel that the government should not be allowed to force a woman to carry to term and give birth to an unwanted child. They support this argument by raising issues of child abuse and neglect against unwanted children. To counter this argument, pro-life advocates support adoption as an alternative. Clearly, there is no easy solution to the question of abortion. The question of when life begins can only be decided by each individual based upon his or her own values and beliefs.[23]

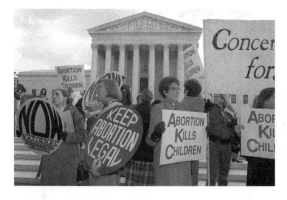

FIGURE 7.12

Political appointments and elections can be won or lost on the issue of abortion.

MATERNAL HEALTH

Maternal health encompasses the health of women in the childbearing years, including those in the pre-pregnancy period, those who are pregnant, and those who are caring for young children (see Figure 7.13). The effect of pregnancy and childbirth on women is an important indicator of their health. Pregnancy and delivery can lead to serious health problems. Maternal mortality rates are the most severe measure of ill health for pregnant women.

The Tenth Revision of the *International Classification of Diseases* (ICD 10) defines a *maternal death* (maternal mortality) as "the death of a women while pregnant or within 42 days of termination of pregnancy, irrespective of the duration and site of the pregnancy, from any cause related to or aggravated by the pregnancy or its management but not from accidental or incidental causes."[28] The *maternal mortality rate* is the number of mothers dying per 100,000 live births in a given year. The number of live births is used in the denominator because the total number of pregnant women is unknown.

In the United States, two to three women die of pregnancy-related complications every day. Between 1970 and 1982, maternal mortality decreased from 21.5 deaths per 100,000 live births to 9.1 deaths per 100,000 live births, more than a 50% decline (see Figure 7.3). However, since 1982 the risk of dying has remained relatively stable, and there has been no marked decrease since that time. This is disturbing because many studies indicate that as many as half of all maternal deaths could be prevented if women had better access to health care and better quality of care, and made changes in health and lifestyle habits. The five leading causes of maternal deaths are hemorrhage, embolism, pregnancy-induced hypertension, sepsis/infection, and anesthesia-related complications.

Additionally, the gap between rates for black and white women remains, with black women being four times more likely than white women to die from pregnancy and its complications. Ensuring early initiation of prenatal care during maternity greatly contributes to reductions in perinatal illness, disability, and death for both the mother and the infant.[29] In addition, a number of underlying causes of high maternal morbidity and mortality rates include poverty, the sociocultural factor, and a limited education.

prenatal health care
medical care provided to a pregnant woman from the time of conception until the birth process occurs

Prenatal Health Care

High-quality **prenatal health care** is one of the fundamentals of a safe motherhood program and includes three major components—risk assessment, treatment for medical conditions or risk reduction, and education.[12,29] Prenatal health care should begin before pregnancy when a couple is considering having a child, and it should continue throughout pregnancy (see Box 7.3). The goals of prenatal care include providing the best care for the pregnant woman and the unborn child, as well as preparing the mother-to-be for the delivery of a healthy baby. During prenatal visits, tests are performed on both the mother and fetus to assess any potential risks, to treat any maternal or fetal complications, and to monitor the growth and development of the fetus. In addition, counseling and guidance are provided regarding the various aspects of pregnancy, including weight gain, exercise, nutrition, and overall health.

Prenatal care is crucial to maternal and infant health. Women who receive early and continuous prenatal health care have better pregnancy outcomes than women who do not. A pregnant woman who receives no prenatal care is

FIGURE 7.13
Maternal health encompasses the health of women in the childbearing years.

OPPORTUNITIES TO REDUCE MATERNAL AND INFANT MORTALITY

Prevention measures that reduce maternal and infant mortality and promote the health of all childbearing women and their newborns should start before conception and continue through the postpartum period. Some of these prevention measures include the following.

Before Conception

- Screen women for health risks and pre-existing chronic conditions such as diabetes, hypertension, and sexually transmitted diseases.
- Counsel women about contraception and provide access to effective family planning services (to prevent unintended pregnancies and unnecessary abortions).
- Counsel women about the benefits of good nutrition; encourage women especially to consume adequate amounts of folic acid supplements (to prevent neural tube defects) and iron.
- Advise women to avoid alcohol, tobacco, and illicit drugs.
- Advise women about the value of regular physical exercise.

During Pregnancy

- Provide women with early access to high-quality care throughout the phases of pregnancy, labor, and delivery. Such care includes risk-appropriate care, treatment for complications, and use of antenatal corticosteroids when appropriate.

- Monitor and, when appropriate, treat pre-existing chronic conditions.
- Screen for and, when appropriate, treat reproductive tract infections, including bacterial vaginosis, group B streptococcus, and human immunodeficiency virus.
- Vaccinate women against influenza, if appropriate.
- Continue counseling against use of alcohol, tobacco, and illicit drugs.
- Continue counseling about nutrition and physical exercise.
- Educate women about the early signs of pregnancy-related problems.

During Postpartum Period

- Vaccinate newborns at age-appropriate times.
- Provide information about well-baby care and the benefits of breastfeeding.
- Warn parents about exposing infants to secondhand smoke.
- Counsel parents about placing infants to sleep on their backs.
- Educate parents about how to protect their infants from exposure to infectious diseases and harmful substances.

Source: Centers for Disease Control and Prevention. Available at http://www.cdc.gov/phtn/tenachievements/mothers1/mb1.htm.

---

low-birth-weight infant one that weighs less than 2,500 grams, or 5.5 pounds, at birth

three times as likely to give birth to a **low-birth-weight infant** (one that weighs less than 5.5 pounds or 2,500 grams) as one who receives the appropriate care, and she is four times as likely to have her baby die in infancy. Getting pregnant women into prenatal care early (during the first three months of pregnancy) is the main policy goal of most publicly funded programs designed to reduce the incidence of low birth weight and infant mortality in the United States. The percentage of women receiving prenatal care during the first trimester was 84.1% in 2003, a slight increase from the 2002 rate of 83.7%, demonstrating a continuing general upward trend toward the *Healthy People 2010* goal of 90%. Non-Hispanic black, Hispanic, and American Indian/Alaska Native women were 2.5 to 3.5 times more likely to begin care late or to receive no prenatal care at all in 2003 (see Figure 7.14). Black, Native American, Hispanic, poorly educated women, and those most likely to be poor and without health insurance are significantly less likely to receive early and comprehensive prenatal care.[29]

INFANT HEALTH

An infant's health depends upon many factors, which include the mother's health and her health behavior prior to and during pregnancy, her level of prenatal care, the quality of her delivery, and the infant's environment after birth. The infant's environment includes not only the home and family environment, but also the availability of essential medical services such as a postnatal physical examination by a *neonatologist* (a medical doctor who specializes in

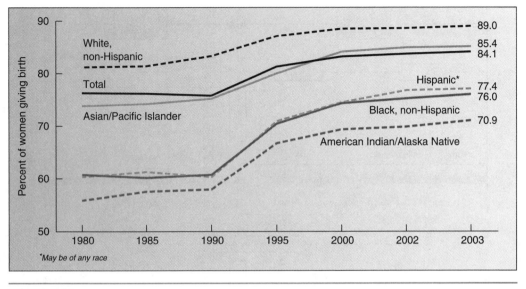

FIGURE 7.14

Mothers beginning prenatal care in the first trimester, by race/ethnicity, 1980–2003. (2003 data are preliminary.)

Source: Centers for Disease Control and Prevention, National Center for Health Statistics, National Vital Statistics System.

the care of newborn children up to 2 months of age), regular visits to a physician, and the appropriate immunizations. The infant's health also depends on proper nutrition and other nurturing care in the home environment. Shortcomings in these areas can result in illness, developmental problems, and even the death of the child.

Infant Mortality

Infant death is an important measure of a nation's health because it is associated with a variety of factors, such as maternal health, quality of access to medical care, socioeconomic conditions, and public health practices.[12] An *infant death* (infant mortality) is the death of a child younger than 1 year (see Figure 7.15). The *infant mortality rate* is expressed as the number of deaths of children younger than 1 year per 1,000 live births.

The infant mortality rate gradually declined from 1980 to 2000 (see Figure 7.2). Decreases in the infant mortality rate during this period have been attributed to improved disease surveillance, advanced clinical care, improved access to health care, better nutrition, the recommendation that infants be placed on their backs when sleeping, and increased educational levels.[12] Since 2000, the infant mortality rate in the United States has shown no further significant decline, maintaining a rate of between 6.8 and 7.0 deaths per 1,000 live births (see Figure 7.2).[30] This is unfortunate, because many of the causes of infant deaths could be eliminated by modifying the behaviors, lifestyles, and conditions that affect birth outcomes, such as smoking, substance abuse, poor nutrition, lack of prenatal care, medical problems, and chronic illness.

The leading causes of infant death include congenital abnormalities, preterm/low birth weight, sudden infant death syndrome (SIDS), problems related to complications of pregnancy, and respiratory distress syndrome.[30]

Infant deaths, or infant mortality, can be further divided into neonatal mortality and postneonatal mortality (see Figure 7.15). *Neonatal mortality* is deaths that occur during the first 28 days after birth. Approximately two-thirds of all infant deaths take place during this period. The most common causes of neonatal death are disorders related to short gestation (premature births) and low birth weight, and congenital birth defects. These causes currently account for

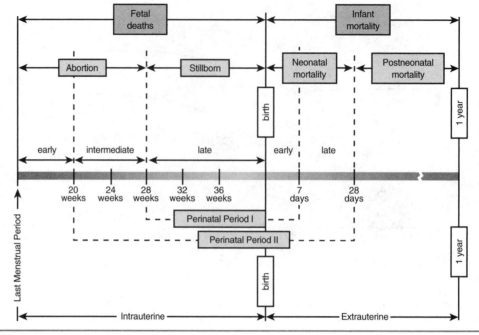

FIGURE 7.15
Important early-life mortality time periods.

approximately one-half of all neonatal deaths. *Postneonatal mortality* is deaths that occur between 28 days and 365 days after birth. The most common causes of postneonatal deaths are sudden infant death syndrome and congenital birth defects.

Improving Infant Health

Due in part to medical research and public health and social services supported by both public and private organizations, infant mortality has declined considerably during the past couple of decades. However, there are many opportunities for decreasing infant deaths and improving infant health even further through reducing risk factors associated with these conditions.

Premature Births

Premature (or preterm) babies are born prior to 37 weeks' gestation. The average length of gestation is 40 weeks, and normal is considered 38 to 42 weeks. The number of babies born prematurely in the United States has been rising steadily since 1981, and in 2005 reached 12.5%, representing one in eight babies being born prematurely.[31] Disorders related to short gestation and low birth weight are the leading causes of neonatal death in the United States. Since premature babies usually have less developed organs than full-term babies, they are more likely to face serious multiple health problems following delivery. Premature babies often require neonatal intensive care, which utilizes specialized medical personnel and equipment. In 2005, the economic burden of preterm births was $26.2 billion, or $51,600 per infant. The majority of the expense was for medical care provided in infancy. Other factors that contribute to the economic burden are maternal care services, early intervention services, special education for preterm infants with learning difficulties, and lost labor productivity.[31,32]

Approximately half of all premature births have no known cause. Known major risk factors associated with preterm labor and birth include a woman's past history of preterm delivery, multiple fetuses, late or no prenatal care, cigarette smoking, drinking alcohol, using illegal drugs, exposure to domestic violence, lack of social support, low income, diabetes, anemia, high blood pressure, obesity, and women younger than 17 or older than 35.[31]

Therefore, although a number of causes of premature birth may have eluded researchers and are currently beyond our control, prenatal care and lifestyle changes can help women reduce their risk of having a premature delivery. Consequently, there is a lot that community health programs can do to assist a woman in reducing her risk of having a premature baby— specifically, educating parents about premature labor and what can be done to prevent it and expanding access to health care coverage so that more women can get prenatal care.

Low Birth Weight

Today, it is widely accepted that low birth weight (LBW) is the single most important factor in neonatal death, as well as being a significant predictor of postneonatal mortality and infant and later childhood morbidity. Most infants weigh 3,400 grams (7 pounds) at birth. LBW infants are those that weigh 2,500 grams, or about 5.5 pounds. LBW infants are 40 times more likely to die in their first year of life than normal-weight babies. LBW babies often require extensive medical attention early in life and subsequently may suffer from a variety of physical, emotional, and intellectual problems. LBW babies have a higher incidence of cerebral palsy, deafness, blindness, epilepsy, chronic lung disease, learning disabilities, and attention deficit disorder.[33]

The percentage of U.S. infants born at LBW has remained relatively stable (between 7.0% and 8.0%) in the last two decades (see Figure 7.16). LBW must continually be aggressively targeted, especially among various racial/ethnic groups, because significant differences exist among these groups (see Chapter 10).

The two factors that are generally recognized to govern infant birth weight are the duration of gestation (premature births) and intrauterine growth rate. Approximately two-thirds of

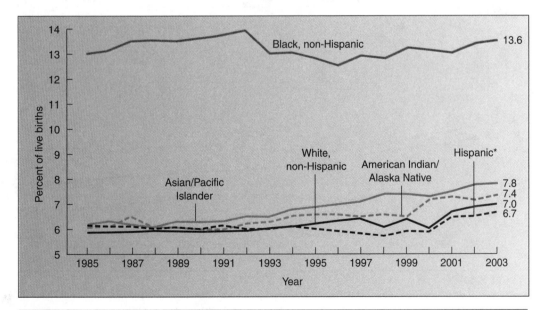

FIGURE 7.16

Percentage of infants born at low birth weight by race/ethnicity, 1985–2003.

*Persons of Hispanic origin may be of any race.

Note: 1985–1988 data are based on race of child; data after 1989 are based on race of mother.

Source: National Center for Health Statistics.

LBW infants are born premature. Therefore, reduction in premature births holds the most potential for overall reduction in LBW. Research on the causes of intrauterine growth retardation (IUGR) leading to LBW babies finds that maternal cigarette smoking during pregnancy is by far the most important risk factor. Other maternal characteristics that are risk factors connected with IUGR include maternal LBW, prior LBW history, low pre-pregnancy weight, drinking alcohol, multiple births, and low pregnancy weight gain.[12] Therefore, all pregnant women should (1) get early, regular prenatal care; (2) eat a balanced diet, including adequate amounts of folic acid; (3) gain enough weight; and (4) avoid smoking and drinking alcohol.[34]

Cigarette Smoking

Research has shown that maternal cigarette smoking during pregnancy is the leading modifiable cause of LBW in the United States, therefore making it an ideal target for intervention. Researchers estimate that smoking during pregnancy is linked to 20% to 30% of LBW infants and 10% of infant deaths.[35] The incidence of LBW infants among mothers who smoke is more than twice that of nonsmokers. The good news is that the percentage of births to women who smoked during pregnancy has been dropping, from 19.5% in 1989 to 10.7% in 2003 (see Figure 7.17). This would seem to indicate that the United States is definitely progressing in the right direction when it comes to reaching its goal of 99% reduction for 2010.

Alcohol and Other Drugs

Prenatal exposure to alcohol can cause a range of disorders, known as fetal alcohol spectrum disorders (FASDs). FASD refers to conditions such as **fetal alcohol syndrome (FAS)**, fetal alchohol effects (FAE), alcohol-related neurodevelopmental disorder (ARND), and alcohol-related birth defects (ARBD) (See Chapter 12). A safe level of alcohol consumption during

fetal alcohol syndrome (FAS) a group of abnormalities that may include growth retardation, abnormal appearance of face and head, and deficits of central nervous system function, including mental retardation, in babies born to mothers who have consumed heavy amounts of alcohol during their pregnancies

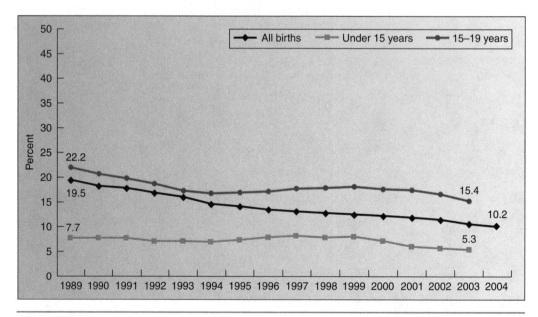

FIGURE 7.17

Percentage of total births to women who smoked during pregnancy, by age of mother, 1989–2004.

Sources: Data for 1970-1999: Eberhardt, M. S., D. D. Ingram, D. M. Makuc, et al. (2001). *Urban and Rural Health Chartbook: Health, United States, 2001.* Hyattsville, MD: National Center for Health Statistics. Data for 2000–2001: National Center for Health Statistics (2003). *Health, United States 2003 with Chartbook on Trends in the Health of Americans.* Hyattsville, MD: Author. Data for 2002: Martin, J. A., P. E. Hamilton, P. D. Sutton, et al. (2003). "Births: Final Data for 2002." *National Vital Statistics Reports,* 52(10). Data for 2004: Hamilton, B. E., J. A. Martin, S. J. Ventura, P. D. Sutton, and F. Menacker (2006). "Births: Preliminary Data for 2004." *National Vital Statistics Reports,* 54(8).

pregnancy has not been determined, but adverse effects are associated with heavy consumption during the first few months of pregnancy.[35] In general, no alcohol during pregnancy is strongly recommended.

Other drug use can also result in a number of deleterious effects on the developing fetus, including impaired fetal growth, that can lead to congenital defects. Crack cocaine use during pregnancy can result in genital and urinary tract malformations in the baby. Marijuana use has also been associated with an increased risk of birth defects. A study showed that infants born to women using marijuana and/or cocaine were significantly smaller than infants of nonusers. Marijuana's effect of increasing maternal heart rate, blood pressure, and carbon monoxide levels may be responsible for impairing the growth of the fetus. Maternal use of cocaine results in lower fetal oxygen levels by inducing uterine contractions.[35]

Breastfeeding

The American Academy of Pediatrics recommends that babies be breast-fed for the first year of life. Breast milk is the ideal food for babies, newborn through 4 to 6 months. Breastfeeding has many advantages for both baby and mother. Breast milk contains substances that help babies resist infections and other diseases. Breast-fed babies have fewer ear infections and colds, less diarrhea, and vomit less often. In addition, breastfeeding has been shown to improve maternal health by reducing postpartum bleeding, allowing for an earlier return to prepregnancy weight and reducing the risk of osteoporosis.[12]

Breastfeeding rates for women of all races have increased in the last decade (see Figure 7.18 and Box 7.4). Breastfeeding rates were highest among women 35 years and older, those who are college educated, and women participating in the Women, Infants, and Children (WIC) dietary supplemental program. Women least likely to breastfeed were those younger than 20 years of age, those not employed, those with low income, and those who were

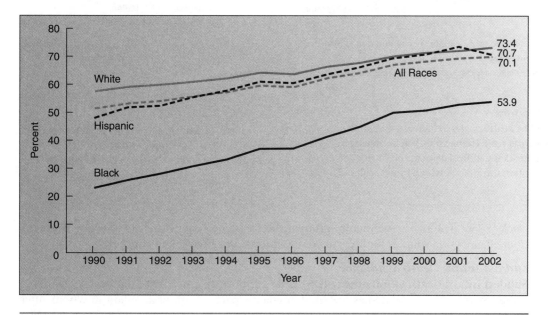

FIGURE 7.18

In-hospital breastfeeding, by race/ethnicity, 1990–2003.

Sources: U.S. Department of Health and Human Services, Health Resources and Services Administration, Maternal and Child Health Bureau. *Women's Health USA 2005.* Rockville, Maryland: U.S. Department of Health and Human Services, 2005; and *Years 1991-1998: Breast Feeding Trends 1998 (1999). Mother's Survey, Years 1999-2003: Unpublished Data.* Ross Products Division. Abbott Laboratories.

BOX
7.4

HEALTHY PEOPLE 2010: OBJECTIVES

Objective 16.19: Increase the proportion of mothers who breastfeed their babies.

Target and baseline:

Objective	Increase in Mothers Who Breastfeed	1998 Baseline	2004 Status	2010 Target
			Percent	
16.19a	In early postpartum period	64	71	75
16.19b	At 6 months	29	36	50
16.19c	At 1 year	16	21	25

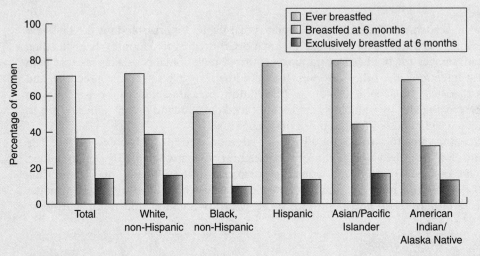

Breastfeeding by race/ethnicity and duration, 2003.

*Persons of Hispanic origin may be of any race.

Source: Centers for Disease Control and Prevention, National Immunization Survey.

For Further Thought

An important public health goal is to increase the number of mothers who breastfeed. Human milk is acknowledged by the American Academy of Pediatrics as the most complete form of nutrition for infants, with a broad realm of benefits for infants' growth and development. What types of programs would you recommend to educate new mothers and their partners and to educate health care providers?

black.[12] Two voluntary community groups, the La Leche League and the Nursing Mother's Council, are good sources for breastfeeding information, advice, and support.

Sudden Infant Death Syndrome

sudden infant death syndrome (SIDS)
sudden unanticipated death of an infant in whom, after examination, there is no recognized cause of death

Sudden infant death syndrome (SIDS) strikes approximately 2,200 babies each year in the United States. SIDS is defined as the sudden unanticipated death of an infant in whom, after examination, there is no recognizable cause of death. Because most cases of SIDS occur when a baby is sleeping in a crib, SIDS has been referred to as *crib death*. SIDS is the third leading cause of infant death. Moreover, after the first month of life, it is the leading cause of infant death (postneonatal mortality), accounting for one-third of deaths during the period.[12,36]

There is currently no way of predicting which infants will die due to SIDS. However, research has shown that sleeping on the side or back rather than the stomach greatly

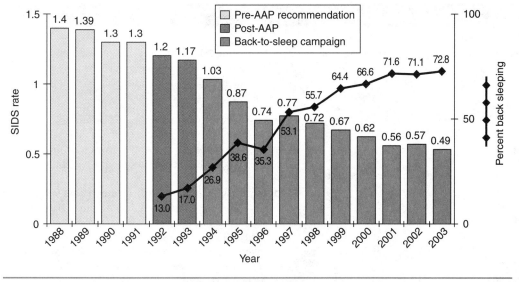

FIGURE 7.19

Rate of sudden infant death syndrome and sleep position: 1988–2003.

Source: National Center for Health Statistics.

decreases the risk of SIDS among healthy full-term infants.[37] In response to this research, the federal government initiated a national "Back to Sleep" campaign in 1992 to educate parents and health professionals with the message that placing babies on their backs or sides to sleep can reduce the risk of SIDS. Since the dissemination of the recommendation, more infants have been put to bed on their backs and sides, and the rate of SIDS has fallen by more than 50% (see Figure 7.19).

CHILD HEALTH

Good health during the childhood years (ages 1–14) is essential to each child's optimal development and America's future. America cannot hope for every child to become a productive member of society if children in this country are allowed to grow up with poverty or live in a violent environment, with mediocre child care, or with no health insurance. Failure to provide timely and remedial care leads to unnecessary illness, disability, and death—events that are associated with much greater costs than the timely care itself. The previous example of the cost of not providing prenatal care given earlier in this chapter presents a vivid example. For those who believe that access to basic care is a standard of justness and fairness in any socialized society, America lingers sadly behind many other nations in the health of her children (see Box 7.5).[38]

Childhood Mortality

Childhood mortality rates are the most severe measure of health in children. The death of a child is an enormous tragedy for family and friends, as well as a loss to the community. As mentioned in the introduction of this chapter, the mortality rates of children have generally declined over the past couple of decades (see Figures 7.5 and 7.6). Unintentional injuries are the leading cause of mortality in children (see Figure 7.20). In fact, unintentional injuries kill more children than all diseases combined. The overwhelming majority of unintentional injury

BOX
7.5

WHERE AMERICA STANDS

Among industrialized nations, the United States ranks:

1st in military technology
1st in military exports
1st in gross domestic product
1st in the number of millionaires and billionaires
1st in health technology
1st in defense expenditures
12th in living standards among our poorest one-fifth of children
13th in the gap between rich and poor children
14th in efforts to lift children out of poverty
16th in low-birth-weight rates
18th in the percent of children in poverty
23rd in infant mortality
Last in protecting our children against gun violence

According to the Centers for Disease Control and Prevention, U.S. children under age 15 are

9 times more likely to die in firearm accident
11 times more likely to commit suicide with a gun
12 times more likely to die from gunfire
16 times more likely to be murdered with a gun than children in 25 other industrialized countries combined

Of all the members of the United Nations, the United States of America and Somalia (which has no legally constituted government) are the only two nations that have failed to ratify the U.N. convention on the Rights of the Child.

Black infant mortality rates in our nation's capital exceed those in 50 nations, including Bahamas, Barbados, Cuba, Dominica, and Oman.

In UNICEF's 2004 *State of the World's Children*, the U.S. ranked lower on maternal mortality than 32 other countries (140 of 172), including Ghana, Lithuania, Croatia, and Syria. We lagged behind 33 other nations (160 of 193) on infant mortality rank.

Source: Children's Defense Fund (2004). *The State of America's Children Yearbook 2004.* Reprinted with permission.

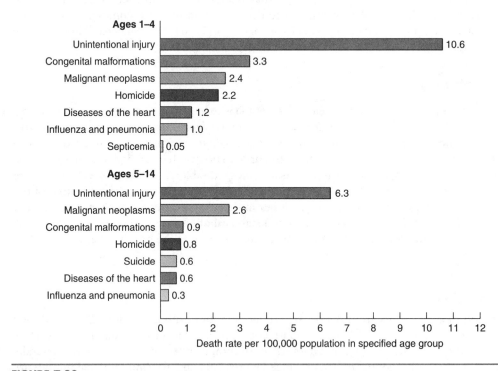

FIGURE 7.20
Leading causes of death in children aged 1 to 14: 2003.
Source: National Center for Health Statistics.

deaths in children are due to motor vehicle crashes. Moreover, the majority of children were not wearing a seatbelt or other restraint.[38] All 50 states have primary child restraint laws. They allow law enforcement officers to stop a driver if a child is not restrained according to the state law. However, the provisions of these laws vary from state to state.

Childhood Morbidity

Although childhood for many children represents a time of relatively good overall health, it is a time when far too many suffer from acute illness, chronic disease, and disabilities. Morbidity statistics on children are more difficult to calculate because they consist of a variety of perspectives. These include unintentional injuries, child maltreatment, and infectious diseases.

Unintentional Injuries

The United States needs to do a better job of protecting its children from unintentional injuries. Even though unintentional injuries are the leading cause of death among children, deaths are a rare event. However, injury-related morbidity is much more prevalent among children (see Figure 7.21). For each childhood death by injury, there are approximately 40 hospitalizations and 1,000 emergency department visits.[39] Every year about one-fourth of all children sustain an injury severe enough to require medical attention, missed school, or bed rest. Moreover, injuries are the leading cause of disability in children, with approximately 100,000 children becoming permanently disabled annually.[39]

In addition to the physical and emotional effects on children and their families, these injuries have enormous financial costs. Injuries requiring medical attention or resulting in restricted activity cost $17 billion annually for medical treatment.[40] Estimates are that 90% of the more than 4,000 unintentional injuries suffered by children each day in a manner seriously enough to require medical treatment could be prevented. Childhood injuries can deprive the country of the child's potential contributions. The injuries incurred in 2000 by children aged 14 and younger will have lasting effects, including total lifetime economic costs of more than $50 billion in medical expenses and lost productivity.[40] (Unintentional injuries are discussed in more detail in Chapter 17.)

Child Maltreatment

Child maltreatment is another source of injury to children. Child maltreatment includes physical abuse, neglect (physical, educational, emotional, and/or medical), sexual abuse, emotional abuse (psychological/verbal abuse and/or mental injury), and other types of maltreatment such as abandonment, exploitation, and/or threats to harm the child. The causes of child maltreatment are not well understood. Child abuse or neglect is often associated with physical injuries and delayed physical growth. However child abuse and neglect is also associated with psychological problems such as aggression and depression. The rate of children maltreated annually has remained between 12 and 15 per 1,000 children over the past decade (see Table 7.1).[41]

The oldest federal agency for children, the Children's Bureau (CB), located in the Administration for Children and Families, has worked to lead the public in taking a more informed and active part in child abuse prevention. The CB has been instrumental in defining the scope of the problem of child maltreatment and in promoting community responsibility for child protection. The CB believes that parents have a right to raise their children as long as they are willing to

FIGURE 7.21
Unintentional injuries are the leading cause of childhood morbidity and mortality.

Table 7.1
Percentage of Children Who Are Victims of Child Maltreatment, and Distribution by Gender, Age, Race, and Hispanic Origin, and Type of Maltreatment, 1990–2004

	1990	1991	1992	1993	1994	1995	1996	1997	1998	1999	2000	2001	2002	2003	2004
Number of victims*	860,577	911,690	994,655	1,026,331	1,032,000	1,005,511	1,011,973	956,711	904,000	829,000	881,000	903,000	896,000	906,000	872,088
Rate per 1,000	13.4	14.0	15.1	15.3	15.2	14.7	14.7	13.8	12.9	11.8	12.2	12.4	12.3	12.4	11.9
Gender (as % of all victims)															
Male	44	45	45	41	41	40	39	40	48	48	48	48	48	48	48
Female	50	52	51	47	46	45	43	44	52	52	52	52	52	52	52
Age of victim (as % of all victims)															
1 year and younger	13	14	13	12	12	11	11	11	14	14	15	16	16	16	17
2–5 years old	24	25	25	23	23	23	22	21	25	24	24	24	24	25	25
6–9 years old	22	23	23	21	20	21	21	21	25	25	24	24	23	23	22
10–13 years old	19	20	19	18	17	17	16	17	20	20	20	21	21	21	20
14–17 years old	14	15	15	14	13	13	13	12	15	15	15	15	15	15	16
18 and older	1	1	1	1	1	1	1	0	1	1	0	0	0	0	0
Type of maltreatment (as % of all victims)															
Neglect	49	46	50	49	52	52	52	55	54	56	60	57	59	61	62
Physical abuse	27	26	23	24	24	24	24	24	23	21	19	19	19	19	18
Sexual abuse	17	16	14	14	14	13	12	12	12	11	10	10	10	10	10
Psychological or emotional abuse	7	6	5	5	5	4	6	6	6	8	8	7	7	5	7
Medical neglect	0	2	3	2	2	3	3	2	2	2	3	2	2	2	2
Other and unknown	10	13	21	17	16	17	19	12	26	28	17	20	19	17	15

*Indicated is a type of investigation disposition that concludes the allegation of maltreatment or risk of maltreatment was supported or founded by state law or state policy and is the highest level of finding by a state agency. Indicated or reason to suspect is an investigation that cannot be substantiated, but there is a reason to suspect that the child may have been maltreated or was at risk of maltreatment. This is applicable only to states that distinguish between substantiated and indicated dispositions. All percentages reported here are based on reporting states; no estimates were made unless otherwise noted.

Sources: Rate per 1,000 for 1990–1999 and number of victims for 1994, 1998, 1999, and 2000: U.S. Department of Health and Human Services, Administration on Children, Youth, and Families. *Child Maltreatment 1999.* Population estimates for 1999: Population Estimates Program, Population Division, U.S. Census Bureau. Internet release date: April 11, 2000. All other estimates for 1990–1999 except rate per 1,000: Trends in the Well-Being of America's Children and Youth 2001. Table HC 2.10 U.S. Department of Health and Human Services. Office of the Assistant Secretary for Planning and Evaluation. Data for 2000: U.S. Department of Health and Human Services, Administration on Children, Youth and Families. *Child Maltreatment 2000* (Washington, DC: U.S. Government Printing Office, 2002). Data for 2001: U.S. Department of Health and Human Services, Administration on Children, Youth and Families. *Child Maltreatment 2001* (Washington, DC: U.S. Government Printing Office, 2003). Population estimates for 2000 and 2001 from original analysis by Child Trends of Bridged Race 2000 and 2001 Population Estimates for Calculating Vital Rates, National Center for Health Statistics, Centers for Disease Control and Prevention, 2003. http://www.cdc.gov/nchs/about/major/dvs/popbridge/popbridge.htm. Data for 2002: U.S. Department of Health and Human Services, Administration on Children, Youth and Families. *Child Maltreatment 2002* (Washington, DC: U.S. Government Printing Office, 2004). Data for 2003: U.S. Department of Health and Human Services, Administration on Children, Youth and Families. *Child Maltreatment 2003* (Washington, DC: U.S. Government Printing Office, 2005). Data for 2004: U.S. Department of Health and Human Services, Administration on Children, Youth and Families. *Child Maltreatment 2004* (Washington, DC: U.S. Government Printing Office, 2006).

protect them. When parents cannot meet their children's needs and keep them from harm, the community has a responsibility to act on behalf of the child. If one suspects a child is being abused or neglected, it is important to call the proper authorities. Any action into the family life should be guided by federal and state laws. According to the CB, the community's responsibility for child protection is based on the following:[42]

- Communities should develop and implement programs to strengthen families and prevent the likelihood of child abuse and neglect.
- Child maltreatment is a community problem; no single agency or individual has the necessary knowledge, skills, resources, or societal mandate to provide the assistance to abused and neglected children and their families.
- Intervention must be sensitive to culture, values, religion, and other differences.
- Professionals must recognize that most parents do not intend to harm their children. Rather, abuse and neglect may be the result of a combination of psychological, social, situational, and societal factors.
- Service providers should recognize that many maltreating adults have the capacity to change their abusive/neglectful behavior, when given sufficient help and resources to do so.
- To help families protect their children and meet their basic needs, the community's response should be nonpunitive, noncritical, and conducted in the least intrusive manner possible.
- Growing up in their own family is optimal for children, as long as the children's safety can be assured.
- When parents cannot or will not meet their child's needs, removal from the home may be necessary. All efforts to develop a permanent plan for a child should be made as quickly as possible.[42]

See Chapter 17 for more detailed information on child abuse and neglect.

Infectious Diseases

In the past, infectious diseases were the leading health concern among children, but increased public health action has resulted in a substantial reduction in both morbidity and mortality rates. Infectious disease control resulted from improvements in sanitation and hygiene and the implementation of universal vaccination programs. Because many vaccine-preventable diseases are more common and more deadly among infants and children, the CDC recommends vaccinating children against most vaccine-preventable diseases early in life. The 2007 recommended immunization schedule is shown in Figure 7.22.

The CDC's immunization schedule for very young children recommends four doses of the diphtheria, tetanus, and pertussis (DTP) vaccine, three or more doses of polio vaccine, one or more doses of measles-mumps-rubella (MMR) vaccine, three or more doses of *Haemophilus influenzae* type b (Hib) vaccine, the hepatitis B vaccine, and the varicella (chickenpox) vaccine. The combined immunization series is referred to as the 4:3:1:3 series. Immunization rates are considered an important indicator of the adequacy of health care for children and of the level of protection a community values related to preventable infectious diseases. The proportion of children aged 19 months to 35 months receiving the recommended combined series has increased from 69% in 1994 to 83% in 2004 (see Figure 7.23).

All children should be immunized at regular health care visits, beginning at birth and continuing to age 6.[43] By immunizing, the community safeguards its children against the potentially devastating effects of vaccine-preventable diseases. No child should ever have to endure the effects of these diseases simply because he or she was not vaccinated on time.

Vaccine ▼ Age ▶	Birth	1 month	2 months	4 months	6 months	12 months	15 months	18 months	19–23 months	2–3 years	4–6 years
Hepatitis B	HepB	HepB			HepB					HepB Series	
Rotavirus			Rota	Rota	Rota						
Diphtheria, Tetanus, Pertussis			DTaP	DTaP	DTaP		DTaP				DTaP
Haemophilus influenzae type b			Hib	Hib	*Hib*	Hib	Hib				
Pneumococcal			PCV	PCV	PCV	PCV				PCV / PPV	
Inactivated Poliovirus			IPV	IPV	IPV						IPV
Influenza					Influenza (Yearly)						
Measles, Mumps, Rubella						MMR					MMR
Varicella						Varicella					Varicella
Hepatitis A						HepA (2 doses)				HepA Series	
Meningococcal										MPSV4	

Range of recommended ages
Catch-up immunization
Certain high-risk groups

FIGURE 7.22

Recommended 2007 immunization schedule for ages 0–6 years: United States, 2007.

Source: Centers for Disease Control and Prevention, National Immunization Program (2006).

Although progress in improving immunization rates has been substantial, about 1 million children in the United States under 2 years of age have not been fully vaccinated with the most critical vaccines. In addition, the National Immunization Survey data showed considerable variation between states and urban areas, indicating that children are not equally well protected in all parts of the United States. This large number of unvaccinated children has been attributed to cost, lack of access to medical care, uneducated parents, and confusion on when to vaccinate children. The U.S. government's Childhood Immunization Initiative includes five strategies: (1) improving immunization services for needy families, especially in public health clinics; (2) reducing vaccine costs for lower-income and uninsured families, especially for vaccines provided in private physicians' offices; (3) building community networks to reach out to families and ensure that young children are vaccinated as needed; (4) improving systems for monitoring diseases and vaccinations; and (5) improving vaccines and vaccine use.[43]

More stringent measures by the medical community are needed to ensure that all children are immunized. Opportunities to vaccinate are frequently missed by health care practitioners in primary care settings that do not routinely inquire about the immunization status of the child. Parents and health practitioners need to work together to ensure that youth are protected from communicable diseases. Timely immunization of children must be accepted as a national obligation because America cannot afford the waste that results from unnecessary illness, disability, and death.[43]

FIGURE 7.23

Percentage of children aged 19 to 35 months receiving the combined series vaccination (4:3:1:3), 1994–2004.

Sources: Data for 1994: Eberhardt, M. S., D. D. Ingram, D. M. Makuc, et al. (2001). *Urban and Rural Health Chartbook: Health, United States, 2001.* Hyattsville, MD: National Center for Health Statistics. Data for 1995–2001: National Center for Health Statistics (2003). *Health, United States 2003 with Chartbook on Trends in the Health of Americans.* Hyattsville, MD: Author. Data for 2002: National Immunization Program (2003). *Immunization Coverage in the U.S.* Results from National Immunization Survey, Centers for Disease Control and Prevention.

COMMUNITY PROGRAMS FOR WOMEN, INFANTS, AND CHILDREN

In the preceding pages, many problems associated with maternal, infant, and child health have been identified. Solutions to many of these problems have been proposed, and in many cases programs are already in place. Some of these programs are aimed at preventing or reducing the levels of maternal and infant morbidity and mortality, whereas others are aimed at the prevention or reduction of childhood morbidity and mortality.

The federal government has over 35 health programs in 16 different agencies to serve the needs of our nation's children. The majority of these programs are well respected and help meet the needs of many children. However, others are **categorical programs,** meaning they are only available to people who can be categorized into a specific group based on disease, age, family means, geography, financial need, or other variables. This means that too many children fall through the cracks and are not served. Some children require services from multiple programs, which complicates the eligibility determination of each child. At times, this can lead to an inefficient system of child health care. Nonetheless, federal programs have contributed to a monumental improvement in maternal, infant, and child health. We discuss some of the more consequential government programs and their past successes and future objectives in the following text.

categorical programs programs available only to people who can be categorized into a group based on specific variables

Maternal and Child Health Bureau

In 1935, Congress enacted Title V of the Social Security Act. Title V is the only federal legislation dedicated to promoting and improving the health of our nation's mothers and children. Since its enactment, Title V-sponsored projects have been incorporated into the ongoing health care system for children and families. Although Title V has been frequently modified over the last couple of decades, the fundamental goal has remained constant: continued progress in the health, safety, and well-being of mothers and children. The most notable landmark achievements of Title V are projects that have produced "guidelines for child health supervision from infancy through adolescence; influenced the nature of nutrition care during pregnancy and lactation; recommended standards for prenatal care; identified successful strategies for the prevention of childhood injuries; and developed health safety standards for out-of-home child care facilities."[44]

In 1990, the Maternal and Child Health Bureau (MCHB) was established as part of the Health Resources and Services Administration in the Department of Health and Human Services to administer Title V funding. This means the MCHB is charged with the responsibility for promoting and improving the health of our nation's mothers and children. MCHB's mission "is to provide national leadership with key stakeholders, to improve the physical and mental health, safety and well-being of the maternal and child health (MCH) population which includes all the nation's women, infants, children, adolescents, and their families, including fathers and children with special health care needs."[45] To fulfill its mission, the MCHB set five broad goals for 2003 to 2007: (1) provide national leadership for maternal and child health, (2) promote an environment that supports maternal and child health, (3) eliminate health barriers and disparities, (4) improve the health infrastructure and systems of care, and (5) assure quality of care.[45]

The MCHB works on accomplishing its goals through the administration of four core public health services: (1) infrastructure-building services, (2) population-based services, (3) enabling services, and (4) direct health care (gap-filling) services. MCHB uses the construct of a pyramid to provide a useful framework for understanding programmatic directions and resource allocation by the bureau and its partners (see Figure 7.24). MCHB continues to strive for a "society that recognizes and fully supports the important role that public health plays in promoting the health of the MCH population, including building, strengthening and assuring MCH health services and infrastructure at all levels."[45]

Women, Infants, and Children Program

WIC
a special supplemental food program for women, infants, and children, sponsored by the USDA

The Women, Infants, and Children (**WIC**) program is a clinic-based program designed to provide a variety of nutritional and health-related goods and services to pregnant, postpartum, and breastfeeding women, infants, and children under the age of 5. The WIC program began as a pilot in 1972 and received permanent federal funding in 1974, in response to growing evidence linking nutritional inadequacies to mental and physical health defects. Congress intended that WIC, unlike other food programs, would serve as "an adjunct to good health care, during critical times of growth and development, to prevent the occurrence of health problems."[46]

The U.S. Department of Agriculture (USDA) administers WIC. The USDA administers grants to the states, where the WIC programs are most often offered through local health departments or state health and welfare agencies (see Figure 7.25). Pregnant or postpartum women, infants, and children up to age 5 are eligible if they meet the following three criteria: (1) reside in the state in which they are applying, (2) meet income requirements (applicant must have a household income below 185% of the federal poverty guideline), (3) are determined to be at "nutritional risk" by a health care professional.[47]

Since WIC's inception as a national nutrition program, it has grown dramatically. In 1974, the average number of monthly WIC participants was 88,000; in 2004 that number was more than 8.5 million women and children (see Figure 7.26).[47] This constitutes half of all infants in America and one-quarter of children between 1 and 5 years of age.

The WIC program has proved to be one of the most effective ways to improve the health of mothers, infants, and young children. Research indicates that participation in the WIC program during pregnancy provides women with a number of positive outcomes, some of which

FIGURE 7.24

MCH pyramid of health services. The conceptual framework for the services of Title V Maternal and Child Health is envisioned as a pyramid with four tiers of services and levels of funding that provide comprehensive services for mothers and children.

Source: U.S. Department of Health and Human Services (2003). *Maternal and Child Health Bureau Strategic Plan: FY 2003–2007.* Washington, DC: Health Resources and Service Administration, Maternal and Child Health Bureau.

include birth to babies with higher birth weights and fewer fetal and infant deaths. The WIC program is also cost effective. USDA research has shown that for every dollar spent on WIC, the taxpayer saves $4 in future expenditures on Medicaid.[47] For this reason, the WIC program continues to possess strong bipartisan support in Congress.

Providing Health Insurance for Women, Infants, and Children

All children deserve to start life on the right track and to have access to comprehensive health services that provide preventive care when they are well and treatment when they are ill or injured. Health insurance provides access to critical preventive medical services as well as acute medical care in the case of illness or injury (see Chapter 14). When compared with children who are privately insured or have governmental insurance, children without health insurance are much more likely to have necessary care delayed or receive no care for health problems, putting

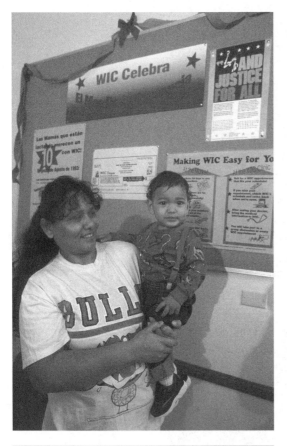

FIGURE 7.25
The WIC program has proven to be extremely effective in improving the health of women, infants, and children in America.

them at greater risk for hospitalization.[48] Therefore, providing health insurance to low-income children is a critical health care safety net.

The government has two principal programs aimed at providing health care coverage to low-income children: the Medicaid program and the State Children's Health Insurance Program (SCHIP). Medicaid, created in 1965, provides medical assistance for certain low-income individuals and families, mostly women and children (see Chapter 14). Children represent slightly more than half of all Medicaid beneficiaries, yet account for only 17% of program spending. A major reason that Medicaid is working well for American children is the multiphase program for preventive health called the Early and Periodic Screening, Diagnostic, and Treatment (EPSDT) for individuals under the age of 21. The Medicaid EPSDT provisions entitle poor children to a comprehensive package of preventive health care and medically necessary diagnosis and treatment.

Although the Medicaid program is a critical health care program for low-income children, being poor does not automatically qualify a child for Medicaid. Medicaid eligibility is determined by each state based on various age and income requirements. As a result, Medicaid coverage varies across the states and leaves a significant number of poor children uninsured. To broaden coverage to low-income children, Congress created SCHIP under provisions in the Balanced Budget Act of 1997 (see Chapter 14). The program targets uninsured children under 19 with family incomes below 200% of poverty who are not eligible for Medicaid or covered by private insurance. Government-funded health insurance is an important source of coverage for children, and its significance has been growing. Medicaid coverage for children increased from 20% of all children in 2000 to 27% in 2005 (see Figure 7.27). During the same time period, the percentage of children with private health insurance coverage decreased from 71% in 2000 to 65% in 2005 (see Figure 7.27). The success in increasing the number of children with coverage is attributable not just to Medicaid but to the combined effects of Medicaid and SCHIP. However, despite these programs, approximately 11% of youth under the age of 19 were uninsured in 2005. Advocates have encouraged state and community decision makers to continue the expansion of Medicaid and SCHIP programs to cover as many uninsured children as possible.

Providing Child Care

Experiences during the first years of childhood significantly influence the health of a child. Research shows that early investments in the nurturing of children provides major advantages for families and society later. While parents should accept the primary responsibility for raising their children, the government can assist families who need help making important investments. Two important investments to the health and welfare of America's children are parenting during the first months of life and the accompanying need for secure relationships with a small number of adults in safe settings as they develop during the first few years of life.

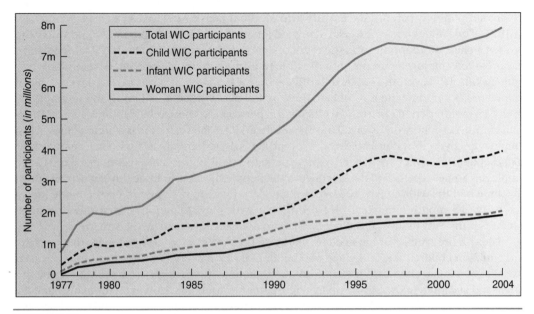

FIGURE 7.26

Trends in WIC program participation, 1977–2004.

Source: National Health Policy Forum, Maternal and Child Health Policy Research Center, based on information from the USDA Web site. Used with permission.

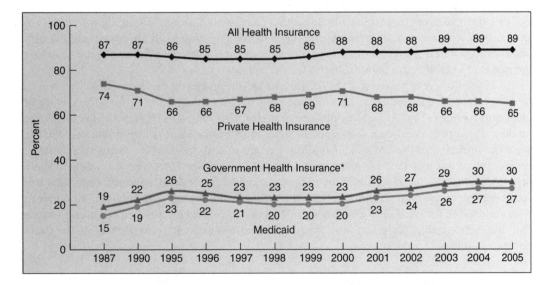

FIGURE 7.27

Percentage of children covered by health insurance, by type of insurance, selected years, 1987–2005.

*Government health insurance consists primarily of Medicaid, but also includes such coverage as Medicare, State Children's Health Insurance Programs (SCHIP), and Medical Care Program of the Uniformed Services (CHAMPUS/Tricare).

Source: Child Trends DataBank (2006). "Health Care Coverage." Available at http://www.childtrendsdatabank.org/indicators/26HealthCareCoverage.cfm.

To support new parents, the **Family and Medical Leave Act (FMLA)** was signed into law in 1993. The FMLA grants 12 weeks of unpaid job-protected leave to men or women after the birth of a child, an adoption, or in the event of illness in the immediate family.[49] This legislation has provided employed parents with the time to nurture their children and develop their parenting skills. However, the FMLA only affects businesses with 50 or more employees. Those employees covered by the law include those who have worked 1,250 hours for an employer over a 12-month period (an average of 25 hours per week). This excludes about 40% of American employees who work in small businesses that do not fall under the law's guidelines. Also, employers covered by the FMLA can exempt key salaried employees who are among their highest paid 10%, if they are needed to prevent "substantial and grievous" economic harm to the employer. Some experts feel the law divides the people by class, helping those who can afford the three months without pay, and bypassing those who cannot. Experts have recommended a six- to twelve-month family care leave program with partial pay for at least three months. America is the only industrialized nation that has not enacted a paid infant-care leave.

Today more families are in need of child care than ever before. Estimates are that as many as 13 million children under the age of 6 are in child care every day. The need for increased use of professional child care has come about as women increasingly are working outside the home and as more children grow up in single-parent households. However, for many families, especially those with low and moderate incomes, high-quality, affordable child care is simply not available. According to a recent study, much of the care we offer children is inadequate, yet a full day of child care costs an average of $4,000 to $10,000 annually per child.[11] These costs are beyond the reach of many working parents, half of whom earn $35,000 or less a year. The lack of high-quality child care prevents children from entering school ready to learn, hinders their success in school, and limits the ability of their parents to be productive workers. Furthermore, after-school care is crucial because juvenile crime peaks between the hours of 3 P.M. and 7 P.M., and school-aged children may be at greater risk of engaging in activities that lead to problems such as violence and teen pregnancy.

In 1988, Congress passed the Family Support Act, which provided funding for child care assistance to welfare parents who are employed or participating in an approved training program. Unfortunately, states must match federal funds for this program, which makes meeting the needs of eligible participants difficult for poor states.

In 1990, Congress passed the Child Care and Development Block Grant (CCDBG), which provides child care subsidies for low-income children and funding to improve the quality of child care services. The "At Risk" Child Care Program, also passed in 1990, provides additional funding to support child care assistance to low-income families at risk of going on welfare. With the initiation of the "At Risk" Child Care Program and the CCDBG, states were able to provide additional assistance to many more low-income families. However, according to state-reported statistics, of the 15 million children eligible for federal support, only 12% are receiving federal help due to limited federal funding.[50] This means that only 1 of 10 children who are eligible for child care assistance under federal law receive any help. Not one state is currently serving all eligible families. This means that too many parents are unable to obtain necessary child care assistance.

Other Advocates for Children

There are numerous groups that advocate for children's health and welfare. Among them are the Children's Defense Fund, UNICEF, and the American Academy of Pediatrics.

Children's Defense Fund (CDF)

Since 1973, the Children's Defense Fund (CDF) has been working to create a nation in which the network of family, community, private-sector, and government supports for children is so tightly intertwined that no child can slip through the cracks. The CDF is a private, nonprofit organization headquartered in Washington, DC, and it is dedicated to providing a voice for the children of America. It has never accepted government funds and supports its programs through donations from foundations, corporate grants, and individuals. The CDF focuses on the needs of poor, minority, and handicapped children and their families. The aim of the CDF is to educate the nation about the needs of children and to encourage preventive investment in children before they get sick or suffer. It provides information and technical assistance to state and local child advocates.

United Nations Children's Fund (UNICEF)

Founded in 1946, the United Nations Children's Fund (UNICEF) is the only organization of the United Nations assigned exclusively to children. This organization works with other United Nations' members, governments, and nongovernmental organizations to improve child conditions through community-based services in primary health care, basic education, and safe water and sanitation in over 140 developing countries. UNICEF gathers data on the health of children throughout the world. UNICEF has assisted in mass vaccinations and been involved in other international health efforts to protect children.

American Academy of Pediatrics (AAP)

The American Academy of Pediatrics (AAP) was founded in 1930 by 35 pediatricians who felt the need for an independent pediatric forum to address children's needs. When the Academy was established, the idea that children have special developmental and health needs was a new one. Preventive health practices now associated with child care, including immunizations and regular health exams, were only just beginning to change the custom of treating children as "miniature adults." The Academy is committed to the attainment of optimal physical, mental, and social health and well-being for all infants, children, adolescents, and young adults. The activities and efforts of the AAP include research, advocacy for children and youth, and public and professional education.

An example of a program that the AAP coordinates is the Healthy Child Care America Campaign. This program is sponsored by the Maternal and Child Health Bureau and the Administration on Children, Youth, and Families. The campaign is based on the principle that families, child care providers, and health care providers working collaboratively can promote the healthy development of young children. The specific goals of the Healthy Child Care America Campaign are to provide:

Safe, healthy child care environments for all children

Up-to-date and easily accessible immunizations for children in child care

Access to quality health, dental, and developmental screening and comprehensive follow-up for children in child care

Health and mental health consultation, support, and education for all families, children, and child care providers

Health, nutrition, and safety education for children in child care, their families, and child care providers

Since the Healthy Child Care America campaign was launched in 1995, many communities around the country have been promoting collaborative partnerships between health and child care professionals to ensure that children receive the best and the highest-quality care possible. By expanding and creating partnerships between families, child care providers, and government, the best care for millions of children continues to occur.

Chapter Summary

- Maternal, infant, and child health are important indicators of a community's overall health. Maternal health encompasses the health of women of childbearing age from pre-pregnancy through pregnancy, labor and delivery, and in the postpartum period. Infant and child health refers to individuals through 14 years of age.

- Families are the primary unit in which infants and children are nurtured and supported regarding healthy development. Significant increases in births to unmarried women in the last two decades, especially among teenagers, are among the many changes in American society that have affected family structure and the economic security of children. Teenage childbearing represents a significant social and financial burden on both the family and the community.

- The establishment of local Family Planning Clinics with Title X funding has resulted in an improvement in maternal and child health indicators for the communities served.

- High-quality prenatal care is one of the fundamentals of a safe motherhood program. Ensuring early initiation of prenatal care during pregnancy greatly contributes to reductions in perinatal illness, disability, and death for the mother and the infant.

Review Questions

1. What has been the trend in infant mortality rates in the United States in the last 30 years? What is the current rate? How does this rate compare with that of other industrial countries?

2. What has been the trend in maternal mortality rates in the United States in the last 30 years? What factors have influenced this trend?

3. Why is prenatal care so important for mothers and infants? What types of services are included?

4. What are the consequences of teen pregnancy to the mother? To the infant? To the community?

5. What is included in family planning? Why is family planning important?

6. Discuss the pro-life and pro-choice positions on the abortion issue.

7. Why was the *Roe v. Wade* court decision so important?

8. What are the leading causes of death in children ages 1 to 4 and ages 5 to 14 years?

9. Why are childhood immunizations so important?

10. What is the WIC program?

11. Why is health insurance important for women, infants, and children?

12. Name three groups that are advocates for the health of children and what they have done to show their support.

Activities

Write a two-page paper summarizing the results and/or information you gain from one of the following activities.

1. Survey 10 classmates and friends and ask them what leads to teen pregnancy. What prompts adolescents to risk pregnancy when they have adequate knowledge of contraception? Ask if they know anyone who became pregnant as an adolescent. Are the reasons given the same as your own? Divide your list into categories of personal beliefs, barriers to action, and social pressure. For example, a comment that might fit under beliefs is "they don't think they can get pregnant the first time"; under barriers, "they are too embarrassed to buy contraception"; and under social pressure, "all the messages in society promoting sex." Which of the three categories had the most responses? Does this surprise you? What implications does this have for programs trying to reduce the incidence of teen pregnancy?

2. Call your local health department and ask for information about the local WIC program. Ask permission to visit and talk to a representative about the program and clientele.

3. Visit, call, or get on the Web site of your state health department and obtain information concerning the number of childhood communicable diseases reported in your state. What are your state laws concerning immunization of children? Does your state provide immunizations free of charge? What qualifications must a person meet to receive free immunizations?

4. Call a local obstetrician's office and ask if he or she accepts Medicaid reimbursement. What is the normal fee for prenatal care and delivery? If he or she does not take Medicaid, ask the obstetrician to whom he or she would refer a pregnant woman with no private insurance.

5. Create a record of your own (or a family member's) immunizations. Find out when and where you were immunized for each of the immunizations listed in Figure 7.22. Are there any immunizations that are still needed? When are you scheduled to get your next tetanus/toxoid immunization?

SCENARIO: ANALYSIS AND RESPONSE

- Good health during the childhood years (ages 1–14) is essential for each child's optimal development and America's future. America cannot hope for every child to become a productive member of society if children in this country are allowed to grow up with poor or mediocre child care, have no health insurance, live in poverty, or live in a violent environment.

- The federal government has over 35 health programs within 16 different agencies helping states to serve the needs of our nation's children. The majority of these programs are well respected and help meet the needs of many children.

We have learned that a lack of prenatal care increases the risk of premature delivery and possible health problems for the infant.

1. If Joan had received prenatal care, how could it have helped in the normal development of the infant? How could the doctor have counseled Joan?
2. How could Joan have found out about opportunities for affordable prenatal care?
3. The cost of treating Joan's infant could run into the hundreds of thousands of dollars, and there is no guarantee that the child will survive. Do you think it would be more cost effective to ensure prenatal care to all women or to continue under the system that is in place now? How would you suggest the United States approach this problem?
4. What programs mentioned in this chapter could have helped Joan?
5. Visit the Web site of the USDA (www.usda.gov) and read about WIC. After reading about WIC, do you think this is something that could help Joan with the raising of her child? Why or why not?

COMMUNITY HEALTH ON THE WEB

The Internet contains a wealth of information about community and public health. Increase your knowledge of some of the topics presented in this chapter by accessing the Jones and Bartlett Publishers Web site at **http://health.jbpub.com/book/communityhealth/6e** and follow the links to complete the following Web activities.

- Maternal and Child Health Bureau
- Women, Infants, and Children Program
- Insure Kids Now!

REFERENCES

1. Pillitteri, A. (2006). *Maternal and Child Health Nursing: Care of the Childbearing and Childrearing Family*, 5th ed. Philadelphia: J. B. Lippincott.

2. U.S. Department of Health and Human Services (2005). *Child Health—USA 2005*. Washington, DC: U.S. Government Printing Office.

3. U.S. Census Bureau, Population Division, Fertility and Family Statistics Branch (2006). *Current Population Survey, Definitions and Explanations*. Available at http://www.census.gov/population/www/cps/cpsdef.html.

4. Friedman, M. (2003). *Family Nursing: Research, Theory and Practice*, 5th ed. Stamford, CT: Appleton & Lange.

5. Terry-Humen, E., J. Manlove, and K. A. Moore (2001). "Births Outside of Marriage: Perceptions vs. Reality." In *Child Trends Research Brief*. Washington, DC: Child Trends.

6. Martin, J. A., B. E. Hamilton, P. D. Sutton, S. J. Ventura, F. Menacker, and S. Kirmeyer (2006). "Births: Final Data for 2004." *National Vital Statistics Reports*, 55(1): 1-31.

7. Martin, J. A., B. E. Hamilton, P. D. Sutton, S. J. Ventura, F. Menacker, and M. Munson (2005). "Births: Final Data for 2003." *National Vital Statistics Reports*, 54(2): 1-30.

8. Ventura, S. J., T. J. Mathew, and B. E. Hamilton (2001). "Births to Teenagers in the United States, 1940-2000." *National Vital Statistics Reports*, 49(10): 1-24.

9. Maynard, R. A. (1997). "The Costs of Adolescent Childbearing." In R. Maynard, ed., *Kids Having Kids: Economic Costs and Social Consequences of Teen Pregnancy*. Washington, DC: The Urban Institute Press, 285-337.

10. United Nations (2005) *Demographic Yearbook, 2002*. New York: United Nations. Available at http://unstats.un.org/unsd/demographic/products/dyb/dybpub2002.htm.

11. Children's Defense Fund (2005). *The State of America's Children 2005*. Washington, DC: Author.

12. U.S. Department of Health and Human Services (2000). *Healthy People 2010* (Conference Edition, in Two Volumes). Washington, DC: Author

13. Jackson, S. (1993). "Opening Session Comments: Laying the Groundwork for Working Together for the Future." *Journal of School Health*, 63(1): 11.

14. Finer, L. B., and S. K. Henshaw (2006). "Disparities in Rates of Unintended Pregnancy in the United States, 1994 and 2001." *Perspectives on Sexual and Reproductive Health*, 38(2): 90-96.

15. Finer, L. B., J. E. Darroch, and J. J. Frost (2001). "U.S. Agencies Providing Publicly Funded Contraceptive Services in 1999." *Perspectives on Sexual and Reproductive Health*, 34(1): 15-24.

16. Henshaw, S. (1998). "Unintended Pregnancy in the United States." *Family Planning Perspectives*, 30(1): 24-29.

17. Chandra, A., G. M. Martinez, W. D. Mosher, J. C. Abma, and J. Jones (2005). "Fertility, Family Planning and Women's Health: Data from the 2002 National Survey of Family Growth." *Vital Health Statistics*, 23(25).

18. "Title X Pregnancy Counseling Act." (1991). *Congressional Digest*, 70(8,9): 195-224.

19. Frost, J. J., L. Frohwirth, and A. Purcell (2004). "The Availability and Use of Publicly Funded Family Planning Clinics: U.S. Trends, 1994-2001." *Perspectives on Sexual and Reproductive Health*, 36(5): 206-215.

20. *Family Planning Annual Report: 2004 Summary* (2005). Submitted to the Office of Population Affairs, Department of Health and Human Services.

21. Alan Guttmacher Institute (2000). *Fulfilling the Promise: Public Policy and U.S. Family Planning Clinics*. New York: Author.

22. Hyde, J., and J. DeLamater (1997). *Understanding Human Sexuality*, 6th ed. Boston: McGraw-Hill.

23. Planned Parenthood Federation of America (2006). *2004-2005 Annual Report*. New York: Author. Available at http://www.planned-parenthood.org/about-us/who-we-are/annual-report.htm.

24. Forrest, J., and R. Samara (1996). "Impact of Publicly Funded Contraceptive Services on Unintended Pregnancies and Implications for Medicaid Expenditures." *Family Planning Perspectives*, 28: 52-59.

25. Frost, J. J., A. Sonfield, and R. B. Gold (2006). *Estimating the Impact of Expanding Medicaid Eligibility for Family Planning Services.* (Occasional Report no. 28). New York: Guttmacher Institute.

26. "Court Reaffirms Roe but Upholds Restrictions." (1992). *Family Planning Perspectives*, 24: 174-185.

27. Strauss, L.T., J. Herdon, J. Change, W. Parker, S. Bowens, and C. Berg (2005). "Abortion Surveillance—United States, 2002." *Morbidity and Mortality Weekly Report*, 54(SS 7): 1-15.

28. World Health Organization (1992). *International Statistical Classification of Diseases and Related Health Problems. Tenth Revision*. Geneva, Switzerland: Author.

29. Centers for Disease Control and Prevention (2000). "Entry into Prenatal Care—United States, 1989-1997." *Morbidity and Mortality Weekly Report*, 49(18): 393-398.

30. Hoyert, D. L., M. P. Heron, S. L. Murphy, and H. C. Kung (2006). "Deaths: Final Data for 2003." *National Vital Statistics Reports*, 54(13): 1-31.

31. Behrman, R. E., and A. Stith Buter, eds. (2006). *Preterm Birth: Causes, Consequences, and Prevention*. Washington, DC: The National Academies Press.

32. March of Dimes (2004). "Premature Birth Rate in U.S. Reaches Historic High." Available at http://www.marchofdimes.com/prematurity/10651_10763.asp.

33. S. Nigel Paneth (1995). "The Problem of Low Birth Weight." *The Future of Children*, 5(1): 35-56.

34. Chomitz, O. R., L. W. Cheung, and E. Lieberman (1995). "The Role of Lifestyle in Preventing Low Birthweight." *The Future of Children*, 5(1): 162-175.

35. Centers for Disease Control and Prevention (1998). "Trends in Infant Mortality Attributable to Birth Defects—United States, 1980-1995." *Morbidity and Mortality Weekly Report*, 47(37): 773-778.

36. Centers for Disease Control and Prevention. "Sudden Infant Death Syndrome (SIDS)." Available at http://www.cdc.gov/SIDS/.

37. Willinger, M., M. J. Hoffman, K. T. Wu, J. R. Hou, R. C. Kessler, S. L. Ward, T. G. Keens, and M. J. Corwin (1998). "Factors Associated with the Transition to Non-prone Sleep Positions of Infants in the United States. The National Infant Sleep Position Study." *Journal of the American Medical Association*, 280: 329-335.

38. National Highway Traffic Safety Administration (2005). *Traffic Safety Facts 2004: Occupant Protection*. Washington, DC: U.S. Department of Transportation.

39. National Center for Injury Prevention and Control (2005). "Childhood Injury Fact Sheet." Available at http://www.cdc.gov/ncipc/factsheets/childh.htm.

40. Finkelstein, E. A., P. S. Corso, and T. R. Miller (2006). *Incidence and Economic Burden of Injuries in the United States*. New York: Oxford University Press.

41. U.S. Department of Health and Human Services, Administration for Children and Families (2006). *Child Maltreatment 2004*. Washington, DC: U.S. Government Printing Office.

42. U.S. Department of Health and Human Services, Administration for Children and Families (2004). "Community Responsibility for Child Protection." Available at http://nccanch.acf.hhs.gov/pubs/otherpubs/commresp.cfm.

43. Centers for Disease Control and Prevention (2000). *Immunization 2000: A History of Achievement, a Future of Promise*. Atlanta, GA: Author.

44. U.S. Department of Health and Human Services, Health Resources and Services Administration (2003). *Understanding Title V of the Social Security Act*. Rockville, MD: Author.

45. U.S. Department of Health and Human Services, Health Resources and Services Administration (2003). *Maternal and Child Health Bureau Strategic Plan: FY 2003-2007*. Available at http://mchb.hrsa.gov/about/stratplan03-07.htm.

46. Special Supplemental Nutrition Program for Women, Infants, and Children (7CFR246) (January 1, 2002). Available at http://frwebgate.access.gpo.gov/cgi-bin/multidb.cgi.

47. U.S. Department of Agriculture, Food and Nutrition Service (2006). "About WIC." Available at http://www.fns.usda.gov/wic/.

48. Institute of Medicine (2002). *Health Insurance Is a Family Matter*. Washington, DC: National Academies Press. Available at http://nap.edu/books/0309085187/html/.

49. Ruhm, C. J. (1997). "The Family and Medical Leave Act." *Journal of Economic Perspectives*, 3: 10-14.

50. U.S. Department of Health and Human Services (2000). "National Study of Child Care for Low-Income Families, State, and Community Substudy." Available at http://acf.dhhs.gov/news/ccstudy.htm.

Chapter 8

Adolescents, Young Adults, and Adults

Chapter Objectives

After studying this chapter, you will be able to:

1 Explain why it is important for community health workers to be aware of the different health concerns of the various age groups in the United States.

2 Define by age the groups of *adolescents and young adults* and *adults.*

3 Briefly describe key demographic characteristics of adolescents and young adults.

4 Explain what the Youth Risk Behavior Surveillance System (YRBSS) and the Behavioral Risk Factor Surveillance System (BRFSS) are and what type of data they generate.

5 Provide a brief behavioral risk profile for adolescents, college students, and adults.

6 Outline the health profiles for the various age groups—adolescents and young adults, and adults—listing the major causes of mortality, morbidity, and risk factors for each group.

7 Give examples of community health strategies for improving the health status of adolescents and young adults, and adults.

SCENARIO

Annie and Latasha are about halfway through their sophomore year at Garber University. Though they came from very different environments—Annie came from a small rural community with a population of about 1,500 and Latasha grew up in large metropolitan area—they have become good friends. This year, as chance would have it, they have similar class schedules and have ended up in the dining hall each morning at about the same time for breakfast.

One morning, while reading the school newspaper over breakfast, Annie came across an article that described an automobile crash involving some university students. Four university students riding in one car collided with a second car driven by a local middle-aged businessman. Annie asked Latasha if she knew any of the students. Latasha asked who they were, and Annie read their names. Latasha did not know them.

Annie said it looked like the students were in big trouble because they had all been drinking alcohol, and no one was 21 years old. When the police tested the driver, her blood alcohol concentration was 0.14%. So not only was she being charged with underage drinking, but also with driving while intoxicated. Luckily, none of the students was injured, but the local businessman was in serious condition in the hospital. The newspaper article indicated that the students were wearing their safety belts, but the businessman was not. Annie told Latasha that she only knew of one similar incident like this back home. She added, "Why would anyone drink and drive?" Latasha replied, "Don't worry about this Annie. It's no big deal. It happens all the time in the city; in fact it is so common this type of news seldom makes the papers."

INTRODUCTION

In this chapter, we will present a profile of the health of Americans in two different groups—adolescents and young adults (15 to 24 years of age) and adults (25 to 64 years of age). Just like the age groups of Americans presented in Chapter 7, each of these groups has its own sets of health risks and problems. Viewing these age group profiles enables public health workers to detect the sources of diseases, injury, and death for specific priority populations and to propose programs to reduce those sources. Effective programs aimed at specific population age groups can reduce the risk factors that contribute to disease, injury, and death for the entire population. We hope that you, the student, will become knowledgeable about the specific health problems of each age group and also become mindful of the subpopulations within these groups that are at special risk.

The years of life between the ages of 15 and 64 are some of the most productive, if not the most productive, of people's lives. Consider all that takes place during these years. Most people complete their formal education, meet and commit to their life-long partners, become parents and raise a family, find and develop their vocation, become owners (or at least mortgage holders) of property, earn their greatest amount of wealth, actively engage in the development of their community, travel more than during any other time in their lives, become aunts or uncles and grandparents, become valued employees, serve as role models and mentors, and plan and save for retirement. It is also a time when they enjoy some of the best health of their lives as well as shape their health (through their lifestyle and health behavior) for their later years.

ADOLESCENTS AND YOUNG ADULTS

adolescents and young adults
those people who fall into the 15- to 24-year-old range

Adolescents and young adults are considered to be those people who fall into the 15- to 24-year-old range. The individuals in this age group are considered very important by our society because they represent the future of our nation. If the United States is going to maintain its standard of living and preeminent position among the countries of the world that it enjoys today, it will depend in large part on these young people.[1]

This period of development of adolescence and young adulthood, often combined when reporting data about young people, can be further split into two subgroups. "Adolescence is generally regarded as the period of life from puberty to maturity."[2] This is not an easy stage of life for most because it is a period of transition from childhood to adulthood. Adolescence "is a time when children psychologically move from areas of relative comfort and emotional security to places and situations that are far more complex and often much more challenging."[3] In addition to the psychological changes, this population of teenagers is also experiencing "hormonal changes, physical maturation, and frequently, opportunities to engage in risk behaviors."[2]

Young adults also face many physical, emotional, and educational changes. For example, young adults complete their physical growth and maturity, leave home, marry and start families, attend postsecondary education, enlist in the military, or begin careers. Couple the demands of these personal changes with the demands of a fast-paced, ever-changing society and it is easy to see why this stage in life is considered one of the most difficult.[1]

The combined period of adolescence and young adulthood is a critical one healthwise. It is during this period in one's life that many health-related beliefs, attitudes, and behaviors are adopted and consolidated.[2,4,5] During this stage of life, young people have increased freedom and access to health-compromising substances and experiences—such as alcohol, tobacco, other drugs, and sexual risk taking—as well as opportunities for health-enhancing experiences such as regularly scheduled exercise and healthful diets.[2,4,5] It is also during this stage that certain lifestyle decisions are made that will have long-term influences on health in later years of life.

Demography

There are several demographic variables that affect the health of this age group, but the three variables that are most important to community health are the number of young people, their living arrangements, and their employment status.

Number of Adolescents and Young Adults

The number of adolescents and young adults peaked in 1979, when the baby boomers swelled their ranks to about 21% of the total population. Since 1979, the proportion of 14- to 24-year-olds has declined. Thus, in 2005 they made up just over 14% of the population, roughly the same proportion they made up in 1960.[6-8]

As we look to the future, the proportion of adolescents and young adults in the general population will continue to increase, and at the same time the racial and ethnic makeup will become increasingly more diverse (see Figure 8.1). In 2005, approximately 66% of the adolescents were white. It is estimated that in 2050, this percentage will decrease to 44%.[2,8]

Living Arrangements

The percentage of children under the age of 18 living in a single-parent family has been on the rise ever since 1965. In fact, the percentage increased sharply in the 1970s and continued to rise slowly through the 1990s. The sharp rise in the 1970s can be attributed to the great increase in the divorce rate.[1] In 2005, almost one-third (32%)[8] of all children lived in single-parent families, versus approximately one-tenth (11%) in 1970.[7] Additionally, more black children (62%) lived in a single-parent home than white children (28%) or Hispanic children (36%).[8]

Family household statistics on single-parent families are only a snapshot of children's living status during a single year. Unfortunately, many children are affected over their lifetimes by growing up in single-parent families. Though the psychological and emotional consequences

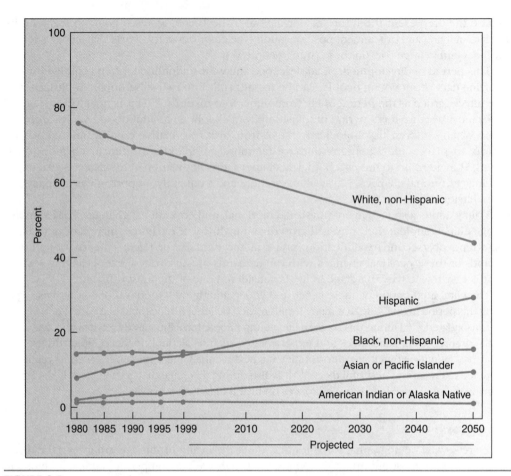

FIGURE 8.1

Race and Hispanic origin of adolescents 10–19 years of age: United States, 1980–2050.

Source: U.S. Department of Commerce, Bureau of the Census, Population Estimates and Projections. In MacKay, A. P., L. A. Fingerhut, and C. R. Duran (2000). *Health, United States, 2000 with Adolescent Health Chartbook.* Hyattsville, MD: National Center for Health Statistics, 27.

of single-parent families are not clear, the economic consequences are indeed. Children living in single-parent families are more likely to experience severe economic disadvantages.[1] These economic disadvantages adversely affect health.

Employment Status

Since the years of 1960 and the early 1980s, when there were significant increases in the participation of young women in the labor force, the proportion of all adolescents and young adults in the labor force has remained relatively constant (see Figure 8.2). However, this age group is beginning to see some significant permanent changes in its labor force participation, particularly 16- to 19-year-old males, mainly due to increased school attendance and enrollment in high school, college, and summer school over the past decade.[9] When the unemployment rates of this age group are separated by race and ethnicity, great differences appear. Regardless of sex, black adolescents and young adults are more likely to be unemployed than whites or Hispanics. White adolescents and young adults have the lowest proportion of unemployment.[10] These proportions, like so many others already discussed, are

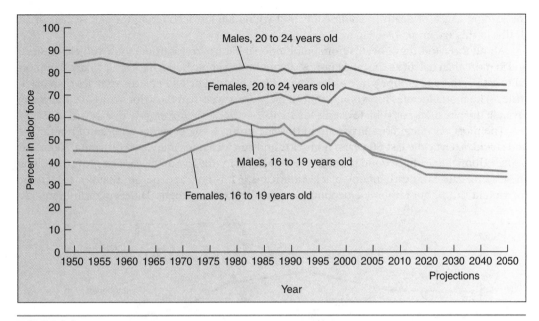

FIGURE 8.2

Labor force participation rate of young adults by sex and age, 1950–2050.

Sources: U.S. Department of Labor, Bureau of Labor Statistics, *Employment and Earnings* (January issues); *Handbook of Labor Statistics,* Bulletin 2217. U.S. Department of Commerce, Bureau of the Census, *Statistical Abstract of the United States, 1956, 1987, and 1999;* and *Current Population Reports,* Series P-50, nos. 31 and 72; and unpublished data. Council of Economic Advisers, *Economic Report of the President,* 1987. Tossi, M. (2006). "A New Look at Long-Term Labor Force Projections to 2050." *Monthly Labor Review Online,* 129(11).

disproportionate by race/ethnicity. These figures are important to community health because most health insurance, and thus access to health care, is connected to employment status.

A Health Profile

With regard to the health profile of this age group, three major areas stand out—mortality, morbidity from specific infectious diseases, and health behavior and lifestyle choices.

Mortality

While, on average, Americans are living longer than ever before, adolescents and young adults suffer their share of life-threatening problems.[1] As it has been with most other age groups, the death rate for adolescents and young adults has significantly declined. Between 1950 and 2003, the death rate of adolescents and young adults declined by 36%, from 128.1 to 81.5 per 100,000.[11] This decline in death rates for adolescents and young adults, like that for children, can be attributed to advances in medicine and injury and disease prevention.[1,11]

Regardless of race or ethnicity, men have higher mortality rates than women.[10] Mortality rates for men and women were highest among black Americans and American Indians/Alaska Natives. The lowest mortality rates of both men and women belong to Asian/Pacific Islanders.[11]

Much of the physical threat to adolescents and young adults stems from their behavior rather than from disease.[1] For young people overall, approximately three-fourths of all mortality can be attributed to three causes—unintentional injuries (mainly motor vehicle crashes) (45%), homicide (16%), and suicide (12%).[11] Mortality from unintentional injuries in this age group declined during the last half-century of the twentieth century. Even so, unintentional injury deaths remain the leading cause of death in adolescents and young adults, accounting for almost half of all deaths in this age group (see Figure 8.3).

About three-fourths of deaths from unintentional injuries result from motor vehicle crashes, and in more than half of all the fatal crashes, alcohol was a contributing factor.[1] Unlike other mortality data in this age group, white males have a higher rate of death in motor vehicles than black males. The mortality rates for women of both races are lower than those for males of either race. Overall, the rate of motor vehicle deaths for 15- to 24-year-olds is lower now than it was in 1950.[2]

The most alarming mortality trend in this age group is the growing number of homicides and suicides. Over the last 50 years, homicide and suicides rates increased between 200% and 300%.[2] Homicide is the second leading cause of death in the 15- to 24-year age group, and it is the leading cause of death among black Americans.[12] It is not race, per se, that is a risk factor for violent death, but rather socioeconomic status and environment. Differences in homicide

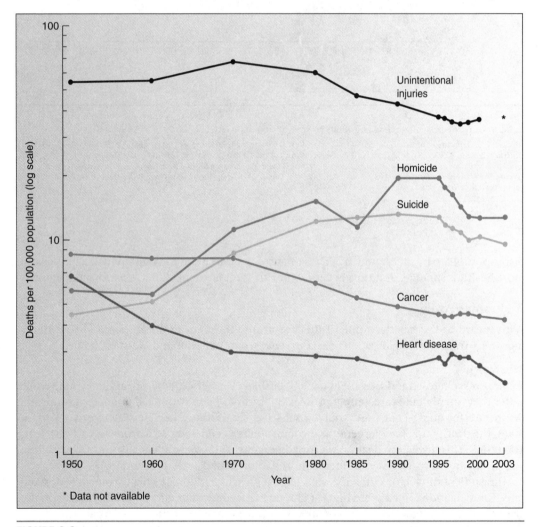

FIGURE 8.3

Death rates for leading causes of death for ages 15 to 24, 1950–2003.

Sources: Fried, V. M., K. Prager, A. P. MacKay, and H. Xia (2003). *Health, United States, 2003, with Chartbook on Trends in Health of Americans*. Hyattsville, MD: National Center for Health Statistics, 50; and National Center for Health Statistics (2006). *Health, United States, 2006, with Chartbook on Trends in the Health of Americans*. Hyattsville, MD: Author.

rates between races are significantly reduced when socioeconomic factors are taken into account. However, alcohol and drugs are involved in about 60% of all homicides and legal interventions.[13]

Suicide is the third leading cause of death in adolescents and young adults, and it is the second leading cause of death of white males in this age group. The rate among black males is about three-fourths that of white males.[11] The suicide rate in females is significantly lower than that for males, although young women attempt suicide more frequently than young men.[14]

Although the number of completed suicides by adolescents and young adults is alarming, it represents only a fraction of all the suicides contemplated. Data from the 2005 Centers for Disease Control and Prevention's Youth Risk Behavior Surveillance System (YRBSS) indicate that approximately one-sixth of ninth to twelfth graders in the United States have thought seriously about attempting suicide (16.9%), while 13% have made a specific plan to attempt suicide, and 8.4% have actually attempted suicide.[14]

Morbidity

Although a higher proportion of adolescents and young adults survive to age 24 than ever before, this group still suffers significantly from a number of different communicable diseases. One of these diseases, measles (rubeola), once thought to be only a childhood disease and close to eradication, made a resurgence in the late 1980s. Measles is a much more severe disease for adolescents and young adults than it is for children. It was first thought that a single vaccination for measles (taken concurrently with mumps and rubella, as the MMR vaccination, at 15 months of age) would confer life-long immunity against the disease. However, measles is much more communicable than once believed, so that a second immunization at the time of first entering school is now recommended. As can be seen in Table 8.1, this change in the immunization schedule has significantly reduced the number of measles cases. The recommendations for measles and other vaccinations are presented in Chapter 7.

The other diseases that are causing considerable morbidity in adolescents and young adults are sexually transmitted diseases (STDs) (see Table 8.1). "Teenagers and young adults are more likely than other age groups to have multiple sex partners, to engage in unprotected sex, and, for young women, to choose sexual partners older than them."[15] While many STDs are completely curable with antibiotics, some viral infections, such as hepatitis, human immunodeficiency virus (HIV), or human papillomavirus (HPV), can be treated but never cured.[16] "The effects of some STDs can last a lifetime; some forms of HPV are the precursor to cervical cancer, and the effects of chlamydia, if untreated, can lead to infertility. As in the case

Table 8.1
Number of Reported Cases (and Incidence Rates) of Selected Communicable Diseases among 15- to 24-Year-Olds, 1981 to 2003

Disease and Age	1981#	1990#	2003
AIDS	—	1,715	2,019 (4.97)
Chlamydia	—	—	630,385 (1,553.06)
Gonorrhea*	617,994	384,490	195,987 (482.85)
Measles	594	5,646	15 (0.04)
Syphilis*	12,965	16,408	1,182 (2.91)
Tuberculosis	2,198	1,867	1,573 (3.88)

Note: # = rates not available. — = data not collected. * = civilian cases only. Incidence rates per 100,000 population.

Sources: U.S. Department of Health and Human Services, Public Health Service, Centers for Disease Control. *Morbidity and Mortality Weekly Report: Annual Summaries,* various years; *HIV/AIDS Supplemental Report, 1998–2002;* and *Reported Tuberculosis in the United States, 2002;* and Centers for Disease Control and Prevention (2005). "Summary of Notifiable Diseases—United States, 2003." *Morbidity and Mortality Weekly Report,* 52(54): 1–85.

of HIV, the precursor to AIDS, the result may even be death."[16] Chlamydia and gonorrhea are the most common curable STDs among this age group.[17] Among teenagers, it is not uncommon to see more than 5% of young men and 5% to 10% of young women infected with chlamydia.[18] "Reported rates for chlamydial and gonococcal infections are higher among female adolescents 15–19 years of age than among male adolescents and adults of either gender."[2] In addition, it is estimated that up to half of all new HIV infections occurring in the United States are found in people under the age of 25.[19] Overall, an estimated 19 million new infections of STDs occur annually in the United States, almost half of them among young people aged 15 to 24 years.[16]

Health Behaviors and Lifestyle Choices of High School Students

While many behavioral patterns begin during the childhood years (ages 1–14), others begin in adolescence and young adulthood. During this period of experimentation, young people are susceptible to developing deleterious behaviors such as the abuse of alcohol and/or tobacco and other drugs, fighting, and weapon carrying.

In 1990, the Centers for Disease Control and Prevention (CDC) initiated the Youth Risk Behavior Surveillance System (YRBSS) to better track selected health behaviors among young people (see Chapter 3 for more information on the YRBSS). This system currently has three complementary components—national school-based surveys, state and local-based surveys, and a national household-based survey. In the spring of 1991, CDC conducted for the first time the national school-based Youth Risk Behavior Survey. This survey continues to be conducted biennially during odd-numbered years among national probability samples of ninth- through twelfth-grade students from private and public schools. Results of the 2005 survey are included in the following sections. In 1990, CDC began offering to each state and to selected local education departments the YRBSS questionnaire and fiscal and technical assistance to conduct the Youth Risk Behavior Survey. During 2005, 40 state and 21 local surveys were conducted.[14] The third component of YRBSS, national household-based surveys, was initiated when the Census Bureau incorporated a Youth Risk Behavior Supplement in the 1992 National Health Interview Survey (NHIS).[20]

In the short period of time the YRBSS has been in operation, it has proved to be very helpful at both the state and local levels. A number of states and local communities have put into place programs and policies to reduce risk behavior in youth. For example, "in Vermont, YRBSS data were used to examine the success of statewide tobacco control programs and promote tobacco prevention programs for youth."[14] Continued support of YRBSS will help monitor and ensure the success of many public health and school health programs.[14]

Behaviors That Contribute to Unintentional Injuries

Five different behaviors of high school students that relate to unintentional injuries are monitored as part of the YRBSS: seat belt use, bicycle helmet use, motorcycle helmet use, riding with a driver who has been drinking alcohol, and driving after drinking alcohol. Since 1991, the numbers of students engaging in these risk behaviors have declined. Yet in 2005, more than one-fourth of students nationwide had, in the 30 days preceding the survey, ridden with a driver who had been drinking alcohol and 9.9% had driven a vehicle after drinking alcohol.[14]

Behaviors That Contribute to Violence

Behaviors that contribute to violence-related injuries of high school students include carrying a weapon (e.g., gun, knife, or club), engaging in a physical fight, engaging in dating violence, having been forced to have sexual intercourse, engaging in school-related violence, suicide ideation, and suicide attempts. Nationwide over one-sixth (18.5%) of high school students reported having carried a weapon during the 30 days prior to the survey, and about one-third (35.9%) of all high school students reported having been in a fight in the past 12 months. It is no wonder that many school districts around the country are taking steps to reduce violent behavior in school. Males are more likely than females to get in a fight or carry a weapon. However, females were more likely than males to have been forced to have sexual intercourse, and to report sadness, suicide ideation, and suicide attempts.[14] (See Chapter 17 for more on violence.)

Tobacco Use

The use of tobacco products represents one of the most widespread, high-risk health behaviors for this group. In 2005, approximately one-fourth of high school students (23.0%) nationwide were current smokers—that is, smoked on at least one day in the past 30 days—which is a significant decrease from 1997, when 36.4% of students were current smokers. Similarly, a significant decrease has been seen among current frequent smokers—those who had smoked on 20 or more days in the past 30 days (2005, 9.4%; 1999, 16.8%). Overall, white students (25.9%) were significantly more likely to report current cigarette use than Hispanic (22.0%) and black (12.9%) students, as well as more frequent use of cigarettes (11.2%, 6.5%, and 3.7%, respectively).[14] The vast majority of people (approximately 90%) who become dependent upon nicotine develop that dependency between the ages of 15 and 24, and most before they reach the age of 18.[21] (See Figure 8.4.)

In addition to cigarette smoking, the use of **smokeless tobacco** or *spit tobacco* (snuff and chewing tobacco) and cigars is a threat to the health of teenagers. In 2005, the overall prevalence of current smokeless tobacco use was 8.0% in high school students, which is a significant decrease from 1995 (11.4%). The prevalence was higher in males (13.6%) than females (2.2%), and higher in whites (10.2%) than Hispanics (5.1%) or blacks (1.7%). White males reported the highest rates of smokeless tobacco use (17.6%). Although the number of students using cigars has significantly decreased since 1997 (22%), approximately one-sixth (14.0%) of students reported current cigar use.

smokeless tobacco snuff and chewing tobacco

Because use of tobacco that begins during adolescence can lead to a lifetime of nicotine dependence and a variety of negative health consequences, the federal government has exerted considerable effort to keep tobacco out of the hands of adolescents. Many believed, and data from the YRBSS verified, that most adolescents have had easy access to tobacco products. During his term of office, President Clinton was proactive in trying to restrict the distribution of tobacco to youth. One piece of legislation that was approved during President Clinton's term included a requirement that retailers must verify the age of persons who purchase cigarettes or smokeless tobacco products.[21] That guideline stated that anyone who appears to be 27 years of age or younger must be "carded" by retailers.

The most sweeping changes related to the sale of cigarettes came in 1998 when 46 state attorneys general agreed to a settlement with tobacco companies. (Florida, Minnesota, Mississippi, and Texas were not included in the settlement because they had already settled individually with the tobacco companies.) The settlement called for the companies to make payments of $206 billion to the states over 25 years beginning in 2000 and to finance antismoking programs in exchange for the states dropping their health care lawsuits for smokers who were treated with Medicaid funds. In addition to paying the states, the tobacco companies agreed to spend $1.7 billion to study youth smoking and to finance antismoking advertising and accept restrictions on marketing practices that appeal to children, such as the use of cartoon characters (e.g., Joe Camel). Although there is significant conclusive evidence that state tobacco prevention and cessation programs work to reduce smoking, save lives, and save money in health care costs, states are failing to

FIGURE 8.4
More than a million teens begin smoking each year.

utilize tobacco settlement dollars to adequately fund tobacco prevention and cessation programs.[22]

Alcohol and Other Drugs

While, for some, the first use of alcohol or other drugs begins during the childhood years, for most experimentation with these substances occurs between the ages of 15 and 24 years. YRBSS data from 2005 indicate that 43.3% of all high school students reported drinking during the previous month. Further, the data indicate that 25.5% have experienced episodic heavy drinking, and 20.2% have used marijuana at least once in the preceding month.[14]

Although one-fifth of all high school students have used marijuana during the preceding month, alcohol use and abuse continue to be major problems for adolescents, particularly among high school dropouts. As was reported earlier in this chapter, alcohol contributes significantly to motor vehicle crashes and violence in this age group.

In addition to the use of marijuana, high school students are reporting the use of other illicit drugs. The 2005 YRBSS data indicated that during the previous 30 days, 4.1% had used a form of cocaine, while during their lifetime 12.4% had used an inhalant, 6.3% had used Ecstasy, 6.2% had used methamphetamines, 4.0% had used steroids without a doctor's prescription, and 2.1% had injected an illegal drug.[14] (Chapter 12 presents a more detailed examination of the problems of alcohol and other drug misuse and abuse.)

Sexual Behaviors That Contribute to Unintended Pregnancy and Sexually Transmitted Diseases

Since the early 1980s, adolescents in the United States have experienced high rates of unintended pregnancies and STDs, including HIV infection.[23] YRBSS data from 2005 show that almost half (46.8%) of all high school students have engaged in sexual intercourse sometime in their lifetime. The prevalence of sexual intercourse ranged between 29.3% for ninth-grade girls to 60.7% for high school senior boys. Furthermore, it was much more likely for black (67.3%) and Hispanic (51.4%) students to have engaged in sexual intercourse than for whites (41.8%).[14] Table 8.2 shows the trends of selected sexual risk behaviors for high school students since 1991.

As you learned in Chapter 7, each year approximately 750,000 women in the United States between the ages of 15 and 19 become pregnant.[24] Although this number is down 36% since its peak in 1990, a significant portion (84%) of these pregnancies are unintended. The teenage pregnancy rate in the United States is substantially higher than in England, France, Canada, and Sweden.[25] In addition to the health risks associated with teenage pregnancies for both mother and child, there are educational, economic, and psychosocial risks as well. Teenage mothers are less likely to get or stay married, less likely to complete high school or college, and more

Table 8.2
Percentage of High School Students Who Reported Selected Sexual Risk Behaviors, by Year—Youth Risk Behavior Survey, United States, 1991, 1999, and 2005

Behavior	1991	1999	2005
Ever had sexual intercourse	54.1	49.9	46.8
Ever had sexual intercourse with four or more partners	18.7	16.2	14.3
Had sexual intercourse during the three months preceding the survey	37.5	36.3	33.9
Used alcohol or drugs before last sexual intercourse	21.6	24.8	23.3
Used or partner used birth control pills at last sexual intercourse	20.8	16.2	17.6
Used or partner used condom at last sexual intercourse	46.2	58.0	62.8

Source: Centers for Disease Control and Prevention (2006). "National Youth Risk Behavior Survey: 1991–2005—Trends in the Prevalence of Sexual Behaviors." Available at http://www.cdc.gov/healthyyouth/yrbs/index.htm.

likely to require public assistance and to live in poverty than their peers who are not mothers.[26]

Physical Activity

Lack of physical activity by young people has increasingly become a concern. In 2005, one-third (31.3%) of students had not participated in sufficient vigorous physical activity (activities that made them sweat and breathe hard for 20 minutes or more on three or more of the seven days preceding the survey) and had not participated in sufficient moderate physical activity (activities that did not make them sweat or breathe hard for 30 minutes or more on five or more of the seven days preceding the survey) during the seven days preceding the survey. Females (38.5%) were more likely than males (24.2%) to not engage in sufficient physical activity. The prevalence of lack of participation in a sufficient amount of physical activity was highest among black students. Nationally, 9.6% of students had not participated in either vigorous or moderate physical activity during the seven days preceding the survey.[14]

Overweight and Weight Control

Much like the concern for insufficient physical activity, the concern regarding students becoming overweight has received significant attention recently (see Figure 8.5). In 2005, approximately one-sixth of students were at risk for becoming overweight (15.7%) or were overweight (13.1%), while 31.5% described themselves as slightly or very overweight. Almost

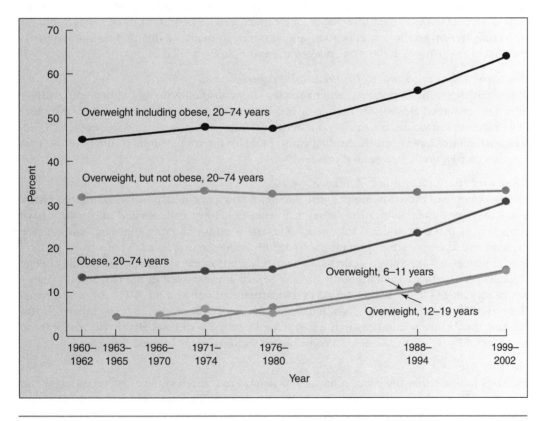

FIGURE 8.5

Overweight and obesity by age: United States, 1960–2002.

Source: National Center for Health Statistics (2005). *Health, United States, 2005, with Chartbook on Trends in the Health of Americans.* Hyattsville, MD: Author.

one-half of students were trying to lose weight (45.6%). Eating less food, fewer calories, or foods low in fat (40.7%) and exercising (60.0%) were commonly documented behaviors for losing weight or avoiding weight gain. The prevalence for engaging in weight loss behaviors and avoiding weight gain behaviors was higher among females (54.8% and 67.4%, respectively) than males (26.8% and 52.9%). Nationally, 12.3% of students had gone without eating for 24 hours or more to lose weight or to keep from gaining weight during the 30 days preceding the survey.[14]

Health Behaviors and Lifestyle Choices of College Students

In 1995, the national college-based survey—the National College Health Risk Behavior Survey (NCHRBS)—was added to the YRBSS process. Prior to that time, the prevalence of health risk behaviors of college students nationwide had not been well characterized.[27] However, the survey did not become a regular component of the YRBSS, and has not been conducted since.

Two currently available data sources regarding the health behaviors of college students are the National College Health Assessment (NCHA)[28] and Monitoring the Future.[29] The NCHA, first implemented in spring 2000, is a national, nonprofit research effort organized by the American College Health Association.[28] Monitoring the Future is conducted at the University of Michigan's Institute for Social Research and, since its inception in 1975, has been funded by the National Institute on Drug Abuse. Monitoring the Future specifically examines drug behaviors and related attitudes of a broad participant age range: eighth, tenth, and twelfth graders to adults through age 40,[29] whereas the NCHA examines a wide range of health behaviors in college students. These data sources, among others, can be helpful to those responsible for delivering health promotion education and services to many of the 17.3 million students enrolled in the nation's 4,200-plus colleges and universities.[30]

Behaviors That Contribute to Unintentional Injuries

Motor vehicle crashes, operating motor vehicles after consuming alcohol, riding with a driver who has consumed alcohol, swimming or boating while using alcohol, and not wearing seat belts are common incidences causing unintentional injuries to college-aged students.[14,27] Unintentional injuries have been the leading cause of death for young adults throughout the past 50 years (see Figure 8.3 presented earlier).[11]

Behaviors That Contribute to Violence

College campuses are communities just like small towns or neighborhoods in large cities. Thus, they have their share of violence. Knowing this, most colleges and universities have programs in place to address this issue. Though weapon carrying, fighting, and suicide ideation and attempts are important public health issues, sexual assault seems to be particularly prevalent among college students. Collectively, approximately one-fifth of female college students reported experiencing some form of sexual abuse/assault in the past school year— sexual touching (11.7%), verbal threats (4.4%), attempted penetration (4.1%), or sexual penetration (2.0%). Additionally, 15.3% of females and 9.8% of males reported being involved in an emotionally abusive relationship in the past school year.[28] Though not all the reasons for these sexual assaults are clear, alcohol is a contributing factor in many of these episodes.

Tobacco Use

Statistics indicate that the more education a person has, the less likely he or she is to use tobacco.[29] Yet in 2005, almost one-fourth (23.8%) of all college students reported being current tobacco users in the previous 30 days,[29] which is consistent with the 23.3% of the total U.S. population who are current smokers.[31] When college students are compared with other young adults one to four years beyond high school, however, significant differences can be seen. Over one-third (35.4%) of others one to four years beyond high school reported being current tobacco users in the previous 30 days.[29] As can be seen in Figures 8.6a and 8.6b, the

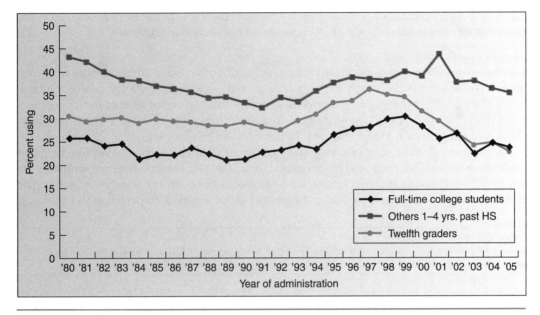

FIGURE 8.6A

Cigarettes: Trends in 30-day prevalence among college students versus others one to four years beyond high school.

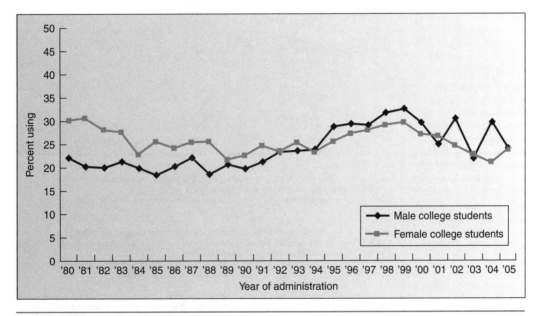

FIGURE 8.6B

Cigarettes: Trends in 30-day prevalence among male versus female college students.

Source: Johnston, L. D., P. M. O'Malley, and J. G. Bachman (2006). *Monitoring the Future National Survey Results on Drug Use, 1975–2005. Vol. II: College Students and Adults Ages 19–45.* Bethesda, MD: National Institute on Drug Abuse.

use of tobacco by college students had been steadily declining until the early 1990s. Since that time, and for some unknown reason, its prevalence has been inconsistent.[29]

Alcohol and Other Drug Use

College and university campuses have long been thought of as places where alcohol and other drugs have been abused. Table 8.3 shows that alcohol is the drug of choice on college campuses, with 67.9% of the students reporting that they had consumed alcohol in the previous thirty days. Table 8.3 also shows that illicit drug use continues to rise, but it is still considerably lower than it was in 1980.[29] Figure 8.7a presents the 25-year trend for alcohol use on college campuses. The figure shows that the number of individuals consuming one or more drinks over the past 30-day period has remained fairly stable for the past 10 years, with approximately 87% of college students having tried alcohol.[29] Although the number of individuals consuming alcohol has decreased over the past 25 years, Figure 8.7b demonstrates the need

---

Table 8.3
Trends in 30-Day Prevalence of Various Types of Drugs among College Students One to Four Years Beyond High School

	Percentage Who Used in Past 30 Days			
	1980	1990	2000	2005*
Approx. wtd. $N =$	1040	1400	1350	1360
Any illicit drug[a]	38.4	15.2	21.5	19.5
Any illicit drug other than marijuana[a]	20.7	4.4	6.9	8.2
Marijuana	34.0	14.0	20.0	17.1
Inhalants[b,c]	1.5	1.0	0.9	0.3
Hallucinogens[c,d]	2.7	1.4	1.4	1.2
LSD	1.4	1.1	0.9	0.1
MDMA (Ecstasy)[e]	NA	0.6	2.5	0.8
Cocaine	6.9	1.2	1.4	1.8
Heroin	0.3	0.0	0.2	0.1
Other narcotics[f,g]	1.8	0.5	1.7	3.1
Amphetamines, adj.[f,h]	NA	1.4	2.9	2.9
Barbiturates[f]	0.9	0.2	1.1	1.3
Tranquilizers[e,f]	2.0	0.5	2.0	2.2
Alcohol[i]	81.8	74.5	67.4	67.9
Cigarettes	25.8	21.5	28.2	23.8

Notes: NA indicates data not available.

[a] "Any illicit drug" includes use of marijuana, hallucinogens, cocaine, or heroin, or other narcotics, amphetamines, sedatives (barbiturates), methaqualone (until 1990), or tranquilizers not under a doctor's orders.

[b] This drug was asked about in four of the five questionnaire forms in 1980-1989 and in three of the six forms in 1999-2005. Total N in 2005 (for college students) is 680.

[c] Unadjusted for known underreporting of certain drugs.

[d] In 2001 the question text was changed on half the questionnaire forms. "Other psychedelics" was changed to "other hallucinogens," and "shrooms" was added to the list of examples. For tranquilizers, "Miltown" was replaced with "Xanax" in the list of examples. Beginning in 2002, the remaining forms were changed to the new wording.

[e] This drug was asked about in two of the five questionnaire forms in 1989, in two of the six questionnaire forms in 1990-2001, and in three of the six questionnaire forms in 2002-2005. Total N in 2005 (for college students) is approximately 680.

[f] Only drug use that was not under a doctor's orders is included here.

[g] In 2002 the question text was changed on half of the questionnaire forms. The list of examples of narcotics other than heroin was updated: Talwin, laudanum, and paregoric—all of which had negligible rates of use by 2001—were replaced by Vicodin, OxyContin, and Percocet. In 2003 the remaining forms were changed to the new wording. The data are based on all forms in 2003 and beyond.

[h] Based on the data from the revised question, which attempts to exclude inappropriate reporting of nonprescription amphetamines.

[i] In 1993 and 1994, the question text was changed slightly in three of the six questionnaire forms to indicate that a "drink" meant "more than just a few sips." Because this revision resulted in rather little change in reported prevalence in the surveys in high school graduates, the data for all forms combined are used in order to provide the most reliable estimate of change. After 1994, the new question text was used in all six of the questionnaire forms.

Source: Johnston, L. D., P. M. O'Malley, J. G. Bachman, and J. E. Schulenberg (2006). *Monitoring the Future National Survey Results on Drug Use, 1975-2005. Vol. II: College Students and Adults Ages 19-45.* Bethesda, MD: National Institute on Drug Abuse.

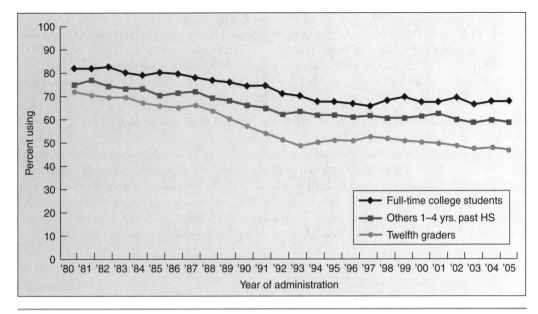

FIGURE 8.7a

Alcohol: Trends in 30-day prevalence among college students versus others one to four years beyond high school.

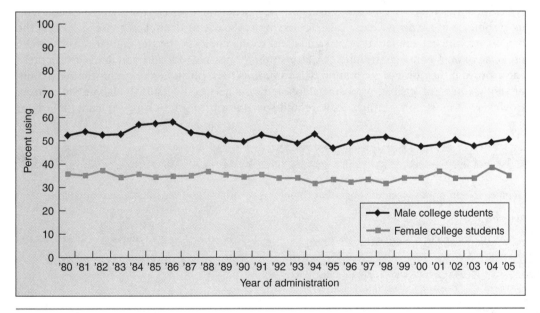

FIGURE 8.7b

Alcohol: Trends in two-week prevalence of five or more drinks in a row among male and female college students.

Source: Johnston, L. D., P. M. O'Malley, and J. G. Bachman (2006). *Monitoring the Future National Survey Results on Drug Use, 1975–2005. Vol. II: College Students and Adults Ages 19–45.* Bethesda, MD: National Institute on Drug Abuse.

for concern regarding the number of college students participating in binge drinking, which is commonly defined as consuming five or more drinks in a row. According to the National College Health Association, 24% of males and 11% of females binge drank three or more times during the two weeks prior to survey administration.[28] Excessive alcohol intake is associated with a number of adverse consequences, including fatal and nonfatal injuries, alcohol poisoning, academic failure, STDs and unintended pregnancy, and various forms of violence.[32]

Sexual Behaviors That Contribute to Unintended Pregnancy and Sexually Transmitted Diseases

Like adolescents, many college students put themselves at risk for unintended pregnancies and infections with STDs through the practice of unprotected sexual activity. Approximately 60% of all gonorrhea cases and three-fourths of all chlamydia cases occur among persons under 25 years of age (see Box 8.1).[33] Only approximately one-quarter (27%) of college students always or mostly used a condom when having intercourse in the 30 days prior to being surveyed, and 18% relied on the withdrawal method or no method for pregnancy prevention.[28]

Community Health Strategies for Improving the Health of Adolescents and Young Adults

There are no easy, simple, or immediate solutions to reducing or eliminating the health problems of adolescents and young adults. As noted in Chapter 1, community health is affected by four major factors—physical factors, community organizing, individual behavior, and social and cultural factors. Of these four, the two that need special attention when dealing with the health problems of adolescents and young adults are social and cultural factors and community organizing. Many health problems originate from the social and cultural environments in which people have been raised and live, and the culture and social norms that have been with us in some cases for many years. Take, for example, the use of alcohol. It is safe to say that the biggest health problem facing adolescents and young adults in the United States today is the use of alcohol. Alcohol contributes to all the leading causes of mortality and morbidity in these age groups. If the norm of a community is to turn its back on adolescents consuming alcohol or young adults (of legal age) abusing alcohol, efforts need to be made to change the culture. However, in most communities, culture and social norms do not change quickly. Efforts to

---

BOX 8.1 | **HEALTHY PEOPLE 2010: OBJECTIVES**

Objective 25-1: Reduce the proportion of adolescents and young adults with *Chlamydia trachomatis* infections.

Target, 2000 status, and baseline:

Objective	Reduction in *Chlamydia trachomatis* infections	1997 Baseline	2004 Status	2010 Target
			Percent	
25-1a.	Females aged 15–24 years attending family planning clinics	5.0	6.9	3.0
25-1b.	Females aged 15–24 years attending STD clinics	12.2	15.3	3.0
25-1c.	Males aged 15–24 years attending STD clinics	15.7	20.2	3.0

For Further Thought

If you were given the responsibility of lowering the incidence of chlamydia in the United States, what community health activities would you recommend?

Source: Centers for Disease Control and Prevention (2006). *Sexually Transmitted Disease Surveillance System, 2005.* Atlanta, GA: Author.

turn these health problems around will need to be community-wide in nature and sustained over a long period of time. By "community-wide," we mean the involvement of all the stakeholders in a community, not just those who are associated with health-related professions—in other words, a community organizing effort is needed. By "sustained over a long period," we mean institutionalizing the change in the culture. For examples of model programs that have been effective in preventing or reducing substance abuse and other related high-risk behaviors in communities and schools, including college campus communities, visit the SAMHSA (Substance Abuse and Mental Health Services Administration) Model Programs Web site at www.modelprograms.samhsa.gov. The programs identified at this Web site have been reviewed by SAMHSA's National Registry of Evidence-based Programs and Practices (NREPP).[34]

To change the culture as it relates to adolescents' use of alcohol, research has shown that alcohol prevention efforts need to be a part of a comprehensive school health education effort and should include components outside the classroom. Thus, prevention programs need to include components that focus on changing norms, interaction among peers, social skills training, and developmental and cultural appropriateness.[35-37]

Many colleges and universities are trying to change the culture on campus as it relates to the use of alcohol. In fact, some schools have signed up for national programs to change campus culture to reduce drinking. Some schools are increasing the number of Friday classes to try to reduce the amount of Thursday-night partying. Others have banned alcohol from campus and toughened penalties for those caught drinking, while still others have restricted tailgating and stadium sales.[38] Almost all schools have developed alcohol education programs that include the following four principles:

1. Legal principle: According to state law you must be 21 years old to consume alcohol.
2. Abstinence principle: If you do not drink alcohol, do not start; it is okay to abstain; many students do abstain.
3. Social norming principle: Not as many of your peers drink alcohol as you think; every college student does not drink.
4. Harm reduction principle: If you do consume alcohol, do so in such a way that you reduce your risk of hazardous outcomes; learn harm reduction skills.

ADULTS

The adult age group (those 25 to 64 years old) represents slightly more than half of the U.S. population. The size of this segment of the overall population is expected to remain stable over the next couple of decades, but in proportion to the rest of the population this segment will become smaller. Therefore, provisions to deal with the health concerns of this age group will need to be maintained.

A Health Profile

The health profile of this age of adults is characterized primarily by mortality from chronic diseases stemming from poor health behavior and poor lifestyle choices made during the earlier years of life.

Mortality

With life expectancy at birth between 75 and 80 years,[11] most Americans can expect to live beyond their 65th birthday. However, many do not. During the 1950s and 1960s, it was revealed that many of the leading causes of death in this age group resulted from preventable conditions associated with unhealthy behaviors and lifestyles. As such, many adults have quit smoking, and more Americans than ever before are exercising regularly and eating healthier diets. These lifestyle improvements, along with successes in public health and advances in medicine, have resulted in a significant decline in the death rate for adults in the last half of the twentieth century, a decline that is projected to continue in the twenty-first century.

In the past, leading causes of death for adults were reported only for the 25- to 64-year-old age group. More recently, the adult years have been subdivided into two groups: 25 to 44 years and 45 to 64 years, with some data being reported in 10-year age spans. In 2003, the death rate for all adults ages 25 to 34 years was 103.6 per 100,000, and for ages 35 to 44 years it was 201.6 per 100,000.[11] The leading causes of death for those in this age group in 2003 were unintentional injuries, malignant neoplasms (cancer), heart disease, suicide, homicide, and HIV. With the exception of HIV, the current leading causes of death were also at the top of the list in 1980.[11] When the mortality data for this age group are broken down by age, race, and ethnicity, some differences appear. For 25- to 34-year-olds, the six leading causes of death are the same, but differ in rank order by race and ethnic group (see Table 8.4). For 35- to 44-year-olds, liver disease and cirrhosis is among the six leading causes for whites and Hispanics, replacing homicide and suicide, respectively, whereas among blacks, the six leading causes include cerebrovascular disease (stroke) rather than suicide.[39]

In 2003, the death rate for 45- to 54-year-olds was 433.2 per 100,000, twice that of the 35-to-44 age group. The death rate for 55- to 64-year-olds was 940.9 per 100,000, more than two times greater than the 45-to-54 age group. The majority of these deaths were the result of noncommunicable health problems. They include cancer, heart disease, unintentional injuries, diabetes, stroke, and chronic lower respiratory disease, which includes emphysema, asthma, and bronchitis. Like with the 25- to 44-year-olds, there are racial and ethnic disparities. Though cancer and heart disease are the first and second causes of death for all three groups presented in Table 8.5, chronic lower respiratory disease appears in the list of the six leading causes for whites, kidney disease appears in the list for blacks, and liver disease and cirrhosis appears in the Hispanic list.[39]

Cancer

Since 1983, the Number 1 cause of death in the adult age group has been cancer (malignant neoplasms). (For a review of malignant neoplasms, see Chapter 4.) Age-adjusted cancer death rates have remained relatively steady since 1950 (193.9 per 100,000 in 1950 compared to 190.1 per 100,000 in 2003). However, the crude death rates have jumped from 139.8 per 100,000 to 191.5 per 100,000 during that same time, reflecting an aging American population.[11]

Three types of cancers account for these large numbers—lung, colorectal, and breast. The leading cause of cancer deaths and the most preventable type of cancer for both men and

Table 8.4
Death Rates, Adults, Ages 25–34 and 35–44 (Rate per 100,000 Population)

	Non-Hispanic White		Non-Hispanic Black		Hispanic	
	25–34 (93.5)	35–44 (186.6)	25–34 (186.8)	35–44 (348.6)	25–34 (79.3)	35–44 (145.8)
Unintentional injuries	32.8	38.1	31.4	39.1	27.6	31.7
Cancer	9.5	34.5	12.3	50.0	6.8	23.2
Heart disease	6.5	27.3	18.4	57.8	4.4	14.7
Suicide	13.6	17.0	9.3	7.6	6.6	7.0
Homicide	5.9	4.8	45.3	23.7	12.3	8.0
HIV	2.2	7.0	20.6	52.8	3.6	13.4
Liver disease and cirrhosis	0.9	7.3	—	5.5	1.1	8.7
Stroke	1.2	4.2	1.7	12.8	1.3	4.4

Source: Anderson, R. N., and B. L. Smith (2005). "Deaths: Leading Causes for 2002." *National Vital Statistics Reports*, 53(17).

Table 8.5
Death Rates, Adults, Ages 45–54 and 55–64 (Rate per 100,000 Population)

	Non-Hispanic White		Non-Hispanic Black		Hispanic	
	45–54 (395.3)	55–64 (902.5)	45–54 (765.8)	55–64 (1565.2)	45–54 (321.3)	55–64 (719.8)
Cancer	118.5	343.3	181.7	485.6	78.2	215.1
Heart disease	84.8	224.5	180.9	442.9	55.3	176.8
Unintentional injuries	36.2	30.7	46.8	41.4	32.0	28.7
Diabetes mellitus	11.7	32.7	30.1	84.2	14.0	52.1
Stroke	11.6	31.4	40.7	88.0	15.3	35.9
Chronic lower respiratory disease	8.4	44.2	—	40.7	—	13.9
Liver disease and cirrhosis	18.1	23.1	20.8	25.5	26.9	38.4
Suicide	17.6	15.0	—	7.6	7.1	7.0
HIV	—	—	53.9	26.1	14.7	9.5
Kidney disease	—	—	—	41.0	—	13.5

Source: Anderson, R.N., and B. L. Smith (2005). "Deaths: Leading Causes for 2002." *National Vital Statistics Reports*, 53(17).

women is lung cancer. This trend is expected to continue as large numbers of smokers continue to age. Of all lung cancer deaths, 87% can be attributed to smoking.[40] The second leading cause of death due to cancer is colorectal cancer. Risk factors for this type of cancer include personal or family history, obesity, lack of physical activity, smoking, alcohol consumption, a diet high in red or processed meats, and a low intake of fruits and vegetables.[40]

Breast cancer is the other cancer of much concern. Until it was surpassed by lung cancer in the mid-1980s, it was the leading cause of cancer deaths in women. Although it is less deadly than lung cancer, the number of cases of breast cancer is more than twice that of lung cancer in women.[40] Because of increased community awareness and the availability of diagnostic screening for breast cancer, survival rates are much higher than for lung cancer. However, breast cancer rates could be reduced even further if a higher percentage of women over 39 years of age complied with the screening recommendations.[40]

To help people understand the prevalence of cancer in their community, the American Cancer Society has created a table that can be used to estimate the number of cancer statistics locally. This information is presented in Table 8.6.

Cardiovascular Diseases
Some of the greatest changes in cause-specific mortality rates in adults are those for the cardiovascular diseases. Age-adjusted mortality rates from diseases of the heart dropped from 586.8 per 100,000 in 1950 to 232.2 per 100,000 in 2003, while deaths from strokes dropped from 180.7 per 100,000 to 53.5 per 100,000 during the same period of time.[11] These figures represent drops of about 60% and 70%, respectively. These changes are due primarily to the public health efforts that have encouraged people to stop smoking, increase their physical activity, and eat more nutritionally. The reduction or postponement of deaths from heart disease has resulted in cancer becoming the leading cause of deaths in adults 45 to 64 years of age.

Health Behaviors and Lifestyle Choices
Many of the risk factors associated with the leading causes of morbidity and mortality in American adults are associated with health behavior and lifestyle choices. Adults have a unique opportunity to take personal action to substantially decrease their risk of ill health, and in recent years, many have taken such action. Today, more than ever before, adults are watching what they eat, wearing their seat belts, controlling their blood pressure, and exercising with regularity.

Table 8.6
How to Estimate Cancer Statistics Locally, 2006

To obtain the estimated number of . . .	Multiply community population by:				
	All Sites	**Female Breast***	**Colon or Rectum**	**Lung**	**Prostate***
New cancer cases	0.0047	0.0014	0.0005	0.0006	0.0016
Cancer deaths	0.0019	0.0003	0.0002	0.0005	0.0002
People who will eventually develop cancer	0.41156	0.1322	0.0566	0.0658	0.1793
People who will eventually die of cancer	0.2110	0.0291	0.0224	0.0537	0.0310

*For female breast cancer multiply by female population, and for prostate cancer multiply by male population.

Note: These calculations provide only a rough approximation of the number of people in a specific community who may develop or die of cancer. These estimates should be used with caution because they do not reflect the age or racial characteristics of the population, access to detection and treatment, or exposure to risk factors. State cancer registries count the number of cancers that occur in localities throughout the state. The American Cancer Society recommends using data from these registries, when it is available, to more accurately estimate local cancer statistics.

Source: American Cancer Society (2006). *Cancer Facts and Figures—2006.* Used with permission of the American Cancer Society, Inc. All rights reserved.

The prevalence of smoking among adults has declined, as has the incidence of drinking and driving. While these are encouraging signs, there is still much more that can be done.

As with the other age groups discussed in this chapter, the National Center for Heath Statistics (NCHS) collects self-reported behavior risk data on adults. These data are collected via the Behavioral Risk Factor Surveillance System (BRFSS). (See Chapter 3 for a discussion about the BRFSS.) One limitation of the data from this system is that they are collected, and usually reported, on all adults over 18 years of age; the data are not broken down by the specific age groups (18–24, 25–44, and 45–64) discussed in this chapter. More detailed information about the health behaviors and lifestyle choices of adults in the United States is presented next.

Risk Factors for Chronic Disease
The best single behavioral change Americans can make to reduce morbidity and mortality is to stop smoking. Smoking is responsible for 30% of deaths in the United States.[41] It is an important risk factor for cancer, heart disease, and stroke. In 2005, over one-fifth (20.9%) of those who were aged 18 years and older smoked.[11] This amounts to about 45 million Americans.[40] The proportion of Americans who smoke has dropped considerably since 1965, when 40% of all Americans smoked. While more men than women (24% versus 18%) smoke,[42] the gap between the genders is decreasing. In general, smoking rates are higher among American Indians and Alaska Natives, people with fewer years of education, and those with lower incomes.[26]

Three other interrelated risk factors that contribute to disease and death in this age group are lack of exercise, failure to maintain an appropriate body weight, and alcohol consumption. Though American adults are exercising more than ever before, few are exercising on a regular basis. The American Heart Association has stated that "24 percent of Americans age 18 or older are not active at all. Fifty-four percent of adults get some exercise, but they don't do it regularly or intensely enough to protect their hearts. Only 22 percent of American adults get enough leisure time exercise to achieve cardiovascular fitness."[43] It was once thought that **intensity** had to be high in order for cardiovascular benefits from exercise to accrue. But now it is believed that even light-to-moderate physical activity can have significant health benefits if done regularly and long term. Such activities include walking, gardening, housework, and dancing.

intensity cardiovascular workload measured by heart rate

Being overweight increases one's chances of a number of health problems, including heart disease, some cancers, hypertension, elevated blood cholesterol, diabetes, stroke, gallbladder disease, and osteoarthritis. In 2004, according to the National Health and Nutrition Examination Surveys, 67% of 20- to 74-year-olds were overweight (including obese), with 34% being obese as defined by **body mass index (BMI)**.[44] Obesity in America is truly an epidemic, with obesity rates increasing by more than 60% in the last 10 years (see Figure 8.8).[45] The trend of weight gain increases with age. The key to maintaining an appropriate weight throughout life is a combination of diet and exercise; total reliance on either factor alone makes it a difficult process.[46]

body mass index (BMI)
the ratio of weight (in kilograms) to height (in meters, squared)

As with other age groups, alcohol consumption often places adults at greater health risk. Approximately 70% of adult Americans consume alcohol. While most do so in moderation, a relatively small percentage develop serious problems with their alcohol use. In 2005, 14.4% of adults reported binge drinking (i.e., consumption of five or more alcoholic beverages on at least one occasion in the previous month).[45] Men are about three times more likely to report binge drinking than women.[45] It is estimated that the 5% who consume the greatest amount of alcohol consume about 36% of all the alcohol consumed in America.[47] These people are at greatest risk for developing a dependence upon alcohol and for developing such alcohol-related health problems as cirrhosis, alcoholism, and alcohol psychosis.

One does not have to become dependent on alcohol to have a drinking problem. Alcohol contributes to society's problems in a great many other ways. As noted in other chapters of this text, alcohol increases the rates of homicide, suicide, family violence, and unintentional injuries such as those from motor vehicle crashes, boating incidents, and falls. The use of alcohol by pregnant women can cause fetal alcohol spectrum disorder, the leading cause of birth defects in children. Clearly, alcohol consumption adversely affects the health and well-being of Americans.

Risk Factors for Personal Injury
Like individuals in the other age groups, adults also put themselves at risk for personal injury by the way they behave. Two such areas of concerns are both related to the operation of motor vehicles—the use of seat belts and the operation of a motor vehicle after drinking alcohol. Most Americans (80%) report wearing seat belts when driving or riding in a motor

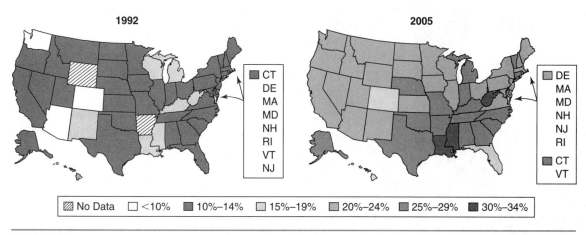

FIGURE 8.8
Obesity trends among U.S. adults.
Note: Obesity is defined as a BMI > 30, or about 30 pounds overweight for a five-foot, four-inch person.
Source: CDC, Behavioral Risk Factor Surveillance System.

vehicle, which is an improvement from 20 years ago, when approximately 60% of the population reported wearing a seat belt when in a motor vehicle.[48] Among drivers 21 years or older, an estimated 15.7% had driven under the influence of alcohol during the past year.[49] The data on both of these behaviors are interesting because both behaviors are regulated by public health laws. This suggests that a society can only be controlled by regulations to the extent that it wants to be.

Awareness and Screening of Certain Medical Conditions

There are a number of regular, noninvasive or minimally invasive health screenings that are recommended for adults to participate in, such as screenings for hypertension, diabetes, high blood cholesterol, and cancer.

hypertension
systolic pressure equal to or greater than 140 mm of mercury (Hg) and/or diastolic pressure equal to or greater than 90 mm Hg for extended periods of time

There is no "ideal" blood pressure. Instead, the acceptable blood pressure falls within a range considered healthy. **Hypertension** exists when systolic pressure is equal to or greater than 140 mm of mercury (Hg) and/or diastolic pressure is equal to or greater than 90 mm Hg for extended periods of time. Statistics show that hypertension is found in about one in three adults in the United States, with one-third of those unaware they have it, making it the most prevalent risk factor for cardiovascular disease in the United States.[50] Fortunately, once detected hypertension is a risk factor that is highly modifiable (see Figure 8.9). The most desirable means of controlling hypertension is through a combination of diet modification, appropriate physical exercise, and weight management. In cases in which these measures prove ineffective, hypertension can usually still be controlled with medication. The keys to reducing morbidity and mortality resulting from hypertension are mass screenings that result in early detection of previously unidentified cases and their appropriate treatment.

Diabetes results from failure of the pancreas to make or use a sufficient amount of insulin. Without insulin, food cannot be properly used by the body. Diabetes cannot be cured, but it

can be controlled through a combination of diet, exercise, medications, and insulin injections. It has already been reported earlier in the chapter that with the exception of 15- to 24-year-olds, diabetes is one of the leading causes of death for all adults. The death rates are highest in American Indians/Alaska Natives and black Americans.[11] However, many deaths resulting from diabetes could be postponed if diabetes was detected and treated appropriately. Approximately 20 million Americans have diabetes, with almost 1.5 million new cases diagnosed in people aged 20 years or older in 2005.[51] The percentage of adults with diagnosed diabetes has increased 61% over the past 10 years (see Figure 8.10).[38] Furthermore, one in three persons with diabetes is unaware that he or she has the disease.[51]

Cholesterol is a soft, fat-like substance that is necessary to build cell membranes. However, elevated cholesterol levels in blood can put people at greater risk for heart disease and stroke. The higher the cholesterol level, the greater the risk.[17] Cholesterol is produced by the liver in sufficient quantities to meet the needs of the body. A person's cholesterol level is also affected by his or her age, heredity, and diet. There is nothing we can do about heredity and age, but diet is something we can modify.

FIGURE 8.9
Hypertension is a highly modifiable risk factor.

Dietary factors are associated with four of the ten leading causes of death in this age group. Many dietary components are involved in the diet-health relationship, but chief among them is the disproportionate consumption of foods high in fat, often at the expense of foods high in complex carbohydrates and dietary fiber. Total dietary fat (saturated

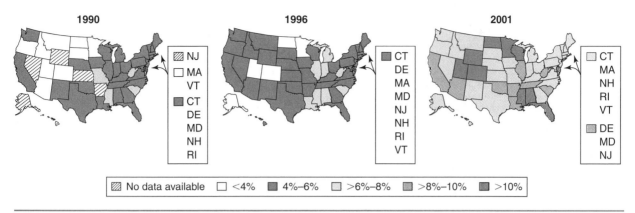

FIGURE 8.10

The percentage of adults with diagnosed diabetes increased 61% from 1990 to 2001. These figures include women with a history of gestational diabetes.

Source: Centers for Disease Control and Prevention, Behavioral Risk Factor Surveillance System.

and unsaturated) accounts for too many total calories consumed in the United States. A diet that contains between 20% and 35% fat, with less than 10% of calories from saturated fats, is recommended.[52] Currently, the largest source of fat in diets comes from cheeses and oils. Diets high in fat and cholesterol are part of the reason why an estimated 50% of American adults have blood cholesterol levels of 200 mg/dL (milligrams per deciliter) and higher, and why about 20% have levels of 240 mg/dL or above.[53] Based on several studies, blood cholesterol levels less than 200 mg/dL in middle-aged adults seem to indicate a relatively low risk of coronary heart disease. In contrast, people with a blood cholesterol level of 240 mg/dL have twice the risk of having a coronary heart attack as people who have a cholesterol level of 200 mg/dL.[53] **Hypercholesterolemia** is the term used for high levels of cholesterol in the blood. Like diabetes, the key to controlling hypercholesterolemia is screening and treatment.

> **hypercholesterol-emia**
> high levels of cholesterol in the blood

The other prevalent medical condition in this age group that should be screened for on a regular basis is cancer. As noted earlier, malignant neoplasms are the leading cause of death in 45- to 64-year-olds. The American Cancer Society recommends a number of screenings for various age groups (see Table 8.7). However, many more adults in the United States could be getting screened. The earlier that cancer is detected, the greater the chance for successful treatment.

Community Health Strategies for Improving the Health of Adults

As noted in the previous pages, adults in the United States are faced with a number of health issues. Even so, for most individuals the years between 25 and 64 are some of the healthiest of their lifetime. A key for keeping these people healthy is to re-emphasize the importance of individual responsibility for health. That is, individuals must engage in behaviors that are health enhancing. From a community health perspective, this means that community health workers must continue to offer primary, secondary, and tertiary prevention programs that are aimed at the needs of this age group. For example, primary prevention programs could include exercise and nutrition programs that help reduce the risks of cancer and cardiovascular disease. Secondary prevention programs that emphasize self or clinical screenings to identify and control disease processes in their early stages, such as mammography, self-testicular exams, and cholesterol screenings, would also be appropriate for this age group. In addition, tertiary prevention programs such as medication compliance to prevent disability by restoring individuals to their optimal level of functioning after the onset of disease or injury could also be useful.

Table 8.7
Summary of American Cancer Society Recommendations for the Early Detection of Cancer in Asymptomatic People

Breast	• Yearly mammograms are recommended starting at age 40. The age at which screening should be stopped should be individualized by considering the potential risks and benefits of screening in the context of overall health status and longevity. • Clinical breast exam should be part of a periodic health exam about every 3 years for women in their 20s and 30s, and every year for women 40 and older. • Women should know how their breasts normally feel and report any breast change promptly to their health care providers. Breast self-exam is an option for women starting in their 20s. • Women at increased risk (e.g., family history, genetic tendency, past breast cancer) should talk with their doctors about the benefits and limitations of starting mammography screening earlier, having additional tests (i.e., breast ultrasound and MRI), or having more frequent exams.
Colon & rectum	Beginning at age 50, men and women should begin screening with 1 of the examination schedules below: • A fecal occult blood test (FOBT) or fecal immunochemical test (FIT) every year • A flexible sigmoidoscopy (FSIG) every 5 years • Annual FOBT or FIT and flexible signoidoscopy every 5 years* • A double-contrast barium enema every 5 years • A colonoscopy every 10 years *Combined testing is preferred over either annual FOBT or FIT, FSIG every 5 years, alone. People who are at moderate or high risk for colorectal cancer should talk with a doctor about a different testing schedule.*
Prostate	The PSA test and the digital rectal examination should be offered annually, beginning at age 50, to men who have a life expectancy of at least 10 years. Men at high risk (African American men and men with a strong family history of 1 or more first-degree relatives diagnosed with prostate cancer at an early age) should begin testing at age 45. For both men at average risk and high risk, information should be provided about what is known and what is uncertain about the benefits and limitations of early detection and treatment of prostate cancer so that they can make an informed decision about testing.
Uterus	**Cervix:** Screening should begin approximately 3 years after a women begins having vaginal intercourse, but no later than 21 years of age. Screening should be done every year with regular Pap tests or every 2 years using liquid-based tests. At or after age 30, women who have had 3 normal test results may be screened every 2 to 3 years. Alternatively, cervical cancer screening with HPV DNA testing and conventional or liquid-based cytology could be performed every 3 years. However, doctors may suggest a woman get screened more often if she has certain risk factors, such as HIV infection or a weak immune system. Women aged 70 and older who have had 3 or more consecutive normal Pap tests in the last 10 years may choose to stop cervical cancer screening. Screening after total hysterectomy (with removal of the cervix) is not necessary unless the surgery was done as a treatment for cervical cancer. **Endometrium:** The American Cancer Society recommends that at the time of menopause all women should be informed about the risks and symptoms of endometrial cancer, and strongly encouraged to report any unexpected bleeding or spotting to their physicians. Annual screening for endometrial cancer with endrometrial biopsy beginning at age 35 should be offered to women with or at risk for hereditary nonpolyposis colon cancer (HNPCC).
Cancer-related checkup	For individuals undergoing periodic health examinations, a cancer-related checkup should include health counseling and, depending on a person's age and gender, might include examinations for cancers of the thyroid, oral cavity, skin, lymph nodes, testes, and ovaries, as well as for some nonmalignant diseases.

Source: American Cancer Society (2007). *Cancer Facts & Figures—2007.* Used with permission of the American Cancer Society, Inc. All rights reserved.

CHAPTER SUMMARY

- Adolescence and young adulthood (15 to 24 years old) and adulthood (25 to 64 years old) are the most productive periods of people's lives. While most people enjoy good health during these years, there is substantial room for improvement.

- The overall health status of these age groups could be improved by reducing the prevalence of high-risk behaviors (e.g., cigarette smoking, excessive alcohol consumption, and physical inactivity) and by increasing participation in health screenings and institutionalizing preventive health care in our society.

- Approximately 75% of adolescent and young adult mortality can be attributed to motor vehicle crashes, other unintentional injuries, homicide and legal intervention, and suicide.

- Adolescents and young adults remain at considerable risk for STD morbidity.

- College students put themselves at considerable risk through unprotected sexual activity, and the use of alcohol, tobacco, and other drugs.

- Mortality rates for older adults (45 to 64 years old) have declined slightly in recent years, but cancer is still the overall leading cause of death, followed by cardiovascular disease.

- Reductions in deaths from cardiovascular diseases in adults have been substantial, but health problems resulting from unhealthy behaviors—like smoking, poor diet, and physical inactivity—can be reduced further if adults are willing to modify their behavior.

- No matter how the health of adolescents and young adults and adults in the United States is broken down and described, it can be summarized by saying that the health of Americans in these age groups has come a long way in the past 50 years, but there is still room for improvement.

REVIEW QUESTIONS

1. Why it is important for community health workers to be aware of the significant health problems of the various age groups in the United States?

2. What ages are included in the following two age groups: adolescents and young adults, and adults? What are the ages of the two subgroups of adults?

3. Why are the number of adolescents and young adults, living arrangements, and employment status such key demographic characteristics of young people in regard to community health? Briefly summarize the data available on these characteristics.

4. What are the leading causes of death for adolescents and young adults, and for adults?

5. What are the Youth Risk Behavior Surveillance System (YRBSS) and the Behavioral Risk Factor Surveillance System (BRFSS), and what type of data do they generate?

6. What are the behaviors that put each of these cohorts— adolescents, college students, and adults—at greatest risk?

7. How would you summarize the health profile of the two cohorts (adolescents and young adults, and adults) presented in this chapter?

ACTIVITIES

1. Obtain a copy of the most recent results of the Youth Risk Behavior Surveillance System (YRBSS) and the Behavioral Risk Factor Surveillance System (BRFSS) for your state. Review the data presented and then prepare a two-page summary on the "Health Behavior Profile of the Adolescents and Young Adults and Adults" of your state.

2. Using the information presented in Table 8.6 and the most recent census data for your community, calculate its estimated cancer statistics.

3. Interview a small group (about 10) of adults (aged 45 to 64) about their present health status. Ask them questions about their health behavior and health problems. Then, summarize the data you collect in writing and compare it to the information in this chapter on this age group. How are the data similar? How do they differ?

4. Pick either adolescents and young adults or adults and write a two-page paper that presents ideas on how the health profile of that age group can be improved in your state.

COMMUNITY HEALTH ON THE WEB

The Internet contains a wealth of information about community and public health. Increase your knowledge of some of the topics presented in this chapter by accessing the Jones and Bartlett Publishers Web site at **http://health.jbpub.com/book/communityhealth/6e** and follow the links to complete the following Web activities.

- Youth Risk Behavior Surveillance System
- Vital Statistics
- Behavorial Risk Factor Surveillance System

REFERENCES

1. Snyder, T., and L. Shafer (1996). *Youth Indicators, 1996* (NCES 96-027). Washington, DC: U.S. Department of Education, National Center for Education Statistics.

2. MacKay, A. P., L. A. Fingerhut, and C. R. Duran (2000). *Health, United States, 2000 with Adolescent Health Chartbook*. Hyattsville, MD: National Center for Health Statistics.

3. American Medical Association (2000). *Talking to Your Teenagers 11-14: Discussion Guide*. Chicago: Author.

4. Seffrin, J. R. (1990). "The Comprehensive School Health Curriculum: Closing the Gap between State-of-the-Art and State-of-the-Practice." *Journal of School Health*, 60(4): 151-156.

5. Valois, R. F., W. G. Thatcher, J. W. Drane, and B. M. Reininger (1997). "Comparison of Selected Health Risk Behaviors between Adolescents in Public and Private High Schools in South Carolina." *Journal of School Health*, 67(10): 434-440.

6. Hobbs, F., and N. Stoops (2002). *Demographic Trends in the 20th Century* (Census 2000 Special Reports, Series CENSR-4). Washington, DC: U.S. Government Printing Office.

7. U.S. Bureau of Census (1999). *Statistical Abstract of the United States, 1999*, 119th ed. Washington, DC: Author.

8. U. S. Census Bureau (2007). The 2007 Statistical Abstract. Available at http://www.census.gov/compendia/statab/population/

9. Toossi, M. (2006). "A New Look at Long-Term Labor Force Projections to 2050." *Monthly Labor Review Online*, 129(11).

10. Sok, E. (2006). "Lower Unemployment in 2005." *Monthly Labor Review Online*, 129(3).

11. National Center for Health Statistics (2006). *Health, United States, 2006, with Chartbook on Trends in the Health of Americans*. Hyattsville, MD: Author.

12. Murphy, S. L. (2000). "Deaths: Final Data for 1998." *National Vital Statistics Reports*, 48(11): 1-105.

13. U.S. Department of Health and Human Services (1991). *Healthy Children 2000: National Health Promotion and Disease Prevention Objectives Related to Mothers, Infants, Children, Adolescents, and Youth* (HHS pub. no. HRSA-M-CH-91-2). Washington, DC: U.S. Government Printing Office.

14. Centers for Disease Control and Prevention (2006). "Youth Risk Behavior Surveillance—United States, 2005." *MMWR Surveillance Summaries*, 55(SS-5).

15. Centers for Disease Control and Prevention (2001). "Tracking the Hidden Epidemics: Trends in STDs in the United States 2000." Available at http://www.cdc.gov/nchstp/dstd/Stats_Trends/Trends2000.pdf.

16. Centers for Disease Control and Prevention (2001). *CDC Fact Book 2000/2001*. Available at http://www.cdc.gov/maso/factbook/main.htm.

17. Centers for Disease Control and Prevention (2005). *Trends in Reportable Sexually Transmitted Diseases in the United States, 2005*.

SCENARIO: ANALYSIS AND RESPONSE

1. What primary prevention measures would have been helpful for the four university students? What primary prevention measures would have helped the businessman?

2. Why do you think that adolescents and young adults and adults engage in high-risk behaviors like those presented in the scenario? If you were a community health worker in this community, what kind of programs would you recommend to lower the health risks of these individuals?

3. Comment on the attitudes of Annie and Latasha toward drunk driving and the automobile crash. Do you agree with one or the other? Why or why not?

4. Do colleges and universities have an obligation to develop prevention programs to keep students out

of situations like the one described in the scenario? Why or why not?

5. Say you were friends with Annie. She got so concerned with the problem of alcohol abuse on campus that she wanted to take action. She thought that maybe she should look into starting a chapter of Boost Alcohol Consciousness Concerning the Health of University Students (BACCHUS). She wanted to see what was on the Web about BACCHUS, but because of a busy afternoon of classes she knew she wouldn't have time to check it, so she asked you if you would do it for her. Go to the Web and use a search engine (e.g., Google) and enter "BACCHUS." What did you find that might be of help to Annie?

Available at http://www.cdc.gov/nchstp/dstd/stats_trends/stats_and_trends.htm.

18. Mertz, K. J., G. M. McQuillan, W. C. Levine, et al. (1998). "A Pilot Study of the Prevalence of Chlamydial Infection in a National Household Survey." *Sexually Transmitted Diseases*, May, 225-228.

19. The Henry J. Kaiser Family Foundation (2000). *National Survey of Teens on HIV/AIDS*. Menlo Park, CA: Author.

20. Kolbe, L. J., L. Kann, and J. L. Collins (1993). "Overview of the Youth Risk Behavior Surveillance System." *Public Health Reports*, 108(1): 2-10.

21. Centers for Disease Control and Prevention (1996). "Tobacco Use and Usual Source of Cigarettes among High School Students—United States,1995." *Morbidity and Mortality Weekly Report*, 45(20): 413-418.

22. American Heart Association, American Cancer Society, Campaign for Tobacco-Free Kids, and American Lung Association (2006). *A Broken Promise to our Children: The 1998 State Tobacco Settlement Eight Years Later*. Available at http://www.tobaccofreekids.org/reports/settlements/2007/fullreport.pdf.

23. Centers for Disease Control and Prevention (1996). "Trends in Sexual Risk Behavior among High School Students—United States—1990, 1991, and 1993." *Morbidity and Mortality Weekly Report*, 44(7): 124-125, 131-132.

24. Ventura, S. J., S. C. Curtin, and T. J. Mathew (2000). "Variations in Teenage Birth Rates, 1991-98: National and State Trends." *National Vital Statistics Reports*, 48(6): 1-16.

25. Darroch, J. E., S. Singh, J. J. Frost, and the Study Team (2001). "Differences in Teenage Pregnancy Rates Among Five Developed Countries: The Role of Sexual Activity and Contraceptive Use." *Family Planning Perspectives*, 33(6): 244-250, 281.

26. U.S. Department of Health and Human Services (2000). *Healthy People 2010: Understanding and Improving Health*. Washington, DC: U.S. Government Printing Office.

27. Centers for Disease Control and Prevention (1997). "Youth Risk Behavior Surveillance: National College Health Risk Behavior Survey—United States, 1995." *Morbidity and Mortality Weekly Report*, 46(SS-6): 1-56.

28. American College Health Association (2004). *National College Health Assessment Web Summary*. Available at http://www.acha.org/projects_programs/assessment.cfm.

29. Johnston, L. D., P. M. O'Malley, and J. G. Bachman (2003). *Monitoring the Future National Survey Results on Drug Use, 1975-2002. Vol. II: College Students and Adults Ages 19-40*. Bethesda, MD: National Institute on Drug Abuse.

30. U.S Department of Education Statistics (2006). *Digest of Education Statistics: 2005*. Available at http://nces.ed.gov/programs/digest/.

31. Shafey, O., S. Dolwick, and G. E. Guindon. eds. (2003). *Tobacco Control Country Profiles 2003*. Atlanta, GA: American Cancer Society.

32. Goldman, M. S., G. M. Boyd, and V. Faden, eds. (March 2002). "College Drinking, What It Is, and What to Do About It: A Review of the State of the Science [Special issue]." *Journal of Studies on Alcohol*, Suppl. 14.

33. Centers for Disease Control and Prevention (2003). *Sexually Transmitted Disease Surveillance, 2002*. Atlanta, GA: Author.

34. Substance Abuse and Mental Health Services Administration. (2005). "SAMHSA Model Programs." Available at http://www.modelprograms.samhsa.gov/model.htm.

35. Lachter, R. B., K. A. Komro, S. Veblen-Mortenson, C. L. Perry, and C. L. Williams (1999). "High School Students' Efforts to Reduce Alcohol Use in their Communities: Project Northland's Youth Development Component." *Journal of Health Education*, 30(6): 330-342.

36. Drug Strategies (1997). *Making the Grade: A Guide to School Drug Prevention Programs*. Washington, DC: Author.

37. Dusenbury, L., and M. Falco (1995). "Eleven Components of Effective Drug Abuse Prevention Curricula." *Journal of School Health*, 65: 420-425.

38. McGinn, D. (27 November 2000). "Scouting a Dry Campus." *Newsweek*, 83-84.

39. Anderson, R. N., and B. L. Smith (2005). "Deaths: Leading Causes for 2002." *National Vital Statistics Reports*, 53(17).

40. American Cancer Society (2001). *Cancer Facts and Figures—2001*. Atlanta, GA: Author.

41. Mokdad, A. H., J. S. Marks, D. F. Stroup, and J. L. Gerberding (2004). "Actual Causes of Death in the United States, 2000." *Journal of the American Medical Association*, 291(10): 1238-1245.

42. Barnes, P., and J. S. Schiller (2006). "Early Release of Selected Estimates Based on Data from the January–June 2006 National Health Interview Survey." National Center for Health Statistics. Available at http://www.cdc.gov/nchs/nhis.htm.

43. American Heart Association (2001). "Physical Activity and Cardiovascular Health: Fact Sheet." Available at http://www.american-heart.org/Health/Lifestyle/Physical_Activity/PAfact.html.

44. Centers for Disease Control and Prevention (2004). "BMI: Body Mass Index." Available at http://www.cdc.gov/nccdphp/dnpa/bmi/.

45. Centers for Disease Control and Prevention (2006). *Behavioral Risk Factor Surveillance System*. Available at http://www.cdc.gov/brfss/index.htm.

46. Centers for Disease Control and Prevention (2006). "Overweight and Obesity: Contributing Factors." Available at http://www.cdc.gov/nccdphp/dnpa/obesity/contributing_factors.htm.

47. Manning, W. G., L. Blumberg, and L. H. Moulton (1995). "The Demand for Alcohol: The Differential Response to Price." *Journal of Health Economics*, 14(2):123-145.

48. Glassbrenner, D., and J. Ye (2006). *Seat Belt Use in 2006—Overall Results*. Washington, DC: NHTSA National Center for Statistics and Analysis.

49. Substance Abuse and Mental Health Services Administration (2006). *The NSDUH Report: Driving Under the Influence among Adult Drivers*. Available at http://www.oas.samhsa.gov/.

50. American Heart Association (2006). "High Blood Pressure." Available at http://www.americanheart.org/.

51. American Diabetes Association (2006). "All About Diabetes." Available at http://www.diabetes.org/.

52. U.S. Department of Health and Human Services (2005). *Dietary Guidelines for Americans*. Washington, DC: Author.

53. American Heart Association (2007). *Am I at Risk?* Dallas, TX: Author.

Chapter 9

Elders

Chapter Outline

Chapter Objectives

After studying this chapter you will be able to:

1 Identify the characteristics of an aging population.

2 Define the following groups—*old, young old, middle old,* and *old old.*

3 Define the terms *aged, aging, elders, gerontology,* and *geriatrics.*

4 Refute several commonly held myths about the elder population.

5 Explain the meaning of an age pyramid.

6 List the factors that affect the size and age of a population.

7 Define fertility and mortality rates and explain how they affect life expectancy.

8 Explain the difference between support and labor-force ratios.

9 Describe older adults with regard to marital status, living arrangements, racial and ethnic background, economic status, and geographic location.

10 Explain how four health behaviors can improve the quality of later life.

11 Briefly outline elder abuse and neglect in the United States.

12 Identify the six instrumental needs of older adults.

13 Briefly summarize the Older Americans Act of 1965.

14 List the services provided for older adults in most communities.

15 Explain the difference between respite care and adult day care.

16 Identify the four different levels of tasks with which elderly need assistance.

SCENARIO

Carl and Sarah have been retired for about five years. Carl retired in good health after 35 years as an insurance agent, and Sarah stopped working outside the home after their children were grown and had families of their own. Upon retirement, they sold their home and paid cash for a condominium that had about half the square footage of their home. This relocation forced them to pare down their belongings to fit into their new and smaller surroundings. As a consequence, though, they felt less tied down to possessions and felt more freedom to do the traveling they had anticipated for several years. Although they now live on a fixed income, the profit from their home has allowed them to live out the retirement they had dreamed about, that is, having the financial resources to sign up for elderhostel programs in other cities, and to visit or host their children and grandchildren over the holidays.

All is not completely rosy for Carl and Sarah, however. Though they enjoy their lives very much, they are faced with an increasing number of health problems. They have accepted this challenge and have begun to do brisk walking on a near daily basis, and Sarah has signed up for a yoga program. Carl is considering joining a Tai Chi program offered at the senior center. They have also suffered the loss of good friends, several of whom have died, and their best friends and neighbors recently moved to be closer to their kids. Carl and Sarah are going to attend an orientation session at the local elementary school to help students read, in hopes of adding more meaning and purpose to their lives and to dwell less on their losses.

They look to the future with a mix of optimism and anxiety. The optimism is based on their consistent ability to meet the challenges of aging, even those losses that are very discouraging in the beginning. The anxiety is based on the unknown: What if their property taxes increase beyond what they can afford? What if their medication costs continue to rise, and the newly passed Medicare prescription legislation turns out to be not as helpful as advertised? Many questions arise, with no definite answers. But Carl and Sarah feel up to the challenge and adventure of aging into the future, and take satisfaction in looking back at lives well lived.

INTRODUCTION

The American population is growing older. The number of elders in America and their proportion of the total population increased dramatically during the twentieth century. In 1950, there were 12 million people (8% of the population) aged 65 years, and by 2005, that number had increased to 37 million (12.4% of the population).[1] For the first time in U.S. history, a significant number of Americans will achieve elder status and, in doing so, live long enough to assume some responsibilities for the care of their aging parents. We need only to look around us to see the change that is taking place (see Figure 9.1). The number of gray heads in restaurants, malls, and movie theaters is increasing. Senior centers, retirement villages, and assisted living facilities are being built in record numbers. And today, more than ever before, many people belong to multigenerational families, where there are opportunities to develop long-lasting relationships with parents, grandparents, and even great-grand-

FIGURE 9.1

The number of elders in the United States is on the rise, and they are more energetic than previous cohorts.

parents. There are now families in which members of three successive generations receive monthly Social Security checks. In the twenty-first century, the economic, social, and health issues associated with the growing proportion of people over the age of 65 in America have become major political concerns. In this chapter, we will define terminology, describe the demographics, and discuss the special needs of and community service for the aging.

Definitions

How old is old? The ageless baseball pitcher Satchel Paige once said, "How old would you be if you didn't know how old you was [sic]?" While his English might be found wanting, Paige's point is important (see Figure 9.2). A person's age might depend upon who measures it and how they define it. For example, while demographers might define old according to chronological years, clinicians might define it by stages of physiological development, and psychologists by developmental stages. Children might see their 35-year-old teacher as old, whereas the 35-year-old teacher might regard her 61-year-old principal as old. Age is and always will be a relative concept.

In the United States and other developed countries, people are considered *old* once they reach the age of 65. But because there are a number of people who are very active and healthy at age 65 and will live a number of productive years after 65, researchers have subdivided old into the *young old* (65–74), the *middle old* (75–84), and the *old old* (85 and over). Interestingly enough, it is this latter group, the old old, that makes up the fastest-growing segment of the elder population.

Also for the purposes of our discussion in this chapter, we will use terms that are associated with aging as they have been defined (and slightly modified) in *Age Words: A Glossary on Health and Aging*.[2]

elders
those 65 years of age and older

aged   The state of being old. A person may be defined as aged on the basis of having reached a specific age; for example, 65 is often used for social or legislative policies, while 75 is used for physiological evaluations.

aging   The changes that occur normally in plants and animals as they grow older. Some age changes begin at birth and continue until death; other changes begin at maturity and end at death.

gerontology   The study of aging from the broadest perspective. Gerontologists examine not only the chemical and biological aspects of aging, but also psychosocial, economic, and historical conditions. Elie Merchmkoff, of the Pasteur Institute in Paris, first used the term in 1903 to describe the biological study of senescence (aging).

geriatrics   The branch of medicine that deals with the structural changes, physiology, diseases, and other medical aspects of old age.

Many terms have been used to describe individuals who are 65 years of age and older, including seniors, "senior citizens, golden agers, retired persons, mature adults, elderly, aged, and old people. There is no clear preference among older people for any of these terms."[2] As Ferrini and Ferrini have stated, "many gerontologists have chosen to adopt the term 'elder' to describe those 65 and older. This term is an attempt to redefine aging in a more positive way that connotes wisdom, respect, leadership, and accumulated knowledge."[2] We agree with Ferrini and Ferrini and the other gerontologists and will frequently use the term **elders** to designate those who have reached their 65th birthday.

FIGURE 9.2

Some would say you are only as old as you think you are. (Satchel Paige remained active in professional baseball long after reaching the age at which others retired.)

MYTHS SURROUNDING AGING

Like other forms of prejudice and discrimination, **ageism** is the result of ignorance, misconceptions, and half-truths about aging and the elderly. Because most people do not interact with older people on a daily basis, it is easy to create a stereotypical image of elders based upon the atypical actions of a few, or negative images in the media.

When you think of older people, who comes to mind? Do you immediately think of a lonely man with a disheveled appearance sitting on a park bench or an older person lying in bed in a nursing home making incomprehensible noises? Or, do you think of Clint Eastwood and Sean Connery (each past 75) in an action-packed, high-suspense thriller?

Ferrini and Ferrini and Dychtwald and Flower have identified a number of commonly held myths about elders.[3,4] They are presented here to remind all that elders are not run-down, worn-out members of our society, but are for the most part independent, capable, and valuable resources for our communities. Do not forget that several U.S. presidents have been eligible for Social Security and Medicare while in office. Here are the myths and the reasons why they are only myths:

1. Myth: "After age 65 life goes steadily downhill."
   Truth: Any chronological age that defines old age is arbitrary. Nonetheless, many gerontologists are substituting age 85 for age 65 as the new chronological definition of old age.
2. Myth: "Old people are all alike."
   Truth: There are more differences among elders than any other segment of the U.S. population.
3. Myth: "Old people are lonely and ignored by their families."
   Truth: Elders are the least likely to be lonely of any age group; and those who live alone are likely to be in close contact, either in person, e-mail, or by telephone, with close friends and/or their family.
4. Myth: "Old age used to be better."
   Truth: It is only in the last half of the twentieth century that a large portion of the U.S. population lived to be 65 years old. If people did live to be old, they were not treated any better than they are today.
5. Myth: "Old people are senile."
   Truth: Senility is the result of disease and only affects about 5% of elders living in noninstitutional settings.
6. Myth: "Old people have the good life."
   Truth: Though elders do gain certain advantages when they retire and when their children leave home, they still face a number of concerns, such as loss of loved ones, loss of health, and loss of value in society.
7. Myth: "Most old people are sickly."
   Truth: Most older people do have at least one chronic health problem, but the majority of elders live active lifestyles.
8. Myth: "Old people no longer have any sexual interest or ability."
   Truth: Sexual interest may or may not diminish with age, but there is an alteration in sexual response. Nonetheless, many elders in reasonably good health have active and satisfying sex lives.
9. Myth: "Most old people end up in nursing homes."
   Truth: Only approximately 4% of those above the age of 65 live in nursing homes, homes for the aged, or other group quarters. Only 1% of those aged 65 to 74 reside in such a place, though the percentage jumps to 19% for the oldest old (those 85 and older). However, this number is still well below half.
10. Myth: "Older people are unproductive."

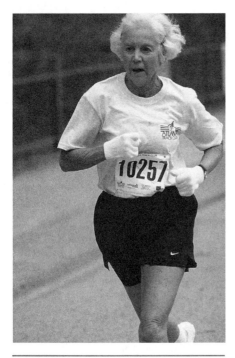

FIGURE 9.3
Many seniors are remaining active well after retirement age.

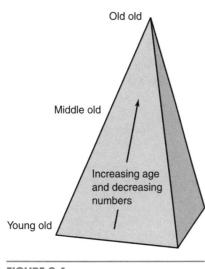

Old old

Middle old

Increasing age and decreasing numbers

Young old

FIGURE 9.4
Symbolic age pyramid.

Truth: Older adults are more likely to be retired, but they are very likely to be productively engaged at home and in the community.

Though a number of issues and concerns facing elders are presented later in this chapter, the majority of elders in the United States today are active and well (see Figure 9.3). In all parts of the country, many elders are still working. Many of the retired elders are (1) attending **elderhostel** programs, (2) remaining politically active (AARP, formerly called the American Association of Retired Persons, is one of the most active lobbying groups in the United States), and (3) volunteering countless hours as tutors at schools, workers for hospices and hospitals, advocates and companions for the mentally and physically ill, intake personnel at crisis centers, and members of community agency boards and churches, to name a few. Elders are an important part of society and play active roles in making communities work.

DEMOGRAPHY OF AGING

Demography is "the study of a population (an aggregate of individuals) and those variables bringing about change in that population."[2] The demography of aging is typically defined as a study of those who are 65 years and over and of the variables that bring about change in their lives. In the following paragraphs, we review some of the demographic features of the elder population, including size, growth rate, and the factors that contribute to this growth. We also discuss other demographic characteristics of this population, such as living arrangements, racial and ethnic composition, geographic distribution, economic status, and housing.

Size and Growth of the Elder Population

The aging of any population can be graphically illustrated with a symbolic age pyramid[5] (see Figure 9.4). The base of this pyramid represents the youngest and largest segment of the population. The sloping sides indicate higher mortality rates and limited life expectancy. Until the mid-1950s, the population pyramid for the United States was not so very different from the traditional age pyramid (see Figure 9.5).

Since the mid-1950s, however, the shape of America's population pyramid has changed. As noted earlier in the chapter, both the number of elders and the proportion of the total population made up of elders grew significantly during the twentieth century. At the beginning of the twentieth century, only 1 in 25 Americans was over the age of 65 years. In 2005, that number had increased to almost 1 in about 8.[1] Demographers' projections suggest that populations will continue to age, not only in this country, but in most other countries as well. In 2011, the *baby boom* generation will begin to turn 65, and by 2030, it is projected that 71 million people (1 in 5) will be age 65 or older.[1] The population aged 85 and older is currently the fastest-growing segment of the older population. It will double in size by 2025 and increase fivefold by 2050.[6,7] During this same time, it is expected that the percentage of

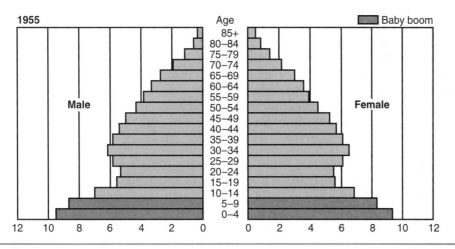

FIGURE 9.5

Population by age and sex: United States, 1955 (in millions).

Source: U.S. Bureau of the Census (1965). "Estimates of the Population of the United States by Single Years of Age, Color, and Sex: 1900 to 1959." *Current Population Reports,* series P-25, no. 311. Washington, DC: U.S. Government Printing Office, 2-5.

elderhostel
education programs specifically for elders, held on college campuses

people aged 18 and younger will remain about the same, around 26%.[6,7] These changes will alter the shape of the population pyramid and make it more like the shape of a population rectangle (see Figure 9.6).

As one might guess, the projected growth of the elder population is expected to raise the **median age** of the U.S. population. In 2006, it was 36.5 (the highest ever recorded).[8] It should peak in 2035 at 38.7 and then decrease to 38.1 by 2050.[9]

demography
the study of a population and those variables bringing about change in that population

median age
the age at which half of the population is older and half is younger

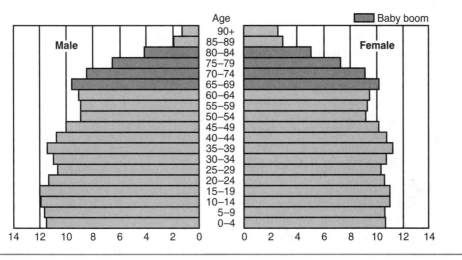

FIGURE 9.6

Projected population by age and sex, 2030 (in millions).

Source: Day, J. C., U.S. Bureau of the Census (1993). "Population Projections of the United States by Age, Sex, Race, and Hispanic Origin: 1993 to 2050." *Current Population Reports,* series P25-1104. Washington, DC: U.S. Government Printing Office (middle series projections), 2-7.

Factors That Affect Population Size and Age

Three factors affect the size and age of a population: its fertility rates, its mortality rates, and its gain or loss from migration of individuals into or out of that population.[2] Though one might assume that all populations will age with time, that is not necessarily true. In fact, a population could get younger with time.[2] If fertility rates and mortality rates are both high, life expectancy would be low, and the age of a population could grow younger. However, this has not been the case in the United States.

Fertility Rates

The *fertility rate* is an expression of the number of births per 1,000 women of childbearing age (15–44) in the population during a specific time period. Fertility rates in the United States were at their highest at the beginning of the twentieth century. Those rates dipped during the Depression years but rebounded after World War II. The period of consistently high fertility rates immediately following World War II has become known as the "baby boom years," hence the name *baby boomers* for those born between 1946 and 1964. During those years, 76 million babies were born. As the baby boomers continue to age, a "human tidal wave" (bulge) will continue to move up the U.S. age pyramid. American society has tried to adjust to the size and needs of the baby boom generation throughout the stages of the life cycle. Just as this generation had a dramatic impact on expanding obstetrics and pediatrics, creating split shifts for students in public schools, and disrupting government policy toward the Vietnam War, the baby boom cohorts will also place tremendous strain on programs and services (e.g., Social Security and Medicare) required of an elderly population. A window of opportunity now exists for planners and policy makers to prepare for the aging of the baby boom generation.[10]

Mortality Rates

The *mortality* or *death rate* (usually expressed in deaths per 100,000 population) also has an impact on the aging population. The annual crude mortality rate in the United States in 1900 was 1,720 per 100,000. Recent data show that that figure has dropped by half to 833.[1] The decrease in the annual mortality rate achieved over the twentieth century was the result of triumphs in medical science and public health practice.

Another demographic variable that interacts with the mortality rate is life expectancy. Although the mortality rate in the United States has been fairly constant for 20+ years, life expectancy has continued to increase. During the twentieth century, there was an overall jump in life expectancy at birth from 47.3 years in 1900 to 77.9 years in 2004.[1] The life expectancy of men and black Americans has always trailed those for women and white Americans, respectively. While the increase in life expectancy in the first half of the twentieth century could be attributed to the decrease in infant and early childhood deaths, the increase in life expectancy since 1970 can be traced to the postponement of death among the middle-aged and elder population.

Migration

net migration
the population gain or loss resulting from migration

The movement of people from one country to another, *migration,* has also contributed to the aging of the population. **Net migration** is the population gain or loss from the movement of migrants in (immigration) and out (emigration) of a country. Historically, in the United States, net migration has resulted in population gain; more people immigrate than emigrate. The greatest immigration in the United States occurred between the end of the Civil War and the beginning of the Great Depression. Most of the immigrants were between the ages of 18 and 35 years—of childbearing age. As these immigrants had children, the population of the United States remained young. However, the decline in immigration following the Depression led to the aging of the American populace as the early immigrants grew old and were not replaced by younger immigrants.

Fortunately, however, the United States continued to absorb young immigrants during the closing decades of the twentieth century. As a consequence, the dependency ratio of workers to older adults in the United States is declining more slowly than in many other developed countries. The future, however, is not so bright. We turn to this topic next.

Dependency and Labor-Force Ratios

Other demographic signs of an aging population are changes in dependency and labor-force ratios. The **dependency ratio** is a comparison between those individuals whom society considers economically unproductive (the nonworking or dependent population) and those it considers economically productive (the working population). Traditionally, the productive and nonproductive populations have been defined by age; the productive population includes those who are 19 to 64. The unproductive population includes both youth (0–19 years old) and the elderly (65+ years). When the dependency ratio includes both youth and the elderly, it is referred to as a **total dependency ratio.** When only the youth are compared to the productive group, the term used is **youth dependency ratio;** when only the elderly are compared, it is called **elderly dependency ratio.**[2]

Changes in dependency ratios "provide an indirect broad indication of periods when we can expect the particular age distribution of the country to affect the need for distinct types of social services, housing, and consumer products."[11] Thus, communities can refer to dependency ratio data as a guide for making the best social policy decisions and as a way to allocate resources. For example, leaders in a community with a relatively high youth dependency ratio compared to the elderly dependency ratio may want to concentrate community resources on programs such as education for the young, health promotion programs for children, special programs for working parents, and other youth-associated concerns. Communities with high elderly dependency ratios might increase programs for elders.

The total dependency ratio (DR) (calculated by adding the number of youth and elderly, divided by the number of persons 20 to 64 years, times 100) in the United States in 1990 was close to its lowest point (DR = 70.5) in the twentieth century, and it is projected to stay at about that same level until about 2010. The total dependency ratio will begin to climb in 2010 and will peak around the year 2035 at about 90 as the baby boomers reach their elder years. At its peak, the total dependency ratio will include a youth dependency ratio of about 50 and an elderly dependency ratio of 40 (see Figure 9.7). It is this big change (from 1990 to 2035) in the elderly dependency ratio that will guide future social policy.

Such an increase in the elderly dependency ratio provides an interesting political scenario because the costs to support youth and the elderly are not the same. Parents pay directly for most of the expenditures to support their children, with the primary exception being public education, which is paid for by taxes. In contrast, much of the support for elders comes from tax-supported programs such as Social Security, Medicare, and Medicaid. In order to meet the impending burden of the elderly, taxes will most certainly need to be raised or benefits reduced. Therefore, the two questions for the future are: Will the productive population be willing to pay increased taxes to support elders? Will services to the elderly be drastically reduced?

While dependency ratio data clearly show one trend, they are merely an estimate and should not be the only accepted estimate. Actually, the dependency ratios presented in Figure 9.7 are based on the assumption that everyone of productive age supports all members of the nonproductive age group. Obviously, this is not the case. Many of those in the productive age group (for instance homemakers, the unemployed, and the disabled) do not partici-

dependency ratio a ratio that compares the number of individuals whom society considers economically unproductive to the number it considers economically productive

total dependency ratio the dependency ratio that includes both youth and elderly

youth dependency ratio the dependency ratio that includes only youth

elderly dependency ratio the dependency ratio that includes only elderly

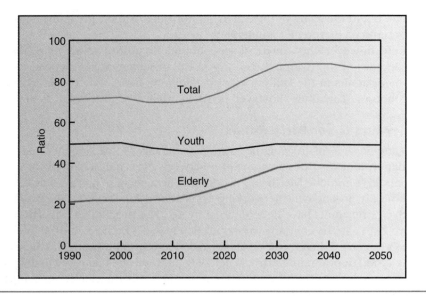

FIGURE 9.7

Total, youth, and elderly dependency ratios, 1990 to 2050.

Source: U.S. Bureau of the Census, 1990 from 1990 Census of Population and Housing, CPH-L-74, "Modified and Actual Age, Sex, Race, and Hispanic Origin Data;" 2050 from "Population Projections of the United States, by Age, Sex, Race, and Hispanic Origin: 1993 to 2050." *Current Population Reports,* series P25-1104. Washington, DC: U.S. Government Printing Office (middle series projections), 1993.

pate in the paid labor force. Conversely, many teenagers and elders do. Thus, dependency ratios, in some situations, could provide misleading figures for decision makers.

Other experts believe that labor-force ratios also need to be considered. **Labor-force ratios** differ from dependency ratios in that they are based on the number of people who are actually working and those who are not, independent of their ages. When labor-force participation rates are used to calculate the labor-force ratios, it is projected that the burden of support for the labor force in the future will be somewhat lighter than that projected through dependency ratios. Nonetheless, under either method of calculation, the ratio of workers to dependents will be lower in the future than it is today.

labor-force ratio a ratio of the total number of those individuals who are not working to the number of those who are

Other Demographic Variables Affecting Elders

Other demographic variables that affect the community health programs of older Americans include marital status, living arrangements, racial and ethnic composition, geographic distribution, economic status, and housing.

Marital Status

Approximately three-fourths of elder men are married, whereas just over half of elder women are married. In addition, elder women are three times more likely than men to be widowed.[10] There are three primary reasons for these differences. First, men have shorter average life expectancies than women and thus tend to precede their wives in death. Second, men tend to marry women who are younger than themselves. Finally, men who lose a spouse through death or divorce are more likely to remarry than women in the same situation. These statistics reveal that most elderly men have a spouse for assistance, especially when health fails, while most women do not. However, "in many ways, the current generation of elderly women are pacesetters as they defy stereotypes of aging. Many have dealt with the shortage of men by developing new interests and friendships. For elderly women (and men) with protective social networks, living alone does not necessarily mean being lonely"[11] (see Figure 9.8).

The number of divorced elderly continues to rise. As the baby boomers move into their older years, the number of divorced elders will grow two- to threefold. These divorced elders represent a new type of need group—those who lack the retirement benefits, insurance, and net worth assets associated with being married.

Living Arrangements

"Like marital status, the living arrangements of America's older population are important because they are closely linked to income, health status, and the availability of caregivers. Older persons who live alone are more likely to be in poverty than older persons who live with their spouses."[12]

FIGURE 9.8

Elder women are three times more likely to be widowed than elder men.

Two-thirds of noninstitutionalized elders live with someone else (spouse, relative, or other nonrelatives), while the remainder live alone.[10] Of those living alone, women are much more likely (almost 2 to 1) to be living alone. The proportion of those living alone is projected to remain about the same, but the numbers are expected to increase dramatically over the next 20 years.[7] Reasons for these increased numbers revolve around the aging of the baby boomers and the improved economic status of the elderly, coupled with their strong desire to live as independently as possible.

Only a small percentage of the elderly population in the United States resides in nursing homes. Recent data show that about 1.5 million of those aged 65 years and over were in nursing homes, representing 4% of the elder population.[1,7] This percentage is down from previous years due in part to the increase in **assisted-living facilities,** which have provided an alternative to long-term care in a nursing home. Of those who do live in nursing homes, older women at all ages have higher usage rates than men. Approximately three-fourths of nursing home residents are women, and over half of all nursing home residents are over 85 years old. As one might expect, the proportion of elders living in a nursing home increases with age.[12]

assisted-living facility a special combination of housing, personalized supportive services and health care designed to meet the needs—both scheduled and unscheduled—of those who need help with activities of daily living

Racial and Ethnic Composition

As the elder population grows larger, it will also grow more diverse, reflecting the demographic changes in the U.S. population as a whole. In 2004, the elder population in the United States was predominantly white. Of the total elder population in 2004, it was estimated that about 82% were white, 8% were black, 6% were of Hispanic origin, 3% were Asian/Pacific Islanders, and less than 1% were American Indian and Alaska Native.[10] By 2050, the elder white population is expected to decline to 61%, while Americans of Hispanic origin will increase to 18%, black Americans will increase to 12%, Asian/Pacific Islanders will increase to 8%, and American Indians and Alaska Natives will stay at less than 1% but will still grow by a rate of 50% (see Figure 9.9).[10] The growth in minority groups will be the result of continued immigration and the higher fertility rates in nonwhites over the past 50 years.

As the older population becomes more ethnically diverse, health professionals will need to become more knowledgeable about the cultural backgrounds of their elder clients. Additional knowledge and improved communication skills can lead to better adherence to health recommendations, and to enhanced health outcomes.[13]

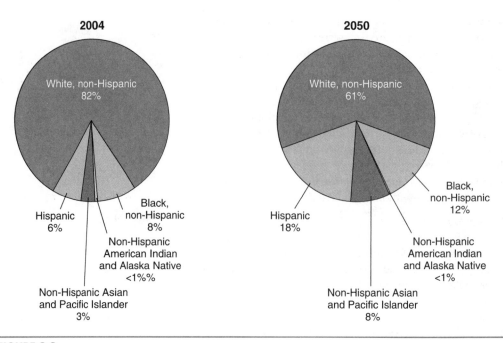

2004

White, non-Hispanic
82%

Hispanic
6%

Black,
non-Hispanic
8%

Non-Hispanic
American Indian
and Alaska Native
<1%%

Non-Hispanic Asian
and Pacific Islander
3%

2050

White, non-Hispanic
61%

Black,
non-Hispanic
12%

Hispanic
18%

Non-Hispanic
American Indian
and Alaska Native
<1%

Non-Hispanic Asian
and Pacific Islander
8%

FIGURE 9.9

Distribution of the population aged 65 and older for 2004 and projected for 2050.

Source: Federal Interagency Forum on Aging Related Statistics (2006). *Older Americans Update 2006: Key Indicators of Well-Being.* Available at http://www.agingstats.gov/.

FIGURE 9.10

Many elders choose to spend their retirement years in states with warm weather.

Geographic Distribution

In 2005, it was estimated that about one-third of America's elders lived in southern states (see Figure 9.10), and just over half lived in the following 10 states: California, Florida, Illinois, Michigan, New Jersey, New York, North Carolina, Ohio, Pennsylvania, and Texas. Each of these states had over 1 million elders. By 2015, Georgia, Virginia, and Washington are expected to join this group. California had the greatest number, with 3.8 million, while Florida had the greatest proportion, with 16.8% (almost 3 million people).[7,12] Some states, including many in the Midwest, have a small total number of elders, but the elders make up a large percentage of their total population.

The populations of some states (such as Florida) "age" because of the inward migration of elders; others (like the Farm Belt states) "age" because their young people leave. Still other states "age" because of low fertility or some combination of factors.[11]

From an ethnic and racial standpoint, the regional concentrations of the elderly are similar to the concentrations of the total population of each group.[11]

Economic Status

The overall economic position of elders has improved significantly since the 1970s.[14] In 1970 about 25% of the elderly lived in poverty, whereas in 2004 the figure had dropped to just less than 10%.[10]

Today, in fact, a smaller percentage of the elderly are impoverished than among those under age 18.[15]

When the sources of income of elders is examined, it is found that 39% of elder income comes from Social Security, almost equal percentages come from asset income (14%), pensions (19%), and earnings (25%), and a small percentage (2%) comes from other miscellaneous sources.[10] Because only one-fourth of elder income comes from work earnings, they are economically more vulnerable to circumstances beyond their control, such as the loss of a spouse; deteriorating health and self-sufficiency; changes in Social Security, Medicare, and Medicaid legislation; and inflation.

Housing

In general, most older Americans live in adequate, affordable housing.[10] Almost 75% live in single-family homes, another 20% live in multiunit structures (mostly apartments), and approximately 6% live in mobile homes (mostly in rural areas).[16] However, millions of elderly continue to live in housing that costs too much, is in substandard condition, or fails to accommodate their physical capabilities or assistance needs.[16] Characteristics of the homes of elders versus those of younger people are that elders have (1) older homes, (2) homes of lower value, (3) homes in greater need of repair, (4) homes less likely to have central heating and air conditioning, and (5) homes less likely to have telephones.[17,18]

For most elders, housing represents an asset because they have no mortgage or rental payments, or they can sell their home for a profit. But for others with low incomes, housing becomes a heavy burden. Approximately 30% of all elderly households pay more for housing than they can afford.[16] The cost of utilities, real estate taxes, insurance, repair, and maintenance have forced many to sell their property or live in a less-desirable residence.

A HEALTH PROFILE OF ELDERS

The health status among elders has improved over the years, both in terms of living longer and remaining functional. The percentage of chronically disabled older persons—those with impairments for three months or longer that impede daily activities—has been slowly falling. However, we do know that the most consistent risk factor of illness and death across the total population is age, and that in general, the health status of elders is not as good as their younger counterparts. In this section of the chapter, we will examine some of the health concerns of aging, including mortality, morbidity, and health behaviors and lifestyle choices.

Mortality

In 2004, the top five causes of death for elders, in order of number of deaths, were heart disease, cancer, stroke, chronic lower respiratory disease (CLRD), and Alzheimer's disease.[1] The top three causes of death were responsible for two-thirds of the deaths.[1] Over the past 50 years, the overall age-adjusted mortality rate for elders has continued to fall. The primary reason for this has been the declining death rates for heart disease and stroke. Despite such drops, heart disease remains the leading cause of death in this age group, and it is responsible for about one-third of the deaths.[1] Unlike the death rates for heart disease and stroke, the cancer death rate has stayed about the same in recent years. The biggest jump in death rates for elders has occurred with diabetes and CLRD.

The U.S. Public Health Service launched *Healthy People 2010* in part to increase the span of healthy life. Many of the objectives, distributed over 28 priority areas, are targeted by age (see Box 9.1).

HEALTHY PEOPLE 2010: OBJECTIVES

.tive 1-9: Reduce the hospitalization rates for three ambulatory-care-sensitive conditions—pediatric asthma, uncontrolled diabetes, and immunization-preventable pneumonia and influenza.

Target and baseline:

Objective	Reduction in Hospitalizations for Ambulatory-Care-Sensitive Conditions	1996 Baseline	2001 Status*	2010 Target
		Admissions per 10,000 Population		
1-9a.	Pediatric asthma—persons under age 18 years	23.0	21.4	17.3
1-9b.	Uncontrolled diabetes—persons aged 18–64 years	7.2	7.7	5.4
1-9c.	Immunization-preventable pneumonia and influenza—persons aged 65 years and older	10.6	11.2	8.0

*No new data at midcourse review.

For Further Thought

If you were given the responsibility for increasing the number of elders who are immunized against preventable pneumonia and influenza, what community health activities would you recommend to get elders to the immunizations?

Morbidity

"The quality of life in later years may be diminished if illness, chronic conditions, or injuries limit the ability of one to care for oneself without assistance. Older persons maintain their independence and eliminate costly caregiving services by, among other things, shopping on their own, cooking their meals, bathing and dressing themselves, and walking and climbing stairs without assistance."[14] Among Medicare enrollees aged 65 and over, about one in five men and one in three women were unable to perform at least one of five physical activities (walking two to three blocks; writing; stooping or kneeling; reaching up over head; lifting something as heavy as 10 pounds).[10] Activity limitations increase with age, and women are more likely than men to have physical limitations.[10] The causes of this reduced activity can be classified into two types—chronic conditions and impairments.

Chronic Conditions

Chronic conditions are systemic health problems that persist longer than three months, such as hypertension, arthritis, heart disease, diabetes, and emphysema. "While not all chronic conditions are life threatening, they are a substantial burden on the health and economic status of individuals, their families, and the nation as a whole."[14] The actual number of chronic conditions increases with age; therefore, limitations from activities become increasingly prevalent with age. In 2004, about 34% of elders reported a limitation of activity due to chronic conditions.[1] Furthermore, many chronic conditions can result in impairments, such as the loss of sight from diabetes. Chronic conditions of elders vary by gender and race. More men experience life-threatening acute illnesses (e.g., heart disease and hypertension-induced stroke), while more women experience physically limiting chronic illness (e.g., osteoporosis and arthritis).

Impairments

Impairments are deficits in the functioning of one's sense organs or limitations in one's mobility or range of motion. Like chronic conditions, impairments are far more prevalent in older adults.

BOX
9.2

HEALTHY PEOPLE 2010: OBJECTIVES

Objective 2-9:   Reduce the proportion of adults with osteoporosis.

Target: 8 percent

Baseline: 10 percent* of adults aged 50 years and older had osteoporosis as measured by low total femur bone mineral density (BMD) in 1988–1994 (age adjusted to the year 2000 standard population).

Status: No measurement since baseline.

*No new data at midcourse review.

For Further Thought

Have you seen any health care facilities in your community that have been advertising that they do bone density testing? How is bone density measured? What are some community health activities that could be carried out in a community to reduce the proportion of adults with osteoporosis?

The four primary impairments are hearing impairments, orthopedic impairments (see Box 9.2), cataracts, and other visual impairments. Another impairment of great concern is memory impairment. "Memory skills are important to general cognitive functioning, and declining scores on tests of memory are indicators of general cognitive loss for older adults. Low cognitive functioning (i.e., memory impairment) is a major risk factor for entering a nursing home."[12]

Like rates for chronic conditions, rates for impairments differ by gender and race. But unlike chronic conditions, impairments are affected by two other variables—previous income level and previous occupational exposure. The smaller the income and the more occupational exposure to health hazards, the greater the number of impairments.

Health Behaviors and Lifestyle Choices

There is no question that health behavior and social factors play significant roles in helping elders maintain health in later life. Some elders believe that they are too old to gain any benefit from changing their health behaviors. This, of course, is not true; it is never too late to make a change for the better.

In interviews, elders generally report more favorable health behaviors than their younger counterparts. They are less likely to (1) consume large amounts of alcohol, (2) smoke cigarettes, and (3) be overweight or obese. However, it should be noted that many of those who abused alcoholic beverages, smoked cigarettes, and were overweight or obese died before age 65 and thus were unavailable for interview.

Even though in general elders report better health behaviors than their younger counterparts, there is still room for improvement. The health behaviors that can affect the health of elders the most are healthy eating, exercise, and immunizations. Healthy eating plays a major role in preventing or delaying the onset of chronic diseases. The dietary quality habits of elders are better than their younger counterparts, but they still leave room for improvement.

The 1996 Surgeon General's Report on Physical Activity and Health reported that inactivity increased with age. While a substantial majority of adults at all age levels did not achieve the recommended level of physical activity, the number of sedentary persons—those who engage in *no* discretionary physical activity at all—increased with age. Only 22.4% of those aged 65 and older report engaging in regular leisure time physical activity, and that percentage drops to 8.4% for those aged 85 and older.[10]

The good news is that walking briskly (about twice as fast as a normal pace) for at least 30 minutes a day most days of the week is almost as beneficial for reducing the death rate as jogging up to 40 miles a week.[19] One study reported that walking four hours per week decreased the risk of future hospitalization for cardiovascular disease.[20] Another study reported that brisk walking three hours a week reduced the incidence of coronary events between 30% and 40%.[21]

Though aerobic conditioning has been considered the exercise of choice for improved cardiorespiratory function, other forms of exercise have proved beneficial as well. Tai chi[22] and resistance exercise,[23,24] for example, provide cardiorespiratory benefits. Resistance exercise, in fact, appears to reduce blood pressure level[25] and cholesterol level,[26,27] outcomes previously obtained primarily through aerobic exercise interventions.

Most people do not think of elders when they hear the word *immunizations*. "But for adults, especially those age 65 and older, getting immunized against certain diseases is important and can prevent thousands of deaths each year."[28] Influenza and pneumonia are the sixth leading cause of death in elders. Vaccinations against these diseases are recommended for elders, especially those who are at increased risk for complications from influenza and pneumonia. Influenza vaccinations are given annually, whereas pneumococcal vaccinations are usually given once in a lifetime, with possible revaccination with severe comorbidity after five years.[8]

Due in large measure to the onset of Medicare reimbursement, the pneumococcal vaccination rate increased dramatically, from 10% in 1989 to 56.8% in 2004.[1,29] Nonetheless, almost half of elders remained unvaccinated, and there was considerable racial disparity. In 2004, 60.9% of whites received pneumonia vaccination, compared with 38.6% of blacks and 33.7% of Hispanics.[10]

Thanks once again to Medicare reimbursement, the influenza vaccination rate also increased dramatically, from 20% in 1989 to 64.6% in 2004.[1,29] While this improvement is dramatic and gratifying to public health officials, almost a third of elders are still not getting an annual flu shot. And among older blacks, the influenza vaccination rate was about 22% lower than among older whites.[10]

Elder Abuse and Neglect

Reports of elder abuse and neglect have increased greatly in recent years. In a 10-year period between the mid-1980s and the mid-1990s, reports of elder abuse in the United States increased by more than 150%.[30] Perhaps a substantial part of the increase in these numbers was due to all 50 states having passed some form of elder abuse prevention laws. Though the laws and definitions of terms vary from state to state, all states have set up reporting systems. Prior to the reporting systems, many incidences of abuse were never recorded. "Generally, adult protective service (APS) agencies receive and investigate reports of suspected elder abuse."[30] According to the first-ever National Elder Abuse Incidence Study, released in 1998, an estimated total of 551,000 elderly persons over age 60 had experienced abuse (physical, emotional/psychological), neglect, or self-neglect in a domestic setting during the year of the study.[31] This study also revealed the following:

- Female elders are abused at a higher rate than men.
- Elders 80 years and older are abused or neglected at two to three times the rate of their proportion of the elderly population.
- In almost 90% of all elder abuse and neglect incidents where a perpetrator is identified, the perpetrator is a family member, and two-thirds of the perpetrators are adult children or spouses.
- Victims of self-neglect are usually depressed, confused, or extremely frail.

Elder abuse and neglect are special problems for elders because they are (1) frail, (2) unable to defend themselves, (3) vulnerable to telemarketing scams and mail-order swindles, and (4) the most common victims of theft of their benefit checks. On a positive note, elder abuse is a problem that has responded well to community monitoring. However, there is still much need for improvement, because only about 16% of elder abuse and neglect incidents are reported.[32]

INSTRUMENTAL NEEDS OF ELDERS

Atchley lists six instrumental needs that determine lifestyles for people of all ages.[33] These are income, housing, personal care, health care, transportation, and community facilities and services. However, the aging process can alter these needs in unpredictable ways. While those elders in the young old group (65–74) usually do not experience appreciable changes in their lifestyles relative to these six needs, elders in the middle old group (75–84) and the old old group (85 and older) eventually do. The rest of this chapter will explore these six needs, discuss their implications for elders, and describe community services for elders.

Income

Though the need for income continues throughout one's life, achieving elder status often reduces the income needs. Perhaps the major reduction occurs with one's retirement. Retirees do not need to purchase job-related items such as special clothing or tools, pay union dues, or join professional associations. Expenses are further reduced because retirees no longer commute every day, buy as many meals away from home, or spend money on business travel. Reaching elder status also usually means that children are grown and no longer dependent, and, as noted earlier, the home mortgage has often been retired. Taxes are usually lower because income is lower. In addition, many community services are offered at reduced prices for elders.

However, aging usually means increased expenses for health care and for home maintenance and repairs that aging homeowners can no longer do themselves. In spite of these increased costs, the overall need for income seems to decrease slightly for people after retirement.

As noted earlier in this chapter, there are five sources of income for elders: Social Security, pensions (e.g., government employee pensions, private pensions, or annuities), earnings from jobs, income from assets (e.g., savings accounts, stocks, bonds, real estate, etc.), and other miscellaneous sources (e.g., public assistance for the poor elders). Social Security benefits account for about two-fifths of income for elders; and asset income, pensions, and personal earnings each provide about one-fifth of total income. In December 2006, the average monthly Social Security payment to retired individuals was $1,044.[34] This amounts to an average of about $12,500 per year. The elders who rely most heavily on Social Security income are the poorest. In 2004, those elders in the lowest income quintile relied on Social Security payments for 83% of their income, whereas those in the highest income quintile only relied on Social Security payments for 19% of their income.[10]

In recent years, the income of elders has improved significantly. When income and other assets of elders are combined, the economic status of elders and those under 65 is not that far apart. However, the fact remains that 10% of the elder population lives in poverty. Certain subgroups of elders have higher rates. Nonmarried women and minorities have the highest poverty rates, ranging from 18% to 22%. Married persons have the lowest poverty rates at 4%.[10]

Housing

Housing, a basic necessity for all, is a central concern for elders in terms of needs and costs. It is an important source of continuity for elders. A home is more than just a place to live. It is a symbol of independence; a place for family gatherings; a source of pleasant memories; and a link to friends, the neighborhood, and the community.[33]

When housing for the elderly is examined, four major needs are discussed. They include appropriateness, accessibility, adequacy, and affordability.[16] These needs are not independent of each other; in fact, they are closely intertwined. Elders may live in affordable housing, but the housing may not be appropriate for their special needs. Or, certain housing may be accessible to the elderly, but it may not be affordable, or there may not be an adequate number available to meet demand.

Housing requirements may change more rapidly than housing consumption during the course of retirement years as a result of changes in household composition, decreasing mobility, and/or increasing morbidity.[18] Thus, the single biggest change in the housing needs of elders is the need for special modifications due to physical disabilities. Such modifications can be very simple—such as handrails for support in bathrooms—or more complex—such as chair lifts for stairs. Sometimes there is need for live-in help, while at other times disabilities may force seniors to leave their homes and seek specialized housing.

The decision to remove elders from their long-term residences is not easily made. Because of the psychological and social value of the home, changing an elder's place of residence has negative effects for both the elder and the family members who help make the arrangements for the move. Recognizing the importance of a home and independence, families often feel tremendous conflict and guilt in deciding to move an elder relative. If the elder does not adjust to the new situation, the guilt continues. Sometimes family members continue to question their decision even after the elder dies. Though moving an elder is very difficult, it is often best for all involved. For example, moving a frail person from a two-story to a one-story home makes good sense, and moving an elder from a very large home to a smaller home or an apartment is logical.

One of the biggest fears associated with relocating an elder is the move to group housing, especially a nursing home. The stereotype that many people have about group housing is not very positive, and most know it can be very expensive: approximately $64,000-plus per year for a total care nursing home. However, just like any other consumer product, good group homes are available. There is some evidence that not-for-profit homes—which constitute about one-third of the nation's 17,000 nursing homes—may be more concerned about quality of care and less concerned about keeping costs down and profits up.[35]

Perhaps the ideal model for long-term care facilities, however, is the Eden Alternative, founded by William Thomas, M.D., in 1991. The basic premise of the Eden Alternative is that nursing homes should treat residents as people who need attentive care in a homelike setting. To accomplish this goal, nursing homes need to contain pets, plants, children, and other amenities that make life worth living.[36] Three hundred nursing homes around the country have incorporated the Eden Alternative into their facilities.

William Thomas, M.D., went one step further than the Eden Alternative; he created the Green House. These houses avoid the institutionalization of larger nursing homes—including those based on the Eden Alternative—by limiting residents in number to about 10 and creating a large home for them rather than a facility. The first Green House, about 6,400 square feet, was constructed in Tupelo, Mississippi, in 2003. Each resident had a private room and bath, and access to a central hearth where cooking and socializing was done. There was a surrounding garden for contemplative walks and for growing vegetables and flowers.

Green Houses promote autonomy. Residents get up, eat, and go to bed when they want. They decide on which foods to eat. Medications are locked in individual rooms, rather than distributed by a cart that is wheeled from room to room. There are few features that are different from the typical home. Green House workers are paid more and are better trained, but the extra costs are offset by employee empowerment that reduces staff turnover and additional training expenses.

People in the first ten Green Houses were selected from nursing homes and represented a typical nursing home population. Of the first 40 residents selected, 12 had advanced dementia, and all Green House residents had the typical array of physical and cognitive limitations associated with the average nursing home resident.[13]

In 2006, the Robert Wood Johnson Foundation provided a $10 million, five-year grant to establish Green Houses around the United States, and to allow other long-term care owners and administrators to replicate them through training support and up to $125,000 in predevelopment loans.

Over the next decade, most elders will not be fortunate enough to have a Green House available to them. To ease the stress and anxiety associated with the relocation of elders, the following are recommended:[37]

retirement communities residential communities that have been specifically developed for those in their retirement years

1. Inform the elder (and family members) that relocation stress is usually temporary.
2. Encourage the elder to endorse the move, because those unwilling to move are most likely to experience stress.
3. Make a new environment predictable to the elder, because it can help to reduce stress.
4. Keep those being moved and their families informed so that stress can be reduced.

The relocation of elders is not always traumatic or done against their will. Many elders are finding housing in communities that have been planned as **retirement communities.** Though these communities are available in all areas of the country, they are most popular in areas with temperate climates (see Figure 9.11). Some of the communities are built as private associations, while others are developed as special areas within larger, already established communities. Legally, the private associations are able to adopt by-laws that put restrictions on the residents, such as a minimum age to move into the area, no children under a certain age living in the residence, and no pets. Retirement communities usually offer a variety of housing alternatives ranging from home or condominium ownership to apartment living. Because these communities are developed to meet the needs of elders, special accommodations are usually made for socializing, recreation, shopping, transportation, and selected educational programs.

continuing-care retirement communities (CCRCs) planned communities for seniors which guarantee a lifelong residence and health care

Two other housing options for elders are **continuing-care retirement communities (CCRCs)** and assisted living residences. CCRCs guarantee the residents a lifelong residence and health care. They work in the following way: The retirees either purchase or term lease (sometimes lifelong) a living unit on a campus-like setting. The living unit could be a single-family dwelling, an apartment, or a room, as in a nursing home. In addition to the living units, the campus usually includes a health clinic and often has either a nursing home or health care center. These other facilities are available to the residents for an additional fee. Residents of the CCRCs can live as independently as they wish but have available to them a variety of services, including housekeeping, meals, transportation, organized recreational and

FIGURE 9.11
The number of planned retirement communities in the United States continues to increase.

social activities, health care, and security. Many living units are equipped with emergency call buttons.

CCRCs are a housing alternative for well-to-do seniors. Unfortunately, CCRCs are beyond the reach of many elders; the purchase or lifelong lease is more than $100,000, and the fee for many of the services is extra. Obviously, seniors who enter into contractual agreements for CCRCs should read their contracts carefully before signing them.

An assisted living residence is a more recent housing option than CCRCs, but it includes many of the same concepts. It is a model of residential care that blends many of the characteristics of the nursing home and community-based long-term care. The Assisted Living Federation of America has defined an assisted living "residence as a special combination of housing, personalized supportive services and health care designed to meet the needs—both scheduled and unscheduled—of those who need help with activities of daily living."[38] Such facilities may include a high-rise apartment complex, a converted Victorian home, or a renovated school.[38] "Residences may be freestanding or housed with other residential options, such as independent living or nursing care. They may be operated by nonprofit or for-profit companies."[38] Most of these facilities offer a variety of services, including the following:[38]

- Three meals a day served in a common dining area
- Housekeeping services
- Transportation
- Assistance with eating, bathing, dressing, toileting, and walking
- Access to health and medical services
- 24-hour security and staff availability
- Emergency call systems for each resident unit
- Health promotion and exercise programs
- Medication management
- Personal laundry services
- Social and recreational activities

Costs for assisted living vary according to facility and parts of the country, but daily basic fees typically "range from approximately $15 to $200—generally less than the cost of home health services and nursing home care."[38]

It has been estimated that there are about 20,000 assisted-living facilities nationwide.[38] In a recent national study, about a fourth of the residents of these facilities received assistance with three or more activities of daily living, such as bathing, dressing, and mobility, and about one-third had moderate to severe cognitive impairment.[39]

Of all the housing problems that confront seniors, the availability of affordable housing is the biggest. Unfortunately, those seniors who are most in need of such housing are often frail and disabled, have low incomes, and live in rural areas. Until recently, many of the needs of this group of elders went unmet. However, during the Clinton presidency, funding was provided for the *Housing Security Plan for Older Americans* administered in the Office of Housing and Urban Development (HUD).[16] This plan embodied three overarching goals:

- "Help seniors remain in their homes and connected to their families and communities.
- Expand affordable housing opportunities for lower income seniors.
- Improve the range and coordination of affordable housing and supportive service combinations available to seniors."[16]

To reach these goals, HUD was working with older homeowners to help them convert the equity in their homes into funds for needed health and safety home improvements, including home rehabilitation loans through HUD's reverse mortgage program. HUD was also providing more money to help build more affordable rental housing for low-income elderly, in addition to helping finance the conversion of some existing housing units to assisted living residencies.[16] With each subsequent administration, however, presidential politics may (and usually does) change funding levels for programs such as this.

Personal Care

While most elders are able to care for themselves, there is a significant minority of elders who require personal assistance for an optimal or even adequate existence. The size of this minority increases as the elders attain middle old (75–84) and old old (85+) status.

Four different levels of tasks have been identified with which seniors may need assistance:

1. Instrumental tasks—such as housekeeping, transportation, maintenance on the automobile or yard, and assistance with business affairs
2. Expressive tasks—including emotional support, socializing and inclusion in social gatherings, and trying to prevent feelings of loneliness and isolation
3. Cognitive tasks—assistance that involves scheduling appointments, monitoring health conditions, reminding elders of the need to take medications, and in general acting as a backup memory
4. Tasks of daily living—such as eating, bathing, dressing, toileting, walking, getting in and out of bed or a chair, and getting outside

Note that this last group of tasks, in addition to being a part of this listing, has special significance. These items have been used to develop a scale, called **Activities of Daily Living (ADLs),** to measure **functional limitations.** Functional limitation refers to the difficulty in performing personal care and home management tasks. However, ADLs do not cover all aspects of disability and are not sufficient by themselves to estimate the need for long-term care. As previously noted, some elders have cognitive impairments that are not measured by ADLs. An additional, commonly used measure called **Instrumental Activities of Daily Living (IADLs)** measures more complex tasks such as handling personal finances, preparing meals, shopping, doing housework, traveling, using the telephone, and taking medications.[14]

When elders begin to need help with one or more of these tasks, it is usually a spouse, adult children, or other family members who first provide the help, thus assuming the role of informal caregivers. An **informal caregiver** has been defined as one who provides unpaid care or assistance to one who has some physical, mental, emotional, or financial need that limits his or her independence. It has been estimated that there are more than 7 million informal caregivers in the United States.[40] An informal caregiver can be either a care provider or care manager.[41] The **care provider** helps identify the needs of the individual and personally performs the caregiving service. Obviously, this can only be done if the person in need and the caregiver live in close proximity to each other. The **care manager** also helps to identify needs, but due to living some distance away or for other reasons, does not provide the service. The care manager makes arrangements for someone else (volunteer or paid) to provide the services.

With the aging of the population, it is now highly probable that many, if not most, adults can expect to have some responsibility as caregivers for their parents (see Figure 9.12). Their role may be as care provider, care manager, or in making the decision to relocate their parents by bringing them into their home, moving them to a smaller home or apartment, or

---

Activities of Daily Living (ADLs) eating, toileting, dressing, bathing, walking, getting in and out of a bed or chair, and getting outside

functional limitations difficulty in performing personal care and home management tasks

Instrumental Activities of Daily Living (IADLs) more complex tasks such as handling personal finances, preparing meals, shopping, doing housework, traveling, using the telephone, and taking medications

informal caregiver one who provides unpaid assistance to one who has some physical, mental, emotional, or financial need limiting his or her independence

care provider one who helps identify the health care needs of an individual and also personally performs the caregiving service

care manager one who helps identify the health care needs of an individual but does not actually provide the health care services

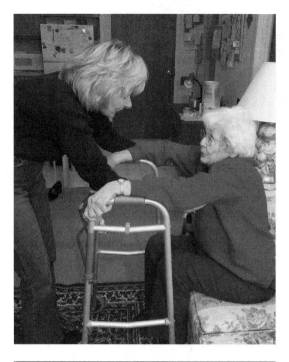

FIGURE 9.12
Adult children are gaining greater responsibility as caregivers.

moving them into a group home. This is a relatively new task because many of the elders of today did not have to care for their parents. Life expectancy was much shorter, and most did not live long enough to be cared for by their adult children.

Caregivers for elders face a number of problems, including decreased personal freedom, lack of privacy, constant demands on their time and energy, resentment that siblings do not share in the caregiving, and an increased financial burden. Many experience feelings of guilt for asking a spouse to help with the care of an in-law, or in knowing that the end of caregiving responsibilities usually means either the elder person's death or placement in a group home. Caregivers often experience a change in lifestyle, especially associated with time for leisure and recreation. Caregiving can also lead to a negative impact on health.[15]

And yet even this onerous task of caregiving has its intimate qualities. One study of older caregivers reported that more than 70% of caregivers had positive feelings toward at least one aspect of caregiving for an older adult.[42] Some of the positive aspects included companionship, fulfillment, enjoyment, and the satisfaction of meeting an obligation. In addition, caregivers are typically not isolated in their role. One study reported that 88% of caregivers had social support from others who helped them with their caregiving responsibilities.[43]

The need for personal care for elders is projected to increase in the coming years. The primary responsibility for providing and financing this care will fall on the family. Due to the financial burden, more families will begin purchasing long-term health care insurance policies. These policies are very expensive if purchased after age 75 but do provide elders with sufficient income protection against the depletion of assets. However, the high premium and co-payment costs of long-term care insurance policies mean that most Americans cannot afford them unless they are willing to purchase them when they are quite young and the costs are considerably more modest. In actuality, though, most policies are bought by people later on in life, when the risk of needing long-term care is great. Not surprisingly, therefore, it is estimated that 50% of long-term care insurance policies lapse due to high premiums.[44] (See the discussion of long-term care insurance in Chapter 14.)

To assist caregivers, federal legislation was passed called the Older Americans Act Amendments of 2000 (Public Law 106-501). This law established the National Family Caregiver Support Program (NFCSP), which has been administered by the Administration on Aging (AoA) of the U.S. Department of Health and Human Services. It was modeled in large part after successful state long-term care programs in California, New Jersey, Wisconsin, Pennsylvania, and others, and after listening to the needs expressed by hundreds of family caregivers in discussions held across the country. The program calls for all states, working in partnership with area agencies on aging and local community-service providers, to have the following five basic services for family caregivers:

- Information to caregivers about available services
- Assistance to caregivers in gaining access to services

- Individual counseling, organization of support groups, and caregiver training to assist them in making decisions and solving problems relating to their caregiving roles
- Respite care to enable caregivers to be temporarily relieved from their caregiving responsibilities
- Supplemental services, on a limited basis, to complement the care provided by caregivers

Health Care

Health care is a major issue for all segments of our society, particularly for elders. Although significant progress has been made in extending life expectancy, a longer life does not necessarily mean a healthier life. Health problems naturally increase with age. With these problems comes a need for increased health care services.

Elders are the heaviest users of health care services. Approximately 25% of elders have 10 or more visits a year to a physician, compared with 13.5% for all people in the United States.[7] They are also hospitalized more often and for longer stays. Although persons 65 years of age and older only represented 12% of the total population in 2004, they accounted for 38% of the roughly 34 million patient discharges from nonfederal short-stay hospitals,[7] and they spend over twice as much per person on prescription drugs as those under 65 years of age.[1] In addition, elders have higher usage rates for professional dental care, vision aids, and medical equipment and supplies than people under age 65. Usage of health care services increases with age, and much of the money spent on health care is spent in the last year of life.

Whereas private sources, such as employer-paid insurance, are the major sources of health care payment for people under age 65, public funds are used to pay for the majority of the health care expenses for elders. Medicare, which was enacted in 1965 and became effective July 1, 1966, provides almost universal health insurance coverage for elders. Medicare coverage, however, is biased toward hospital care, while chronic care health needs such as eyeglasses (see Figure 9.13), hearing aids, and most long-term services are not covered.

On January 1, 2006, Medicare Part D, a medication reimbursement program, was launched. It is too soon to tell how effective this program will be. A major component of this legislation is the mandated middlemen, private insurers, and it is difficult for beneficiaries to figure out which private plan among many is best for them. Also, Medicare Part D does not allow the federal government to negotiate lower prices directly from drug manufacturers, and drug prices rose sharply over the rate of inflation after the drug benefit went into effect. There is also a "donut hole," that is, an uncovered gap in medication costs in which the beneficiary bears full costs. (See Chapter 14 for more information on Medicare Part D.)

In 2005, the Medicare program had 42.5 million enrollees and expenditures of just over $336 billion.[1] With the increasing cost of health care and the aging population, these numbers will only grow. Of those elders covered in 2005, less than 10% were covered by Medicare only, while the others were covered by both Medicare and a private

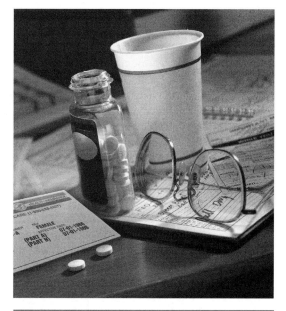

FIGURE 9.13

Medicare provides almost universal health insurance for elders.

insurance to supplement their Medicare coverage.[1] This private insurance is referred to as *Medigap,* because it helps to fill the gaps in health care cost that Medicare leaves. In addition, Medicaid, a federal-state program that was also approved in 1965, helps to cover the health care costs of poor elders, primarily for nursing home care (continuing care), home health care, and prescription drugs. In 2003, almost 8% of the elders were covered by both Medicare and Medicaid.[1] (See Chapter 14 for a complete discussion of Medicare, Medicaid, and Medigap.)

All indications are that the health care costs for elders will continue to escalate because of the aging population and rising health care costs. In an effort to try to help offset the increasing costs of Medicare, a change was made to the premium structure for Medicare Part B (see Chapter 14 for a discussion of Part B). Beginning in 2007, about 4% of the enrollees—those with higher incomes (>$80,000)—were charged higher premiums for Part B. This is one small step and by no means the end to change for Medicare. Future legislators will be forced to choose from among the following alternatives: (1) raising taxes to pay for the care, (2) reallocating tax dollars from other programs to pay for care, (3) cutting back on coverage presently offered, (4) offering care to only those who truly cannot afford it otherwise (also known as *means testing*), or (5) completely revamping the present system under which the care is funded.

In the meantime, the importance of instilling in Americans the value of preventing the onset of chronic diseases through healthy living cannot be overstated. While it is not possible to prevent all chronic health problems, encouraging healthy behaviors is a step in the right direction.

Transportation

The National Institute on Aging estimates that 600,000 people aged 70 and older give up their driving each year. On average, elders live about 10 years after they stop driving.[45] There is little guidance, however, not only on when to stop driving, but also on how to compensate for no longer having personal control over one's transportation.

Transportation is of prime importance to elders because it enables them to remain independent. "Housing, medical, financial and social services are useful only to the extent that transportation can make them accessible to those in need."[46] The two factors that have the greatest effect on the transportation needs of elders are income and health status. Some elders who have always driven their own automobiles eventually find that they are no longer able to do so. The ever-increasing costs of purchasing and maintaining an automobile sometimes become prohibitive on a fixed income. Also, with age comes physical problems that restrict one's ability to operate an automobile safely. In addition, those with extreme disabilities may find that they will need a modified automobile (to accommodate their disability) or specialized transportation (e.g., a vehicle that can accommodate a wheelchair) in order to be transported.

With regard to transportation needs, elders can be categorized into three different groups: (1) those who can use the present forms of transportation, whether it be their own vehicle or public transportation, (2) those who could use public transportation if the barriers of cost and access (no service available) were removed, and (3) those who need special services beyond what is available through public transportation.[33]

The unavailability of transportation services has stimulated a number of private and public organizations that serve elders (e.g., churches, community services, and local area agencies on aging) to provide these services. Some communities even subsidize the cost of public transportation by offering reduced rates for elders. While these services have been helpful to elders, mobility is still more difficult for elders than for other adults. Try to imagine what it would be like if you had to depend constantly on someone else for all your transportation needs.

The ideal solution to the transportation needs of elders, according to Atchley, would include four components: (1) fare reductions or discounts for all public transportation, including that for interstate travel, (2) subsidies to ensure adequate scheduling and routing of present public transportation, (3) subsidized taxi fares for the disabled and infirm, and (4) funds for senior centers to purchase and equip vehicles to transport seniors properly, especially in rural areas.[33]

An innovative response to the challenge for older adults who give up driving is the Independent Transportation Network. Older adults who agree to stop driving trade in their cars, and the value is booked into an account from which they can draw to receive rides. About $8 is deducted for each car ride given by a paid driver, less when scheduling rides in advance or for sharing a ride.

The Independent Transportation Network program was started by Katherine Freund, whose son was hit by an elderly driver in Portland, Maine. Pilot programs are being started in several cities. For more information, contact www.itnportland.org.

Community Facilities and Services

As has been mentioned previously, one of the most common occurrences of the aging process is loss of independence. Even some of the most basic activities of adults become major tasks for elders because of low income, ill health, and lack of transportation. Because of the limitations of elders and the barriers they must face, they have special needs in regard to community facilities and services. If these needs are met, the lifestyles of elders are greatly enhanced. If not, they are confronted with anything from a slight inconvenience to a very poor quality of life.

With a view toward improving the lives of elders, Congress enacted the **Older Americans Act of 1965 (OAA)** and has amended it several times. Among the programs created by key amendments are the national nutrition program for elders, the State and Area Agencies on Aging, and other programs (e.g., the caregiver program discussed earlier) to increase the services and protect the rights of elders.

Though the initial act was important, the services and facilities available to elders were greatly improved after the passage of the 1973 amendments, which established the State Departments on Aging and Area Agencies on Aging. These systems inform, guide, and link older persons to available, appropriate, and acceptable services in order to meet their needs. The amendments were written to provide the state and area agencies with the flexibility to develop plans that allow for local variations. In 2007, there were 56 State Units on Aging. "Most states are divided into planning and service areas (PSAs), so that programs can be tailored to meet the specific needs of older persons residing in those areas. Area Agencies on Aging are the agencies designated by the state to be the focal point for OAA programs within a PSA."[46]

With each part of the country—and for that matter each community—having its own peculiarities, the services available to elders can vary greatly from one community to another. Even the names of the local agencies (few of which are called Area Agency on Aging) can vary a great deal, and it may require a phone call to the National Association of Area Agencies on Aging (202-872-0888) to locate your local Area Agency on Aging.

It is important to keep in mind, however, that the growth in our nation's elder population, combined with this population's financial ability to pay for service, has created an entrepreneurial atmosphere surrounding adult care services. In some larger communities, or in those communities with a large number of elder residents, the range of services can be astonishing. In the following text, we provide brief descriptions of facilities and services available in many communities.

Older Americans Act of 1965 federal legislation to improve the lives of elders

Meal Service

The 1972 amendments to the Older Americans Act outlined a national nutrition program for elders and provided funds for communities to establish meal services. Today's meal services are provided through home-delivered meal and congregate meal programs. The concept of the home-delivered meal programs (often known as **Meals on Wheels**) is the regular delivery of meals—usually once a day, five days per week—to elders in their homes. These meals are prepared in a central location, sometimes in a hospital, school, or senior center, and are delivered by community volunteers.

Congregate meal programs are provided for individuals who can travel to a central site, often within senior centers or publicly funded housing units. Usually, it is the noon meal that is provided. Generally, these meals are funded by federal and state monies and make use of commodity food services. In recent years, congregate meal programs seem to be gaining favor over home-delivered meal programs because they also provide social interaction (see Figure 9.14) and the opportunity to tie in with other social services.[33] However, there will always be a segment of the population requiring home-delivered meals because of their homebound status.

Both types of meal programs are strictly regulated by federal and state guidelines to ensure that the meals meet standard nutritional requirements. The cost of the meals varies by site and client income level. Elders may pay full price, pay a portion of the cost, or just make a voluntary contribution.

Homemaker Service

For a number of elders, periodic homemaker services can be the critical factor enabling them to remain in their own homes. For these elders, physical impairment restricts their ability to carry out normal housekeeping activities such as house cleaning, laundry, and meal preparation. The availability of these services allows many elders to live semi-independently and delays their moving in with relatives or into group housing.

Chore and Home Maintenance Service

Chore and home maintenance service includes such services as yard work, cleaning gutters and windows, installing screens and storm windows, making minor plumbing and electrical repairs, maintaining furnaces and air conditioners, and helping to adapt a home to any impairments seniors might have. This adaptation may include provisions for wheelchairs and installing ramps or special railings to assist elders to move from one area to another.

Visitor Service

Social interaction and social contacts are an important need for every human being, regardless of age. **Visitor services** amount to one individual taking time to visit with another person who is **homebound,** or unable to leave his or her residence. This service is usually done on a voluntary basis, many times with elders doing the visiting, and serves both the homebound and those who are institutionalized. It is not uncommon for church or social organizations to conduct a visitor program for homebound members.

Adult Day Care

Adult day care programs provide care during the daytime hours for elders who are unable to be left alone. These services are modeled after child day care. Most programs offer meals, snacks, and social activities for the clients. Some either provide or make arrangements for the clients to receive therapy, counseling, health education, or other health services. Other day care programs are designed for elders with special needs, such as Alzheimer clients, the blind, or veterans. Adult day care programs allow families to continue with daytime activities while still providing the primary care for a family member.

Respite Care

Respite care is planned, short-term care. Such care allows families who provide primary care for an elder family member to leave their elder in a supervised care setting for anywhere from a day to a few weeks. Respite services provide full care, including sleeping quarters, meals, bathing facilities, social activities, and the monitoring of medications.[2] This is the service most frequently requested by informal caregivers. (See the section on personal care earlier in chapter.) Such a program allows primary caregivers to take a vacation, visit other relatives, or to be otherwise relieved from their constant caregiving responsibilities.

Home Health Care

Home health care "is an important alternative to traditional institutional care. Services such as medical treatment, physical therapy, and homemaker services often allow patients to be cared for at lower cost than a nursing home or hospital and in familiar surroundings of their home."[14] These programs, run by official health agencies like the local health department, hospitals, or private companies, provide a full range of services, including preventive,

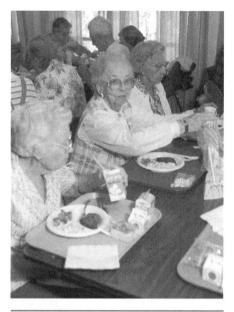

FIGURE 9.14
Congregate meals programs are not only valuable because of the enhanced nutrition but also because of the social interaction.

primary, rehabilitative, and therapeutic services, in the client's home. The care is often provided by nurses, home health aides, and personal care workers (licensed health care workers). A decreasing percentage of home health care expenditures have been paid for by Medicare over the past decade, and a significant portion is being paid for by families out of pocket. Other means of paying for this care could include long-term care insurance policies, Medicaid, or reimbursement by Medigap.

Senior Centers

The enactment of the Older Americans Act of 1965 provided funds to develop multipurpose senior centers, facilities where elders can congregate for fellowship, meals, education, and recreation. More recently, a number of communities have built senior centers with local tax dollars. Senior centers are widespread in the United States and are the most common community facility aimed at serving seniors.[34] However, they are found much less commonly in rural areas.

In addition to the traditional services (meals, fellowship, and recreation) offered at senior centers, some communities use the centers to serve as a central location for offering a variety of other senior services, including legal assistance, income counseling, income tax return assistance, program referrals, employment services, and other appropriate services and information.

Other Services

There are many other services available to seniors in some communities. Usually, larger communities and those with more seniors provide a greater variety of services. The types of services provided in any one community are limited only by the creativity of those providing the service. In some communities, "service packages" are being offered. Such packages allow seniors to pick several services they need and to pay for them as if they were a single service.

respite care
planned short-term care, usually for the purpose of relieving a full-time informal caregiver

home health care services
health care services provided in the patient's place of residence

CHAPTER SUMMARY

- The median age of the U.S. population is at an all-time high and will continue to increase through the first third of this century.

- There are many myths about the elderly population.

- The increasing median age is affected by decreasing fertility rates, declining mortality rates, and the decline in immigration.

- We are now at a point in history when a significant portion of Americans will assume some responsibility for the care of their aging parents.

- One of the most common occurrences of the aging process is the reduction in independence.

- An aging population presents the community with several concerns, which means legislators and taxpayers will be faced with decisions about how best to afford the costs (Social Security, government employee pensions, Medicare, etc.) of an ever-increasing elderly dependency ratio.

- Communities will also need to deal with the special needs of income, housing, personal care, health care, transportation, and community facilities and services for elders.

- All projections indicate that the incomes of seniors will remain lower than those of the general population, that the need for affordable and accessible housing will increase, that there will be increased needs for personal services and care, that health care needs and costs will increase, and that the demand for barrier-free transportation will increase for elders.

- The growth in our nation's elder population, combined with this population's financial ability to pay for service, has created an entrepreneurial atmosphere surrounding adult care services.

REVIEW QUESTIONS

1. What are some signs, visible to the average person, that the U.S. population is aging?

2. What years of life are defined by each of the following groups—old, young old, middle old, and old old?

3. What is meant by the terms *aged, aging, elder, gerontology,* and *geriatrics*?

4. Why is there a myth that old people are sickly?

5. What are demographers? What do they do?

6. Why does a pyramid represent the age characteristics of the U.S. population of the 1950s?

7. What are the three factors that affect the size and age of a population?

8. How have life expectancy figures changed over the years in the United States? What were the major reasons for the change in the first half of the twentieth century? The second half?

9. Why are dependency and labor-force ratios so important?

10. How are dependency and labor-force ratios calculated?

11. Are all elders the same with regard to demographic variables?

12. How do the income needs of people change in retirement?

13. Why do adults feel guilty when they have to relocate their aged parents?

14. What is the difference between a care provider and a care manager?

15. What are some of the major problems caregivers face?

16. Why are continuing-care retirement communities attractive to elders?

17. What is an assisted living residence?

18. What is the difference between Activities of Daily Living and Instrumental Activities of Daily Living?

19. What are the most frequently occurring health problems of elders?

20. From what financial sources do elders normally pay for health care?

21. What does the term *Medigap* mean?

22. How do income and health status affect the transportation needs of elders?

23. What is the ideal solution for the transportation needs of elders?

24. What are State Departments on Aging and Area Agencies on Aging?

25. Why is a visitor service so important for homebound and institutionalized persons?

26. What is the difference between adult day care and respite care?

ACTIVITIES

1. Make arrangements with a local long-term care facility to visit one of their residents. Make at least three one-hour visits to a resident over a six-week period of time. Upon completion of the visits, write a paper that answers the following questions:

   What were your feelings when you first walked into the facility?

   What were your feelings when you first met the resident?

What did you learn about the elderly that you did not know before?

What did you learn about yourself because of this experience?

Did your feeling about the resident change during the course of your visits? If so, how?

If you had to live in a long-term care facility, would you be able to adjust to it? What would be most difficult for you in your adjustment? What character traits do you have that would help you adjust?

2. Interview a retired person over the age of 65. In your interview, include the following questions. Write a two-page paper about this interview.

What are your greatest needs as an elder?

What are your greatest fears connected with aging?

What are your greatest joys at this stage in your life?

If you could have done anything differently when you were younger to affect your life now, what would it have been?

Have you had any problems getting health care with Medicare? If so, what were they? Do you have a Medigap policy? If so, has your Medigap policy been worth the cost?

In what ways are you able to contribute to your community?

3. Spend a half-day at a local senior center. Then, write a paper that (a) summarizes your experience, (b) identifies your reaction (personal feelings) to the experience, and (c) shares what you have learned from the experience.

4. Review a newspaper obituary column for 14 consecutive days. Using the information provided in the obituaries: (a) demographically describe those who died, (b) keep track of what community services are noted, and (c) consider what generalizations can be made from the group as a whole.

COMMUNITY HEALTH ON THE WEB

The Internet contains a wealth of information about community and public health. Increase your knowledge of some of the topics presented in this chapter by accessing the Jones and Bartlett Publishers Web site at **http://health.jbpub.com/book/communityhealth/6e** and follow the links to complete the following Web activities.

- AARP
- Administration on Aging
- National Institute on Aging

REFERENCES

1. National Center for Health Statistics (2006). *Health United Sates, 2006 with Chartbook on Trends in Health of Americans*. Hyattsville, MD: Author.

2. U.S. Department of Health and Human Services (1986). *Age Words: A Glossary on Health and Aging* (NIH pub. no. 86-1849). Washington, DC: U.S. Government Printing Office.

3. Ferrini, A. F., and R. L. Ferrini (2000). *Health in the Later Years*, 3rd ed. Boston: McGraw-Hill Higher Education.

4. Dychtwald, K., and J. Flower (1989). *Age Wave: The Challenges and Opportunities of an Aging America*. Los Angeles: Jeremy P. Tarcher.

5. Thomlinson, R. (1976). *Population Dynamics: Causes and Consequences of World Demographic Change*. New York: Random House.

6. U.S Census Bureau (2004). *U.S. Interim Projections by Age, Sex, Race, and Hispanic Origin*. Available at http://www.census.gov/ipc/www/usinterimproj/.

7. U.S Census Bureau (2007). *The 2007 Statistical Abstract: The National Data Book*. Available at http://www.census.gov/.

8. U.S. Central Intelligence Agency (2007). "Median Age." In *The World Factbook 2007*. Available at https://www.cia.gov/cia/publications/factbook/fields/2177.html.

9. Day, J. C. (1996). *Population Projections of the United States by Age, Sex, Race, and Hispanic Origin: 1995 to 2050* (Current Population Reports P25-1130). Washington, DC: U.S. Bureau of the Census.

10. Federal Interagency Forum on Aging Related Statistics (2006). *Older Americans Update 2006: Key Indicators of Well-Being*. Available at http://www.agingstats.gov/.

SCENARIO: ANALYSIS AND RESPONSE

1. Based upon what you read in this chapter, how would you predict that Carl and Sarah's lives might progress over the next 20 years? Consider the six instrumental needs presented in the chapter.

2. What could Carl and Sarah have done when they were working to better plan for their retirement?

3. If you had to give Carl and Sarah two pieces of health care advice, what would they be?

11. U.S. Bureau of the Census (1996). *65 in the United States* (Current Population Reports P23-190). Washington, DC: U.S. Government Printing Office.

12. Federal Interagency Forum on Aging-Related Statistics (2001). *Older Americans 2000: Key Indicators of Well-Being.* Available at http://www.agingstats.gov/chartbook2000/default.htm.

13. Haber, D. (2005). "Cultural Diversity among Older Adults: Addressing Health Education." *Educational Gerontology*, 31: 683-697.

14. Kramarow, E. H., H. Lentzner, R. Rooks, J. Weeks, and S. Saydah (1999). *Health and Aging Chartbook: Health United States, 1999* (HHS pub. no. PHS-99-123-1). Hyattsville, MD: National Center for Health Statistics.

15. Hooyman, N., and H. Kiyak (2005). *Social Gerontology: A Multidisciplinary Perspective*, 7th ed. Boston: Allyn and Bacon.

16. U.S. Department of Housing and Urban Development, Office of Policy Development and Research (1999). *Housing Our Elders.* Washington, DC: Author.

17. U.S. Department of Health and Human Services (1991). *Aging America: Trends and Projections* (HHS pub. no. FCOA-91-28001). Washington, DC: U.S. Government Printing Office.

18. Naifeh, M. L. (1993). *Housing of the Elderly: 1991* (Current Housing Reports Series H123/93-1). Washington, DC: U.S. Government Printing Office.

19. Blair, S., et al. (2001). "Physical Fitness and All-Cause Mortality: A Prospective Study of Healthy Men and Women." *Journal of the American Medical Association*, 262: 2395-2401.

20. LaCroix, A., et al. (1996). "Does Walking Decrease the Risk of Cardiovascular Disease Hospitalization and Death in Older Adults?" *Journal of the American Geriatrics Society*, 44: 113-120.

21. Manson, J., et al. (1999). "A Prospective Study of Walking as Compared with Vigorous Exercise in the Prevention of Coronary Heart Disease in Women." *New England Journal of Medicine*, 341: 650-658.

22. Lan, C., et al. (1999). "The Effect of Tai Chi on Cardiorespiratory Function in Patients with Coronary Artery Bypass Surgery." *Medical Science Sports Exercise*, 31: 634-638.

23. Tanassescu, M., et al. (2002). "Exercise Type and Intensity in Relation to Coronary Heart Disease in Men." *Journal of the American Medical Association*, 288: 1994-2000.

24. Vincent, K., et al. (2002). "Resistance Exercise and Physical Performance in Adults Aged 60 to 83." *Journal of the American Geriatrics Society*, 50: 1100-1107.

25. Kelley, G., and K. Kelley (2000). "Progressive Resistance Exercise and Resting Blood Pressure: A Meta-analysis of Randomized Controlled Trials." *Hypertension*, 35: 838-843.

26. Kraus, W., et al. (2002). "Effects of the Amount and Intensity of Exercise on Plasma Lipoproteins." *New England Journal of Medicine*, 347: 1483-1492.

27. Prabhakaran, B., et al. (1999). "Effect of 14 Weeks of Resistance Training on Lipid Profile and Body Fat Percentage in Premenopausal Women." *British Journal of Sports Medicine*, 33: 190-195.

28. Brooks, J. (May 2000). "Immunizations: Not Just for the Young." *Closing the Gap*, 10-12.

29. Haber, D. (2007). *Health Promotion and Aging: Practical Applications for Health Professionals*, 4th ed. New York: Springer Publishing.

30. Administration on Aging (2006). "Elder Abuse Prevention." Available at http://www.aoa.gov/press/fact/alpha/fact_elder_abuse_pf.asp.

31. Administration on Aging (2001). *The National Elder Abuse Incidence Study*. Available at http://www.aoa.gov/abuse/report/Cexecsum.htm.

32. Haber, D. (2007). "Elder Abuse." Personal communication.

33. Atchley, R. C. (1994). *Social Forces and Aging: An Introduction to Social Gerontology*, 7th ed. Belmont, CA: Wadsworth.

34. Social Security Administration (2007). "Monthly Statistical Snapshot, December 2006." Available at http://www.ssa.gov/policy/docs/quickfacts/ stat_snapshot/index.html.

35. Harrington, C., et al. (2001). "Does Investor Ownership of Nursing Homes Compromise the Quality of Care?" *American Journal of Public Health*, 91: 1452-1455.

36. Thomas, W. (1995). *The Eden Alternative*. Acton, MA: VanderWyk & Burnham.

37. Borup, J. H. (1981). "Relocation: Attitudes, Information Network and Problems Encountered." *The Gerontologist*, 21: 501-511.

38. The Assisted Living Federation of America (2004). "What Is Assisted Living?" Available at http://www.alfa.org/public/articles/details.cfm?id=126.

39. Hawes, C., M. Rose, and O. S. Phillips (1999). *A National Study of Assisted Living for the Frail Elderly. Executive Summary: Results of a National Survey of Facilities*. Available at http://aspe.os.dhhs.gov/daltcp/reports/facreses.htm.

40. Oxendine, J. (May 2000). "Who Is Helping the Care Givers?" *Closing the Gap*, 4.

41. Archbold, P. G. (1983). "Impact of Parent-Caring on Women." *Family Relations*, 32: 39-45.

42. Cohen, C., et al. (2002). "Positive Aspects of Caregiving: Rounding Out the Caregiver Support System." *The Gerontologist*, 35: 489-497.

43. Penrod, et al. (1995). "Who Cares? The Size, Scope, and Composition of the Care Giver Support System." *The Gerontologist*, 35: 489-497.

44. Weiner, J., and L. Illston (1996). "Financing and Organization of Health Care." In R. Binstock and L. George, eds., *Handbook of Aging and the Social Sciences*, 4th ed. San Diego: Academic Press.

45. Foley, D., et al. (2002). "Driving Life Expectancy of Persons Aged 70 Years and Older in the United States." *American Journal of Public Health*, 92: 1284-1289.

46. Administration on Aging. (2007). "How to Find Help." Available at http://www.aoa.gov/eldfam/How_To_Find/Agencies/Agencies.asp.

Chapter 10

Community Health and Minorities

Chapter Outline

Chapter Objectives

After studying this chapter, you should be able to:

1 Explain the concept of diversity as it describes the American people.

2 Explain the impact of a more diverse population in the United States as it relates to community health efforts.

3 Explain the importance of the 1985 landmark report *The Secretary's Task Force Report on Black and Minority Health.*

4 List the racial and ethnic categories currently used by the U.S. government in statistical activities and program administration reporting.

5 List some limitations related to collecting racial and ethnic health data.

6 Identify some of the sociodemographic and socioeconomic characteristics of minority groups in the United States.

7 List some of the beliefs and values of minority groups in the United States.

8 List and describe the six priority areas of the *Race and Health Initiative.*

9 Define *socioeconomic gradient* and provide an example as it relates to minority health.

10 Define *cultural sensitivity* and *cultural and linguistic competence* and the importance of each related to minority community health.

11 Identify the three kinds of power associated with empowerment and explain the importance of each related to minority community health.

SCENARIO

Tom just returned from a cross-country business trip that took him from New York City to Miami, to San Antonio, to Los Angeles, and back to his Midwest hometown, Middletown, U.S.A. When his curious teenage children asked him to tell them about the people who live in the "big cities," he began by saying, "There seem to be more minorities and foreigners in the cities than before. I heard at least five or six different languages spoken. Signs in the hotels and in the storefronts are written in at least two, and sometimes three or four languages.

"Another thing that always amazes me is the number of ethnic restaurants. Here, we have just one Mexican, one Italian, and one Chinese restaurant, but in New York City and other big cities there are hundreds of restaurants serving foods from other cultures. I get the feeling that the United States is more culturally diverse than at anytime in its past, even when it was considered the 'melting pot' for the world's populations."

INTRODUCTION

The strength and greatness of America lies in the diversity of its people. Over the centuries, wave after wave of immigrants have come to America to start new lives. They have brought with them many of their traditions and cultures. However, it is recognized that even as America rapidly becomes the world's first truly multiracial democracy, race relations remains an issue that too often divides the nation and keeps the American dream from becoming a reality for all Americans. In 1997, former President Bill Clinton announced "One America in the 21st Century: The President's Initiative on Race."[1] This initiative was a critical element in an effort to prepare the country to live as one America in the twenty-first century and was based on opportunity for all, responsibility for all, and one community for all Americans. The goal of Clinton's Initiative on Race was to strengthen our shared foundation as Americans so we can all live in an atmosphere of trust and understanding. Every American must invest in creating One America, so that as a nation, people can effectively act together to fulfill the promise of the American dream in the twenty-first century. As we progress through the twenty-first century, we must continue to recognize that the strength and greatness of America lies in the diversity or differences of its people (see Figure 10.1). The failure to understand and appreciate these differences can have serious implications not only with race relations, but also when it comes to improving the health of diverse communities.

majority
those with characteristics that are found in over 50% of a population

minority groups
subgroups of the population that consist of less than 50% of the population

Today in the United States, the **majority** of Americans (67%) are referred to as "white, non-Latino." The remaining 33% of the U.S. population are members of what is traditionally viewed as racial or ethnic **minorities** (see Figure 10.2). Accordingly, **minority health** refers to the morbidity and mortality of American Indians/Alaska Natives, Asian Americans and Pacific Islanders, black Americans, and Hispanics in the United States. Current projections suggest that the U.S. population will become increasingly diverse. By 2050, nearly one-half of the U.S. population will be composed of racial minorities (see Figure 10.3).[2] The impact of a more diverse population in the United States in relation to community health efforts connected with minorities will be important based on what we learned about our past. "The health status of the nation as a whole has improved significantly during the twentieth century. Advances in medical technology, lifestyle improvements,

FIGURE 10.1

The strength and greatness of America lies in the diversity of its people.

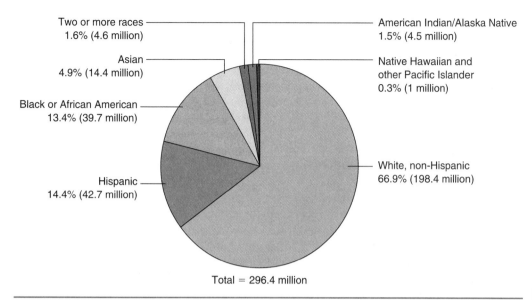

FIGURE 10.2

Percent distribution of U.S. population by race/ethnicity, 2005.

Note: Percentages do not add up to 100% due to rounding and because Hispanics may be any race and are therefore counted under more than one category.

Source: U.S. Census Bureau, National Population Estimates.

minority health
refers to the morbidity and mortality of American Indians/Alaska Natives, Americans of Hispanic origin, Asians and Pacific Islanders, and black Americans in the United States

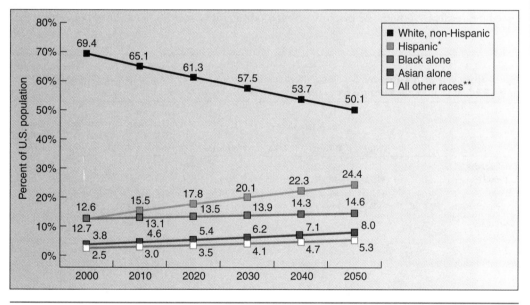

FIGURE 10.3

Projected U.S. population by race and Hispanic origin, selected years.

Note: Percentages for 2000 are actual.

*Hispanics can be of any race. Totals do not equal 100% for this reason.

**"All other races" includes American Indian and Alaska Native alone, Native Hawaiian and Other Pacific Islander alone, and two or more races.

Source: U.S. Census Bureau, Population Division (2004). *U.S. Interim Projections by Age, Sex, Race, and Hispanic Origin.* Available at http://www.census.gov/ipc/www/usinterimproj/.

and environmental protections have all led to health gains. Yet these changes have not produced equal benefit in some racial and ethnic populations. This is the continuing challenge to public health professionals and the standard we must keep in mind when measuring our progress: what is the health status of the least empowered among us?"[3] As the racial and ethnic minority groups currently experiencing poorer health status grow in proportion to the total U.S. population, the future health of all Americans will be influenced by the success in improving the health of these groups. It is the nature of health disparities among the least empowered (primarily minorities) that is the main focus of this chapter.

A landmark 1985 report, *The Secretary's Task Force Report on Black and Minority Health,* first documented the health status disparities of minority groups in the United States.[4] This report provided substantial data documenting that minority populations, compared to the nation as a whole, experience higher rates of morbidity and mortality. Specifically, the report identified six causes of death that accounted for more than 80% of the excess mortality observed among black Americans, Hispanics, Asian Americans and Pacific Islanders, and Native Americans. These six causes were infant mortality, cancer, cardiovascular disease and stroke, diabetes, homicide and accidents, and chemical dependency. *The Secretary's Task Force Report on Black and Minority Health* contributed significantly to the development of a number of *Healthy People 2000* objectives.[5] Work toward these objectives via the community health initiatives concentrated on minority populations produced some measurable decreases in age-adjusted death rates for seven specific causes of death (see Table 10.1). In an attempt to further document racial and ethnic changes over time in important Health Status Indicators (HSI), the index of disparity is provided in Table 10.2 for 1990 and 1998. The index of disparity summarizes differences among racial and ethnic minority groups' rates to the total group. "This statistic provides a basis for comparing the degree of difference in race and ethnic specific rates in 1990 with the disparity in race/ethnic rates in 1998."[6] As shown in Table 10.2,

Table 10.1
Age-Adjusted Death Rates for Selected Causes of Death by Race and Hispanic Origin, 1990 and 1998, and Percent Change from 1990 to 1998: United States

	Total	Non-Hispanic		Hispanic	American Indian or Alaska Native	Asian or Pacific Islander	Ratio Highest/ Lowest[2]
		White	Black				
Total deaths							
1990[1]	518.0	483.7	785.2	395.2	441.7	295.5	2.7
1998	471.7	452.7	710.7	342.8	458.1	264.6	2.7
Percent change, 1990–98	−8.9	−6.4	−9.5	−13.3	3.7	−10.5	
Heart disease							
1990[1]	151.3	145.3	211.8	101.5	106.0	78.0	2.7
1998	126.6	123.6	188.0	84.2	97.1	67.4	2.8
Percent change, 1990–98	−16.3	−14.9	−11.2	−17.0	−8.4	−13.6	
Stroke							
1990[1]	27.5	25.1	47.8	20.7	19.1	24.7	2.5
1998	25.1	23.3	42.5	19.0	19.6	22.7	2.2
Percent change, 1990–98	−9.0	−7.2	−11.1	−8.2	2.6	−8.1	
Lung cancer							
1990[1]	39.8	39.8	50.9	15.7	19.6	17.6	3.2
1998	37.0	38.3	46.0	13.6	25.1	17.2	3.4
Percent change, 1990–98	−7.0	−3.8	−9.6	−13.4	28.1	−2.3	
Female breast cancer							
1990[1]	23.0	23.0	27.3	14.0	9.9	9.9	2.8
1998	18.8	18.7	26.1	12.1	10.3	9.8	2.7
Percent change, 1990–98	−18.3	−18.7	−4.4	−13.6	4.0	−1.0	

Table 10.1   (Continued)

	Total	Non-Hispanic White	Non-Hispanic Black	Hispanic	American Indian or Alaska Native	Asian or Pacific Islander	Ratio Highest/ Lowest[2]
Motor vehicle crash							
1990[1]	18.4	18.1	18.3	19.2	33.0	12.5	2.6
1998	15.6	15.7	17.2	14.9	31.8	8.6	3.7
Percent change, 1990-98	−15.2	−13.3	−6.0	−22.4	−3.6	−31.2	
Suicide							
1990[1]	11.5	12.5	7.0	7.2	12.4	6.0	2.1
1998	10.4	11.8	6.1	6.0	13.4	5.9	2.3
Percent change, 1990-98	−9.6	−5.6	−12.9	−16.7	8.1	−1.7	
Homicide							
1990[1]	10.2	4.1	39.6	17.5	11.1	5.2	9.7
1998	7.3	3.2	26.1	9.9	9.9	3.7	8.2
Percent change, 1990-98	−28.4	−22.0	−34.1	−43.4	−10.8	−28.8	

[1]Age-adjusted death rates for 1990 were calculated based on population estimates for July 1, 1990. Rates published elsewhere for 1990 are based on the enumerated population on April 1, 1990, for the year in which the decennial census was taken. Rates for noncensus years are based on July 1 (midyear) populations. In order to measure changes over time, rates based on the July 1 populations are used.
[2]Ratio of the highest race/ethnic-specific rate to the lowest race/ethnic-specific rate for each year.

Source: Keppel, K. G., J. N. Pearcy, and D. K. Wagener (January 2002). *Trends in Racial and Ethnic-Specific Rates for the Health Status Indicators: United States 1990-1998* (Healthy People Statistical Notes no. 23). Hyattsville, MD: National Center for Health Statistics.

Table 10.2
Index of Disparity among Five Racial/Ethnic Groups for the Health Status Indicators: United States, 1990, 1998, and Percent Change

	Index of Disparity 1990	Index of Disparity 1998	Percent Change 1990–98 Decrease	Percent Change 1990–98 Increase
Infant mortality rates	38.9	36.4	−6.4	
Low birth weight (percent)	28.4	23.0	−19.0**	
No prenatal care in first trimester (percent)	46.9	43.5	−7.2**	
Live birth rates for women aged 15-17 years	65.4	67.7		3.5**
Total death rates	27.9	25.8	−7.5**	
Heart disease death rates	31.1	30.9	−0.6**	
Stroke death rates	29.6	26.4	−10.8**	
Lung cancer death rates	39.0	35.4	−9.2**	
Female breast cancer death rates	34.3	33.6	−2.0	
Motor vehicle crash death rates	23.6	32.8		39.0**
Suicide death rates	28.2	33.8		19.9**
Homicide death rates	95.5	86.8	−9.1**	
Work-related injury death rates (1993-98)[1]	6.3	22.1		250.8[a]
Tuberculosis case rates	160.4	170.3		6.2[a]
Primary and secondary syphilis case rates	175.3	153.1	−12.7[a]	
Children under age 18 years in poverty (percent)[2]	64.7	56.2	−13.1	
Percentage with poor air quality (1992-1998)	31.1	29.5	−5.1[a]	

**The difference in the index of disparity is statistically significant at the 0.05 level.
[a]The statistical significance of the difference in the index of disparity was not tested. Methods for assessing the reliability of the underlying rates are not available.
[1]The index of disparity for work-related injury deaths is not strictly comparable with the index of disparity for the other indicators because the data are available for the following groups: white, black, Hispanic, American Indian, Aleut and Eskimo, and Asian or Pacific Islanders. Persons of Hispanic origin may be of any race.
[2]The index of disparity for the percentage of children in poverty is not strictly comparable with the index of disparity for the other indicators because the data are available for the following groups: white non-Hispanic, black, Hispanic, and Asian or Pacific Islander.

Source: Keppel, K. G., J. N. Pearcy, and D. K. Wagener (January 2002). *Trends in Racial and Ethnic-Specific Rates for the Health Status Indicators: United States 1990-1998* (Healthy People Statistical Notes no. 23). Hyattsville, MD: National Center for Health Statistics.

there was a decline in 12 of the 17 HSIs. However, in some instances the disparities remained the same or in some cases widened, as evidenced by an increase in 5 of the 17 HSIs.

In 1998, then-President Clinton declared that the United States would continue to commit to a national goal of eliminating racial and ethnic health disparities by the year 2010.[7] Following this announcement, the *Initiative to Eliminate Racial and Ethnic Disparities in Health*, or the *Race and Health Initiative*, was launched. The purpose of this national effort was to enhance efforts in (1) preventing disease, (2) promoting health, and (3) delivering care to racial and ethnic minority communities. One of the primary aims of this initiative consists of consultation and collaboration among federal agencies; state, local, and tribal governments; and community professionals to research and address issues of education, income, environment, and other socioeconomic factors that affect health outcomes. Accordingly, the *Race and Health Initiative* is a paramount part of *Healthy People 2010*'s broad health goal to "eliminate health disparities among Americans."[8] This initiative will be addressed in more detail after a brief discussion on how racial and ethnic populations are classified.

RACIAL AND ETHNIC CLASSIFICATIONS

It is standard practice for the federal government to describe participants and populations in terms of "race" or "ethnicity." The racial and ethnic categories are used in statistical activities and program administration reporting, including the monitoring and enforcement of civil rights. In the 1980s, the regulations used for the statistical classification of racial and ethnic groups by federal agencies were based on the 1978 publication by the Office of Management and Budget (OMB) of Directive 15 titled "Race and Ethnic Standards for Federal Statistics and Administrative Reporting."[9] This directive presented brief rules for classifying persons into four racial categories (American Indian or Alaskan Native, Asian or Pacific Islander, black, and white) and two ethnic categories (of Hispanic origin or not of Hispanic origin) (see Appendix 2). It required the categorization of blacks and whites into one of the two ethnic categories. Directive 15 was not intended to be scientific or anthropological in nature, but rather a way to **operationalize** race and ethnicity. The operational definitions detailed in Directive 15 provided the standards by which federal government agencies collected and classified racial and ethnic data in the 1980s and 1990s.

operationalize (operational definition) provide working definitions

In the early 1990s, this classification system came under increasing criticism from those who asserted that the minimum categories set forth in Directive 15 did not reflect the increasing diversity of our nation's population. In response to those criticisms, OMB committed to a comprehensive review process in the mid-1990s in collaboration with the Interagency Committee for the Review of the Racial and Ethnic Standards that would enhance the accuracy of the demographic information collected by the federal government. In 1997, revised standards were issued.[10] These revised standards were used in the year 2000 decennial census. (See Appendix 3 for a listing of the operational definitions that were used by the Bureau of Census to collect the 2000 decennial census.) One of the first federal programs to support and adopt the revised standards was the Department of Health and Human Services (HHS). In October 1997, the Secretary of the HHS issued a policy supporting the inclusion of the new revised federal standards for racial and ethnic data for employment in the HHS data systems and consequently in developing and measuring *Healthy People 2010* objectives.

The 1997 classification standards expanded race from four to five categories by separating the "Asian or Pacific Islander" category into two categories—"Asian" and "Native Hawaiian or Other Pacific Islander." Additionally, the term "Hispanic" was changed to "Hispanic or Latino" and "Negro" can be used in addition to "Black or African American." Finally, the reporting of more than one race for multiracial persons was strongly encouraged, along with specifying that the Hispanic origin question should precede the race question. The Census 2000 form best illustrates these changes (see Figure 10.4). There are 15 check box response categories and three write-in areas on the Census 2000 questionnaire for indicating race and ethnicity. The Hispanic origin question (Question 7) is asked before the race question (Question 8), and "Asian and Pacific Islander" has been divided into two categories—"Asian" and "Native Hawaiian and Other Pacific Islander." There are six designated Asian and three specified Pacific Islander categories, as well as "Other Asian" and "Other Pacific Islander." Finally, the category "some other race," which was intended to gain responses such as Mulatto, Creole, and Mestizo, has a write-in area.

FIGURE 10.4
U.S. Census 2000 form questions for race and ethnicity.

It is important to consider a couple of aspects related to the collecting of data on race and ethnicity. First, the categories of race are more of a social category than a biological one.[11] Although race historically has been viewed as a biological construct, it is now known to be more accurately characterized as a social category that has changed over time and varies across societies and cultures.[11,12] As you will read later in this chapter, numerous studies have shown that racial disparities in health generally do not mirror biologically determined differences in these groups.[13] Second, self-reported data regarding race and ethnicity may be unreliable because individuals of varied cultures and heritage and multiple races can have difficulty classifying their racial or ethnic identity on standardized forms. Third, many nonfederal health data systems do not collect self-reported race or ethnicity data, or in some cases, it may be uncertain who recorded the race and ethnicity data. For example, in a medical care setting the information may be entered by clerical staff or hospital personnel. This can make analyzing health information concerning the health status of minorities a challenging task.

HEALTH DATA SOURCES AND THEIR LIMITATIONS

The reporting of accurate and complete race and ethnicity data provides essential information to target and evaluate public health inventions aimed at minority populations.[14] However, because of the diversity in America's population, community health professionals and researchers have long recognized many crucial issues in the way that racial and ethnic variables are assessed in the collection, analysis, and dissemination of health information.[15] In the same manner, the HHS is aware of the serious gaps in its own information systems and databases regarding racial and ethnic data. For example, in a recent longitudinal study completed by the Centers for Disease Control and Prevention's National Electronic Telecommunications System for Surveillance, it was found that data regarding a patient's race and ethnicity were received in only one-half of the cases of selected notifiable diseases.[14] In comparison, data on age and sex were reported between 95% to 99% of the time during that same period. According to the authors of the study, race and ethnicity may not be reported by health care providers for at least four reasons:[14]

1. Providers may not know what the federal standards for data collection are about race and ethnicity on their patients for surveillance purposes.
2. If a health care provider forgets or is reluctant to ask a patient's racial/ethnic background, this information may not be recorded.
3. Patients may choose not to provide information about their race and ethnicity.
4. Clinical laboratory staff may not report race and ethnicity data because they do not have access to that information.

In addition to incomplete data collection, there are many cases of *bias analysis.* Bias analysis occurs when two separate data reporting systems are used to obtain rates by race and Hispanic origin. An illustration of analysis bias that is currently happening is the misreporting of race and Hispanic origin in the numerator of deaths on death certificates combined with the underreporting in the denominator of the population subgroups.[16] As a consequence of the combined effect of numerator and denominator biases, it has been estimated that death rates for the white population are overestimated by about 1% and by 5% for the black American population. At the same time, death rates are underestimated for the American Indian or Alaska Native population by nearly 21%, by 11% for Asian or Pacific Islanders, and by 2% for Hispanics.[16]

Collecting appropriate racial and ethnic data is a significant challenge facing public health. The HHS has developed a long-term strategy for improving the collection and use of racial and ethnic data throughout the department and its agencies and, more specifically, for the *Race and Health Initiative.*[17] The diversified aspects of this plan will require time and resources by the department and its agencies. One national health objective for 2010, which the HHS is overseeing, is the upgrading of data collection on race and ethnicity in public health surveys that use the self-reported race of the respondent. In addition, the HHS is working with health data systems that do not collect self-reported race or ethnicity on individuals, to do so. Increasing both the reliability and amount of data will assist in monitoring and assessing the outcomes related to meeting the proposed goal of eliminating racial and ethnic health disparities in *Healthy People 2010.* A standard data table will be used to display the baseline status of each subpopulation group by race and ethnicity (*American Indian* or *Alaska Native, Asian American, Pacific Islander, Black* or *African American, White, Hispanic* or *Latino,* or *Not Hispanic* or *Latino*) for each objective listed in *Healthy People 2010.*[8] Data will be presented for all minorities, whether or not a disparity exists when compared to the total population. It is believed that this approach will better identify missing data on racial and ethnic minorities and encourage further attempts by the appropriate agencies or community advocate groups to collect this information. For example, 157 (36%) of the 434 population-based *Healthy People 2010* objectives and subobjectives did not have data available for Hispanics in 2000.

Recognizing some of the limitations and gaps in collecting racial/ethnic data is important. Knowing that in some cases data are not available or the available data are not as precise as we would like, we present the best information about the community health issues faced by the primary minority groups. However, as you continue to read this chapter please be reminded of the limitations of the data on racial and ethnic minority groups. Finally, please note that throughout the remainder of the chapter we use the terms *Americans of Hispanic origin, Asian Americans, Pacific Islanders, black Americans, Native Americans,* and *white Americans,* unless there is a direct quotation or extrapolation from data or documents that use other terminology (e.g., *American Indians* in lieu of *Native Americans*).

Next, in order to gain a better understanding of minority groups in the United States, we will briefly review several sociodemographic and socioeconomic characteristics along with broad general health beliefs for each group. These characteristics will eventually be used later in the chapter to discuss why health disparities exist in minority groups. Furthermore, all cultural and ethnic groups hold concepts related to health and illness and associated practices for maintaining well-being or providing treatment when it is indicated. However, caution is needed to avoid stereotyping. There is a considerable amount of heterogeneity within these groups, and therefore making summary statements of cultural beliefs is difficult and can be questionable. The world's 210 nations are well represented in the United States, and these diverse cultures are continually being integrated and intermixed. Additionally, members of a cultural or ethnic group who are younger or more **acculturated** into mainstream America society may not adhere to popular and folk health beliefs.

acculturated
cultural modification of an individual or group by adapting to or borrowing traits from another culture

AMERICANS OF HISPANIC ORIGIN

As we begin our discussion of Americans of Hispanic origin, readers are reminded that Hispanic origin is an ethnicity classification, not a race. The term *Hispanic* was introduced by the OMB in 1977, creating an ethnic category that included persons of Mexican, Puerto Rican, Cuban, Central America, South America, or some other Spanish origin.[9] In 1997, the term *Hispanic* was changed to "Hispanic or Latino."[10] For the purposes of data collection, the only ethnic distinction that the U.S. government makes is "Hispanic" or "non-Hispanic." Therefore, all Americans of Hispanic origin are also classified by a race. Nearly all Hispanics are classified as white Americans (96%) in the United States.

In 2005, Americans of Hispanic origin numbered approximately 42.7 million and constituted 14.4% of the total U.S. population, making them the largest minority group in the nation (see Figure 10.2). Since 1990, the Hispanic population has been the most rapidly growing ethnic group in the United States (see Figure 10.3). People of Mexican origin are the largest Hispanic group in the United States, representing nearly 64% of the country's Hispanic population.[2] Additionally, approximately 10% of Americans of Hispanic origin are of Puerto Rican background, with about 3% each of Cuban, Salvadoran, and Dominican origins. The remaining are of some other Central American, South American, or other Hispanic or Latino origins.

As mentioned earlier, disparities in health statistics among minorities can be traced to differences in education and income. A high school education is considered an essential basic training requirement to enter the labor force. The high school educational attainment level of Hispanic youth has been consistently lower when compared with other groups (see Figure 10.5).[18] However, the high school completion rate has increased over the last couple of decades, from 57% in 1980 to 69.9% in 2004. Linked with education is earning power. The median income of Hispanic families is significantly lower than that of Asian/Pacific Islanders and whites (see Figure 10.6).[19] Poverty rates for persons of Hispanic origin averaged 22%, nearly three times the rate for white Americans (see Figure 10.7).[20]

Traditional health beliefs of Mexican Americans and other Latin cultures include the "role of God."[21] Good health is seen as a matter of fortune or reward from God for good behavior. Maintaining harmony and balance with God is linked to the concept of good health, and warding off evil spirits is important to maintain this balance. *Curanderismo* is the most common form of Mexican American folk medicine.[21] A *curandera*'s, or healer's, ability includes a varied repertoire of religious belief systems (mainly Catholicism), herbal knowledge, witchcraft, and scientific medicine.

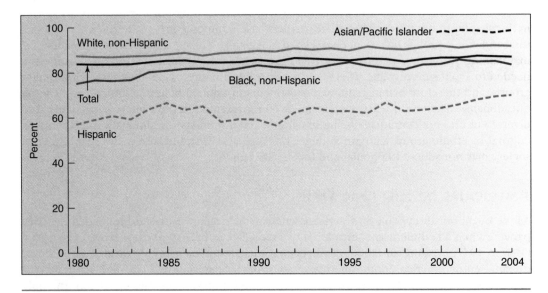

FIGURE 10.5

Percentage of adults ages 18 to 24 who have completed high school, by race and Hispanic origin, 1980 to 2004.

Note: Percentages are based only on those not currently enrolled in high school or below. Prior to 1992, this indicator was measured as completing four or more years of high school rather than the actual attainment of a high school diploma or equivalent.

Source: U.S. Census Bureau (2006). *Current Population Survey, October Supplement.* Tabulated by the U.S. Department of Education, National Center for Education Statistics.

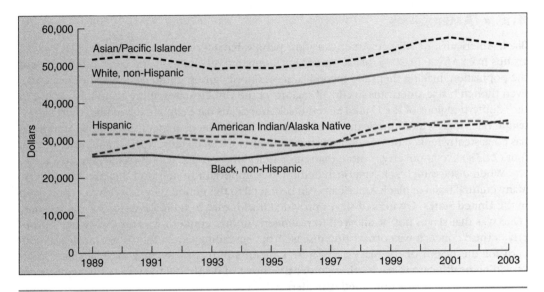

FIGURE 10.6

Median income (in constant 2003 dollars) of households, by race/ethnicity: 1989 to 2003.

Note: The 2003 Current Population Survey (CPS) offered respondents the option of choosing more than one race. The 2002 and 2001 CPS recorded only one race for each respondent. The three-year averages are based on combining the 2003 CPS race categories with the relevant single-race categories of White, Black, American Indian or Alaska Native, or Asian and Pacific Islander recorded in the 2002 and 2001 CPS.

Source: U.S. Census Bureau (2005). *Current Population Survey, 1989–2000,* and annual *Social and Economic Supplements,* 2000 to 2004. Washington, DC: U.S. Government Printing Office.

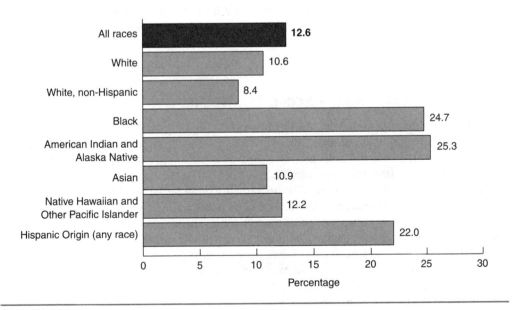

FIGURE 10.7

Poverty rates by race and Hispanic origin: three-year averages, 2003 to 2005.

Note: Federal surveys now give respondents the option of reporting more than one race. Therefore, two basic ways of defining a race group are possible. A group such as Asian may be defined as those who reported Asian and no other race (the race-alone or single-race concept) or as those who reported Asian regardless of whether they also reported another race (the race-alone-or-in-combination concept). This figure shows data using the first approach (race alone).

Source: U.S. Census Bureau (2006). *Current Population Survey, 2004–2006. Annual Social and Economic Supplements.* Washington, DC. U.S Government Printing Office.

BLACK AMERICANS

Black Americans, or African Americans, are people having origins in any of the black racial groups from Africa. In 2005, black Americans numbered 39.7 million and constituted 12.3% of the population, making them the second largest minority group in the nation (see Figure 10.2). Even though black Americans live in all regions of the United States, more than one-half live in the southern regions of the United States. Black Americans have slightly lower high school graduation rates than white Americans (see Figure 10.5).[18] The median income for black Americans has consistently ranked below all racial and ethnic groups (see Figure 10.6),[19] and nearly one in four (24.7%) live in poverty,[20] more than three times the rates for whites (see Figure 10.7).

When discussing black American culture, it is important to mention the effect of slavery. Many cultural traits of black Americans can be traced to the period when slavery was practiced in the United States. Owners of slaves provided health care to their slaves for several reasons. "One was that slaves not be allowed to malinger; another concern was for the owner's property; a third concern was preventing disease from spreading; and a fourth was an actual concern for the health of the slaves."[22] These concerns plus the law that forbade slaves from providing health care to each other, under the threat of death, led to an underground system of health care by mostly untrained providers.

After the Civil War, poverty, discrimination, and poor living conditions led to a high prevalence of disease, disability, and death among black Americans.[23] Racial discrimination limited this group's access to adequate health care through the middle of the twentieth century, much as it did to education and voting rights. This discrimination continues to have an impact on the health status of black Americans today. Many black Americans still find it difficult to gain access to health care because of discrimination. Lacking access to more formalized American health care, first by slavery and then by segregation and discrimination, many black Americans implemented traditional health methods.[24] These traditional methods include curing illnesses with roots, herbs, barks, and teas by an individual knowledgeable about their use. Many black Americans continue to use traditional health methods today because they are acceptable, available, and affordable.

ASIAN AMERICANS AND PACIFIC ISLANDERS

As we begin our discussion of Asian Americans and Pacific Islanders, it is important to remind readers about the 1997 "Revisions to the Standards for the Classification of Federal Data on Race and Ethnicity." The most distinct change was separating Asian Americans and Pacific Islanders (see Figure 10.4 and Appendix 3).

In June 1999, former President Clinton signed Executive Order 13125 to improve the quality of life of Asian Americans and Pacific Islanders through increased participation in federal programs where they may be underserved (e.g., health, human services, education, housing, labor, transportation, and economic and community development).[25] One important goal of the order is collecting separate data on each group. Asian and Pacific Islanders are really two distinct groups, and combining the data tended to conceal substantial socioeconomic and health differences among these groups.[26] However, even by 2001, most federal agencies were still not collecting separate data on these two groups, citing methodological and funding constraints.[27] Accordingly, the following data on Asian Americans and Pacific Islanders is presented in aggregate, unless otherwise noted.

In 2005, Asians numbered approximately 14.4 million and constituted 4.9% of the population, and native Hawaiians and other Pacific Islanders numbered 990,000, or 0.3% of the population (see Figure 10.2). Asian American populations are generally concentrated in the western states, the Northeast, and parts of the South. Native Hawaiian and other Pacific Islanders

(NHOPIs) live throughout the United States, but their populations are most concentrated in the western mainland states and Hawaii.[2]

When education and income are reported in aggregate for Asians and NHOPIs, they appear well off (see Figures 10.5 and 10.6). The high school completion rates of 18- through 24-year-olds and the median incomes were the highest compared with all other racial and ethnic groups. Unfortunately, these aggregated data mask the large variation within this population group.[28] According to Yoon and Chien, the education and income of Asians and NHOPIs form a *bipolar distribution* (skewed toward each extreme with few in the middle).[29] To better understand this concept, consider the following: Among people aged 25 years and older, Asians and NHOPIs are more likely than white Americans (42% vs. 28%) to have earned a college degree; however, they are also more likely than white Americans (8% vs. 5%) to have less than a ninth-grade education.[30] Additionally, 33% of Asians and NHOPIs had incomes of $75,000 or more, compared with 29% of white families, while at the same time more Asians and NHOPIs had incomes under $25,000 than whites (21% vs. 19%). This deceptive view, formed by aggregate data only, has led to the myth that Asians and NHOPIs are a "model community" when in fact they suffer from as many disparities as other racial and ethnic minority groups.[29]

As mentioned previously, Asian Americans and Pacific Islanders are two discrete groups. Therefore, we now proceed with a brief overview of each. The term *Asian American* refers to people of Asian descent who are American citizens. Immigration is an integral part of Asian American community growth, as many are seeking better economic and employment opportunities and/or are reuniting with family members. They or their ancestors came from more than 20 different Asian countries, including Cambodia, China, India, Japan, Korea, Malaysia, Pakistan, the Philippine Islands, Thailand, and Vietnam.[30] Among these groups, the Chinese and Filipinos are the two largest subgroups. Even among those who have come from the same country, immigration to America may have occurred at different times, and thus there are generational differences. For example, some families may have immigrated well over a hundred years ago as laborers, while those coming today carry with them professional degrees.[31] These differences contribute to a substantial diversity in socioeconomic status among these groups, thus creating the myth discussed earlier that Asian Americans are a "model group."

Although variations among Asian Americans is the norm, many share similarities based on their religious background and the belief of equilibrium or balance.[32] The concept of balance is related to health, and imbalance is related to disease. This balance or imbalance is highly related to diet, which influences people's daily activities of living within their environment. Therefore, to achieve health and avoid illness, people must adjust to the environment in a holistic manner.

The term *Pacific Islander* (PI) includes peoples of Hawaii, Guam, Samoa, or other Pacific Islands and their descendants.[30] The Native Hawaiian population forms the majority of PIs. In contrast to Asian Americans, there is no large-scale immigration of PIs into the continental United States. Because Hawaii is the state in which the majority of PIs live, this will be our main focus. Similar to other minority groups, there are many health disparities among PIs.[33] Two key health issues for Native Hawaiians include health care allocation and the question of reimbursement for medical care.

Nearly 90% of Hawaii's land mass is federally designated as rural. Approximately 20% of Native Hawaiians live in rural Hawaii. However, the majority of the state's health care resources are fixed in the capitol city of Honolulu. As a result of this imbalance of health care resource allocation, there is an inadequate number of health care professionals on the neighboring islands.[34] Additionally, transportation issues between the islands make it more difficult to access health care in Honolulu. Even public transportation on the separate islands is unreliable, so local access to medical care is challenging. The second medical care issue deals with the Native Hawaiian health belief, which suggests that the healer cannot be reimbursed directly for his or her therapeutic work. According to Blaisell,[35] such healer skill is not a question of learning but rather a question of righteousness. Therefore, it is not considered appropriate to be paid for doing what is right.

AMERICAN INDIANS AND ALASKA NATIVES

The American Indian and Alaska Native (AI/AN) population, the original inhabitants of America, numbered nearly 4.5 million in 2005, or 1.5% of the total population (see Figure 10.2). It has been estimated that prior to the arrival of European explorers, 12 million AI/ANs lived and flourished throughout what is now the United States. Exposure to diseases and ecological changes introduced by explorers and colonists decimated the AI/AN population. Although many of the descendants were assimilated by intermarriages or successfully adapted to the new culture, as a group the AI/ANs became economically and socially disadvantaged, and this status is reflected in their relatively poor health status.[36,37] The 2003–2005 average poverty rate for AI/ANs was 25.3%, which is the highest among all racial and ethnic groups (see Figure 10.7). Similarly, their median income and high school completion rates were among the lowest of any racial and ethnic group (see Figures 10.5 and 10.6).

Native Americans comprise many different American Indian tribal groups and Alaskan villages. Each of these tribes/villages has distinct customs, language, and beliefs. The majority, however, share the same cultural values that have been identified by Edwards and Egbert-Edwards:[38]

- Appreciation of individuality with emphasis upon an individual's right to freedom, autonomy, and respect.
- Group consensus in tribal/village decision making.
- Respect for all living things.
- Appreciation, respect, and reverence for the land.
- Feelings of hospitality toward friends, family, clanspeople, tribesmen, and respectful visitors.
- An expectation that tribal/village members will bring honor and respect to their families, clans, and tribes. Bringing shame or dishonor to self or tribe is negatively reinforced.
- A belief in a supreme being and life after death. Indian religion is the dominant influence for traditional Indian people.

Central to Native American culture is that the people "strive for a close integration within the family, clan and tribe and live in harmony with their environment. This occurs simultaneously on physical, mental, and spiritual levels; thus, individual wellness is considered as harmony and balance among mind, body, spirit and the environment."[38] This concept is not congruent with the medical model approach or public health approach that is generally accepted by the majority of Americans. As a result, in many Native American communities there is conflict between the medical/public health approach and the approaches used by Native American healers (see Table 10.3).[38] Providing appropriate health care for Native Americans usually involves resolving conflicts between the two approaches in such a way that they complement each other.

U.S. Government, Native Americans, and the Provision of Health Care

Though classified by definition and for statistical purposes as a minority group, Native Americans are unlike any other subgroup in the United States. Some (but not all) tribes are sovereign nations, based in part upon their treaties with the U.S. government. Tribal sovereignty, which is perhaps the most important Native American issue, creates a distinct and special relationship between various tribes and the U.S. government. This sovereignty came about when the tribes transferred vir-

Table 10.3
A Comparison of Indian Medicine and Modern Medicine

Indian Medicine	Modern Medicine
Behavior-oriented	Complaint-oriented
Whole-specific	Organ-specific
Imbalance	Caused
Visionary diagnosis	Technical diagnosis
Wellness-oriented	Illness-oriented

Source: Garrett, J. T. (1990). "Indian Health: Values, Beliefs, and Practices." In M. S. Harper, ed., *Minority Aging: Essential Curricula Content for Selected Health and Allied Health Professionals* (HHS pub. no. HRS-P-DV90-4). Washington, DC: U.S. Government Printing Office.

tually all the land in the United States to the federal government in return for the provision of certain services. The U.S. government agreed to manage the land, water, agriculture, and mineral and timber resources, and to provide education and health services to tribe members. Each of these services is owed to them, and if they become indignant when people suggest they are getting them free, it is a rightful indignation.[39]

Provisions of education for Native Americans date back to the Civilization Act of 1819, while provisions for health services began in 1832.[36] The first medical efforts were carried out by Army physicians who vaccinated Native Americans against smallpox and applied sanitary procedures to curb other communicable diseases among tribes living in the vicinity of military posts. The health services provided for Native Americans after the signing of the early treaties were limited. It was common for the U.S. government, through the treaties, to impose time limits of 5 to 20 years on the provisions of health care.[40]

The original government agency overseeing the welfare of Native Americans was the Bureau of Indian Affairs (BIA). When this bureau was transferred from the War Department to the Department of the Interior in 1849, physician services were extended to Native Americans. Over the next 70+ years, health care services were continually improved, with the first Native American hospital built in 1882. However, comprehensive health services were still lacking. It was not until 1921, when the Snyder Act created the BIA Health Division, that more emphasis was given to providing health services to Native Americans. In 1954 with the passage of Public Law 83-568, known as the Transfer Act, the responsibility of health care for Native Americans was transferred from the Department of Interior's BIA to the Public Health Service (PHS). It was at this time that the Indian Health Service (IHS) was created. With this act, the health needs of Native Americans were finally met in a comprehensive way.

In keeping with the concept of tribal sovereignty, the Indian Self-Determination and Education Assistance Act (PL 93-63) of 1975 authorized the IHS to involve tribes in the administration and operation of all or certain programs under a special contract. It authorized the IHS to provide grants to tribes, on request, for planning, development, and operation of health programs.[36] Today, a number of programs are managed and operated under contract by individual tribes.[37]

Indian Health Service

The IHS, an agency within the HHS, is responsible for providing federal health services to Native Americans and Alaska Natives.[37] This agency is organized into 12 areas throughout the United States (see Figure 10.8) and operates hospitals, clinics and health stations, and a variety of other programs. The goal of the IHS is to raise the health status of American Indians and Alaska Natives to the highest possible level. To attain this goal, the IHS

1. Assists Indian tribes in developing their health programs through activities such as health management training, technical assistance, and human resource development

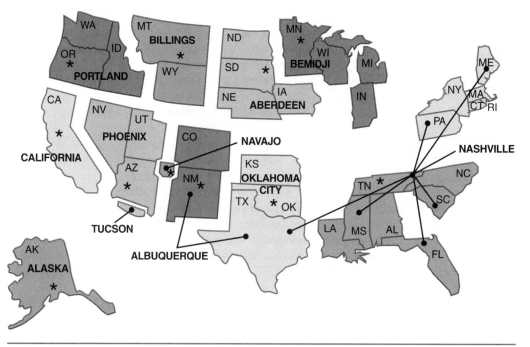

FIGURE 10.8

Indian Health Service (IHS) structure.

Note: Texas is administered by Nashville, Oklahoma City, and Albuquerque.

*Area office

Source: U.S. Department of Health and Human Services (2000). "Regional Differences in Indian Health 1998–99." Indian Health Services, Program Statistics Team, 31. Available at http://www.ihs.gov/publicinfo/publications/trends98/region98.asp.

refugee
a person who flees one area or country to seek shelter or protection from danger in another

2. Facilitates and assists Indian tribes in coordinating health resources available through federal, state, and local programs, in operating comprehensive health care services and in health program evaluation
3. Provides comprehensive health care services, including hospital and ambulatory medical care, preventive and rehabilitative services, and development of community sanitation facilities
4. Serves as the principal federal advocate for Indians in the health field to ensure comprehensive health services for American Indian and Alaska Native people[37]

immigrant
individuals who migrate from one country to another for the purpose of seeking permanent residence

REFUGEES: THE NEW IMMIGRANTS

In this section we introduce several new terms that describe people who have arrived in the United States relatively recently. Because of their status as new arrivals, these people sometimes share similar health problems. The first term, **refugees,** means people who flee one area, usually their home country, to seek shelter or protection from danger. Refugees arriving in the United States may be seeking political asylum, refuge from war, or escape from famine or other environmental disaster. The second term, **immigrants,** describes individuals who migrate here from another country for the purpose of seeking permanent residence and hopefully a better life. **Aliens** are people born in and owing allegiance to a country other than the one in which they live. Thus, aliens are not citizens and are only allowed to stay in a foreign country for a specified period of time defined by law or policy. Many aliens, including college students, although in the United States legally, are not permitted to work. Sometimes, how-

alien
a person born in and owing allegiance to a country other than the one in which he/she lives

ever, they violate this provision and find employment illegally. Lastly, **illegal aliens** are those who enter this country without any permission whatsoever. Most of these illegal aliens have entered from Mexico simply by crossing the Rio Grande river at night.

illegal alien
an individual who entered this country without permission

Although all refugees who enter this country can be classified into one of the existing racial/ethnic categories used by our government, as a single group they present many special concerns not seen in minorities who are born and raised in the United States. Most of the refugees currently entering the United States arrive from *developing countries,* countries with meager economic resources. These refugees usually settle in urban areas, even though they may have a rural orientation. Many refugees are poor, have low levels of formal education, and have few marketable work skills. Many arrive with serious health problems, including undernourishment or starvation, physical and emotional injuries from hostile action or confinement in refugee camps, poor health care, and overcrowdedness.[41] A majority of the refugees are young, many of the women are of childbearing age, and most come from Latin American and Southeast Asian countries.

The arrival of such refugees places additional strains on both public and private health and social services. Some of the problems that have surfaced include the following:

- Lack of jobs to fit the skills of the refugees
- New competition for the lower socioeconomic groups in the United States for work and housing
- Strain on the budgets of the public education systems to meet the needs of the non-English-speaking refugee children
- Further burden on the human, health, and mental health services provided mostly by minority communities
- Cultural barriers to using the U.S. health care system, including lack of financial resources, cultural ignorance of health care providers, lack of bilingual health care workers, distrust and unfamiliarity with Western medicine, poor understanding of the etiology of certain diseases, difficulties of accessing services, and ignorance of available services

This immigration has resulted in growing backlash movements against refugees in some areas of the country. Examples include the "only English" movement and the Immigration Reform and Control Act of 1986 that requires employers to prove the identity and work authorization for every prospective employee—the logic of which is based on the perception of work as a privilege associated with citizenship and, by extension, with legal residence.[41]

The difficulties facing refugees in the United States, including finding employment and obtaining access to education and appropriate human, health, and mental health services, represent significant barriers to the social integration of refugees into American society. Like most of the other minority groups in the United States, refugees may become a part of those disadvantaged in this country. There is, however, one bright note to the increase of refugees in this country—the enrichment of the U.S. culture. Until 1970, the United States was primarily composed of only black and white Americans. In the last 30+ years, this country has been significantly enriched by the cultures of those coming from other countries, and as noted earlier, the minority groups are the fastest-growing segments of the U.S. population.[42]

RACE AND HEALTH INITIATIVE

As mentioned previously, in 1998, former President Clinton committed the nation to an ambitious goal by the year 2010: Eliminate health disparities among racial and ethnic minority populations in six areas of health while maintaining the progress on overall health of the American people.[7] The *Race and Health Initiative*'s six priority areas are (1) infant mortality, (2) cancer screening and management, (3) cardiovascular disease, (4) diabetes, (5) HIV/AIDS, and (6) adult and child immunization.

The *Race and Health Initiative* reaffirms the government's extensive focus on minority health issues by emphasizing key areas that are representative of the larger minority health picture.[7] The six health issues account for a substantial burden of disease that is highly modifiable if appropriate interventions are applied. In addition, enough current data exist in each major area to be able to measure improvement and progress. Thus, the *Race and Health Initiative* is intertwined with *Healthy People 2010* and the goals of the nation for the next decade.[8]

It is important to note that *Healthy People 2010* will continue to pursue other areas of concern related to minority health that are not directly covered under these six major areas. Similarly, we acknowledge that disparities exist in many other areas of minority health; however, this chapter will present data on the six health areas identified in the *Race and Health Initiative*. We will begin by providing data documenting the disparities that exist in each of the categories, as well as data related to major risk factors that contribute to each of the conditions. As you continue to read, it is important not to stereotype any group, for it is known that each health concern cuts across all racial and ethnic groups.

Infant Mortality

As noted in Chapter 7, infant mortality is defined as the death of an infant before his or her first birthday. The infant mortality rate correlates highly to the general health and well-being of the nation. The United States made significant improvement in the twentieth century regarding infant health. However, while the vast majority of infants born in America today are healthy at birth, many are not. As a result, many industrialized nations report infant mortality rates that are better than those of the United States (see Figure 7.4). Additionally, infant mortality data within the United States are characterized by a long-standing and serious disparity among racial and ethnic minorities (see Figure 10.9). Infant death rates among black Americans, American Indians and Alaska Natives, and Americans of Hispanic origin have all been above the national average of approximately seven deaths per 1,000 live births. The greatest disparity exists for black Americans, whose infant death rate is more than two times that of white American infants.

There are many reasons associated with higher infant mortality rates among black Americans. Two of the more important explanations include lack of prenatal care and giving birth to low-birth-weight (LBW) babies. Prenatal care is crucial to maternal and infant health (see Chapter 7). Women who receive early and continuous prenatal health care have better pregnancy outcomes than woman who do not. Black American, Native American, and Hispanic women are less likely to receive early and comprehensive prenatal care (see Figure 7.14).[43] In the same manner, black Americans and Native Americans are more likely to give birth to LBW babies (see Figure 10.10).

Cancer Screening and Management

Approximately 1.4 million new cases of invasive cancer are diagnosed in the United States annually.[44] Nearly half of those who develop cancer will die from it. Cancer is the second leading cause of death in the United States, accounting for more than 550,000 deaths annually (see Chapter 4 and Chapter 8). From 1998 to 2002, cancer incidence rates per 100,000 population were 682.6 among black Americans, 556.4 among white Americans, 420.7 among Hispanics, 383.5 among Asian/Pacific Islanders, and 259.0 among American Indian/Alaska Natives

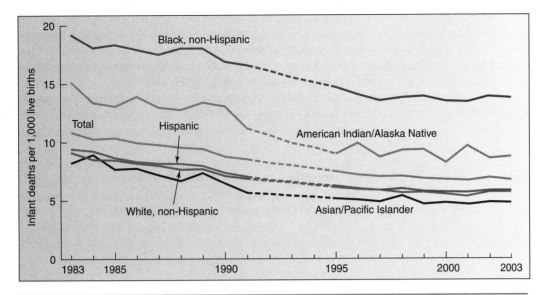

FIGURE 10.9

Infant mortality rates by race and Hispanic origin of mother: selected years, 1983 to 2003.

Note: Data are available for 1983–1991 and 1995–2003. Infant deaths are deaths before a child's first birthday.

Source: Centers for Disease Control and Prevention, National Center for Health Statistics, National Linked File of Live Births and Infant Deaths.

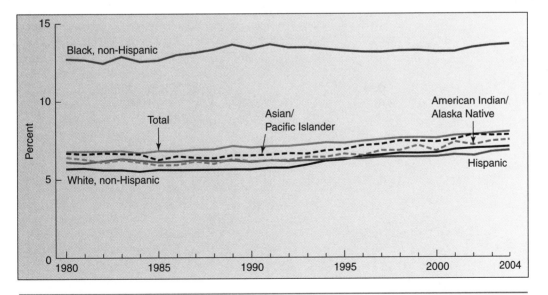

FIGURE 10.10

Percentage of infants born of low birth weight, by mother's race and Hispanic origin, 1980 to 2004.

Source: Centers for Disease Control and Prevention, National Center for Health Statistics, National Vital Statistics System.

(see Table 10.4). During the same period of time, cancer death rates per 100,000 population were 339.4 among black Americans, 247.5 among white Americans, 171.4 among Hispanics, 148.0 among Asian/Pacific Islanders, and 159.7 among American Indian/Alaska Natives (see Table 10.4). A number of these disparities in cancer incidence and death rates among minorities are attributed to lifestyle factors, late diagnosis, and access to health care.[45]

The good news is that cancer is preventable. Primary cancer prevention refers to preventing the occurrence of cancer. The American Cancer Society estimates that approximately 60% of all

Table 10.4
Incidence and Mortality Rates of Cancer by Site, Race, and Ethnicity: United States, 1998–2002

	White	African American	Asian American and Pacific Islander	American Indian and Alaska Native	Hispanic/ Latino*
Incidence					
All sites					
Males	556.4	682.6	383.5	255.4	420.7
Females	429.3	398.5	303.6	220.5	310.9
Breast (female)	141.1	119.4	96.6	54.8	89.9
Colon & rectum					
Males	61.7	72.5	56.0	36.7	48.3
Females	45.3	56.0	39.7	32.2	32.3
Lung & bronchus					
Males	76.7	113.9	59.4	42.6	44.6
Females	51.1	55.2	28.3	23.6	23.3
Prostate	169.0	272.0	101.4	50.3	141.9
Stomach					
Males	10.7	17.7	21.0	15.9	17.2
Females	5.0	9.6	12.0	9.1	10.1
Liver & intrahepatic bile duct					
Males	7.4	12.1	21.4	8.7	14.1
Females	2.9	3.7	7.9	5.2	6.1
Uterine cervix	8.7	11.1	8.9	49.4	15.8
Mortality					
All sites					
Males	242.5	339.4	148.0	159.7	171.4
Females	164.5	194.3	99.4	113.8	111.0
Breast (female)	25.9	34.7	12.7	13.8	16.7
Colon & rectum					
Males	24.3	34.0	15.8	16.2	17.7
Females	16.8	24.1	10.6	11.8	11.6
Lung & bronchus					
Males	75.2	101.3	39.4	47.0	38.7
Females	41.8	39.9	18.8	27.1	14.8
Prostate	27.7	68.1	12.1	18.3	23.0
Stomach					
Males	5.6	12.8	11.2	7.3	9.5
Females	2.8	6.3	6.8	4.1	5.3
Liver & intrahepatic bile duct					
Males	6.2	9.5	15.4	7.9	10.7
Females	2.7	3.8	6.5	4.3	5.1
Uterine cervix	2.5	5.3	2.7	2.6	3.5

Note: Rates are per 100,000, age-adjusted to the 2000 U.S. standard population.

*Hispanic/Latinos are not mutually exclusive from whites, African Americans, Asian Americans and Pacific Islanders, and American Indians and Alaska Natives.

Source: Ries, L. A. G., M. P. Eisner, C. L. Kosary, et al., eds. (2003). *SEER Cancer Statistics Review, 1975–2002.* Bethesda, MD: National Cancer Institute.

cancers in the United States could be prevented through lifestyle behavior changes (i.e., avoiding smoking, avoiding excessive sun exposure, and eating nutritiously).[44] Smoking is the most preventable cause of lung cancer death in our society. The death rate for lung cancer is 25% higher in black Americans than white Americans (see Table 10.4). Paralleling this death rate is the fact that black Americans have a higher incidence of smoking than white Americans.

Secondary cancer prevention refers to early detection of cancer through screening tests. The earlier a cancer is detected, the greater the chances one will survive. The disparity in lower survival rates among black Americans is reflected in Table 10.5, which shows that black Americans are less likely to have their cancers detected in a localized stage. One particular cancer of significant interest related to the *Race and Health Initiative* is breast cancer. Breast cancer is the second leading cause of cancer death among women. Most deaths from breast cancer can be reduced through early detetction. Breast cancer survival rates are significantly increased if the cancer is detected early through monthly self-examination and/or periodic mammograms (breast X-rays). Despite the importance of mammography, it is underutilized as an early detection procedure by many minority women (see Box 10.1). The goal of *Healthy People 2010* is to have at least 70% of women from all racial or ethnic groups aged 40 and older receiving a mammogram within the preceding two years.[8]

Table 10.5
Stage at Diagnosis of Colorectal, Breast, Prostate, and Cervical Cancer, by Race and Ethnicity, 1996–2000

	Localized		Regional		Distant	
	Rate	**%**	**Rate**	**%**	**Rate**	**%**
Colorectal						
White	21.4	42	19.7	39	9.6	19
African American	22.4	39	21.0	36	14.2	25
Hispanic/Latino	14.6	39	14.4	39	7.9	22
American Indian and Alaska Native	11.8	35	13.2	40	8.5	25
Asian American and Pacific Islander	18.9	42	17.9	40	7.7	18
Breast (female)						
White	90.2	66	39.8	29	7.5	5
African American	65.6	55	40.6	36	10.6	9
Hispanic/Latino	50.7	57	29.2	35	6.2	7
American Indian and Alaska Native	32.4	56	19.9	36	4.8	8
Asian American and Pacific Islander	63.1	65	28.2	30	4.3	5
Prostate*						
White	145.2	95			8.2	5
African American	225.9	93			20.0	7
Hispanic/Latino	112.1	93			9.7	7
American Indian and Alaska Native	42.6	88			7.2	12
Asian American and Pacific Islander	84.9	92			8.0	8
Uterine cervix						
White	5.0	58	2.9	33	0.8	9
African American	5.5	51	4.4	39	1.2	10
Hispanic/Latino	8.1	57	5.8	34	1.6	9
American Indian and Alaska Native	3.3	57	2.5	36	0.5	7
Asian American and Pacific Islander	5.0	54	3.8	38	0.9	8

Note: Rates are per 100,000, age-adjusted to the 2000 U.S. population. Hispanics/Latinos are not mutually exclusive from whites, African Americans, Asian Americans and Pacific Islanders, and American Indians and Alaska Natives.

*The rate and percentage for localized stage represent local and regional stages combined.

Source: Ries, L. A. G., M. P. Eisner, C. L. Kosary, et al., eds. (2003). *SEER Cancer Statistics Review, 1975–2000.* Bethesda, MD: National Cancer Institute.

BOX
10.1

HEALTHY PEOPLE 2010: OBJECTIVE

Objective 3.13: Increase the proportion of women aged 40 years and older who have received a mammogram within the preceding two years.

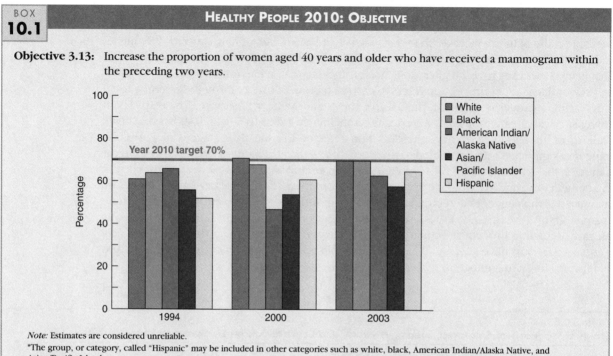

Note: Estimates are considered unreliable.

*The group, or category, called "Hispanic" may be included in other categories such as white, black, American Indian/Alaska Native, and Asian/Pacific Islander.

Source: National Center for Health Statistics. National Health Interview Survey in *Health, United States, 2005 with Chartbook on Trends in the Health of Americans.*

For Further Thought

Research indicates that mortality due to breast cancer can be reduced through the use of mammography. Data for 2003 show that 70% of white and black women received mammograms, whereas American Indian/ Alaska Native, Asian/Pacific Islander, and Hispanic women were less likely to have had a mammogram. What type of program could be implemented to further increase the percentage of these minority women who participate in mammograms?

Cardiovascular Diseases

Cardiovascular disease (CVD), primarily in the form of coronary heart disease and stroke, kills more Americans annually than any other disease. In fact, CVD claims more lives each year than the next five leading causes of death combined. Death rates from coronary heart disease and stroke vary widely among racial and ethnic groups (see Figures 10.11 and 10.12). Black Americans suffer disproportionately higher rates of death from coronary heart disease and stroke than other racial and ethnic groups.

One of the major modifiable risk factors for coronary artery disease and stroke is hypertension.

One in five Americans aged 60 and older suffers from hypertension. The prevalence of hypertension varies noticeably according to race/ethnicity, with the highest prevalence among black Americans (see Figure 10.13).[46] In addition, black Americans tend to develop hypertension earlier in life than whites. The reasons for this are unknown. In fact, the cause of 90% to 95% of the cases of hypertension in all races and ethnic groups is unknown. Therefore, secondary prevention or screening for hypertension is essential. Hypertension is easily detected and normally controllable. However, because hypertension presents no symptoms, approximately one-third of people with high blood pressure do not know they have it.

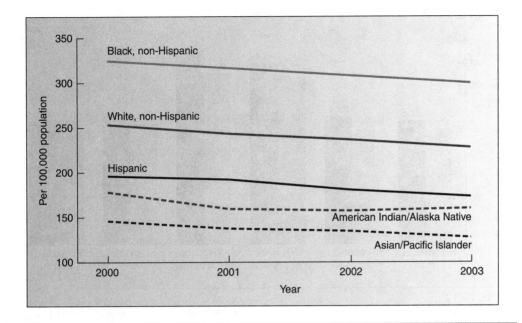

FIGURE 10.11

Death rates for diseases of the heart (age adjusted to the year 2000 standard population).

Source: CDC, NCHS, National Vital Statistics System.

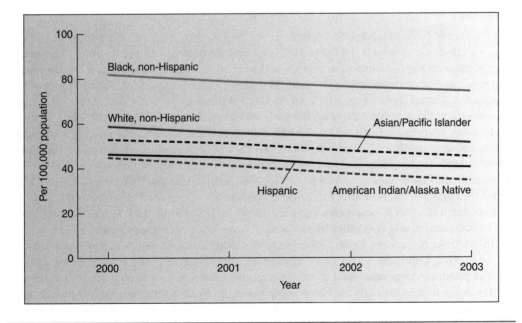

FIGURE 10.12

Death rates for cerebrovascular diseases (age adjusted to the year 2000 standard population).

Source: CDC, NCHS, National Vital Statistics System.

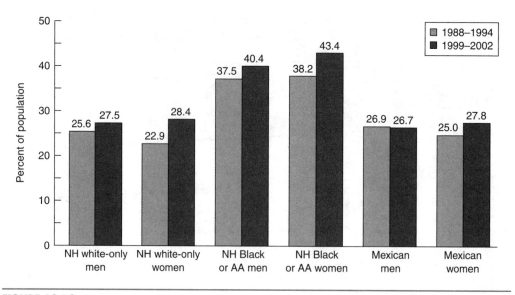

FIGURE 10.13

Prevalence of hypertension among adults aged 20 and older by race/ethnicity and gender in the United States, 1988–1994 and 1999–2002.

Note: NH = non-Hispanic; AA = Asian American.

Source: Centers for Disease Control and Prevention, National Center for Health Statistics (2005). *Health, United States, 2004, with Chartbook on Trends in the Health of Americans.* Washington, DC: U.S. Government Printing Office.

Diabetes

Approximately 9.6% of adults 20 years or older population (21.6 million people) have diabetes—a condition in which the body does not produce or properly use insulin.[47] The prevalence of diabetes has risen in recent years, and this trend is projected to continue. Furthermore, the prevalence of diabetes in people aged 20 years or older is varied in minority groups. Hispanics are 1.7 times more likely, black Americans 1.8 times more likely, and American Indians 2.2 times more likely to have diabetes than whites of similar age (see Figure 10.14).

In 2003, diabetes contributed to 78,815 deaths in the United States, making it the sixth leading cause of death in the United States.[48] Furthermore, the adjusted death rate for deaths related to diabetes has increased by approximately 40% in the last two decades. This increase in age-adjusted death rates occurred in all racial and ethnic groups. However, diabetes death rates do vary considerably among racial and ethnic groups. Compared to white non-Hispanics, diabetes death rates were nearly two and a half times higher among black Americans and American Indians, and nearly two times higher among Americans of Hispanic origin.[47]

In addition to causing death, other serious complications from diabetes include heart disease, stroke, blindness, and kidney disease. In fact, diabetes is the leading cause of new cases of blindness in people aged 20 to 74, and the leading cause of end-stage renal disease (ESRD), accounting for nearly half of all new cases. In 2002, a total of 153,730 people with ESRD due to diabetes were living on chronic dialysis or with a kidney transplant.[47] Between 1984 and 2002, ESRD attributable to diabetes was greatest among black men and women and lowest among white women (see Figure 10.15). Inpatient hospitalization care is one of the most expensive venues for diabetes care. Hospital admissions for long-term care of diabetes are highest among black Americans and Hispanics.

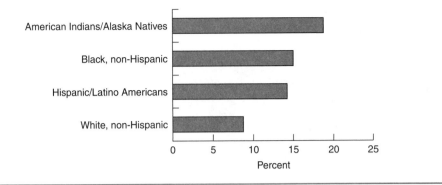

FIGURE 10.14

Age-adjusted total prevalence of diabetes in people aged 20 years or older, by race/ethnicity: United States, 2005.

Source: National Diabetes Information Clearinghouse (2007). *National Diabetes Statistics.* Available at http://diabetes.niddk.nih .gov/dm/pubs/statistics/index.htm.

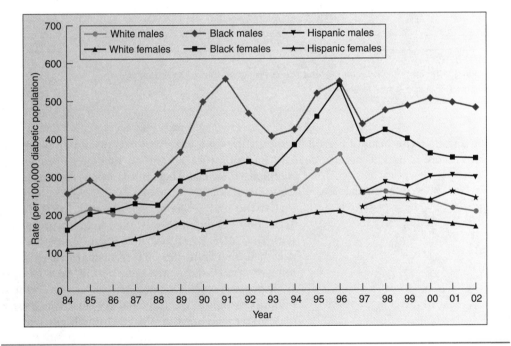

FIGURE 10.15

Age-adjusted incidence of end-stage renal disease related to diabetes per 100,000 diabetic population, by race, ethnicity, and sex: United States, 1984 to 2002.

Source: Centers for Disease Control and Prevention, National Diabetes Surveillance System. "Data and Trends: End-Stage Renal Disease." Available at http://www.cdc.gov/diabetes/statistics/esrd/Fig5.htm.

HIV Infection/AIDS

AIDS stands for *acquired immune deficiency syndrome*, a disorder first documented in the United States in 1981, through which the body's immune system is impaired to varying degrees. The cause of AIDS is a virus known as human immunodeficiency virus, or HIV. An HIV infection is a chronic condition that progressively damages the body's immune system,

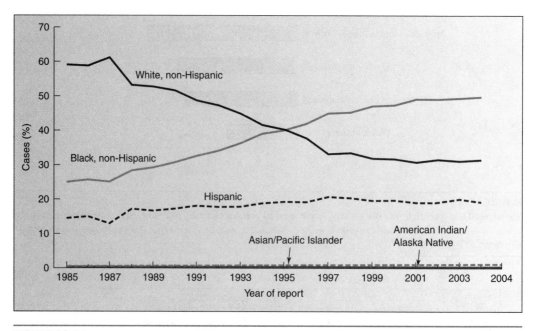

FIGURE 10.16

Proportion of AIDS cases, by race/ethnicity and year of diagnosis, 1985 to 2004, United States.

Source: Centers for Disease Control and Prevention.

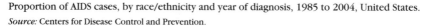

FIGURE 10.17

Race/ethnicity of persons (including children) with HIV/AIDS diagnosed during 2004.

Note: Based on data from 35 areas with long-term, confidential, name-based HIV reporting.

Source: Centers for Disease Control and Prevention (April 2006). "A Glance at the HIV/AIDS Epidemic [Fact sheet]." Available at http://www.cdc.gov/hiv/resources/factsheets/At-A-Glance.htm.

making an otherwise healthy person less able to resist a variety of infections and disorders. Presently, there is no known cure for HIV infection or AIDS and no vaccine to prevent it. Additionally, no major cure breakthroughs are expected for years to come.

At the end of 2003, an estimated 1,039,000 to 1,185,000 persons in the United States were living with HIV/AIDS.[48] An estimated 529,113 people of all ages had died from the opportunistic diseases stemming from AIDS during the same period. AIDS has had a disproportionate impact on racial and ethnic minority groups in the United States since the disease was first recognized in 1981. Through the end of 2004, well over half of all identified cases since 1981 were reported among racial and ethnic groups. In fact, the proportional distribution of AIDS cases among racial and ethnic groups has shifted since the beginning of the epidemic (see Figure 10.16). The proportion of cases has increased among black Americans and Hispanics and decreased among whites. In 2004, black Americans and Hispanics, who represented less than half of the population, accounted for more than one-half of the estimated number of HIV/AIDS cases diagnosed (see Figure 10.17). Consistent with the AIDS case rates are higher AIDS death rates for black Americans and Hispanics.[49]

Part of the reason for the disproportionate numbers of HIV and AIDS cases in black Americans and Americans of Hispanic origin has been attributed to a higher prevalence of unsafe or risky health behaviors (e.g., unprotected sexual intercourse and intravenous drug use), existing co-conditions (e.g., genital ulcer disease), and the lack of access to health care that would provide early diagnosis and treatment. A prevailing barrier to HIV/AIDS prevention may be that this condition is not being viewed as among the highest priorities in some minority communities when compared with other life survival problems.[50] With no cure for HIV/AIDS in sight, better health education to reduce and eliminate unsafe behaviors and increased access to medical resources for existing cases are essential to prevention.

Child and Adult Immunization Rates

As a result of widespread immunization practices, many infectious diseases that were once common have been significantly reduced. Childhood immunization rates provide one measure of the extent to which children are protected from dangerous vaccine-preventable illnesses. An important immunization rate for children aged 19 to 35 months is the 4:3:1:3:3:1 vaccine series that includes DTP/DT/DTaP; poliovirus vaccine; measles, mumps, and rubella vaccine (MMR); *Haemophilus influenzae* type b vaccine; hepatitis B vaccine; and varicella vaccine. In 2005, coverage estimates for the 4:3:1:3:3:1 vaccine series did not vary significantly by race or ethnicity among children aged 19 to 35 months, ranging from 79.5% for children of multiple races to 77.1% for Asians, 76.3% for blacks, 76.0% for whites, and 75.6% for Hispanics.[51] During 2002 to 2004, coverage for the 4:3:1:3:3:1 vaccine series was lower among black compared with white children (see Figure 10.18). The overall rise must continue in order to achieve the *Healthy People 2010* target of 90% coverage for all recommended childhood immunizations in all populations.[8]

Immunization does not end with childhood. It is important for adults, especially those 65 years and older, to become immunized against certain infectious diseases that can cause illness, disability, or death. Figure 10.19 shows the 2006–2007 adult immunization schedule

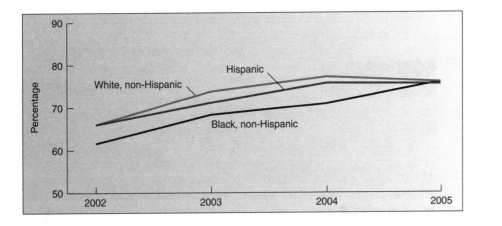

FIGURE 10.18

Vaccination coverage with four or more diphtheria-tetanus-pertussis doses (DTP/DT).

Note: The 4:3:1:3:3:1 vaccine series consists of four or more doses of diphtheria and tetanus toxoids and pertussis vaccines, diphtheria and tetanus toxoids vaccine, or diphtheria and tetanus toxoids vaccine and any acellular pertussis vaccine (DTP/DT/DTaP); three or more doses of poliovirus vaccine; one or more dose of measles, mumps, and rubella (MMR) vaccine; three or more doses of *Haemophilus influenzae* type b vaccine; three or more doses of hepatitis B vaccine; and one or more dose of varicella vaccine.

Source: Centers for Disease Control and Prevention (2006). "National, State, and Urban Area Vaccination Coverage among Children Aged 19 to 35 Months—United States, 2005." *Morbidity and Mortality Weekly Report*, 55(36): 988–993.

Vaccine	Age group		
	19–49 years	50–64 years	≥ 65 years
Tetanus, diphtheria, pertussis (Td/Tdap)	1-dose Td booster every 10 yrs		
	Substitute 1 dose of Tdap for Td		
Human papillomavirus (HPV)	3 doses (females)		
Measles, mumps, rubella (MMR)	1 or 2 doses	1 dose	
Varicella	2 doses (0, 4–8 wks)	2 doses (0, 4–8 wks)	
Influenza	1 dose annually	1 dose annually	
Pneumococcal (polysaccharide)	1–2 doses		1 dose
Hepatitis A	2 doses (0, 6–12 mos, or 0, 6–18 mos)		
Hepatitis B	3 doses (0, 1–2, 4–6 mos)		
Meningococcal	1 or more doses		

Vaccine	Indication							
	Pregnancy	Congenital immuno-deficiency, leukemia, lymphoma, generalized malignancy, cerebrospinal fluid leaks, therapy with alkylating agents, anti-metabolites, radiation, or high-dose, long-term corticosteroids	Diabetes, heart disease, chronic pulmonary disease, chronic alcoholism	Asplenia (including elective splenectomy and terminal complement component deficiencies)	Chronic liver disease, recipients of clotting factor concentrates	Kidney failure, end-stage renal disease, recipients of hemodialysis	Human immuno-deficiency virus (HIV) infection	Health care workers
Tetanus, diphtheria, pertussis (Td/Tdap)	1-dose Td booster every 10 yrs							
	Substitute 1 dose of Tdap for Td							
Human papillomavirus (HPV)	3 doses for women through age 26 yrs (0, 2, 6 mos)							
Measles, mumps, rubella (MMR)			1 or 2 doses					
Varicella			2 doses (0, 4–8 wks)					2 doses
Influenza	1 dose annually		1 dose annually	1 dose annually				
Pneumococcal (polysaccharide)	1–2 doses	1–2 doses						1–2 doses
Hepatitis A	2 doses (0, 6–12 mos, or 0, 6–18 mos)				2 doses (0, 6–12 mos, or 0, 6–18 mos)			
Hepatitis B	3 doses (0, 1–2, 4–6 mos)				3 doses (0, 1–2, 4–6 mos)			
Meningococcal	1 dose		1 dose		1 dose			

For all persons in this category who meet the age requirements and who lack evidence of immunity (e.g., lack documentation of vaccination or have no evidence of prior infection)

Recommended if some other risk factor is present (e.g., on the basis of medical, occupational, lifestyle, or other indications)

Contraindicated

FIGURE 10.19

Recommended adult immunization schedule, United States, 2006-2007, by age group and medical condition.

Source: Centers for Disease Control and Prevention.

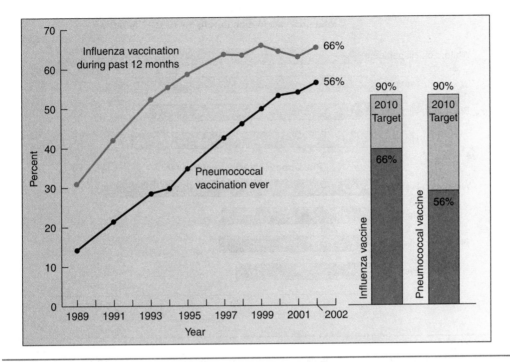

FIGURE 10.20

Influenza and pneumococcal vaccination among adults 65 years of age and over: United States, 1989 to 2002.

Note: Data are for the civilian noninstitutionalized population and are age adjusted.

Source: Centers for Disease Control and Prevention, National Center for Health Statistics, National Health Interview Survey.

recommended by the CDC's National Immunization Program. Two important adult immunizations included on the schedule, as well as among the infectious disease objectives stated in *Healthy People 2010,* are immunizations for influenza and pneumoccocal diseases.[8] The goal is to increase the number of noninstitutionalized adults 65 and older who are immunized annually against influenza and who have ever received an immunization against pneumoccocal disease to 90% (see Figure 10.20). Increased immunization rates of influenza and pneumoccocal diseases would significantly lower the number of infectious deaths caused in elders. Annually an estimated 40,000 adults over 65 die from influenza and pneumoccocal infections, making it the fifth leading cause of death among the elder population.[48] Immunization rates among minorities for influenza and pneumococcal infections are substantially lower than for white Americans (see Figure 10.21).[52] Therefore, even though these two immunization rates among all adults have shown a significant increase since 1989, in order to reach the goal of 90% by 2010, increased efforts must be focused on minority populations.[8]

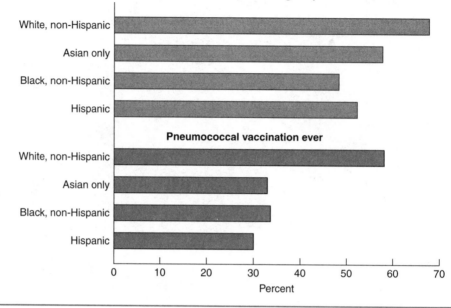

FIGURE 10.21
Influenza and pneumococcal vaccination among adults 65 years of age and over, by race and Hispanic origin: United States, 2000 to 2002.

Source: Fried, V. M., K. Prager, A. P. MacKay, and H. Xia (2004). *Chartbook on Trends in the Health of Americans: Health, United States, 2004.* Hyattsville, MD: National Center for Health Statistics.

SOCIOECONOMIC STATUS AND RACIAL AND ETHNIC DISPARITIES IN HEALTH

socioeconomic status
relating to a combination of social and economic factors

Preceding our discussion of the *Race and Health Initiative,* we acknowledged that disparities exist in many other areas of minority health. However, we limited our focus to the six health areas identified in the initiative. In like manner, there are many factors that contribute to these disparities. These include economics, education, and behavioral factors—such as lifestyle and health practices—as well as cultural, legal, and political factors (see Figure 10.22). We will focus our discussion on **socioeconomic status**, which has been considered the most influential single contributor to premature morbidity and mortality by many public health researchers.[13] However, it is important to emphasize that the association between SES and race and ethnicity is complicated and cannot fully explain all disparities in health status. Furthermore, many of these factors are not always direct in nature—they are what are referred to as *indirect causal associations* or *intermediary factors.* For example, poverty by itself may not cause disease and death; however, by precluding adequate nutrition, preventive medical care, and housing, it leads to increased morbidity and premature mortality.

As we stated earlier, the categories of race are more of a social category than a biological one. Racial disparities in health generally do not reflect biologically determined differences.[13] In fact, biological differences between racial groups are small compared with biological differences within groups.[53] More than 90% of the differences in genetic makeup occur within racial and ethnic groups rather than between the groups. Such disparities in health status among minority groups are much better understood in terms of the groups' living circumstances.[54] A group's living circumstances may be referred to as its socioeconomic status (SES). Common SES factors studied include level of education, level of income, and poverty.

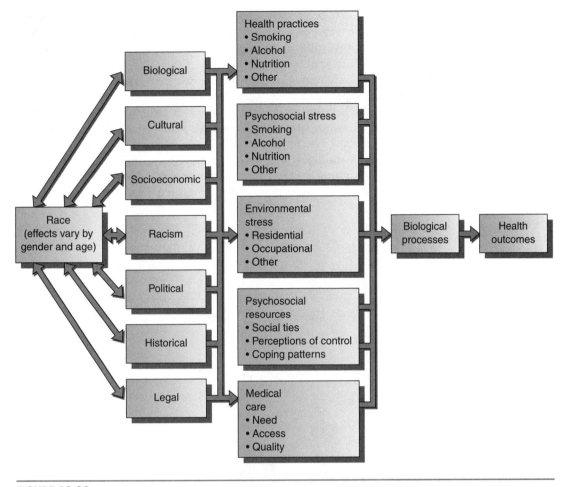

FIGURE 10.22

A framework for understanding the relationship between race and health.

Source: Williams, D. R. (1993). "Race in the Health of America: Problems, Issues and Directions," *MMWR,* 42(RR-10): 9.

Public health research has long studied SES factors and their relationship to health. These studies have shown that better health is associated with more years of education and having more income, a more prestigious job, and living in superior neighborhoods. Similarly, elevated levels of morbidity, disability, and mortality are associated with less education, lower income, poverty, unemployment, and poor housing. An extensive amount of research documents that SES factors play a significant role in the association of race and ethnicity with health.[8] Furthermore, research in the last couple of decades indicates that the relationship between SES and health occurs at every socioeconomic level and for a broad range of SES indicators.[55] This relationship between SES and health can be described as a gradient. For example, research has documented that the more family income increases above the poverty threshold, the more health improves, and that the greater the gap in income, the greater the gap in health.

This gradient effect between SES and health has important implications that are related to the gap between the privileged and nonprivileged, or the "haves and have-nots." In the United States, many inequalities still exist between all racial and ethnic groups related to level of education, income, and poverty (see Figures 10.5, 10.6, and 10.7). Minority groups often occupy the lowest socioeconomic rankings in the United States. These low rankings become a significant community health concern when one recognizes that progress toward the *Healthy*

People 2000 objectives was found to be greatest among higher SES groups and least among the lower SES groups.[5] Next, we will concentrate on the overlap between race, ethnicity, and SES by illustrating a few examples of health disparities across various levels of education and income within racial and ethnic groups.

Level of education is an important indicator related to health status because it appears to lead to better health indirectly—presumably because it increases knowledge about health and the beliefs that develop and assert health-promoting behaviors to maintain health and participate in prevention activities.[8] Two important health indices related to reducing infant morbidity and mortality include prenatal care for pregnant women and avoiding cigarette smoking if pregnant (see Chapter 7). As shown in Figures 10.23 and 10.24, level of education is a strong indicator of use of early prenatal care and cigarette smoking during pregnancy. The more educated mothers are, the more likely they are to receive prenatal care in every race and

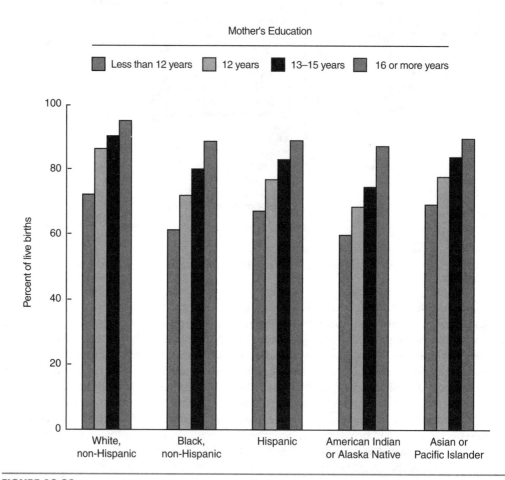

FIGURE 10.23

Prenatal care use in the first trimester among mothers 20 years of age and over by mother's education, race, and Hispanic origin in the United States, 1996.

Source: Pamuk, E., D. Makuc, K. Heck, C. Reuben, and K. Lochner (1998). *Socioeconomic Status and Health Chartbook, Health, United States, 1998* (HHS pub. no. PHS 98-1232). Hyattsville, MD: National Center for Health Statistics.

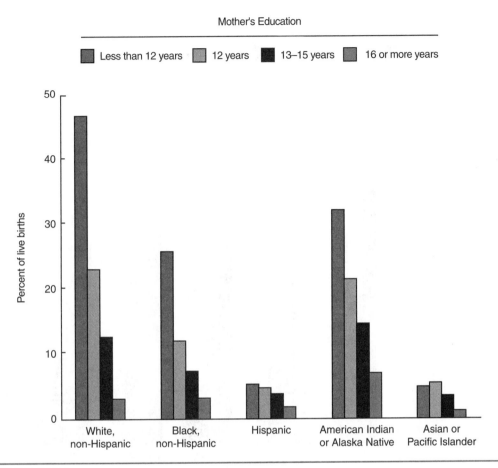

FIGURE 10.24

Cigarette smoking during pregnancy among mothers 20 years of age and over by mother's education, race, and Hispanic origin in the United States, 1996.

Source: Pamuk, E., D. Makuc, K. Heck, C. Reuben, and K. Lochner (1998). *Socioeconomic Status and Health Chartbook, Health, United States, 1998* (HHS pub. no. PHS 98-1232). Hyattsville, MD: National Center for Health Statistics.

ethnic group. Likewise, the more educated a woman is, the less likely she is to smoke during pregnancy.[56]

A number of studies have demonstrated that self-assessed health can be a valid and reliable index of a person's overall health.[57] Respondents are asked to assess their general health by selecting "excellent," "very good," "good," "fair," or "poor." Figure 10.25 demonstrates that there is a strong SES gradient among white Americans, non-Hispanic black Americans, and Americans of Hispanic origin. The poorer people are, the more likely they are to assess their health status as poor. Similarly, the poorer people are, the less likely they are to have health insurance coverage (see Figure 10.26) and the less likely they are to have physician contact (see Figure 10.27).

These examples of SES disadvantage contribute to a better understanding of racial and ethnic health disparities and provide direction toward possible intervention strategies that may help narrow the differences. Ultimately, closing the gaps between racial and ethnic minority health disparities will require altering socioeconomic conditions.[58]

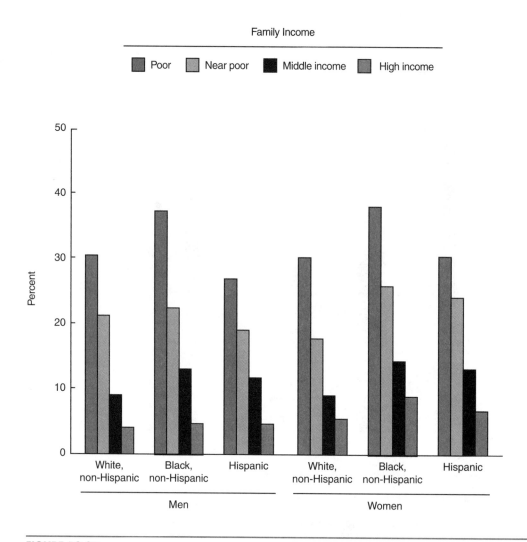

FIGURE 10.25

Fair or poor health among adults 18 years of age and over by family income, race, and Hispanic origin in the United States, 1995.

Source: Pamuk, E., D. Makuc, K. Heck, C. Reuben, and K. Lochner (1998). *Socioeconomic Status and Health Chartbook, Health, United States, 1998* (HHS pub. no. PHS 98-1232). Hyattsville, Maryland: National Center for Health Statistics.

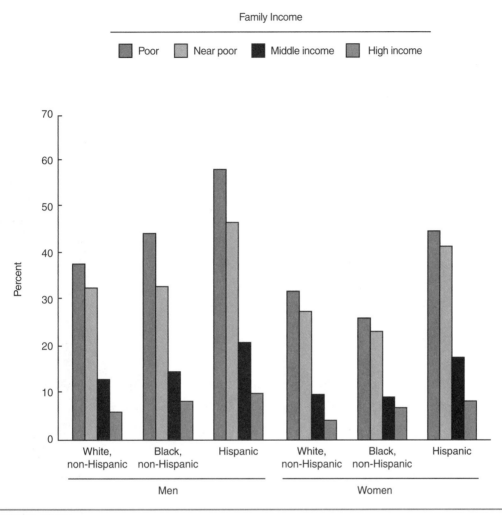

FIGURE 10.26

No health insurance coverage among persons 18 to 64 years of age by family income, race, and Hispanic origin in the United States, average annual 1994–1995.

Source: Pamuk, E., D. Makuc, K. Heck, C. Reuben, and K. Lochner (1998). *Socioeconomic Status and Health Chartbook, Health, United States, 1998* (HHS pub. no. PHS 98-1232). Hyattsville, Maryland: National Center for Health Statistics.

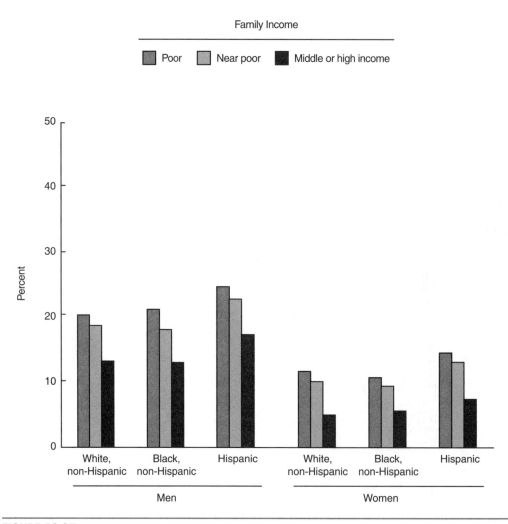

FIGURE 10.27

No physician contact within the past year among adults 18 to 64 years of age by family income, race, and Hispanic origin in the United States, average annual 1994–1995.

Source: Pamuk, E., D. Makuc, K. Heck, C. Reuben, and K. Lochner (1998). *Socioeconomic Status and Health Chartbook, Health, United States, 1998* (HHS pub. no. PHS 98-1232). Hyattsville, Maryland: National Center for Health Statistics.

EQUITY IN MINORITY HEALTH

One of the primary aims of the *Race and Health Initiative* consists of consultation and collaboration among federal agencies; state, local, and tribal governments; and community professionals to research and address issues of education, income, environment, and other socioeconomic factors that affect health outcomes. We know that many health problems faced by minorities are attributable not to race or ethnic origin but to social or economic conditions or disenfranchisement. These health problems are inseparable from a variety of other social problems, making simple solutions unlikely. We also know that multiple resources will be required to resolve these social and economic problems, and that solutions to these problems for one group may not work for another. Americans of Hispanic origin, Asian Americans, Pacific Islanders, black Americans, and Native Americans each have unique cultural traditions that must be respected if the solutions are to be successful. In other words, we must operationally integrate an understanding of the culture of the target population; solutions must be *culturally sensitive.* In a more general sense, significant strides in the improvement of health in minority groups can be achieved if community health professionals become more culturally competent and are able to empower local communities.

Cultural Competence

In this chapter's introduction, we stated that the strength and greatness of America lies in the diversity of its people and their cultures. However, cultural differences can and do present major obstacles to implementing effective community health programs and services. The demographic shifts in minority populations and the resulting diversity in health providers treating more patients has increased interest among health professionals to increase culturally appropriate services that lead to improved outcomes, efficiency, and satisfaction for their clients.[59] This increased interest is not only being found among health care providers but also among patients, policy makers, educators, and accreditation and credentialing agencies. In March 2001, the HHS and the Office of Minority Health published standards for culturally and linguistically appropriate services (CLAS) in health care (see Box 10.2).[59] These criteria are the first comprehensive and nationally recognized standards of cultural and linguistic competence in health care service delivery that have been developed. In the past, national organizations and federal agencies independently developed their own standards and policies. The result was a wide spectrum of ideas about what constitutes culturally appropriate health services. The CLAS report went further and defined **cultural and linguistic competence** as

> cultural and linguistic competence
> a set of congruent behaviors, attitudes, and policies that come together in a system, agency, or among professionals that enables effective work in cross-cultural situations

> A set of congruent behaviors, attitudes, and policies that come together in a system, agency, or among professionals that enables effective work in cross cultural situations. *Culture* refers to integrated patterns of human behavior that include language, thoughts, communications, actions, customs, beliefs, values, and institutions of racial, ethnic, religious or social groups. *Competence* implies having the capacity to function effectively as an individual and an organization within the context of the cultural beliefs, behaviors, and needs presented by consumers and their communities.[59]

Based on this definition, culture is a vital factor in both how community health professionals deliver services and how community members respond to community health programs and preventive interventions. In a society as culturally diverse as the United States, community health educators need to be able to communicate with different communities and understand how culture influences health behaviors.[60] It is important that community health promotion/disease prevention programs be understandable and acceptable within the cultural framework of the population to be reached. Lee has published the following list of 10 principles related to cultural competency that are considered important for community health practitioners to understand when planning and implementing health promotion/disease prevention programs:[61]

1. Having a self understanding of race, ethnicity, and power
2. Understanding the historical factors that impact the health of minority populations, such as racism and immigration patterns
3. Understanding the particular psycho-social stressors relevant to minority participants (such as socioeconomic status and migration)
4. Understanding the cultural differences within minority groups
5. Understanding the minority client within a family life cycle and in an intergenerational conceptual framework
6. Understanding the differences between the "culturally acceptable" behaviors of psycho-pathological characteristics of different minority groups.

1. Health care organizations should ensure that patients/consumers receive from all staff members effective, understandable, and respectful care that is provided in a manner compatible with their cultural health beliefs and practices and preferred language.

2. Health care organizations should implement strategies to recruit, retain, and promote at all levels of the organization a diverse staff and leadership that are representative of the demographic characteristics of the service area.

3. Health care organizations should ensure that staff at all levels and across all disciplines receive ongoing education and training in culturally and linguistically appropriate service delivery.

4. Health care organizations must offer and provide language assistance services, including bilingual staff and interpreter services, at no cost to each patient/consumer with limited English proficiency at all points of contact, in a timely manner during all hours of operation.

5. Health care organizations must provide to patients/consumers in their preferred language both verbal offers and written notices informing them of their right to receive language assistance services.

6. Health care organizations must assure the competence of language assistance provided to limited English proficient patients/consumers by interpreters and bilingual staff. Family and friends should not be used to provide interpretation services (except on request by the patient/consumer).

7. Health care organizations must make available easily understood patient-related materials and post signage in the languages of the commonly encountered groups and/or groups represented in the service area.

8. Health care organizations should develop, implement, and promote a written strategic plan that outlines clear goals, policies, operational plans, and management accountability/oversight mechanisms to provide culturally and linguistically appropriate services.

9. Health care organizations should conduct initial and ongoing organizational self-assessments of CLAS-related activities and are encouraged to inte-grate cultural and linguistic competence-related measures into their internal audits, performance improvement programs, patient satisfaction assessments, and outcomes-based evaluations.

10. Health care organizations should ensure that data on the individual patient's/consumer's race, ethnicity, and spoken and written language are collected in health records, integrated into the organization's management information systems, and periodically updated.

11. Health care organizations should maintain a current demographic, cultural, and epidemiological profile of the community as well as a needs assessment to accurately plan for and implement services that respond to the cultural and linguistic characteristics of the service area.

12. Health care organizations should develop participatory, collaborative partnerships with communities and utilize a variety of formal and informal mechanisms to facilitate community and patient/consumer involvement in designing and implementing CLAS-related activities.

13. Health care organizations should ensure that conflict and grievance resolution processes are culturally and linguistically sensitive and capable of identifying, preventing, and resolving cross-cultural conflicts or complaints by patients/consumers.

14. Health care organizations are encouraged to regularly make available to the public information about their progress and successful innovations in implementing the CLAS standards and to provide public notice in their communities about the availability of this information.

Note: The standards are organized by three themes.
 1. Culturally competent care (Standards 1–3)
 2. Language access services (Standards 4–7)
 3. Organizational supports for cultural competence (Standards 8–14)

Source: U.S. Department of Health and Human Services, Office of Minority Health (2001). *National Standards for Culturally and Linguistically Appropriate Services in Health Care: Final Report.* Washington, DC: Author.

7. Understanding the indigenous healing practices and the role of religion in the treatment of minority patients
8. Understanding the cultural beliefs of health and help seeking patterns of minority individuals
9. Understanding the health service resources for minority patients
10. Understanding the public health policies and its impact on minorities and communities

For community health educators whose role it is to educate groups and communities of diverse cultural backgrounds, cultural competence is critical (see Appendix 4). Additionally, successful community health intervention and educational activities should be firmly grounded in an understanding and appreciation of the cultural characteristics of the target group. *Healthy People 2010* is firmly devoted to the principle that "every person in every community across the Nation deserves equal access to comprehensive, culturally competent, community-based health care systems that are committed to serving the needs of the individual and promoting community health."[8]

Empowering the Self and the Community

Another principle deeply etched in *Healthy People 2010* with respect to achieving equity is the ideal that the "greatest opportunities for reducing health disparities are in *empowering* individuals to make informed health care decisions and in promoting community-wide safety, education, and access to health care."[8] One reason why minority groups lack the resources to eliminate community health problems is their lack of empowerment. To *empower* means to give power or authority; to enable or permit. With reference to our discussion, it means to enable people to work to solve their community health problems. Simply put, to acquire better health and health care services, a community must be empowered to do so.

Friedman identified three kinds of power associated with empowerment—social, political, and psychological.[62] An increase in social power brings with it access to "bases" of production such as information, knowledge and skills, participation in social organizations, and financial resources. Increased productivity enables greater influence on markets, which in turn can influence change.

A social power-base is needed to gain political power. Political power is more than just being able to vote; it is also the power of voice and of collective action. In a democracy, seldom does a single voice effect change; it is the collective voice that can make things happen. The early labor movement in this country that led to the establishment of unions is a good example.

Psychological power is best described as an individual sense of potency demonstrated in self-confident behavior. It is often the result of successful action in the social and political domains. With the investiture of all three types of power, empowerment can take place. Empowerment replaces hopelessness with a sense of being in control and a sense that one can make a difference. Once people are empowered, the power then needs to be transferred to the communities. When communities are empowered, they can cause change and solve problems. See Chapter 5 for a discussion of community organization as a means of empowering a community.

The process of empowerment may seem abstract because of the theoretical concepts that are involved, but it is not. Follow the process in this example. A group of people, a community, lacks access to the appropriate health care. For this group to be empowered, they must build a foundation with social power. To do this, the group must gain access to the bases of production. They must acquire information about available health care programs and obtain the knowledge and skills to access care. Some in the group need to become members of social organizations that are concerned with health care (such as health departments or voluntary agencies), and the group has to obtain the necessary financial resources to enable them to be noticed in the marketplace as a consumer group. To gain such social power, it is imperative that the group be literate and have the appropriate education. Many groups never gain social power because they do not possess the education to access the bases of production.

When the group has attained social power, a subgroup is able to work toward political power. The subgroup can be heard in the marketplace with its vote and voice. Members of this subgroup can organize to present a united front for collective action. Minority groups have the potential to have a loud voice if united. Once united, they are in a position to influence decision makers at various governmental levels. In the specific case in which the goal is greater access to health care, this could mean getting the local health department to expand the types and numbers of available clinics.

Increased political power can lead to psychological power. Such power would give this particular group the confidence that the expansion of health department clinics is just the first of many achievements. Therefore, through this same process, other community improvements also can be made.

CHAPTER SUMMARY

- One of the great strengths of the United States has been, and remains, the diversity of its people.
- The federal government has recently categorized the U.S. population into five racial groups (American Indian or Alaska Native, Asian, black or African American, Native Hawaiian or Other Pacific Islander, and white) and two ethnic groups (Hispanic or Latino and non-Hispanic or Latino).
- The reporting of accurate and complete race and ethnicity data provides essential information to target and evaluate public health inventions aimed at minority populations.
- All cultural and ethnic groups hold concepts related to health and illness and associated practices for maintaining well-being or providing treatment when it is indicated.
- The *Race and Health Initiative* includes six priority areas: (1) infant mortality, (2) cancer screening and management, (3) cardiovascular disease, (4) diabetes, (5) HIV/AIDS, and (6) adult and child immunization. These key areas are representative of the larger minority health picture and account for a substantial burden of disease that is highly modifiable if the appropriate interventions are applied.
- Socioeconomic status (SES) has been considered the most influential single contributor to premature morbidity and mortality by many public health researchers. Research in the last couple of decades indicates that the relationship between SES and health occurs at every socioeconomic level and for a broad range of SES indicators. This relationship between SES and health can be described as a gradient.
- Significant strides in the improvement of health in minority groups can be achieved if community health professionals become more culturally sensitive and competent.

- Minority groups must be empowered to solve their own problems through the processes of social, political, and psychological empowerment.

REVIEW QUESTIONS

1. Why is it said that the United States was built on diversity?
2. What is the Office of Management and Budget's Directive 15?
3. Why is it important for community health workers to be aware of the significant health disparities among various minority groups in the United States?
4. What were the significant findings of the 1985 landmark report *The Secretary's Task Force Report on Black and Minority Health?*
5. List and explain the six priorities areas in the *Race and Health Initiative.*
6. What role does socioeconomic status play in health disparities among racial and ethnic minority groups?
7. Why is it important for community health professionals and workers to be culturally sensitive and competent?
8. List each of the three kinds of power associated with empowerment. What is the importance of each in empowering individuals and communities?

ACTIVITIES

1. Using the most recent census report (available in your library or on the Web), create a demographic profile of the state and county in which you live. Locate the following information—population; racial/ethnic composition; percentage of people represented by the different age groups, gender breakdown, and marital status; and percentage of people living in poverty.
2. Make an appointment with an employee of the health department in your hometown. Find out the differences

in health status between the racial/ethnic groups in the community by obtaining the race/ethnicity-specific morbidity and mortality data. Discuss these differences with the health department employee, then summarize your findings in a one-page paper.

3. In a two- to three-page paper, present the proposal you would recommend to the President of the United States for closing the health status gap between the races and ethnic groups.

4. Identify a specific racial/ethnic minority group and select a health problem. Study the topic and present in a three-page paper the present status of the problem, the future outlook for the problem, and what could be done to reduce or eliminate the problem.

5. Write a two-page position paper on "Why racial/ethnic minority groups have a lower health status than the majority white Americans."

COMMUNITY HEALTH ON THE WEB

The Internet contains a wealth of information about community and public health. Increase your knowledge of some of the topics presented in this chapter by accessing the Jones and Bartlett Publishers Web site at **http://health.jbpub.com/book/communityhealth/6e** and follow the links to complete the following Web activities.

• Office of Minority Health

• Eliminating Racial and Ethnic Disparities in Health

• Indian Health Service

REFERENCES

1. The White House (1999). Available at http://www.whitehouse.gov/Initiatives/OneAmerica/america.html.

2. U.S. Census Bureau, Population Division (2004). *U.S. Interim Projections by Age, Sex, Race, and Hispanic Origin*. Available at http://www.census.gov/ipc/www/usinterimproj/.

3. Centers for Disease Control and Prevention (1997). *Minority Health Is the Health of the Nation*. Washington, DC: U.S. Government Printing Office.

4. U.S. Department of Health and Human Services (1988). *Report of the Secretary's Task Force on Black and Minority Health*. Washington, DC: Author.

5. U.S. Department of Health and Human Services (1990). *Healthy People 2000: National Health Promotion Disease Prevention Objectives* (HHS pub. no. PHS 90-50212). Washington, DC: U.S. Government Printing Office.

6. Keppel, K. G., J. N. Pearcy, and D. K. Wagener (2002). *Trends in Racial and Ethnic-Specific Rates for the Health Status Indicators: United States 1990-1998* (Healthy People Statistical Notes no. 23). Hyattsville, MD: National Center for Health Statistics.

7. U.S. Department of Health and Human Services (2000). *Race and Health Initiative*. Available at http://raceandhealth.hhs.gov/.

8. U.S. Department of Health and Human Services (2000). *Healthy People 2010: Understanding and Improving Health*, 2nd ed. Washington, DC: U.S. Government Printing Office.

9. Office of Management and Budget (1978). "Directive 15: Race and Ethnic Standards for Federal Statistics and Administrative Reporting." In U.S. Department of Commerce, Office of Federal Statistical Policy and Standards, *Statistical Policy Handbook*. Washington, DC: Author, 37-38.

10. Office of Management and Budget (1997). "Revisions to the Standards for the Classification of Federal Data on Race and Ethnicity." *Federal Register*.

11. Nelson, H., and R. Jurmain (1998). *Introduction to Physical Anthropology*, 4th ed. St. Paul, MN: West Publishing.

12. Williams, D. R., R. Lavizzo-Mourey, and R. C. Warren (1994). "The Concept of Race and Health Status in America." *Public Health Reports*, 109: 26-41.

13. Senior, P. A., and R. Bhopa (1994). "Ethnicity as a Variable in Epidemiological Research." *British Medical Journal*, 309: 327-330.

14. Centers for Disease Control and Prevention (1999). "Reporting Race and Ethnicity Data—National Electronic Telecommunications System for Surveillance, 1994-1997." *Morbidity and Mortality Weekly Report*, 48(15): 305-312.

15. Centers for Disease Control and Prevention (1993). "Use of Race and Ethnicity in Public Health Surveillance: Summary of the CDC/ATSDR Workshop." *Morbidity and Mortality Weekly Report*, 42(10): 1-17.

16. Rosenberg, H. M., J. D. Maurer, and P. D. Sorlie (1999). "Quality of Death Rates by Race and Hispanic Origin: A Summary of Current Research." *Vital Statistics Reports*, 2:128.

17. U.S. Department of Health and Human Services (1999). *Improving the Collection and Use of Racial and Ethnic Data in HHS*. Available at http://aspe.os.dhhs.gov/datacncl/racerpt/.

18. U.S. Census Bureau (2006). *Current Population Survey, October Supplement*. Washington, DC: U.S. Department of Education, National Center for Education Statistics.

19. U.S. Census Bureau (2005). *Current Population Survey, 1989-2000*, and annual *Social and Economic Supplements*, 2000 to 2004. Washington, DC: U.S. Government Printing Office.

SCENARIO: ANALYSIS AND RESPONSE

1. Do you agree with Tom when he says the United States is more culturally diverse than at any time in the past? Why or why not? Do you see this as a strength or weakness for the country?

2. What signs are there in your community that the United States is becoming more internationalized and that minority groups are growing?

3. What strengths do you see as a result of an increasingly diverse population in the United States? What weaknesses?

4. Do you agree with the major health priorities as outlined in the *Race and Health Initiative* regarding the community you live in? Why or why not?

20. U.S. Census Bureau (2006). *Current Population Survey, 2004–2006*. Annual *Social and Economic Supplements*. Washington, DC. U.S Government Printing Office.

21. Fishman, B., L. Bobo, K. Kosub, and R. Womeodu (1993). "Cultural Issues in Serving Minority Populations: Emphasis on Mexican Americans and African Americans." *American Journal of the Medical Sciences*, 306: 160–166.

22. U.S. Department of Health and Human Services (1993). "Advance Report of Final Mortality Statistics, 1990." *Monthly Vital Statistics Report*, 41(9): 42.

23. Satcher, D., and D. J. Thomas (1990). "Dimensions of Minority Aging: Implications for Curriculum Development for Selected Health Professions." In M. S. Harper, ed., *Minority Aging: Essential Curricula Content for Selected Health and Allied Health Professions* (HHS pub. no. HRS-P-DV 90-4). Washington, DC: U.S. Government Printing Office, 23–32.

24. Airhihenbuwa, C. O., and I. E. Harrison (1993). "Traditional Medicine in Africa: Past, Present and Future." In P. Conrad and E. Gallagher, eds., *Healing and Health Care in Developing Countries*. Philadelphia: Temple University Press.

25. President's Advisory Commission on Asian Americans and Pacific Islanders (2001). *A People Looking Forward: Action for Access and Partnerships in the 21st Century*. Interim Report to the President. Available at http://www.aapi/gov/intreport.htm.

26. President's Advisory Commission on Asian Americans and Pacific Islanders (2003). *Asian Americans and Pacific Islanders Addressing Health Disparities: Opportunities for Building a Healthier America*. Available at http://www.aapi.gov/Commission_Final_Health_Report.pdf.

27. Ghosh, C. (2003). "Healthy People 2010 and Asian Americans/Pacific Islanders: Defining a Baseline of Information." *American Journal of Public Health*, 93: 2093–2098.

28. Mayeno, L., and S. M. Hirota (1994). "Access to Health Care." In N. W. S. Zane, D. T. Takeuchi, and K. N. J. Young, eds., *Confronting Critical Health Issues of Asian and Pacific Islander Americans*. Thousand Oaks, CA: Sage Publications.

29. Yoon, E., and E. Chien (1996). "Asian American and Pacific Islander Health: A Paradigm for Minority Health." *Journal of the American Medical Association*, 275, 736–737.

30. Humes, K., and J. McKinnon (2000). "The Asian and Pacific Islander Population in the United States." In U.S. Census Bureau, *Current Population Reports* (Series P20-529). Washington, DC: U.S. Government Printing Office.

31. Kitano, H. H. L. (1990). "Values, Beliefs, and Practices of Asian-American Elderly: Implications for Geriatric Education." In M. S. Harper, ed., *Minority Aging: Essential Curricula Content for Selected Health and Allied Health Professions* (HHS pub. no. HRS-P-DV 90-4). Washington, DC: U.S. Government Printing Office, 341–348.

32. Frye, B. A. (1995). "Use of Cultural Themes in Promoting Health among Southeast Asian Refugees." *American Journal of Health Promotion*, 9: 269–280.

33. Aiu, P. (June/July, 2000). "Comparing Native Hawaiians' Health to the Nation." *Closing the Gap*, 8–9.

34. Jiang, S. (June/July 2000). "Correcting the Visions of Paradise." *Closing the Gap*, 4.

35. Blaisdell, R. K. (1989). "Historical and Cultural Aspects of Native Hawaiian Health." In E. Wegner, ed., *Social Process in Hawai'i*. Honolulu: University of Hawai'i Press, 32.

36. Garrett, J. T. (1990). "Indian Health: Values, Beliefs and Practices." In M. S. Harper, ed., *Minority Aging: Essential Curricula Content for Selected Health and Allied Health Professionals* (HHS pub. no. HRS-P-DV90-4). Washington, DC: U.S. Government Printing Office, 179–191.

37. U.S. Department of Health and Human Services, Indian Health Services, Program Statistics Team (2000). "Regional Differences in Indian Health 1998–99." Available at http://www.his.gov/publicinfo/publications/trends98/region98.asp.

38. Edwards, E. D., and M. Egbert-Edwards (1990). "Family Care and Native American Elderly." In M. S. Harper, ed., *Minority Aging: Essential Curricula Content for Selected Health and Allied Health Professions* (HHS pub. no. HRS-P-DV90-4). Washington, DC: U.S. Government Printing Office, 145–163.

39. Rhoades, E. R. (1990). "Profile of American Indians and Alaska Natives." In M. S. Harper, ed., *Minority Aging: Essential Curricula Content for Selected Health and Allied Health Professions* (HHS pub. no. HRS-P-DV90-4). Washington, DC: U.S. Government Printing Office, 45–62.

40. U.S. Department of Health and Human Services (1992). *Comprehensive Health Care Program for American Indians and Alaska Natives*. Washington, DC: U.S. Government Printing Office.

41. Uba, L. (1992). "Cultural Barriers to Health Care for Southeast Asian Refugees." *Public Health Reports*, 107(5): 544–548.

42. Sotomayor, M. (1990). "The New Immigrants: The Undocumented and Refugees." In M. S. Harper, ed., *Minority Aging: Essential Curricula Content for Selected Health and Allied Health Professions* (HHS pub. no. HRS-P-DV 90-4). Washington, DC: U.S. Government Printing Office, 627–637.

43. Lewitt, E. M., et al. (Spring 1995). "The Direct Cost of Low Birth Weight." *The Future of Children*, 5(1): 35–56.

44. American Cancer Society (2006). "Cancer Statistics 2006." *CA: A Cancer Journal for Clinicians*, 56: 106–130.

45. Freeman, H. P. (2004). "Poverty, Culture, and Social Injustice: Determinants of Cancer Disparities" *CA: A Cancer Journal for Clinicians*, 54(2): 72–77.

46. U.S. Department of Health and Human Services (2003). *Seventh Report of the Joint National Committee on Prevention, Evaluation, and Treatment of High Blood Pressure* (NIH pub. no. 03-5233). Bethesda, MD: National Institutes of Health.

47. American Diabetes Association (2006). "Diabetes Facts and Figures." Available at http://www.diabetes.org/ada/facts.asp.

48. Centers for Disease Control and Prevention (2006). *HIV/AIDS Surveillance Report*, 17: 1–37.

49. National Center for Health Statistics (2006). "Deaths: Final Data for 2003." *National Vital Statistics Reports*, 54(13): 1–35.

50. U.S. Department of Health and Human Services (1995). *Progress Report for: Black Americans*. Washington, DC: U.S. Government Printing Office.

51. Centers for Disease Control and Prevention (2006). "National, State, and Urban Area Vaccination Coverage among Children Aged 19 to 35 Months—United States, 2005." *Morbidity and Mortality Weekly Report*, 55(36): 988–993.

52. Centers for Disease Control and Prevention (2006). "Influenza and Pneumococcal Vaccination Levels among Persons Aged 65 Years and Older, United States, 2004–2005." *Morbidity and Mortality Weekly Report*, 55(39): 1065–1068.

53. Shiver, M. D. (1997). "Ethnic Variation as a Key to the Biology of Human Disease." *Annals of Internal Medicine*, 127: 401–403.

54. Navarro, V. (1990). "Race or Class Versus Race and Class: Mortality Differentials in the United States" *Lancet*, 336: 1238–1240.

55. Adler, N., and J. Ostrove (2000) "Socioeconomic Status and Health: What We Know and What We Don't." *Annals of the New York Academy of Sciences*, 896: 3–15.

56. Pamuk, E., D. Makuc, K. Heck, C. Reuben, and L. Lochner (1998). *Socioeconomic Status and Health Chartbook, Health, United States, 1998* (HHS pub. no. PHS 98-1232). Hyattsville, MD: National Center for Health Statistics.

57. Idler, E. L., and S. V. Kasl (1995). "Self-Ratings of Health: Do They Also Predict Change in Functional Ability?" *Journal of Gerontology*, 50B(6): S344–S353.

58. Pappas, G. (1994) "Elucidating the Relationships between Race, Socioeconomic Status, and Health." *American Journal of Public Health*, 84(6): 892–893.

59. Office of Minority Health (2000). "Assuring Cultural Competence in Health Care: Recommendations for National Standards and an Out-comes-Focused Research Agenda." Available at http://www.omhrc.gov/inetpub/wwwroot/clas/indexfinal.htm.

60. Loustaunau, M. (2000). "Becoming Culturally Sensitive: Preparing for Service as a Health Educator in a Multicultural World." In S. Smith, ed., *Community Health Perspectives*. Madison, WI: Coursewise Publishing, 33–37.

61. Lee, E. (2000). *Working with Asian Americans*. New York: Guilford Press.

62. Friedmann, J. (1992). *Empowerment: The Politics of Alternative Development*. Cambridge, MA: Blackwell.

Chapter 11

Community Mental Health

Chapter Objectives

After studying this chapter, you will be able to:

1 Define *mental health* and *mental disorders.*

2 Explain what is meant by the *DSM-IV-TR.*

3 Identify the major causes of mental disorders.

4 Explain why mental health is one of the major community health problems in the United States.

5 Define *stress* and explain its relationship to physical and mental health.

6 Briefly trace the history of mental health care in America, highlighting the major changes both before and after World War II.

7 Define the term *deinstitutionalization* and list and discuss the propelling forces that brought it about.

8 Describe the movement toward community mental health centers.

9 Explain what is meant by *Community Support Program* and list some of the services provided by successful programs.

10 Identify the major mental and physical problems of the homeless.

11 Define *primary, secondary,* and *tertiary prevention* as they relate to mental health care services and give an example of each.

12 List and briefly describe the three basic approaches to treatment for mental disorders.

13 Define *self-help groups,* give examples, and explain how they are helpful to their members.

14 Explain the purpose of the Substance Abuse and Mental Health Services Administration.

15 Define what is meant by *behavioral health care services.*

16 Define *evidenced-based practices* in behavioral health interventions.

17 Explain what is at issue when the phrase *parity* in *health care services* is used in reference to health care services for those with mental illness.

SCENARIO

Maria Sanchez, her husband, and their three children had lived in their apartment building for about two years when they noticed a new person moving in on the floor below them. New families moved in from time to time, but this person didn't have a family and kept to herself. After asking around, Maria learned from a neighbor downstairs that the new person's name was Lynn and that she was not currently employed, but hoped to find work soon, perhaps as a salesperson or a custodian. Maria hasn't found her very friendly so far—Lynn tends to look away without saying anything when Maria passes her in the hallway. Maria also learned that Lynn was recovering from a recent bout of mental illness and that she was pleased to be living independently once again.

Maria noticed that every few days a regular visitor arrived at the building in a van from the mental health center to spend an hour or so with Lynn in her apartment. Maria worries that people who see the mental health center van might think those in the van were visiting Maria's family. She knew that people with mental illness needed to live somewhere, but why did it have to be in her building? Would other recovering mental patients rent the next vacant apartment in her building? Would people begin loitering in front of the building or behaving strangely? Would Maria's children be safe? Would the value of their apartment begin to decline?

INTRODUCTION

Mental illness is one of the major health issues facing every community. It is the leading cause of disability in the United States, Canada, and western Europe (see Figure 11.1).[1] Approximately 22% to 23% of American adults (about 44 million people) have diagnosable mental disorders during a given year. Another 6% have addictive disorders, and another 3% have both mental and addictive disorders. Thus, about 28% to 30% of the adult population have either a mental or addictive disorder.[2] About 5 million adults in the United States have serious mental illness, that is, illness that interferes with some aspect of social functioning.[2,3] Only between one-fourth to one-third of those diagnosed with a mental disorder receive treatment.[2] Some of these people require only minimal counseling, followed by regular attendance of supportive self-help group meetings to remain in recovery, while others suffer repeated episodes of disabling mental illness. These individuals have conditions for which they require more frequent medical treatment and more significant community support. Finally, there are the most severely disturbed individuals, who require repeated hospitalization.

College students and youth also experience a variety of mental and addictive disorders. A study of client problems seen by a university counseling center revealed that, in addition to the occurrence of typical problems such as relationship problems and development issues, more severe problems such as anxiety, depression, suicidal ideation, sexual assault, and personality disorders were often diagnosed. During the 13-year period of the study, depression had doubled and the number of suicidal students had tripled.[4] Approximately four million children and adolescents suffer from a major mental illness that results in significant impairment at home, at school, and with peers.[2] While 1 in 10 youths has an impairing mental illness, only 1 in 5 receives mental health services in a given year.[5]

Because the needs of the mentally ill are many and diverse, the services required to meet these needs are likewise diverse and, as we will explain, include not only therapeutic services but social services, too. Because many mental disorders are chronic in nature, significant community resources are required to meet the continuing demands for care.

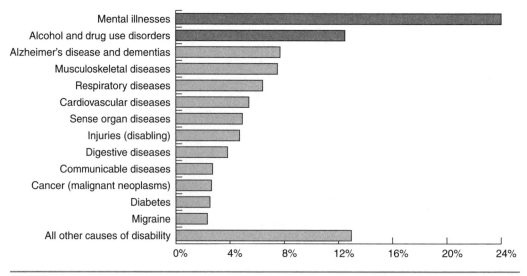

FIGURE 11.1

Causes of disability for all ages combined: United States, Canada, and western Europe, 2000.

Note: Measures of disability are based on the number of years of "healthy" life lost with less than full health (i.e., YLD: years lost due to disability) for each incidence of disease, illness, or condition.

Source: President's New Freedom Commission on Mental Health (2003). *Achieving the Promise: Transforming Mental Health Care in America.* Rockville, MD: Author, 20.

mental health
emotional and social well-being, including one's psychological resources for dealing with day-to-day problems of life

Definitions

Mental health is the "state of successful performance of mental function, resulting in productive activities, fulfilling relationships with other people, and the ability to adapt to change and to cope with adversity."[2] Characteristics of people with good mental health include possessing a good self-image, feeling right about other people, and being able to meet the demands of everyday life.

Good mental health can be expressed as emotional maturity. In this regard, adults who have good mental health are able to:

mental illness
a collective term for all diagnosable mental disorders

1. Function under adversity
2. Change or adapt to changes around them
3. Maintain control over their tension and anxiety
4. Find more satisfaction in giving than receiving
5. Show consideration for others
6. Curb hate and guilt
7. Love others

mental disorders
health conditions characterized by alterations in thinking, mood, or behavior (or some combination thereof) associated with distress and/or impaired functioning

"**Mental illness** is a term that refers collectively to all diagnosable mental disorders. **Mental disorders** are health conditions that are characterized by alterations in thinking, mood, or behavior (or some combination thereof) associated with distress and/or impaired functioning."[2] People with mental illness have organic or metabolic (biochemical) disorders that prevent them from functioning effectively and happily in society. Many people with mental illness can be treated successfully with medications and are thus able to live successfully in our communities.

Classification of Mental Disorders

It is important to keep in mind that classification systems of human origin are imperfect attempts to arrange natural phenomena into carefully constructed, but sometimes arbitrary, categories. Such is the case with the classification of mental disorders, which are for the most part based on descriptions of behavioral signs and symptoms. The most often cited reference for the classification of mental disorders is the *Diagnostic and Statistical Manual of Mental Disorders,* 4th edition, text revision (*DSM-IV-TR*).[6] The *DSM-IV-TR,* published by the American Psychiatric Association, represents the best current thinking on the diagnosis and classification of mental disorders but does not in all cases describe the causes of these disorders.

One criterion for classifying mental disorders is age of onset. The onset of some disorders occurs in infancy, others in adulthood. Examples of mental disorders that are first evident at an early age include developmental disorders (such as mental retardation), behavioral disruptive disorders (such as attention-deficit hyperactivity), and gender-identity disorders of childhood. Disorders of adolescence and adulthood include psychoactive substance abuse disorder, schizophrenia, and mood disorders. Each of these disorders can be mild, moderate, or severe, and each may result in mild to severe impairments of social functioning. Disorders classified in the *DSM-IV-TR* are listed in Table 11.1.

Origins and Causes of Mental Disorders

The origins of mental disorders, while not always fully understood, can usually be attributed to either hereditary or environmental factors or to a combination of both. When such is not the case, disorders may be referred to as *idiopathic* (of unknown origin).

There are several causes of mental disorders, including mental deficiency at birth, physical (or physiological) impairment, and psychological causes. Mental deficiency at birth can be inherited (genetic causes), have an idiopathic (unknown) origin, or be the result of maternal exposure to physical, chemical, or biological agents. Two-thirds of mental retardation cases are traceable to environmental factors such as poor prenatal care, poor maternal nutrition, or

Table 11.1
Diagnostic Categories of Mental Disorders

Category	Example
Disorders usually first evident in infancy, childhood, or adolescence	Mental retardation; attention-deficit hyperactivity disorder
Organic mental disorders	Alzheimer's disease; dementia associated with alcoholism or chronic drug use
Psychoactive substance use disorders	Alcohol, nicotine, cocaine, or other drug dependence
Schizophrenia	Paranoid schizophrenia
Delusional (paranoid) disorder	Persecutory delusional (paranoid) disorder
Miscellaneous psychotic disorders	Brief reactive psychosis
Mood disorders	Major depression; bipolar disorder
Anxiety disorders	Panic disorder; obsessive compulsive disorder; post-traumatic stress disorder
Somatoform disorders	Conversion disorder; hypochondriasis
Dissociative disorders	Multiple personality disorder
Sexual disorders	Paraphilias (exhibitionism, fetishisms); sexual dysfunctions
Sleep disorders	Insomnia disorder; dream anxiety disorder
Impulse control disorders	Kleptomania; pathological gambling
Adjustment disorders	Anxious mood; withdrawal
Personality disorders	Avoidant; dependent; obsessive

maternal exposure to alcohol, tobacco, or other drugs; as such, they are preventable. For example, fetal alcohol spectrum disorder, a condition that includes mental deficiency, is the result of maternal (and fetal) exposure to excessive amounts of alcohol during gestation. One recent study revealed that an estimated 423,000 women used alcohol during their pregnancies, while 413,000 used cigarettes and 97,000 used at least one illicit drug.[7]

Inherited causes of mental disorders can be present at birth or appear later in life. For example, an imbalance in the levels of neurotransmitters in the brain could appear during adolescence or young adulthood. Abnormal neurotransmitter levels, which often have a genetic origin, can result in such **affective (mood) disorders** as **bipolar disorder** and **major depression** (see Box 11.1).

Mental disorders can also occur from postnatal exposure to physical, chemical, and biological agents. Brain function impairment can be caused by trauma, such as a car crash or bullet wound, or by disease, such as syphilis, cancer, or stroke. Mental impairment can also be caused by such environmental factors as chronic nutritional deficiency or by lead poisoning.

Psychological sources of mental disorders include dysfunctional family environments. Children reared in abusive, neglectful, or violent family environments can develop mental dis-

affective mood disorder
a mental disorder characterized by a disturbance of mood, either depression or elation (mania); examples: bipolar disorder, major depression

bipolar disorder
an affective disorder characterized by distinct periods of elevated mood alternating with periods of depression

---

BOX 11.1

CRITERIA FOR MAJOR DEPRESSIVE EPISODE

A. Five (or more) of the following symptoms have been present during the same two-week period and represent a change from previous functioning. At least one of the symptoms is either (1) depressed mood or (2) loss of interest or pleasure.
Note: Do not include symptoms that are clearly due to a general medical condition, or mood-incongruent delusions or hallucinations.

(1) Depressed mood most of the day, nearly every day, as indicated by either subjective report (e.g., feels sad or empty) or observation made by others (e.g., appears tearful). Note: In children and adolescents, can be irritable mood

(2) Markedly diminished interest or pleasure in all, or almost all, activities most of the day, nearly every day (as indicated by either subjective account or observation made by others)

(3) Significant weight loss when not dieting or weight gain (e.g., a change of more than 5% of body weight in a month), or decrease or increase in appetite nearly every day. Note: In children, consider failure to make expected weight gains

(4) Insomnia or hypersomnia nearly every day

(5) Psychomotor agitation or retardation nearly every day (observable by others, not merely subjective feelings of restlessness or being slowed down)

(6) Fatigue or loss of energy nearly every day

(7) Feelings of worthlessness or excessive or inappropriate guilt (which may be delusional)

nearly every day (not merely self-reproach or guilt about being sick)

(8) Diminished ability to think or concentrate, or indecisiveness, nearly every day (either by subjective account or as observed by others)

(9) Recurrent thoughts of death (not just fear of dying), recurrent suicidal ideation without a specific plan, or a suicide attempt or a specific plan for committing suicide

B. The symptoms do not meet criteria for a Mixed Episode.

C. The symptoms cause clinically significant distress or impairment in social, occupational, or other important areas of functioning.

D. The symptoms are not due to the direct physiological effects of a substance (e.g., a drug of abuse, a medication) or a general medical condition (e.g., hypothyroidism).

E. The symptoms are not better accounted for by bereavement, that is, after the loss of a loved one, the symptoms persist for longer than two months or are characterized by marked functional impairment, morbid preoccupation with worthlessness, suicidal ideation, psychotic symptoms, or psychomotor retardation.

Source: Adapted from American Psychiatric Association (2000). *Diagnostic and Statistical Manual of Mental Disorders,* 4th ed., text revision. Washington, DC: American Psychiatric Association.

orders (see Figure 11.2). The prevalence of child abuse and neglect has reached epidemic proportions in America. Each year there are more than 900,000 confirmed victims of maltreatment in the United States, according to the Children's Defense Fund.[8]

It is estimated that 1 in 5 youths has some sort of diagnosable disorder. Furthermore, the prevalence of serious emotional disturbance in youth (9 to 17 years old) ranges from 5% to 13%. Thus, a minimum of 1 in 20 to a maximum 1 in 7.7 youths suffers from emotional disturbances that include functional impairment[2,3] (see Figure 11.3).

The negative influences of unhealthy neighborhoods, deviant peer groups (such as gangs), and challenging economic conditions or growing up in dysfunctional families may further increase the risk that these young people will develop mental disorders. Broken families add to the burden on our nation's mental health services, leading children's advocates to question the priorities of federal programs that provide more money to the states for foster care than for programs designed to strengthen families. The U.S. Department of Health and Human Services estimates that there were 523,000 children in foster care in 2003.[8]

FIGURE 11.2
A dysfunctional family environment can increase one's risk for mental illness.

MENTAL ILLNESS IN AMERICA

Health and social statistics clearly indicate that mental illness constitutes one of our nation's most pervasive public health problems. For many healthy Americans, exposure to stressful lifestyles represents an increased risk of mental illness.

major depression
an affective disorder characterized by a dysphoric mood, usually depression, or loss of interest or pleasure in almost all usual activities or pastimes

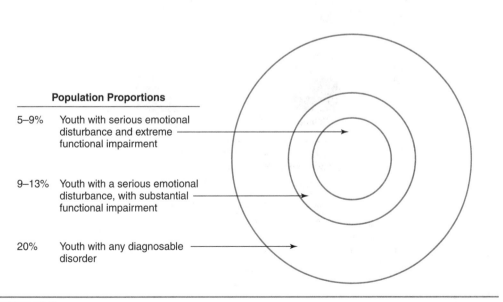

Population Proportions

5–9%   Youth with serious emotional disturbance and extreme functional impairment

9–13%   Youth with a serious emotional disturbance, with substantial functional impairment

20%   Youth with any diagnosable disorder

FIGURE 11.3
Prevalence of serious emotional disturbance in 9- to 17-year-olds.

Source: Center for Mental Health Services (1996). *Mental Health, United States, 1996.* Mandersheid, R. W., and M. A. Sonnenschein, eds. (HHS pub. no. SMA 96-3098). Washington, DC: U.S. Government Printing Office, 83.

Statistical Indicators of Mental Illness

the federal agency,
housed within the
Department of Health
and Human Services'
Substance Abuse and
Mental Services
Administration, that is
the nation's leading
mental health
services agency

Center for Mental Health Services (CMHS)
the federal agency, housed within the Department of Health and Human Services' Substance Abuse and Mental Services Administration, that is the nation's leading mental health services agency

The **Center for Mental Health Services (CMHS)** in the Substance Abuse and Mental Health Services Administration estimates that 4.8 million American adults had a severe and persistent mental illness during the 1990 calendar year and 5.6 million adults had a serious mental illness during that same period.[2] It has been estimated that 15.4% of the U.S. population 18 years of age and older have had at least one incident that would meet the criteria of a mental health or substance abuse disorder within the past 30 days.[2] About 35% of the population aged 15 to 54 have had a mental disorder in their lifetime. Of these, 39% also had substance abuse/dependence. Among those with a mental disorder in the past year, 21% also had abuse/substance dependence (see Figure 11.4).[9] Frequently, these mental disorders are chronic in nature; approximately half of those admitted to mental institutions have had previous admissions. On any given day, 3.4 million Americans are in specialty mental health treatment, and another 944,000 are in substance abuse treatment.[9]

Social Indicators of Mental Illness

The social statistics that reflect the depth and breadth of the mental illness problem in our society are staggering. There are approximately 30,000 suicides each year in the United States.

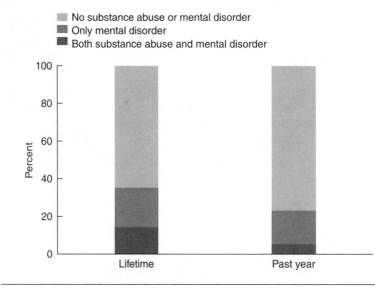

Percent of the population with a mental disorder with and without substance abuse/dependence, ages 15 to 54, 1991

	Percent of population		Percent of persons with mental disorder	
	Lifetime	Past year	Lifetime	Past year
Any mental disorder	**35.1%**	**22.9%**	–	–
Only mental disorder	21.4	18.2	61%	79%
Both substance abuse and mental disorder	13.7	4.7	39	21

FIGURE 11.4

Percentage of the population with a mental disorder with or without substance abuse/dependence, ages 15 to 54, 1991.

Source: Rouse, B. A., ed. (1995). *Substance Abuse and Mental Health Statistics Sourcebook* (HHS pub. no. SMA 95-3064). Washington, DC: U.S. Government Printing Office, 39.

In 2001, the Number 2 and Number 3 leading causes of death in youth aged 15 to 24 were homicide (including legal intervention) and suicide, respectively (see Chapter 8).[10] One of the objectives of *Healthy People 2010* aimed at improving the mental health status of Americans is to reduce the suicide rate. During the first four years (1999–2003), little progress was made in reducing suicide rates in most population subgroups (see Box 11.2). Perhaps another social

---

BOX
11.2

HEALTHY PEOPLE 2010: OBJECTIVES

Objective 18-1:   Reduce the suicide rate.

	Baseline Year	Baseline	2003	Target 2010
	1999	a\10.5	10.8	b\4.8
Race and ethnicity				
American Indian or Alaska Native	1999	a\10.1	10.0	b\4.8
Asian or Pacific Islander	1999	a\6.0	5.6	b\4.8
Asian	1999	a\DNC	DNA	b\4.8
Native Hawaiian or other Pacific Islander	1999	a\DNC	DNA	b\4.8
Black or African American	1999	a\5.6	5.2	b\4.8
White	1999	a\11.3	11.8	b\4.8
Hispanic or Latino	1999	a\5.9	5.5	b\4.8
Not Hispanic or Latino	1999	a\11.0	11.4	b\4.8
Black or African American, not Hispanic/Latino	1999	a\5.7	5.4	b\4.8
White, not Hispanic or Latino	1999	a\12.0	12.7	b\4.8
Gender				
Female	1999	a\4.0	4.2	b\4.8
Male	1999	a\17.8	18.0	b\4.8
Education level (persons aged 25 to 64 years)				
Less than high school	1999	a,1\17.7	2\20.8	b\4.8
High school graduate	1999	a,1\18.4	2\21.0	b\4.8
At least some college	1999	a,1\9.4	2\10.2	b\4.8
Select populations				
Age groups				
Persons aged 10–14 years (not age adjusted)	1999	a\1.2	1.2	NA
Persons aged 15–19 years (not age adjusted)	1999	a\8.0	7.3	NA
Persons aged 20–24 years (not age adjusted)	1999	a\12.3	12.1	NA

Note: Data may include revisions and may differ from those shown previously. Any displayed age-adjusted data are adjusted to the 2000 standard population.
—- = Data are not available. DNA = Data have not been analyzed. DNC = Data for specific population are not collected.
DSU = Data do not meet the criteria for statistical reliability, data quality, or confidence. NA = Not applicable.
a\Baseline has been revised.
b\Target has been revised.
c\New baseline. Objective was previously developmental.
1\Total of 46 reporting states and the District of Columbia.
2\Total of 43 reporting states and the District of Columbia.
3\Respondents were asked to select one or more races and identify one race as best representing their race.

Source: CDC (2006). *DATA2010 . . . The Healthy People 2010 Database—June, 2006 Edition.* Available at http://wonder.cdc.gov.

For Further Thought

Think about the relationship between alcohol and other drug use and depression. If the rates of binge drinking and illicit drug use by teenagers were to decline during this decade, how would it affect the suicide rate?

(continued)

BOX 11.2	Healthy People 2010: Objectives (continued)

Objective 18-2: Reduce the suicide attempts by adolescents (grades 9 through 12).

	Baseline Year	Baseline 1999	2003	Target
Race and ethnicity				
American Indian or Alaska Native only	1999	DSU	DSU	1.0%
Asian or Pacific Islander only	1999	DNC	DNC	1.0%
Asian only	1999	DNA	DNA	1.0%
Native Hawaiian or other Pacific Islander only	1999	DSU	DSU	1.0%
Black or African American only	1999	DNA	DNA	1.0%
White only	1999	DNA	DNA	1.0%
Two or more races	1999	DSU	DSU	1.0%
American Indian or Alaska Native; White	1999	DSU	DSU	1.0%
Black or African American; White	1999	DSU	DSU	1.0%
Hispanic or Latino	1999	3.0%	5.0%	1.0%
Not Hispanic or Latino	1999	2.6%	2.4%	1.0%
Black or African American only, not Hispanic/Latino	1999	2.9%	3.7%	1.0%
White only, not Hispanic or Latino	1999	1.9%	1.7%	1.0%
Gender				
Female	1999	3.1%	3.2%	1.0%
Male	1999	2.1%	2.4%	1.0%
Parent's education level				
Less than high school	1999	DNC	DNC	1.0%
High school graduate	1999	DNC	DNC	1.0%
At least some college	1999	DNC	DNC	1.0%
Sexual orientation	1999	DNC	DNC	1.0%

Note: Data may include revisions and may differ from those shown previously. Any displayed age-adjusted data are adjusted to the 2000 standard population.
—- = Data are not available. DNA = Data have not been analyzed. DNC = Data for specific population are not collected. DSU = Data do not meet the criteria for statistical reliability, data quality, or confidence. NA = Not applicable.
a\Baseline has been revised.
b\Target has been revised.
c\New baseline. Objective was previously developmental.
1\Total of 46 reporting states and the District of Columbia.
2\Total of 43 reporting states and the District of Columbia.
3\Respondents were asked to select one or more races and identify one race as best representing their race.

Source: CDC (2007). *DATA2010 . . . The Healthy People 2010 Database—June, 2006 Edition.* Available at http://wonder.cdc.gov.

indicator of mental illness in America is the proportion of failed marriages. One in five marriages is disrupted in 5 years; one in three in 10 years.[11]

The prevalence of alcohol, tobacco, and other drug abuse in this country is yet another social indicator of the mental illness problem. For example, 40% of the college-aged young adults and 28% of high school seniors interviewed had drunk at least five or more drinks in a row in the past two weeks.[12,13] The percentage of twelfth graders reporting the use of any illegal drug in the past 30 days increased to 25% in 2002.[12] These figures, which will be discussed in more detail in Chapter 12, are further evidence that many of our youth lack the necessary psychological resources for coping with life's problems.

Stress: A Contemporary Mental Health Problem

Stress can be defined as one's psychological and physiological response to stressors—stimuli in the physical and social environment that produce feelings of tension and strain. Stress, as a contributor to mental health problems, is likely to remain important as life becomes increasingly complex. Even Americans who believe they have good mental health carry out their everyday activities under considerable stress. Stressors can be subtle—such as having to wait in line, getting stuck in traffic, or having to keep an appointment—or they can be major life events such as getting married or divorced or losing a loved one. Coping with a physical health problem such as hypertension, obesity, or other disease can increase stress and raise one's risk of developing a mental disorder. While some exposure to stressors is good, perhaps even essential to a satisfying life, chronic exposure to stressors that exceed one's coping resources—biological, psychological, and social—can undermine one's health. Holmes and Rahe actually classified and ranked various stressors and found a relationship between these stressors and physical health.[14]

The process through which exposure to stressors results in health deficits has been described by Selye[15] and Sarafino.[16] According to Selye's model, which he called the **General Adaptation Syndrome (GAS),** confrontation with a stressor results in a three-stage physiological response: (1) an alarm reaction stage, (2) a stage of resistance, and finally (3) a stage of exhaustion (see Figure 11.5). In the alarm reaction stage, the body prepares to strongly resist the stressor. Various hormonal changes in the body increase the individual's heart rate, respiration, and blood pressure. This is the **fight or flight reaction,** a response that the body cannot maintain for very long. Continued presence of the stressor produces a stage of resistance. In this stage, the body tries to adapt to the stressor. The level of physiological arousal declines somewhat but still remains above normal. During the stage of resistance, the body begins to replenish the hormones released in the alarm reaction stage, but the body's ability to resist new stressors is impaired. As a result, the person is increasingly vulnerable to certain health problems that are referred to as **diseases of adaptation.** Such diseases include ulcers, high blood pressure, coronary heart disease, asthma, and other diseases related to impaired immune function.[16]

The third stage of Selye's GAS is the stage of exhaustion. Prolonged physiological arousal produced by continual or repeated stress can deplete energy stores until one's physical ability to resist is very limited. During this stage, physiological damage, physical diseases, mental health problems, and even death can occur.

General Adaptation Syndrome (GAS) the complex physiological responses resulting from exposure to stressors

fight or flight reaction an alarm reaction that prepares one physiologically for sudden action

diseases of adaptation diseases that result from chronic exposure to excess levels of stressors, which produce a General Adaptation Syndrome response

FIGURE 11.5

General Adaptation Syndrome.

Source: Sarafino, E. P. (1990). *Healthy Psychology: Biopsychosocial Interactions.* New York: John Wiley & Sons, 84. Reprinted with permission.

Evidence suggests that stress can affect health either directly by way of physiologic changes in the body or indirectly through a change in a person's behavior. The clearest connection between stress and disease is demonstrated by the release of hormones by the endocrine system during the alarm reaction stage of the GAS. During this stage, both the cardiovascular and immune systems of the body are affected. Hormones produce fast or erratic beating of the heart, which can be fatal. The same hormones have been associated with increases in levels of blood lipids. High blood lipids cause a buildup of plaque on the blood vessel walls and greatly increase the likelihood of hypertension, stroke, and heart attack.[17,18] The release of certain hormones also impairs the functioning of the immune system.[19,20] These hormones reduce the activity of T cells and natural killer cells, making it more difficult for the immune system to fight cancer and other diseases.[21] Table 11.2 provides a list of psychophysiological disorders that have been found to be associated with stress.

The indirect effects of stress on health occur when those who experience high levels of stress respond with unhealthy behaviors. For example, it has been shown that individuals under more stress drink more alcohol and smoke more cigarettes than those under less stress.[22,23] Use of these substances has been associated with higher risks for heart disease and cancer, as well as injury and death from unintentional injuries.

The relationship between stress and mental illness is complicated. The effects of severe stress, such as that experienced under military combat conditions and by children who are sexually and physically abused, have been well documented. It stands to reason that even exposure to less intense stressors would likewise result in stress and affect one's health adversely.

Avoiding stressful situations is always preferable to managing stress. Effective time management, goal setting, and prioritizing tasks are ways individuals can reduce the stress that comes with approaching deadlines. Procrastination, on the other hand, can increase stress. Also, taking a realistic view of one's abilities and what one expects to accomplish is important. "Perfectionism leads to undue stress because perfection is an unattainable goal."[24]

Stress management is primarily a personal, rather than a community, health matter. Experts recommend a combination of physical, social, environmental, and psychological approaches to managing stress.[24] Physical approaches to stress reduction include good nutrition and adequate sleep and aerobic exercise. Healthy social interaction and optimizing environmental factors such as noise, lighting, and living space can also reduce one's stress. Finally, a variety of psychological techniques have proven effective in reducing stress for some people. These include guided imagery and visualization, biofeedback, progressive relaxation, and meditation and hypnosis.[24] Among the many resources available to help people deal with the stress in their lives is the American Institute of Stress Web site at www.stress.org.

Community support for those experiencing excessive stress in their lives can be found in local mental health associations, local offices of comprehensive mental health centers, and

---

Table 11.2
Psychophysiological Disorders Associated with Stress

Allergies (asthma, tissue inflammation, rheumatoid arthritis)	Gastrointestinal problems (colitis, stomach ulcers)
Cancer	
Cardiovascular conditions	Headaches (muscle-contraction and migraine)
Coronary artery disease	Infectious diseases (colds and influenza)
Depression	Hypertension
Dysmenorrhea (painful menstruation)	Irritable bowel syndrome
Exhaustion	Skin disorders (eczema, hives, psoriasis)

other more specialized agencies, such as A Better Way, for battered spouses and children. College and university counseling and psychological service centers provide help for students. Relief from stress for some might be as close as the nearest church, synagogue, or mosque. Religious leaders are often experienced in helping people suffering from stress; also, the social interactions available in these settings can be comforting. Finally, there are community service organizations such as Rotary, Kiwanis, Lions, and many others that provide opportunities for socialization. In a college or university setting, similar opportunities are available for joining in social or service clubs.

HISTORY OF MENTAL HEALTH CARE IN AMERICA

Before discussing our nation's current response to mental illness, we present a brief history of past efforts to confront this issue. The collective response to mental illness in America has been a cyclic phenomenon, marked by enthusiastic reform movements followed by periods of national ambivalence toward those suffering from mental disorders. The following reform movements we discuss began when an existing system for caring for those with mental illness became intolerable for society and ended when their economic burden became unbearable.

Mental Health Care before World War II

In Colonial America, when communities were sparsely populated, people experiencing mental illness were cared for by their families or private caretakers. Those "distracted" persons or "lunatics," as they were called, who were not cared for by their families usually became the responsibility of the local community. In the eighteenth century as the size and complexity of communities grew, institutionalization of the insane first appeared. This often took place in undifferentiated poorhouses or almshouses where, along with those who had mental retardation, those with physical disabilities, the homeless, and the otherwise deviant were also housed.[25]

moral treatment treatment for mental illness based on belief that mental illness was caused by moral decay

As America's population grew in the late eighteenth and early nineteenth centuries, so did the number of people who were unable to live independently. Gradually, as the situation in the poorhouses and almshouses worsened, efforts were made to separate people by their type of disability. One of the first efforts was that of Dr. Thomas Bond, who in 1751 built Pennsylvania Hospital, the first institution in America specifically designed to care for those with mental illness.[26] Conditions in the hospital were harsh (see Figure 11.6), and treatments, which consisted of "blood letting, blistering, emetics, and warm and cold baths," were unpleasant.[27]

The Moral Treatment Era

Philippe Pinel of France developed a more humane approach that he called *traitement moral,* or in English, "moral treatment," based upon the assumption that environmental changes could affect an individual's mind and thus alter behavior.[25] In America, William Tuke put **moral treatment** into practice beginning in 1792. This treatment was based on his belief that the causes of mental illnesses were moral deterioration, exemplified by "infidelity, overwork, envy, gluttony, drinking, sexual excesses, and the like."[27] In a peaceful rural setting, people with mental illness were removed from the everyday life stressors of their home environments and given "asylum" in a quiet country environment. They

FIGURE 11.6

Treatment for mental illness in the eighteenth and nineteenth centuries was often inhumane and unsuccessful.

FIGURE 11.7
Dorothea Dix helped to establish public mental hospitals in many states.

received a regimen of rest, light food, exercise, fresh air, and amusements. While actual recovery rates are debatable, this approach, at the time, was deemed successful and became widely accepted as the ideal form of treatment for relatively well-to-do persons with mental illness in small, relatively homogeneous, New England Protestant communities of that era.[28]

The apparent successes of the moral treatment approach in the private sector led to attempts to adapt this model of mental health care to the public sector. However, by the 1840s, because of massive immigration and rapid urbanization, there was such a heterogeneous mass of people with mental illnesses that the capacity of the public asylums was soon overcrowded. The majority of those who were mentally and socially unfit again ended up in the urban almshouses, which were chronically underfunded and overpopulated. This was the state of affairs when Dorothea Lynde Dix undertook her campaign to close down county-run almshouses and establish state-run hospitals.

Dorothea Dix (1802–1897) (see Figure 11.7) was a Sunday-school teacher from Cambridge, Massachusetts, who worked tirelessly for 45 years advocating decent care for indigents with mental illness. It was her belief that it was the responsibility of the state to care for those with mental illness. When her lobbying for a federal law failed, Dix lobbied on a state-by-state basis. Her efforts were in most cases successful; all in all, Dix was personally involved in the founding of 32 public mental hospitals.[29]

The State Hospitals

The state mental hospitals were supposed to provide an environment in which medical care would be provided by professional staff, trained to work with each patient individually (see Figure 11.8). Initially, the upper limit of patients was set at 250 so that treatment could occur within the bonds of close personal relationships between caregiving staff members and patients, as prescribed in the methods of the moral treatment.

FIGURE 11.8
The state mental hospital was at one time viewed as the appropriate public response to the needs of those with mental illness.

Unfortunately, even as new state hospitals continued to be built, the deterioration of those already in existence had begun. The chronic nature of mental illness was a large part of the problem. It became increasingly apparent that long-term or even lifetime stays were the norms for many patients.[29] "Maximum capacities" were quickly reached, exceeded, and repeatedly revised upward. The ability to provide personalized care was lost, as was the promise of significant medical treatment. Staff members were unable to reward patients for efforts at self-control, and physical restraints became more practical, especially in large wards.[26] As funding for these institutions became increasingly susceptible to state budget cuts, the level of care also diminished until all that remained was custodial care. The institutions at that point had become little more than places to "warehouse" people with mental illness. It became increasingly difficult to find dedicated staff to work at the unrewarding jobs in these institutions, and the turnover rate was high. Administration became more of a bureaucracy, and treatment and cure became almost nonexistent.

The Mental Hygiene Movement

The next movement in mental health care in the United States was the **mental hygiene movement,** which occurred during the first decades of the twentieth century. One of the prominent figures in the reform movement was *Adolf Meyer* (1866–1950), a psychiatrist who felt that psychiatrists should provide acute care for patients with mental illness in new psychopathic hospitals, after which the same patients would be remitted to community-based aftercare. The psychopathic hospitals would receive, diagnose, treat, and release patients, or in certain cases, remand them over to the state hospitals. Some of the receiving hospitals that were established during this period, such as Bellevue in New York and Boston Psychopathic Hospital, remain in operation today.[26]

Another name associated with the mental hygiene movement is that of *Clifford W. Beers* (1876–1943). Clifford Beers (see Figure 11.9) was a graduate of Yale University who suffered from a bipolar mood disorder that resulted in repeated hospitalizations throughout his life.[30] His book, *A Mind That Found Itself,* published in 1908, described his illness and experiences in mental hospitals. He was able to enlist the support of others in his cause to improve conditions and to promote research on the prevention and treatment of mental illness. He founded the National Committee on Mental Hygiene, which in 1950 became the National Association of Mental Health and in 1979 changed its name to the **National Mental Health Association (NMHA).** While Meyer and Beers contributed to mental health education in many ways, the mental hygiene movement did little to advance institutional reform of state mental facilities.

By 1940 the population in state mental institutions had grown to nearly one half million, many of whom were elderly and senile. Budget cuts continued, and caseloads per worker in the institutions became so large that only subsistence care was possible.

At about this time two new treatments began to gain prominence in psychiatric medicine—electroconvulsive shock therapy and the lobotomy. **Electroconvulsive therapy (ECT)** evolved from several earlier types of shock therapy, including fever shock therapy, insulin shock therapy, and chemical shock therapy. Shock therapy was practiced after it was observed that mental patients experienced improvements in their conditions after suffering convulsions and that there were very few people who suffered from both schizophrenia and epilepsy. In ECT, electric current is used to produce convulsions in the patient. The practice was introduced into the United States in 1939 and grew in popularity until the 1960s, when it became apparent that in too many cases ECT was being used to control mental patients for the convenience of hospital staff, rather than to help the patient recover from illness.[31] However, during the late 1980s and early 1990s, ECT use experienced a resurgence because of the recognition of its utility, cost-effectiveness, and short hospital stays. The procedure remains an important treatment option and is reimbursable by Medicare.[32]

The **lobotomy,** the surgical severance of nerve fibers of the brain by incision, was introduced at about the same time. First developed and used in dogs in Germany in 1890 and a couple of years later on schizophrenic patients in Switzerland, the procedure was popularized by a Portuguese neuropsychiatrist, Dr. Antônio Egas Moniz. In the United States the procedure was popularized by Dr. Walter Freeman, who invented the so-called ice-pick lobotomy. Between 1939 and 1951, the procedure was carried out on more than 18,000 patients in the United States[33] (Figure 11.10). The popularity of the lobotomy procedure was undoubtedly prolonged when, in 1949, Dr. Moniz was awarded the Nobel Prize for Medicine and Physiology. However, by 1950 voices of opposition to the procedure began to gather strength. It

mental hygiene movement
a movement based on the belief that mental illness can be cured if identified and treated early

National Mental Health Association
a voluntary health agency, with state and local affiliates, that sponsors education and prevention programs

electroconvulsive therapy (ECT)
method of treatment for mental disorders involving the administration of electric current to induce a coma or convulsions

lobotomy
surgical severance of nerve fibers of the brain by incision

FIGURE 11.9
Clifford Beers founded the National Committee on Mental Hygiene and led the fight for those with mental illness.

FIGURE 11.10

A team of doctors and nurses prepares to demonstrate the procedures involved in electroconvulsive therapy (shock treatment), 1942.

was shown that following the surgery, only one-third of patients demonstrated improvement, while another one-third became worse off. Also, the surgery was not reversible. The appearance of new antipsychotic and antidepressive drugs in the 1950s made the widespread use of lobotomies unnecessary.[33]

Mental Health Care after World War II

In the postwar 1940s, a number of alliances formed to urge greater federal involvement in mental health care. One of these groups was the National Mental Health Foundation (NMHF), founded by a group of conscientious objectors (COs), people who objected to serving in the military on religious grounds. In place of military duty, many COs had spent their war years working in these mental institutions. Through the NMHF, the COs publicized the deterioration of the state mental hospitals and lobbied for improvements. The mood of the country, together with testimony before Congress by both military and civilian experts, soon resulted in the passage of the *National Mental Health Act of 1946,* which established the

National Institute of Mental Health (NIMH). Modeled after the National Cancer Institute, established in 1937, NIMH came under the umbrella of the National Institutes of Health. The purposes of NIMH were (1) to foster and aid research related to the cause, diagnosis, and treatment of neuropsychiatric disorders; (2) to provide training and award fellowships and grants for work in mental health; and (3) to aid the states in the prevention, diagnosis, and treatment of neuropsychiatric disorders.[29] In 1950, a council of state governments suggested that more support was needed for research into the etiology and treatment of those with mental illness so that these people could be discharged from mental institutions. During the early 1950s, public distress about the conditions in state mental hospitals continued to grow until the necessity of finding a new approach to caring for those with mental illness was clear and inescapable.[27]

Deinstitutionalization

The term **deinstitutionalization** has been used to describe the discharging of thousands of patients from state-owned mental hospitals and the resettling and maintaining of these discharged persons in less restrictive community settings. The magnitude of the process can be documented with the following statistics. In 1955 there were 558,922 resident patients in state and county mental institutions.[34] By 1970 the number had dropped to 337,619, by 1980 to 150,000, and by 1990 to between 110,000 and 120,000.[34,35] Deinstitutionalization, which began in the 1950s and continued through the 1980s, was not a preplanned policy. Rather, it occurred as a result of social and economic forces that had built up for more than half a century.

Deinstitutionalization was propelled by four forces: (1) economics, (2) idealism, (3) legal considerations, and (4) the development and marketing of antipsychotic drugs.[27] Economically, there was not only a push, there was also a pull. The push was the states' need to reduce expenditures for mental hospitals so that more could be spent on the other three major state budgetary items—education, roads, and welfare. Meanwhile, a pulling economic force began to germinate with the prospect of profits from providing outpatient and inpatient services to those with mental illness. This prospect became brighter with changes in federal legislation (Medicare and Medicaid) enabling payment for these services with federal funds. (For more information about Medicare and Medicaid, see Chapter 14.)

In the early 1960s questions began to be raised about the legality of keeping people locked up, especially if no real effort was being made to treat them. The American Bar Association

National Institute of Mental Health (NIMH) the nation's leading mental health research agency, housed in the National Institutes of Health

deinstitutionalization the process of discharging, on a large scale, patients from state mental hospitals to less restrictive community settings

chlorpromazine (Thorazine) the first and most famous antipsychotic drug, introduced in 1954 under the brand name Thorazine

Thorazine (see chlorpromazine)

published a study in 1961 of the laws relating to this issue. One of the points raised in its review was that mental patients, even when institutionalized, had certain rights, including the right to treatment. That same year, Congressional hearings were held on the commitment procedures operating in Washington, DC. These hearings focused on broad issues, including the constitutional rights of patients. The fundamental issue discussed was "whether society, which is unable or unwilling to provide treatment, has the right to deprive a patient of his liberty on the sole grounds that he is in need of care."[34]

Over the ensuing decade, there was a subtle change in how the courts viewed civil commitment. There was more concern for the rights of individuals with mental illness—who were viewed as needing the courts' protection from inappropriate involuntary commitment—and less concern for society's right to be protected from these individuals.[27] Eventually, the test for involuntary civil commitment became one of whether these individuals could be considered dangerous to themselves or others.

While economics, idealism, and legal considerations all helped to launch deinstitutionalization, another force expedited it—new antipsychotic drugs. The most widely used drug was **chlorpromazine**, introduced as **Thorazine** by Smith, Kline, and French in 1954. Chlorpromazine was termed **neuroleptic** because it appeared to reduce nervous activity. When used in the institutional setting, the purpose of Thorazine and the other phenothiazines introduced later was to make patients more amenable to other forms of therapy. The drug did produce a remarkably calming effect in psychotic patients, and as a result, patients became more cooperative and hospital psychopathic wards became much quieter. So unusual were the effects of chlorpromazine that the drug in many cases became the *only* form of treatment provided. In these situations, a "**chemical straitjacket**" was said to have been substituted for a physical one.

In the haste to put this drug into use, some of its acute and chronic side effects were overlooked. Acute side effects (such as blurred vision, weight gain, and constipation) can cause compliance failures resulting in relapses or in attempts to self-medicate with other drugs, including drugs of abuse. Long-term use of chlorpromazine can result in deleterious consequences for the central nervous system. The most grave of these chronic side effects is **tardive dyskinesia**—the irreversible, involuntary, and abnormal movements of the tongue, mouth, arms, and legs.[26] In spite of these deleterious effects, Thorazine and the other phenothiazines are still used extensively to treat psychotic patients.

Community Mental Health Centers

In 1961 the report of the Joint Commission on Mental Illness and Health (JCMIH) was released. The JCMIH, established in the 1950s, was made up of representatives of both the American Medical Association and the American Psychiatric Association along with members of several volunteer citizen groups. Among the JCMIH's recommendations was that acute mental illness be treated in community-based settings. Treatment in these settings was viewed as a form of secondary prevention, in which the development of more serious mental breakdowns would be prevented.

President John Kennedy read the commission's report, and in February 1963, he addressed the issue of mental health care in a speech to Congress.[24] The **Mental Retardation Facilities and Community Mental Health Centers (CMHC) Act** was passed later that year and was signed on October 31, 1963. Funding for the legislation was not completed until 1965, and it did not go into effect until 1966.

The original goal of the CMHC Act was to provide one fully staffed, full-time **community mental health center (CMHC)** in each of 1,499 designated catchment areas constituted to cover essentially 100% of the geographic territory in the United States (Figure 11.11). Community mental health centers can meet the requirements for Medicare reimbursement by providing four core services: (1) outpatient services to the elderly, children, and the

neuroleptic drugs drugs that reduce nervous activity; another term for antipsychotic drugs

chemical straitjacket a drug that subdues a mental patient's behavior

tardive dyskinesia irreversible, involuntary, and abnormal movements of the tongue, mouth, arms, and legs, which can result from long-term use of certain antipsychotic drugs (such as chlorpromazine)

Mental Retardation Facilities and Community Mental Health Centers (CMHC) Act a law that made the federal government responsible for assisting in the funding of mental health facilities and services

community mental health center (CMHC) a fully staffed center originally funded by the federal government that provides comprehensive mental health services to local populations

FIGURE 11.11
Between 1966 and 1989, 750 community mental health centers were established.

severely mentally ill; (2) 24-hour-a-day emergency care; (3) day treatment or other partial hospitalization services; and (4) screenings to determine whether to admit patients to state mental facilities.[36]

Although the CMHCs did provide mental health care services to residents in the communities in which they were built, they did not live up to their original expectations of serving those deinstitutionalized persons with chronic mental illness. The latter arrived in communities that in most cases could not provide the type of comprehensive social service network they needed. The necessary funding and services for this were simply not there.

Meanwhile, many older patients with chronic mental illness were never truly deinstitutionalized. Instead, they were **transinstitutionalized** to nursing homes, where the cost of their care was now paid for with federal, rather than state, funds and where the cost of the care turned out to be higher. Many younger patients were also transinstitutionalized when they ended up in jails for major or minor offenses. This problem continues today and is discussed in further detail later in this chapter.

Despite all of the problems that have been attributed to deinstitutionalization, there have been some positive outcomes. One is that a majority of released mental patients surveyed have stated a preference for life in the community over life in an institution. Also, in some communities, halfway houses and support services were forthcoming once the need for these became clear. Finally, the quality of inpatient stays has improved and their duration has been shortened.

The Community Support Movement

The response of NIMH to the criticism that the CMHCs were not meeting the need of deinstitutionalized people with chronic mental illness was the **Community Support Program (CSP)** of 1977. This program offered grants to communities to develop needed social support systems to assist people with chronic mental illness. A goal of Community Support Services is to promote "recovery" in people with serious and persistent mental disorders. Recovery, in this sense, does not mean cure, but rather the achievement of nearly normal life by individuals with chronic mental illness, where a reasonably full range of lifestyle choices is possible.

CSPs have been considered a novel approach because for the first time they recognize that the problems of those with chronic mental illness are—first and foremost—social welfare problems. CSPs arose with the recognition of the fact that many of those with serious mental illness also suffer from deficits in the resources necessary for successful independent living— namely, income, housing, food, medical care, transportation, vocational training, and opportunities for recreation.[37] Thus, CSPs offer an array of services, including housing support,[38] employment support,[39] and education support,[40] all which taken together can be considered *psychosocial rehabilitation*.[37] In summary, the focus of CSPs is on services, not on facilities as was true of the CMHC movement. Between 1986 and 1994, the use of CSPs by people with severe persistent mental disorders more than doubled.

One of the best-known and successful models of psychosocial rehabilitation is the Madison (Wisconsin) Model, also called Assertiveness Community Training (ACT). Support services provided by ACT staff include "domestic skills, medication, finances, housing and advocacy with other providers."[37] Studies have shown that ACT reduces both hospital use and costs. As the Madison Model becomes disseminated into more communities and tested, its role in comprehensive community health care will become clearer.[37,41]

transinstitutionalization
transferring patients from one type of public institution to another, usually as a result of policy change

Community Support Program (CSP)
a federal program that provides funds to communities to develop a social support system for those with mental illness

MENTAL HEALTH CARE CONCERNS IN AMERICA TODAY

Perhaps the most disappointing observation that can be made about community mental health today is that America still has no national mental health program. Although progress in providing appropriate care and support for people with mental illness has been made in some communities, the availability of such care and services is by no means universal. Significant challenges remain: (1) how to provide services to homeless people with serious mental illness and/or co-occurring substance use disorders, (2) resolving the problem of the more than one million people with mental illness incarcerated in American jails and prisons, and (3) making mental health care services available to all who need them at an affordable cost.

Serious Mental Illness in People Who Are Homeless

More than 637,000 people are homeless during any given week in America, and 2.1 million adults experience homelessness over the course of a year.[42] It is estimated that 80% of these homeless individuals are temporarily homeless, 10% are episodically homeless, and 10% are chronically homeless (see Figure 11.12).

"Though only about five percent of people with serious mental illnesses are homeless at any given point in time, as many as two-thirds of all people with serious mental illnesses have experienced homelessness or have been at risk of homelessness at some point in their lives."[44]

Mental Health Problems among People Who Are Homeless

The prevalence of mental health problems among people who are homeless ranges from 2% to 90%, alcohol problems from 4% to 86%, and other drug problems from 1% to 70%. About one-third of adult homeless people have mental problems. Severe and disabling disorders such as schizophrenia, dementia, mental retardation, antisocial personality disorder, and multiple coexisting disorders were higher in homeless persons than in persons included in a household population. However, conditions such as anxiety disorders, major affective disorders, and substance abuse disorders were more common in the domiciled population.[43] In one study, homeless people were 38 times more likely to have schizophrenia, 22 times more likely to have antisocial personality disorder, and 5 times more likely to be cognitively impaired than those who were not homeless.

Approximately one-fifth of the homeless are women; many of those with mental illness do not receive the necessary care.[44] Homeless children are also more likely than their domiciled peers to experience developmental delays, emotional problems, abuse, and mental problems.[43]

Homeless people, including those who have mental illness, are more exposed to environmental factors such as extremes in temperature, moisture, burns, crowding, assaults, and motor vehicle–related injuries than their domiciled counterparts. The effects of these environmental factors may be worsened by anxiety about where to find the next meal and safe shelter and, sometimes, by the effects of chronic alcohol or drug abuse.[45]

Substance Use Disorders in People Who Are Homeless

About half of all adults who are homeless have substance use disorders, and many have co-occurring mental illness as well. The problem of co-occurring disorders (serious mental illness and disordered substance use) as they relate to homelessness has been recognized by the U.S. Department of Health and Human Services, which in 2003 pledged $1.6 billion over the next five years to reduce drug use, build treatment capacity, and increase access to

FIGURE 11.12

As many as two-thirds of all people with serious mental illness have experienced homelessness or been at risk for homelessness at some point in their lives.

services that promote recovery from substance use among the homeless.[42] This federal effort, described in *Blueprint for Change: Ending Chronic Homelessness for Persons with Serious Mental Illnesses and/or Co-occurring Substance Use Disorders,* is meant to work hand-in-hand with state and community comprehensive plans to end homelessness.[42]

The New Asylums: Mental Health Care in Our Jails and Prisons

Are local jails, and state and federal prisons, the most appropriate site for housing and treating people with mental illness in this country? Although the answer is almost certainly no, data suggest that this is what is occurring. According to a 2006 Department of Justice report, more than half of all prison and jail inmates have mental health problems.[46] This includes 705,600 inmates in state prisons, 70,200 in federal prisons, and 479,900 in local jails. These figures represent 56% of state prisoners, 45% of federal prisoners, and 64% of jail inmates (see Table 11.3). Furthermore, approximately 24% of jail inmates, 15% of state prisoners, and 10% of federal prisoners reported at least one symptom that meets the criteria for a psychotic disorder.[46]

A study published in 2004 revealed that rapid growth in the number of state prison facilities and the prison population has outstripped the slower growth of mental health services.[47] The number of state prisons in 1988 was 757; this number grew to 1,097 by 2000, a 44.9% increase. During that same period, the number of prisoners grew from 505,712 to 1,084,625, a 114.5% increase.[47] The study found that although mental health services were available in more prisons, the percentage of prisons performing psychiatric testing and assessment had declined. Thus, mental health services became less available to the prison population during that period.

In Ohio, 16% of state prison inmates require hospitalization for mental disorders.[48] In some cases, persons who were originally arrested for relatively minor crimes, such as trespassing or stealing a bicycle, remain in prison for years beyond their original sentence because they do not meet the good conduct guidelines required for release or parole (Figure 11.13). Mental illness (paranoid schizophrenia, bipolar disorder, or other serious mental disorder) may preclude inmates' compliance with their prescribed medication schedules. Without these medications, inmates with mental illness may be incapable of "good behavior," a prerequisite for parole or release. In fact, they may become candidates for placement in more isolated and restrictive prison units.[48]

For those whose mental illness is controlled with medication, and who remain on that medication, release is possible. Upon their release, these people are provided with enough medication for a short period (usually a two-week supply). However, it can take up to three months to schedule an appointment with a physician to obtain a prescription for their needed

---

Table 11.3
Prevalence of Mental Health Problems among Inmates in American Prisons and Jails, 2005

Mental Health Problem	State Prison Inmates		Federal Prison Inmates		Local Jail Inmates	
	Number	Percentage	Number	Percentage	Number	Percentage
Any mental health problem*	705,600	56.2	70,200	44.8	479,900	64.2
No mental health problem	549,000	43.8	86,500	55.2	267,600	35.8
Estimated number of inmates (June 30, 2005)	1,255,514	100.0	156,643	100.0	747,529	100.0

*Details do not add to totals because of rounding.

Source: Table developed from data provided in: James, D. J., and L. E. Glaze (2006). *Mental Health Problems of Prison and Jail Inmates.* Bureau of Justice Statistics Special Report (NCJ pub. no. 213600). Available at www.ojp.usdoj.gov/bjs/pub/.

medication. For this and other reasons, many of those released find it difficult to remain in compliance with their release documents. Whereas some, who are released directly to well-functioning community support programs or halfway houses, may experience extended periods of recovery, others find that it is all too easy to stop taking their medications. Their mental condition deteriorates, and their behavior becomes such that they end up back in prison. It has been said that it is easier for a mentally ill person without financial means to obtain treatment for mental illness in the prison system than on the outside.[48]

Two other populations at high risk for developing mental illness are citizens exposed to disasters and soldiers returning from combat zones. For example, 20% of Manhattan residents living near the World Trade Center at the time of the attacks of September 11, 2001, had symptoms consistent with post-traumatic stress disorder (PTSD) five to eight weeks after the attack, and nearly 10% suffered from depression, which occurred most often in those who had suffered losses as a result of the attack.[49] The police officers and firefighters of New Orleans who responded following Hurricane Katrina were exposed to both physical injuries and illnesses and to psychological stressors. Approximately 19% of police officers and 22% of firefighters reported symptoms of PTSD, and 26% of police officers and 27% of firefighters reported symptoms of major depression.[50]

Military service in a combat zone increases one's risk of experiencing PTSD, major depression, or other mental health problems (see Figure 11.14). A 2006 study found a high rate of mental health services utilization among veterans of Operation Iraqi Freedom. The study noted that the prevalence rates of mental health problems were consistently higher among those deployed to Iraq (19%) than those deployed to Afghanistan (11%). Thirty-five percent of veterans returning from Iraq accessed mental health services in the year after returning home.[51] These findings have implications for estimating the level of mental health services that may be needed in our communities.

FIGURE 11.13

Many prison inmates with mental illness remain in prison years beyond their original sentence because they are unable to conform to good conduct requirements of the prison system.

MEETING THE NEEDS OF THOSE WITH MENTAL ILLNESS: PREVENTION AND TREATMENT

Meeting the needs of people with mental illness represents a significant challenge for many communities as they strive to provide effective and economical prevention and treatment services to this segment of the population.

Prevention

The basic concepts of prevention in community health were presented in Chapter 4. The concepts of primary, secondary, and tertiary prevention can be applied to community mental health. Application of prevention strategies is considered much more cost-effective than treatment.[52]

Primary prevention in community mental health has as its goal forestalling the onset of mental illness. Two examples are training in cognitive problem solving to prevent failure in school and social support groups for the newly widowed to prevent depression.

FIGURE 11.14

Military troops returning from duty in combat zones are heavy users of mental health services when these services are accessible.

Effective primary prevention reduces the incidence (rate of new cases) of mental illness in the community.

Secondary prevention, while not reducing the incidence of mental illness, can reduce its prevalence by shortening the duration of episodes, through case finding and prompt intervention. Employee assistance programs, juvenile delinquency diversion programs, and crisis intervention programs are all examples of secondary prevention of mental illness.

Tertiary prevention, treatment, and rehabilitation do not actually reduce the prevalence of mental illness in the community. Instead, they ameliorate the illness and prevent further problems for the individual and the community. Supported living programs, previously discussed in "The Community Support Movement" section, are examples of tertiary prevention.[52]

Preventive Services

Communities today are challenged with a difficult task in providing mental health care services for their members. These services need to be comprehensive, including primary, secondary, and tertiary prevention services.

The task of providing primary prevention services falls mainly on the private voluntary agencies, such as the National Mental Health Association and its state and local affiliates. These agencies provide educational speakers, videos, books, and pamphlets about mental health, mental illness, and services. They also may offer workshops on stress management, self-esteem development, and coping-skills development. Some sponsor support groups for parents of children who are emotionally disabled or suffer from some other behavioral disorder. These agencies also act as referral agencies for those in crisis.

The needs of those in the community who require mental health care (secondary prevention) are met by an assortment of providers, including treatment providers in private clinics, CMHCs, hospital emergency rooms, and social service providers in Social Security, welfare, veterans, and housing offices. For securing the necessary services, this hodgepodge of federal, state, and local offices and social programs is overwhelming even to someone in good mental health.

While some would say that community mental health services are improving by and large, significant problems still remain. For example, a significant gap persists in the availability and quality of care for insured and uninsured patients. Continued federal and state budget constraints suggest that this gap will continue to widen.

Treatment Approaches

psychotherapy
a treatment that involves verbal communication between the patient and a trained clinician

Treatment goals for mental disorders are (1) to reduce symptoms, (2) to improve personal and social functioning, (3) to develop and strengthen coping skills, and (4) to promote behaviors that make a person's life better. The two basic approaches to treating mental disorders are *psychotherapy* and *psychopharmacology*.[2]

Psychotherapy

cognitive-behavioral therapy
treatment based on learning theory in which a patient learns adaptive skills through rewards and satisfaction

Psychotherapy or psychosocial therapy involves treatment through verbal communication. Three common types are used—supportive, psychodynamic, and cognitive-behavioral therapy. The first two types involve face-to-face discussions with therapists who are trained to listen, interpret, define, and resolve the troubling personal problems of the patient (see Figure 11.15). There are numerous approaches to psychotherapy, including interpersonal, couple, group, and family approaches. Psychodynamic psychotherapy examines current problems as they relate to earlier experiences, even from childhood, while cognitive psychotherapy focuses on faulty or distorted thinking patterns. Psychotherapy is most likely to be successful in less severe cases of emotional distress or when used in conjunction with other approaches (such as psychopharmacologic therapy). **Cognitive-behavioral therapy** is a type of therapy that involves the use of learning theory in which a patient learns adaptive skills through rewards and satisfaction. Cognitive-behavioral therapy usually involves the cooperation of persons important to the patient, such as other family members. Included in behavioral therapy are biofeedback, stress management, and relaxation training. This type of therapy can also be used together with medication.

Psychopharmacology

Psychopharmacological therapy involves treatment with medications. This treatment is based upon the recognition that mental illnesses are medical illnesses just like hypothyroidism or diabetes and as such are treatable with drugs. Since the introduction of chlorpromazine in 1954, there has been a significant increase in the number and types of approved medications for the treatment of mental disorders. Conditions for which medications exist are schizophrenia, bipolar disorder, major depression, anxiety, panic disorder, and obsessive-compulsive disorder. Because of the seriousness of the side effects of some of these drugs, and because of the nature of mental illness itself, compliance failures (failure to adhere to the prescribed schedule for taking the drug) are common.

Another form of biomedical therapy is ECT, formerly known as shock therapy. In ECT, which was discussed earlier in this chapter, alternating electric current passes through the brain to produce unconsciousness and a convulsive seizure. This form of treatment is sometimes used for major depression, selected cases of schizophrenia, or overwhelming suicide ideation, especially when the need for treatment is seen as urgent. Contemporary ECT methods employ low doses of electric shock to the brain. General anesthetics are provided to reduce the unpleasant side effects.

FIGURE 11.15
Psychotherapy is usually only one of the services needed by persons who are suffering from mental illness.

One of the objectives of *Healthy People 2010* is to increase the proportion of adults with mental disorders who are receiving treatment (see Box 11.3). Unfortunately, the same force that is driving most of the other types of health care decisions, namely cost, also drives decisions about treatment for mental disorders. Thus, treatment goals are becoming more and more outcome based. An "effective outcome" is defined in terms that "balance employers' needs and interests with those of patients: alleviating a patient's symptoms of distress (to reduce overall medical expenditures), improving functioning (to boost job productivity), and enhancing employees' sense of well-being (to promote positive attitudes, job satisfaction and high morale)."[53]

psychopharmaco-logical therapy treatment for mental illness that involves medications

Self-Help Support Groups

Another approach or adjunct to successful treatment is **self-help support groups,** groups of concerned members of the community who are united by a shared interest, concern, or deficit not shared by other members of the community. The shared characteristic is often stigmatizing or isolating and viewed as something not normal by the rest of the members of the community.[52] Self-help support groups usually operate without professional leadership; instead, leadership responsibilities are often shared by members of the group. The roles of help-giver and help-receiver are entirely interchangeable. These groups serve to replace the community that was "lost" through stigmatization or isolation. Self-help support groups also reduce vulnerability and supply feedback and guidance to their members. They also provide their

self-help support groups groups of concerned members of the community who are united by a shared interest, concern, or deficit not shared by other members of the community (Alcoholics Anonymous, for example)

BOX
11.3
HEALTHY PEOPLE 2010: OBJECTIVES

Objective 18-9: Increase the proportion of adults with mental disorders who receive treatment.

Objective	Increase in Adults with Mental Disorders Receiving Treatment	Baseline Year 2002 (unless noted)	2010 Target
		Percentage	
18.9a	Adults aged 18 to 54 with serious mental illness	62	68
18.9b	Adults aged 18 years and older with recognized depression	58	64
18.9c	Adults aged 18 years and older with schizophrenia	60 (1981)	75
18.9d	Adults aged 18 years and older with generalized anxiety disorder	60	79

Source: CDC (2006). *DATA2010 . . . The Healthy People Database—June 2006 Edition.* Available at http://wonder.cdc.gov.

For Further Thought

Less than one in four adults with recognized depression receives treatment. What reasons can you think of that contribute to this statistic?

National Alliance for the Mentally Ill (NAMI) a national self-help group that supports the belief that major mental disorders are brain diseases that are of genetic origin and biological in nature and are diagnosable and treatable with medications

members with a philosophy and an outlook on their affliction.[52] Examples of self-help groups are the **National Alliance for the Mentally Ill (NAMI),** Recovery, Inc., and Alcoholics Anonymous (AA). For more information on NAMI, see Box 11.4.

Federal Initiatives for Mental Health Care

Until recently, the federal government's leadership in community mental health has been spotty. While federal funds have been made available for research, surveillance, and goal setting for mental health, there has been less support for prevention, early intervention, and treatment for those with mental illness. The "decade of the brain" culminated in 1999 when the U.S. Department of Health and Human Services issued *Mental Health: A Report of the Surgeon General.* This comprehensive report attempted to put mental health and mental illness

---

BOX
11.4
NATIONAL ALLIANCE FOR THE MENTALLY ILL

The National Alliance for the Mentally Ill (NAMI) "is the nation's largest grassroots mental health organization dedicated to improving the lives of persons living with serious mental illness and their families. Founded in 1979, NAMI has become the nation's voice on mental illness, a national organization including NAMI organizations in every state and in over 1,100 local communities across the country who join together to meet the NAMI mission through advocacy, research, support, and education."

According to its mission statement, "NAMI is dedicated to the eradication of mental illnesses and to the improvement of the quality of life of all whose lives are affected by these diseases." NAMI members, leaders, and friends share the agency's mission of "support, education, advocacy, and research for people living with

mental illness through various activities" that include maintaining a Web site and toll-free help line, sponsoring a Mental Illness Awareness Week, and maintaining a public education speakers bureau.

NAMI also provides a cadre of educational programs and a network of support groups. NAMI "advocates on the federal level to ensure nondiscriminatory and equitable federal and private-sector policies are in place as well as a commitment to research for the treatment and cures for mental illness." As with other voluntary health organizations, NAMI is involved in fund-raising, and does so with events such as NAMI Walks and an annual black-tie event, the Unmasking Mental Illness Science and Research Gala, held in Washington, DC.

More information about NAMI is available at their Web site: www.NAMI.org.

"front and center" among America's public health problems. It was more than just a status report, although it provided many useful statistics. It was an excellent compilation of mental health care services, service needs, and barriers to receiving these services. According to the foreword, "The report lays down a challenge to the Nation—to our communities, our health and social service agencies, our policy makers, employers, and citizens—to take action."[2]

In 2002 President George W. Bush created the New Freedom Commission on Mental Health. The commission's report, *Achieving the Promise: Transforming Mental Health Care in America,* is available at the commission's Web site, www.mentalhealthcommission.gov/. The commission recognizes that mental illnesses are the leading cause of disability in the United States, Canada, and western Europe and that they carry a high financial cost—$79 billion in the United States alone. Further, the report notes the problems of fragmentation and gaps in care for children, adults, and older adults with serious mental illness and the "lack of national priority for mental health and suicide prevention."[1]

As its title indicates, the commission's report calls for a transformed mental health care system; it establishes six goals, with recommendations for achieving each goal. The commission envisions a mental health system in which (1) Americans understand that mental health is essential to overall health, (2) mental health care is consumer and family driven, (3) disparities in mental health services are eliminated, (4) early mental health screening, assessment, and referral to services are common practices, (5) excellent mental health care is delivered and research is accelerated, and (6) technology is used to access mental health care and information. Although the commission did not propose any new programs or agencies to assist the nation in achieving these broad goals, it did cite a number of successful "model" programs as examples that could be followed by other communities. The report does a good job of identifying the burden of mental illness and the challenges America faces in transforming the systems involved in intervention, prevention, and treatment of mental disorders. Likewise, the commission's vision of a "transformed system" is praiseworthy. However, the report stops short of describing a road map or scheme for the transformation, and certainly doesn't recommend the expenditure of any federal funds to achieve the stated goals.

The federal agencies with primary responsibilities for mental health issues in the Department of Health and Human Services are the National Institute of Mental Health (NIMH), one of the National Institutes of Health, and the **Substance Abuse and Mental Health Services Administration (SAMHSA).** The mission of NIMH is "to reduce the burden of mental illness and behavioral disorders through research on mind, brain and behavior."[54]

Within SAMHSA are three centers: the Center for Substance Abuse Treatment (CSAT), the Center for Substance Abuse Prevention (CSAP), and the Center for Mental Health Services (CMHS), mentioned earlier. The mission of the CMHS is to "improve the availability and accessibility of high quality community-based services for people with or at risk for mental illness and their families."[55]

Community Mental Health and Managed Care

Currently, all eyes in the mental health care field are watching the dramatic effects that managed care organizations (MCOs) are producing in community mental health care. One effect has been to reduce the cost of mental health services.[2] This reduction is achieved by removing overutilization, such as unnecessary hospitalization. For MCOs, the cost of providing care is of prime importance, and in each case cost must be justified by an outcome that is effective. The risks of cost containment are that it will diminish either access to care or quality of care.

The term created by the managed care industry that applies to mental health and substance abuse care services is **behavioral health care services.**[56] Under managed care programs, medical services are provided only when a condition is serious enough that care is considered "medically necessary." Whether this requirement has been met may be difficult to

Substance Abuse and Mental Health Services Administration (SAMHSA) the parent agency within the Department of Health and Human Services that contains the Center for Mental Health Services

behavioral health care services the managed care term for mental health and substance abuse/dependence care services determine in cases when a patient with mental illness presents with a "behavioral health" condition. Some MCOs issue separate contracts to specialized vendors known as **managed behavioral health care organizations (MBHOs).** This process has come to be known as a "carve-out."

Furthermore, in treating "behavioral health" problems, there is rarely a consensus among the stakeholders as to what constitutes a good outcome. One important trend in behavioral health care today is the application of **evidence-based practices.** That is, only those interventions for which there is evidence of effectiveness are to be used. In an effort to document the effectiveness of interventions for substance abuse and mental health disorders, the Office of Managed Care in the Center for Mental Health Services has published a report describing cost-effective behavioral health interventions.[57] The report recommends six services for consideration by MCOs or MBHOs. These are prenatal and infancy home visits, smoking cessation education and counseling, targeted short-term mental health therapy, self-care education for adults, presurgical educational intervention for adults, and brief counseling and advice to reduce alcohol use. It remains to be seen whether MCOs and MBHOs will embrace this report and provide these recommended services.

Another issue in mental health care coverage is parity. **Parity** refers to the effort to treat mental health care financing on the same basis as financing for general health care services. Proponents for parity suggest it is simply a matter of fairness. In the past, care for mental illnesses has often not been provided or has been reimbursed at a lower level than that for other medical conditions. In 1996 the Mental Health Parity Act was passed. This act was implemented in 1998 but fell short of requiring complete parity between medical coverage and mental health care coverage.[2]

In 1999, President Clinton directed the Office of Personnel Management (OPM) to ensure parity of mental health and substance abuse benefits for the Federal Employees Health Benefits (FEHB) program. Through the OPM, federal employees who enroll can select from more than 350 health insurance products. Beginning January 1, 2001, the OPM required parity of coverage for mental health and substance abuse care. That is, the plans had to be "identical with regard to traditional medical care deductibles, coinsurance, co-pays, and day and visit limitations."[58]

To accomplish this, the OPM encouraged the plans to employ managed care techniques. Many of the plans contracted with MBHOs to help control costs. An analysis of this program noted that use of mental health and substance abuse services increased after implementation of the parity plan, but that during the same time period use also increased in comparison (control) plans without parity. Thus, it was determined that access to mental health care services neither increased nor decreased under parity. The analysis failed to detect any decrease in the quality of care, but out-of-pocket expenditures by beneficiaries were reduced.[58] It remains to be seen whether parity in coverage will spread to the wider marketplace.

Changes in the practice of mental health care are part of the reason that parity in insurance coverage is now possible. Twenty to thirty years ago, long-term psychotherapy was a common form of treatment. Today, many mental health care providers use primarily short-term or time-limited psychotherapeutic strategies and/or psychopharmacologic therapies; long-term treatment in inpatient settings is rare.[59]

It is difficult to determine whether the nation, states, and local communities will respond to the needs of those with mental illness in the future. It will depend on economics, on the degree to which taxpayers have been personally touched by mental illness, or on the degree to which they are willing to tolerate the spectacle of homeless people with mental illness in their communities and in their jails and prisons. A key task facing communities is to find ways to unite formal services and informal supports to promote recovery by people who are coping with mental disorders.

CHAPTER SUMMARY

- Mental illness constitutes a major community health concern because of its chronicity, prevalence, and the demands it places on community resources.

- Americans are afflicted with a variety of mental disorders, caused by genetic factors, environmental factors, or a combination of both. These disorders, which can range from mild to severe, are often chronic and may limit the ability of those afflicted to live independently.

- Stress, resulting from social and environmental forces, can have a detrimental influence on both physical and mental health.

- Over the years, society's response to the needs of those with mental illness has been characterized by long periods of apathy interrupted by enthusiastic movements for new and enlightened approaches to care.

- Deinstitutionalization, in which thousands of mental patients housed in state and county hospitals were discharged and returned to their communities, was the most prominent movement of the twentieth century. The origins of many of the current problems in community mental health care, such as a large number of homeless people and prison inmates with mental illness, can be traced to this movement.

- Community support programs for those living in our communities with mental illness, such as the Madison Model, show promise that with community support, many individuals can achieve the level of recovery necessary for them to be successfully integrated into local communities.

- Combat-zone military veterans and survivors of and responders to natural and human-made disasters are at especially high risk for developing mental disorders.

- The basic concepts of prevention in community health (primary, secondary, and tertiary prevention) can be applied to the prevention and treatment of mental disorders.

- Among the most common treatment approaches are psychotherapy, including cognitive-behavioral therapy, and psychopharmacology, which is based on the use of medications.

- While there is no national program to provide treatment for those with mental illness, there have been several federal initiatives aimed at improving prevention and treatment.

- *Healthy People 2010* objectives include reducing the suicide rate among Americans and increasing the proportion of those with mental disorders who receive treatment.

- Important issues face those concerned with providing services for those with mental disorders. One is finding ways to provide a variety of preventive, intervention, and treatment services to a heterogeneous group of clients, such as the homeless, in a climate of cost containment under managed care. Another is finding a way to achieve parity in coverage and cost of service reimbursement between mental health care services and services for other types of medical conditions.

REVIEW QUESTIONS

1. What is meant by the term *mental health?*

2. What are the characteristics of a mentally healthy person?

3. What is a mental disorder?

4. Name and give examples of the different causes of mental disorders.

5. What evidence is there that mental illness is one of our most pervasive public health problems in the United States?

6. What is stress? Give some examples of stressors.

7. How can stress cause physical illness?

8. What is the relationship between stress and mental health?

9. How were those with mental illness cared for in Colonial America?

10. What was included in Tuke's therapy known as "moral treatment"?

11. What role did Dorothea Dix play in the treatment of indigent people with mental illness?

12. How would you characterize the treatment of those with mental illness in state hospitals prior to World War II?

13. When did the mental hygiene movement occur in the United States? What was the focus of this movement?

14. Who founded the National Committee on Mental Hygiene, which later became the National Mental Health Association?

15. What piece of legislation resulted in the establishment of the National Institute of Mental Health, and what were the purposes of the Institute?

16. Define the word *deinstitutionalization.* When did it start in the United States? What caused it?

17. What is a "chemical straitjacket"?

18. Why was there a movement toward community mental health centers in the early 1960s?

19. What services are provided by community mental health centers?

20. Why is the Community Support Program considered a novel approach?

SCENARIO: ANALYSIS AND RESPONSE

1. Let's assume that Maria Sanchez is not alone in her concerns about Lynn, her new neighbor. Another neighbor, Paul, has called for a meeting of the residents to discuss this "new type" of resident. You are a resident too, and he is expecting you to attend. What is your response?
2. What worries might residents express regarding their new neighbor?
3. Would it make any difference to you whether Lynn found a job and was away at work during a good part of the day?
4. Do you suppose the landlord knew about Lynn's medical history when he or she rented the unit to her? Can landlords refuse to rent to someone like Lynn?
5. Are you aware of any federal laws, such as the Fair Housing Act or the Americans with Disabilities Act (ADA), that could bear on this matter?
6. If you were Maria, what would be your response? What would you do?

Resource: Substance Abuse and Mental Health Services Administration Resource Center to Address Discrimination and Stigma. "Combating NIMBYism in Providing Housing to People Who Have Mental Illness." Available at http://www.stopstigma.samhsa.gov/archtel_pdfs/combatingNIMBY.pdf.

---

21. What types of support are provided by Community Support Programs?
22. Approximately what percentage of the homeless are living with mental illness? What percentage of state prison inmates have mental health problems?
23. Describe primary, secondary, and tertiary prevention of mental illness and give an example of a service for each level of prevention.
24. What is involved in psychotherapy for mental illness? In cognitive-behavioral therapy? In psychopharmacological therapy?
25. What are self-help support groups? How do they increase treatment effectiveness?
26. What is the mission of the National Institute for Mental Health?
27. What is the mission of the Center for Mental Health Services?
28. What does the term *behavioral health* mean with regard to mental health care?
29. What are evidence-based practices with regard to the care for those with mental illness?
30. What are some issues surrounding managed care for the mentally ill?
31. What does *parity* mean with regard to health care services for the mentally ill?

ACTIVITIES

1. Make a list of all the stressors you have experienced in the last two weeks. Select two of the items on the list and answer the following questions about them:
Did you realize the stressor was a stressor when you first confronted it? Explain.
What physiological responses did you notice that you had when confronted with the stressor?
Have you confronted the stressor before? Explain your answer.
What stress mediators (coping responses) do you have to deal with each of the stressors?
Do you feel you will some day fall victim to a disease of adaptation?

2. Using a local telephone book or one from your hometown, identify the organizations in the community that you believe would provide mental health services. Then create a list of the agencies/organizations. Divide the list into three sections based upon the type of service (primary, secondary, tertiary prevention) offered. If you are not sure what type of services are offered, call the agency/organization to find out. After you have completed your list, write a paragraph or two about what you feel to be the status of mental health care in your community.

3. Make an appointment with someone in the counseling and psychological service center on your campus for an orientation to the services offered by the center. Most mental health services range from stress management to test anxiety to individual counseling. Find out what your school has to offer and write a one-page summary of available services.

4. Call agencies or service groups in your community to find out what services are needed for the homeless. Also find out how serious the homeless situation is in the community and what plans there are to deal with the problem. Summarize your findings in a two-page paper. Agencies or services to call include the American Red Cross, the local police department, the Salvation Army, the local soup kitchen, a community mental health center, local hospitals, local homeless shelters, and other shelters.

5. Look through your local phone book or call the community information/crisis center to locate a mental health or substance abuse self-help support group. Call the group's number and find out what kinds of open meetings or public education activities they have.

COMMUNITY HEALTH ON THE WEB

The Internet contains a wealth of information about community mental health. Increase your knowledge of some of the topics presented in this chapter by accessing the Jones and Bartlett Publishers Web site at **http://health.jbpub.com/book/communityhealth/6e** and follow the links to complete the following Web activities.

- Center for Mental Health Services
- National Institute of Mental Health
- National Alliance on Mental Illness

REFERENCES

1. President's New Freedom Commission on Mental Health (2003). *Achieving the Promise: Transforming Mental Health Care in America*. Rockville, MD: Author.

2. U.S. Department of Health and Human Services (1999). *Mental Health: A Report of the Surgeon General*. Rockville, MD: Substance Abuse and Mental Health Services Administration.

3. Manderscheid, R. W., and M. A. Sonnenschein, eds. (1996). *Mental Health, United States, 1996* (DHHS pub. no. SMA 96-3098). Washington, DC: U.S. Government Printing Office.

4. Benton, S. A., J. M. Robertson, W. C. Tseng, F. B. Newton, and S. L. Benton (2003). "Changes in Counseling Center Client Problems across 13 Years." *Professional Psychology: Research and Practice*, 34(1): 66–72.

5. Office of the Surgeon General, U.S. Department of Health and Human Services (3 January 2001). "Surgeon General Releases a National Action Agenda on Children's Mental Health." *HHS News*. Available at http://www.hhs.gov/surgeongeneral/news/pressreleases/pressreleasechildren.htm.

6. American Psychiatric Association (2000). *Diagnostic and Statistical Manual of Mental Disorders*, 4th ed., text revision. Washington, DC: Author.

7. Substance Abuse and Mental Health Services Administration. (2006). *Results from the 2005 National Survey on Drug Use and Health: National Findings* (Office of Applied Studies, NSDUH Series H-30; DHHS pub. no. SMA 06-4194). Rockville, MD: Author. Available at http://www.oas.samhsa.gov/NSDUH/2k5NSDUH/2k5results.htm.

8. Children's Defense Fund (2005). *The State of Children in America's Union 2005*. Washington, DC: Author. Available at http://www.childrensdefense.org.

9. Rouse, B. A. (1995). *Substance Abuse and Mental Health Statistics Sourcebook* (DHHS pub. no. SMA 95-3064). Washington, DC: U.S. Government Printing Office.

10. Miniño, A. M., M. Heron, and B. L. Smith (2006). "Deaths: Preliminary Data for 2004." *National Vital Statistics Report*, 54(19): 1–52.

11. Bramlett, M. D., and M. D. Mosher (2002). *Cohabitation, Marriage, Divorce, and Remarriage in the United States* (Vital and Health Statistics no. 23). Hyattsville, MD: National Center for Health Statistics. Available at http://www.cdc.gov/nchs/releases/02news/div_mar_cohab.htm.

12. Johnston, L. D., P. M. O'Malley, J. G. Bachman, and J. E. Schulenbert (2006). *Monitoring the Future National Survey Results on Drug Use 1975–2005. Vol. I: Secondary School Students* (NIH pub. no. 06-5883).

Rockville, MD: National Institute on Drug Abuse. Available at http://www.monitoringthefuture.org/pubs/.

13. Johnston, L. D., P. M. O'Malley, J. G. Bachman, and J. E. Schulenbert (2006). *Monitoring the Future National Survey Results on Drug Use 1975–2005. Vol. II: College Students and Adults Ages 19–40* (NIH pub. no. 06-5884). Rockville, MD: National Institute on Drug Abuse. Available at http://www.monitoringthefuture.org/pubs/.

14. Holmes, T. H., and R. H. Rahe (1967). "The Social Readjustment Rating Scale." *Journal of Psychosomatic Research*, 11: 213–218.

15. Selye, H. (1946). "The General Adaptation Syndrome and Disease of Adaptation." *Journal of Clinical Endocrinology and Metabolism*, 6: 117–130.

16. Sarafino, E. P. (1990). *Health Psychology: Biopsychological Interactions*. New York: John Wiley & Sons.

17. McKinney, M. E., P. J. Jofschire, J. C. Buell, and R. S. Eliot (1984). "Hemodynamic and Biochemical Responses to Stress: The Necessary Link between Type A Behavior and Cardiovascular Disease." *Behavioral Medicine Update*, 64(4): 16–21.

18. Scheiderman, N. (1983). "Animal Behavior Models of Coronary Heart Disease." In D. S. Krantz, A. Baum, and J. E. Singer, eds., *Handbook of Psychology and Health*, vol. 3. Hillsdale, NJ: Erlbaum.

19. Jemmott, J. B., and S. E. Locke (1984). "Psychosocial Factors, Immunologic Mediation, and Human Susceptibility to Infectious Diseases. How Much Do We Know?" *Psychological Bulletin*, 95: 78–108.

20. Schleifer, S. J., B. Scott, M. Stein, and S. E. Keller (1986). "Behavioral and Developmental Aspects of Immunity." *Journal of the American Academy of Child Psychiatry*, 26: 751–763.

21. Wimbush, F. B., and M. L. Nelson (2000). "Stress, Psychosomatic Illness, and Health." In V. H. Rice, ed., *Handbook of Stress, Coping and Health: Implications for Nursing Research, Theory and Practice*. Thousand Oaks, CA: Sage Publications.

22. Baer, P. E., L. B. Garmezy, R. J. McLaughlin, A. D. Pokorny, and M. J. Wernick (1987). "Stress, Coping, Family Conflict, and Adolescent Alcohol Use." *Journal of Behavioral Medicine*, 10: 449–466.

23. Conway, T. L., R. R. Vickers, H. W. Ward, and R. H. Rahe (1981). "Occupational Stress and Variation in Cigarette, Coffee, and Alcohol Consumption." *Journal of Health and Social Behavior*, 22: 155–165.

24. Payne, W. A., D. B. Hahn, and E. B. Lucas (2006). *Understanding Your Health*, 9th ed. New York: McGraw-Hill Higher Education.

25. Grob, G. N. (1994). *The Mad among Us: A History of the Care of America's Mentally Ill*. New York: The Free Press.

26. Johnson, A. B. (1990). *Out of Bedlam: The Truth about Deinstitutionalization*. New York: Basic Books, 306.

27. Gerhart, U. C. (1990). *Caring for the Chronic Mentally Ill*. Itasca, IL: F. E. Peacock, 5.

28. Mosher, L. R., and L. Burti (1989). *Community Mental Health*. New York: W. W. Norton.

29. Foley, H. A., and S. S. Sharfstein (1983). *Madness and Government*. Washington, DC: American Psychiatric Press.

30. Dain, N. (1980). *Clifford Beers: Advocate for the Insane*. Pittsburgh, PA: University of Pittsburgh Press.

31. Sabbatini, R. M. E. (1997). "The History of Shock Therapy in Psychiatry." *Brain and Mind Magazine—Electronic Magazine on Neuroscience*. Available at http://www.epub.org.br/cm/n04/ historia/shock_i.htm.

32. Rosenbach, M., R. Hermann, and R. Dorwart (1997). "Use of Electroconvulsive Therapy in the Medicare Population between 1987 and 1992." *Psychiatric Services*, 48(12): 1537–1542.

33. Sabbatini, R. M. E. (1997). "The History of Lobotomy." *Brain and Mind Magazine—Electronic Magazine on Neuroscience*. Available at http://www.epub.org.br/cm/n02/historia/psicocirg_i.htm.

34. Grob, G. N. (1991). *From Asylum to Community*. Princeton, NJ: Princeton University Press.

35. Peele, R. (1991). "Can a Public Psychiatric Administrator Be Ethical?" In S. L. Keill, ed., *Administrative Issues in Public Mental Health*. San Francisco: Jossey-Bass, 41–50.

36. Centers for Medicare and Medicaid Services (2002). "Medicare Expands Crackdown on Waste, Fraud, and Abuse in Community Mental Health Centers [Press release]." Available at http://www.cms.hhs.gov/media/press/release.asp?Counter589.

37. Levine, M., P. A. Toro, and D. V. Perkins (1993). "Social and Community Interventions." *Annual Review of Psychology*, 44: 525-558.

38. Carling, P. J. (1993). "Housing and Supports for Persons with Mental Illness: Emerging Approaches to Research and Practice." *Hospital and Community Psychiatry*, 44(5): 439-449.

39. Bond, G. R., R. E. Drake, K. T. Mueser, and D. R. Becker (1997). "An Update on Supported Employment for People with Severe Mental Illness." *Psychiatric Services*, 48(3): 335-346.

40. Mowbray, C., T. D. Bybee, and W. Shriner (1996). "Characteristics of Participants in a Supported Education Program for Adults with Psychiatric Disabilities." *Psychiatric Services*, 47(12): 1371-1377.

41. Dixon, L. (2000). "Gold Award: A Community Treatment Program, Mendota Mental Health Institute, Madison, Wisconsin." *Psychiatric Services*, 51(6): 755-758.

42. U.S. Department of Health and Human Services, Substance Abuse and Mental Health Services Administration (2003). *Blueprint for Change: Ending Chronic Homelessness for Persons with Serious Mental Illnesses and/or Co-occurring Substance Use Disorders* (DHHS pub. no. SMA-04-3870). Rockville, MD: Author.

43. Fischer, P. J., R. E. Drake, and W. R. Breakey (1992). "Mental Health Problems among Homeless Persons: A Review of Epidemiological Research from 1980 to 1990." In R. H. Lamb, L. L. Bachrach, and F. I. Kass, eds., *Treating the Homeless Mentally Ill: A Report of the Task Force on the Homeless Mentally Ill*. Washington, DC: American Psychiatric Association, 75-93.

44. Robertson, M. J., and M. A. Winkleby (1996). "Mental Health Problems of Homeless Women and Differences across Subgroups." *Annual Review of Public Health*, 17: 311-336.

45. Brickner, P. W. (1992). "Medical Concerns of Homeless Patients." In R. H. Lamb, L. L. Bachrach, and F. I. Kass, eds., *Treating the Homeless Mentally Ill: A Report of the Task Force on the Homeless Mentally Ill*. Washington, DC: American Psychiatric Association, 249-261.

46. James, D. J., and L. E. Glaze (2006). *Mental Health Problems of Prison and Jail Inmates* (NCJ pub. no. 213600). Available at http://www.ojp.usdoj.gov/bjs/pub/pdf/mhppji.pdf.

47. Mandersheid, R. W., A. Gravesande, and I. S. Goldstrom (2004). "Growth of Mental Health Services in State Adult Correctional Facilities, 1988 to 2000." *Psychiatric Services*, 55(8): 869-872.

48. Frontline (2005). *The New Asylums*. PBS Video. Boston: WGBH Educational Foundation. Available at http://www.pbs.org.

49. Galea, S., J. Ahern, H. Resnick, D. Kilpatrick, M. Bucuvalas, J. Gold, and D. Vlahov (2002). "Psychological Sequelae of the September 11 Terrorist Attacks in New York City." *New England Journal of Medicine*, 346(13): 982-1087.

50. Centers for Disease Control and Prevention (2006). "Health Hazard Evaluation of Police Officers and Firefighters after Hurricane Katrina—New Orleans, Louisiana, October 17-28 and November 30-December 5, 2005." *Morbidity and Mortality Weekly Report*, 55(16): 456-458.

51. Hoge, C., J. Auchterlonie, and C. Milliken (2006). "Mental Health Problems, Use of Mental Health Services, and Attrition from Military Service after Returning from Deployment to Iraq and Afghanistan." *Journal of the American Medical Association*, 295(9): 1023-1032.

52. Levine, M., D. D. Perkins, and D. V. Perkins (2004). *Principles of Community Psychology: Perspectives and Applications*, 3rd ed. New York: Oxford University Press.

53. National Institute of Mental Health (1998). "Mental Illness in America: The National Institute of Mental Health Agenda." Available at http://www.nimh.gov/research/amer.htm.

54. National Institute of Mental Health. "About the National Institute of Mental Health." Available at http://www.nimh.nih.gov/about/nimh.cfm.

55. Substance Abuse and Mental Health Services Administration. "SAMHSA: Who We Are." Available at http://www.samhsa.gov/about/content/0500whoweare.htm.

56. Edmunds, M., R. Frank, M. Hogan, D. McCarty, R. Robinson-Beale, and C. Weisner, eds. (1997). *Managing Managed Care: Quality Improvement in Behavioral Health*. Washington, DC: National Academy Press.

57. Dorfman, S. (2000). *Preventive Interventions under Managed Care: Mental Health and Substance Abuse Services* (DHHS pub. no. SMA 00-3437). Rockville, MD: Substance Abuse and Mental Health Services Administration.

58. Goldman, H. R. F., A. Burnam, H. Huskamp, S. Ridgely, S. Normand, A. Young, C. Barry, V. Azzone, C. Lichtenstein, and M. Basinsky (2006). "Behavioral Health Insurance Parity for Federal Employees." *New England Journal of Medicine*, 354(13): 1378-1386.

59. Glied, S., and A. Cuellar (2006). "Better Behavioral Health Care Coverage for Everyone." *New England Journal of Medicine*, 354(13): 1415-1416.

Chapter 12

Alcohol, Tobacco, and Other Drugs: A Community Concern

Chapter Objectives

After studying this chapter, you will be able to:

1 Identify personal and community consequences of alcohol and other drug abuse.

2 Describe the trends of alcohol and other drug use by high school students.

3 Define *drug use, misuse,* and *abuse.*

4 Define *drug dependence.*

5 List and discuss the risk factors for the abuse of alcohol and other drugs.

6 Explain why alcohol is considered the Number 1 drug abuse problem in America.

7 Describe the health risks of cigarette smoking.

8 Define the terms *over-the-counter* and *prescription drugs* and explain the purposes of these drugs and how they are regulated.

9 Define the terms *controlled substances* and *illicit (illegal) drugs* and provide examples.

10 Characterize recent trends in the prevalence of drug use among American high school seniors.

11 List and explain four elements of drug abuse prevention and control.

12 Give an example of primary, secondary, and tertiary prevention activities in drug abuse prevention and control programs.

13 Summarize the federal government's drug abuse control efforts.

14 List and describe an effective community and an effective school drug abuse prevention program.

15 List the five facets of a typical workplace substance abuse prevention program.

16 Name some voluntary health agencies and self-help support groups involved in the prevention, control, and treatment of alcohol, tobacco, and other drug abuse.

SCENARIO

Larissa started doing methamphetamine at 17. She had seen all of the TV ads about "your brain on drugs," but did not see herself in that role. She would sneak out to party with friends, at first on weekends, and then almost every night, and then every night. But that didn't make her an addict, she thought. She didn't sleep or eat much at home, but pretended to be asleep when her parents, who worked almost all of the time, were at home. If her parents left her food, she would put it in the garbage disposal so they would think she had eaten it. When they noticed her weight loss, she told them she had developed an eating disorder, but was correcting it.

Eventually meth became the most important thing in Larissa's life. She dropped out of school and moved in with her friend Dustin, who was cooking meth. The cooking made a mess and smelled, so she and Dustin kept moving to different motels. They even lived outside in the woods for a while. They had no money.

When Larissa became pregnant, she stopped using and moved back with her parents. Two months after her son Jarod was born, Larissa met Dustin and began using again. She left Jarod with her parents; she cared only about methamphetamine. She began injecting meth and developed abscesses on her arms. Dustin was gone a lot now, and she began to feel hopeless. She decided to end her life. One day, while Larissa was thinking about how to end her life, the police arrived and arrested her. She weighed 95 pounds and looked like a ghost. As she sat in jail, she realized that she was just the same as all of the other addicts she'd seen. She decided to enter a rehabilitation program.

INTRODUCTION

The use, misuse, and abuse of mind-altering substances undoubtedly predates our recorded history. It is perhaps part of human nature to wish to experience strange and unusual feelings or changes in mood and perceptions. Early civilizations may have used drugs as a vehicle to communicate with spirits. Even today, drugs are used for this purpose in some cultures.

For many Americans, drug-taking is experimental or social, a temporary departure from a natural, nondrugged physical and mental state. For many others, it is a misguided attempt to self-medicate or to cope with personal problems such as depression, loneliness, guilt, or low self-esteem. For a small but significant segment of the population, drug-taking ceases to be a matter of conscious choice; these people have become chronic drug abusers or drug dependent. In most cultures, chronic alcohol or other drug abuse or dependence is regarded as destructive behavior, both to oneself and to the surrounding community. Community members whose lives center around drug acquisition and use usually provide little benefit to their communities and often detract from their communities.

Scope of the Current Drug Problem in the United States

It is difficult to argue with those who state that the abuse of alcohol, tobacco, and other drugs is the nation's number 1 community health problem. According to a recent study, more deaths, illnesses, and disabilities can be attributed to substance abuse than to any other preventable health condition.[1] One-fourth of the 2 million deaths each year are due to alcohol, tobacco, or illicit drug use (see Table 12.1). Estimates of the economic cost of substance abuse in the United States vary in range between $414 billion and $487 billion per year.[1,2] These estimates include direct costs (such as health care expenditures, premature death, and impaired productivity) and indirect costs, which include the costs of crime and law enforcement, courts, jails, and social work. Of the $487 billion annual drug bill, the cost of alcohol abuse and alcoholism is estimated at $220 billion, drug abuse at $110 billion, and smoking at $157 billion

Table 12.1
The Annual Cost in Lives and Dollars Attributable to Alcohol, Tobacco, and Illicit Drug Abuse in the United States

Type of Drug	Estimated Number of Deaths Each Year	Economic Cost to Society (in Billions)
Alcohol	100,000	$220
Tobacco	430,000	$157
Illicit drugs	16,000	$110
TOTAL	546,000	$487

Sources: Horgan, C., K. C. Skwara, and G. Strickler (2001). *Substance Abuse: The Nation's Number One Health Problem.* Princeton, NJ: Robert Wood Johnson Foundation; and National Center on Addiction and Substance Abuse at Columbia University (2006). *The Commercial Value of Underage and Pathological Drinking to the Alcohol Industry: A CASA White Paper.* Available at http://www.casacolumbia.org/absolutenm/templates/Home.aspx.

(see Table 12.1). Clearly, the abuse of alcohol and other drugs is one of America's most expensive community health problems.

Those abusing alcohol and other drugs represent serious health threats to themselves, their families, and their communities. They are a threat to themselves and their families because they put themselves and their families at risk for physical, mental, and financial ruin. The habitual drug user may develop a psychological and/or **physical dependence** on the drug and thus experience great difficulty in discontinuing use, even in the face of deteriorating physical and mental health and erosion of financial resources. If the drug is an illegal one, its use constitutes criminal activity and may carry with it the added risks of arrest and incarceration.

Abusers of alcohol and other drugs represent a serious threat to the community because they have greater health care needs, suffer more injuries, and are less productive than those who do not. Community consequences range from loss of economic opportunity and productivity to social and economic destruction (see Table 12.2). Additionally, those who abuse drugs may perpetrate more violent acts that result in economic loss, injury, and death. The violence associated with the abuse of alcohol and other drugs is depicted in Figure 12.1.

physical dependence a physiological state in which discontinued drug use results in clinical illness

Table 12.2
Personal and Community Consequences of Drug Abuse

Personal Consequences	Community Consequences
Absenteeism from school or work	Loss of productivity and revenue
Underachievement at school or work	Lower average SAT scores
Scholastic failure/interruption of education	Loss of economic opportunity
Loss of employment	Increase in public welfare load
Marital instability/family problems	Increase in number of broken homes
Risk of infectious diseases	Epidemics of sexually transmitted diseases
Risk of chronic or degenerative diseases	Unnecessary burden on health care system
Increased risk of accidents	Unnecessary deaths and economic losses
Financial problems	Defaults on mortgages, loans/bankruptcies
Criminal activity	Increased cost of insurance and security
Arrest and incarceration	Increased cost for police/courts/prisons
Risk of adulterated drugs	Increased burden on medical care system
Adverse drug reactions or "bad trips"	Greater need for emergency medical services
Drug-induced psychoses	Unnecessary drain on mental health services
Drug overdose	Unnecessary demand for medical services
Injury to fetus or newborn baby	Unnecessary use of expensive neonatal care
Loss of self-esteem	Increase in mental illness, underachievement
Suicide	Damaged and destroyed families
Death	

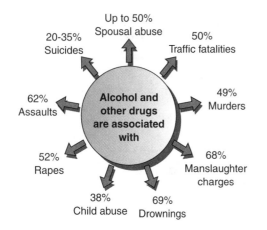

FIGURE 12.1

Violence associated with the use of alcohol and other drugs.

Source: National Clearinghouse for Alcohol and Drug Information (1995). *Making the Link* [Fact sheets]. Rockville, MD: Author.

According to the annual Monitoring the Future surveys on drug use among those in grades 8, 10, and 12, drug use declined steadily until 1992 and then rose again until 1996 or 1997, depending upon the grade. Overall illicit drug use began to decline gradually among eighth graders, while holding steady for older students, until 2002, when a general decline was noted.[3,4] The decline continued through 2005 but usage still remained above the 1992 levels. For example, in 2005 the use of marijuana (in the past 30 days) was reported by 19.8% of high school seniors, compared with 22.4% in 2001, but only 11.9% in 1992. Use of any illicit drug other than marijuana (in the past 30 days) also showed a slight decline in recent years, from 11.0% in 2001 to 10.3% in 2005, but remained well above the 1992 figure of just 6.3%. Thirty-day use of one drug, MDMA (Ecstasy), declined significantly among high school seniors, however, from a high of 3.6% in 2000 to 1.0% in 2005.[4] It is interesting to note that college students report lower levels of usage of virtually all illicit drugs than high school seniors,[4] suggesting that drug-using high school seniors are less likely to attend college than their non-drug-using classmates.

When the words *drug abuse* are mentioned, most people think of illicit drugs, such as heroin, LSD, cocaine, and other illegal substances. While the abuse of illicit drugs is certainly a major problem in America, abuse of alcohol and tobacco products are, perhaps, more serious challenges to America's health. Tobacco use by high school seniors has increased since 1992, while alcohol use remained high during the same period (see Figure 12.2).

drug
a substance other than food that when taken in small quantities alters one's physical, mental, or emotional state

psychoactive drugs
drugs that alter sensory perceptions, mood, thought processes, or behavior

drug use
a non-evaluative term referring to drug-taking behavior in general; any drug-taking behavior

drug misuse
inappropriate use of prescription or nonprescription drugs

Table 12.3
Percentage of High School Seniors Who Have Used Drugs

	Class of 1992			Class of 2005		
	Ever Used	Past Month	Daily Use	Ever Used	Past Month	Daily Use
Alcohol	87.5%	51.3%	3.4%	75.1%*	47.0%	3.1%
Cigarettes	61.8	27.8	17.2	50.0	23.2	13.6
Marijuana	32.6	11.9	1.9	44.8	19.8	5.0
Amphetamines	13.9	2.8	0.2	14.6	3.9	†
Inhalants	16.6	2.3	0.1	11.4	2.0	†
Cocaine	6.1	1.3	0.1	8.0	2.3	†
Tranquilizers	6.0	1.0	†	9.9	2.9	†
LSD	8.6	2.1	0.1	3.5	0.7	†
MDMA	—	—	—	5.4	1.0	†
Crack	2.6	0.6	0.1	3.5	1.0	†
PCP	2.4	0.6	0.1	2.4	0.7	†
Heroin	1.2	0.3	†	1.5	0.5	†

*More than just a few sips.
†Less than 0.05%.
— No data.

Sources: For 1992 data: Johnston, L. D., P. M. O'Malley, and J. G. Bachman (1993). *Monitoring the Future National Survey Results on Drug Use, 1975-1992. Vol. I: Secondary School Students* (NIH pub. no. 93-3597). Bethesda, MD: National Institute on Drug Abuse. For 2005 data: Johnston, L. D., P. M. O'Malley, J. G. Bachman, and J. E. Schulenbert (2006). *Monitoring the Future National Survey Results on Drug Use 1975-2005. Vol. I: Secondary School Students* (NIH pub. no. 06-5883). Rockville, MD: National Institute on Drug Abuse. Available at http://www.monitoringthefuture.org/pubs/.

America has been trying to solve the problem of drug abuse for decades. Most adults who abuse drugs eventually "mature out" of the behavior, but there is a constant supply of potential drug users among America's children. This "generational forgetting" means that drug prevention education is never finished. Instead, drug prevention efforts must become a permanent part of our culture. That is, we must teach our children about the dangers of experimental drug use in the same way we teach them to look both ways before they cross the street.

Definitions

We begin a discussion of alcohol, tobacco, and other drugs as a community health problem by defining some terms. A **drug** is a substance, other than food or vitamins, that upon entering the body in small amounts alters one's physical, mental, or emotional state. **Psychoactive drugs** are drugs that alter sensory perceptions, mood, thought processes, or behavior.

In this chapter, the term **drug use** is a non-evaluative term referring to drug-taking behavior in general, regardless of whether the behavior is appropriate. **Drug misuse** refers primarily to the inappropriate use of legally purchased prescription or nonprescription drugs. For example, drug misuse occurs when one discontinues the use of a prescribed antibiotic before the entire prescribed dose is completed or when one takes four aspirin rather than two as specified on the label. **Drug abuse** can be defined in several ways depending upon the drug and the situation. Drug abuse occurs when one takes a prescription or nonprescription drug for a purpose other than that for which it is medically approved. For example, drug abuse occurs when one takes a prescription diet pill for its mood altering effects (stimulation). The abuse of legal drugs such as nicotine or alcohol is said to occur when one is aware that continued use is detrimental to one's health. Because illicit drugs have no approved medical uses, any illicit drug use is considered drug abuse. Likewise, the use of alcohol and nicotine by those under the legal age is considered drug abuse.

Drug (chemical) dependence occurs when a user feels that a particular drug is necessary for normal functioning. Dependence may be **psychological,** in which case the user experiences a strong emotional or psychological desire to continue use of the drug even though clinical signs of physical illness may not appear; or it can be physical, in which discontinuation of drug use results in clinical illness. Usually, both psychological and physical dependence are present at the same time, making the discontinuation of drug use very difficult. Such is frequently the case with cigarette smoking.

FACTORS THAT CONTRIBUTE TO ALCOHOL, TOBACCO, AND OTHER DRUG ABUSE

The factors that contribute to the abuse of alcohol, tobacco, and other drugs are many, and the decision to use drugs lies ultimately with the individual; it's a matter of choice. However, studies have determined that individuals are differentially at risk for engaging in drug-taking behavior.[5] Factors that increase the probability of drug use are called *risk factors;* those that lower the probability of drug use are called *protective factors.* People with a high number of risk factors are said to be vulnerable to drug abuse or dependence, while those who have few risk factors and more protective factors are said to be resistant to drug abuse.

FIGURE 12.2

The prevalence of alcohol use among American high school seniors in the middle and late 1990s remained high, while cigarette smoking rose dramatically.

drug abuse
use of a drug when it is detrimental to one's health or well-being

drug (chemical) dependence
a psychological and sometimes physical state characterized by a craving for a drug

psychological dependence
a psychological state characterized by an overwhelming desire to continue use of a drug

Risk and protective factors can be either genetic (inherited) or environmental. Numerous studies have concluded that inherited traits can increase one's risk of developing dependence on alcohol, and it is logical to assume that susceptibility to other drugs might also be inherited. Environmental risk factors, such as one's home and family life, school and peer groups, and society and culture, have also been identified.

Inherited Risk Factors

The vast majority of the data supporting the notion that the risk of drug dependence can be inherited comes from studies on alcoholism. Evidence for the heritability of risk for alcoholism is provided by numerous studies,[6-8] which have been reviewed by Tabakoff and Hoffman[9] in the *Seventh Special Report to the U.S. Congress on Alcohol and Health,* from the Secretary of Health and Human Services.[10] Studies of alcoholics' families have found that there are at least two types of inherited alcoholism,[7] now referred to as Type I (or milieu-limited), and Type II (or male-limited) alcoholism.[10] These observational studies of alcoholics' families are supported by research using genetic and biological markers in animal models. Some of these markers predispose an individual biochemically to increased susceptibility to developing alcohol-related problems, while others may actually be protective in nature. For example, genes that code for enzymes that inhibit the normal metabolism of alcohol could cause one to respond positively to the effects of alcohol and thus to drink more, or respond negatively to alcohol and thus drink less or not at all.[9] A study has provided evidence in support of the idea that genes also influence cigarette smoking.[11] The heritability of susceptibility to other drugs is still under investigation.

Environmental Risk Factors

There are a great many environmental factors, both psychological and social, that influence the use and abuse of alcohol and other drugs. Included are personal factors such as the influences of home and family life, school and peer groups, and other components of the social and cultural environment.

Personal Factors

Personal factors include personality traits, such as impulsiveness, depressive mood, susceptibility to stress, or possibly personality disturbances. Some of these factors have been reviewed by Needle and colleagues.[12] While models that involve personal factors provide frameworks for research and theorizing about the etiology of alcohol and drug abuse, they have their limitations. It is difficult to determine the degree to which these factors are inherited or are simply the product of the family environment. For example, one's choice to use alcohol or drugs in response to a stressful situation (and the outcome of that decision) could be the result of either inherited characteristics, learned behavior, or a combination of these factors.

Home and Family Life

The importance of home and family life on alcohol and drug abuse has been the subject of numerous studies, some of which have been reviewed by Meller[13] and by Needle and colleagues.[12] Research demonstrates that not all family-associated risk is genetic in origin. Family structure, family dynamics, quality of parenting, and family problems can all contribute to drug experimentation by children and adolescents (see Figure 12.3). Family turmoil (deaths and divorces) have been associated with the initiation of alcohol

FIGURE 12.3
Influences of home and family life can affect one's decisions about alcohol, tobacco, and other drugs.

and other drug use.[12] In this sense, alcohol and drug use are a symptom of personal and/or family problems, not a cause.[14]

The development of interpersonal skills, such as communication skills, independent living skills, and learning to get along with others, is nurtured in the home. The failure of parents to provide an environment conducive to the development of these skills can result in the loss of self-esteem and increase in delinquency, nonconformity, and sociopathic behavior, all personal risk factors for alcohol and drug abuse.[10]

Finally, family attitudes toward alcohol and drug use influence adolescents' beliefs and expectations about the effects of drugs. These expectations have been shown to be important factors in adolescents' choices to initiate and continue alcohol use.[10] The age of first use of alcohol, tobacco, and illicit drugs is correlated to later development of alcohol and drug problems, especially if use begins before age 15.[15]

FIGURE 12.4
Peers can influence one's expectations of the effects of a drug.

School and Peer Groups

Perceived and actual drug use by peers influences attitudes and choices by adolescents (see Figure 12.4). Some studies have shown that perceived support of drinking by peers is the single most important factor in an adolescent's choice to drink.[10] Peers can also influence expectations for a drug. Alcohol may be perceived as "a 'magic elixir' that can enhance social and physical pleasure, sexual performance and responsiveness, power and aggression and social competence."[10] It is interesting to note that these are precisely the mythical qualities about alcohol portrayed in advertisements for beer and other alcoholic beverages.

Sociocultural Environment

The notion of environmental risk includes the effects of sociocultural and physical settings on drug-taking behavior. The study of the effects of the physical and social environment upon the individual is termed *social ecology*.[16] Environmental risk for drug-taking can stem from one's immediate neighborhood or from society at large. For example, living in the inner city—with its sordidness, physical decay, and threats to personal safety—could set into motion a variety of changes in values and behaviors, including some related to alcohol or drug use.

Opportunities for community interventions exist, though. For example, federal, state, and local drug-prevention education programs, law enforcement successes, and treatment availability can improve the social environment and reduce the prevalence of drug abuse. Also, increasing taxes on tobacco products and alcoholic beverages and developing zoning ordinances that limit the number of bars and liquor stores in certain neighborhoods can be effective in reducing the alcohol, tobacco, and other drug problems in a community.

TYPES OF DRUGS ABUSED AND RESULTING PROBLEMS

Almost any psychoactive drug available is subject to abuse by at least some segment of the population. Classification systems of drugs of abuse are many, but none of them is perfect. Problems of classification arise because all drugs have multiple effects and because the legal status of a drug can depend upon its formulation and strength, and in some cases, upon the age of the user. In this chapter, our classification system includes legal drugs and illegal drugs. Legal (licit) drugs include alcohol, nicotine, and nonprescription and prescription drugs. Illegal (illicit) drugs can be classified further on the basis of physiological effects as stimulants, depressants, narcotics, hallucinogens, marijuana, and other drugs.

Legal Drugs

Legal drugs are drugs that can be legally bought and sold in the marketplace, including those that are closely regulated, like morphine; those that are lightly regulated, like alcohol and tobacco; and still others that are not regulated at all, like caffeine.

Alcohol

Alcohol is the Number 1 problem drug in America by almost any standard of measurement—the number of those who abuse it, the number of injuries and injury deaths it causes, the amount of money spent on it, and its social and economic costs to society through broken homes and lost wages. Alcohol is consumed in a variety of forms, including beer, wine, fortified wines and brandies, and distilled spirits. While many people view distilled spirits as the most dangerous form of alcohol, it is now recognized that the form of alcohol involved in most heavy-episodic drinking is beer. Much of this beer is drunk by high school and college students, and much of this drinking is **binge drinking** (consuming five or more drinks on a single occasion for males and four or more drinks for females).

binge drinking
consuming five or more drinks in a row for males and four or more drinks in a row for females

A major community health concern is underage drinking, that is, drinking by those younger than 21 years. An analysis has revealed that nearly 26% of underage drinkers meet clinical criteria for alcohol abuse or dependence, compared with 9.6% of adult drinkers.[2] Underage drinkers, many of them children and teenagers, can destroy their own lives and the lives of others through reckless driving, risky sexual behavior that can lead to disease transmission and unintentional pregnancies, and the commission of other violent and injurious acts. At issue is the fact that an estimated $22.5 billion, or 17% of all money spent on alcohol, can be accounted for by underage drinking. The alcohol industry would take a huge hit if underage drinking were to stop. The industry relies on underage drinkers for two reasons: the amount of alcohol consumed by them and the fact that many pathological underage drinkers will become pathological adult drinkers, a group that accounts for $25.8 billion, or 20.1%, of the consumer expenditures for alcohol.[2]

problem drinker
one for whom alcohol consumption results in a medical, social, or other type of problem

Drinking by high school and college students continues to be very widespread despite the fact that it is illegal for virtually all high school students and for most college students to purchase these beverages. In 2005, 75.1% of high school seniors reported having drunk alcohol (more than a few sips) at least once in their lifetime, with 68.6% in the past year, and 47.5% in the past 30 days. Thirty percent (nearly one in three high school seniors) reported having been drunk in the past 30 days.[4] Twenty-eight percent of high school seniors reported occasions of binge drinking at least once in the prior two-week period. College students reported an even higher prevalence of binge drinking; 40% stated that they had consumed five or more drinks in a row in the past two-week period. The rate of binge drinking among college students has not changed in the past four years.[4]

alcoholism
a disease characterized by impaired control over drinking, preoccupation with drinking, and continued use of alcohol despite adverse consequences

Most of those who experiment with alcohol begin their use in a social context and become light or moderate drinkers. Alcohol use is reinforcing in two ways: It lowers anxieties and produces a mild euphoria. For many people, alcohol use does not become a significant problem, but for about 10% of those who drink, it does. Some of these people become **problem drinkers;** that is, they begin to experience personal, interpersonal, legal, or financial problems because of their alcohol consumption. Still others lose control of their drinking and develop a dependence upon alcohol. Physical dependence on alcohol and the loss of control over one's drinking are two important characteristics of **alcoholism.** According to the *Journal of the American Medical Association:*

> *Alcoholism* is a primary, chronic disease with genetic, psychosocial, and environmental factors influencing its development and manifestations. The disease is often progressive and fatal. It is characterized by impaired control over drinking, preoccupation with the drug alcohol, use of

alcohol despite adverse consequences, and distortions in thinking, most notably denial. Each of these symptoms may be continuous or periodic.[18]

The cost of alcohol abuse and alcoholism in the United States was estimated for 2005 to be $220 billion.[2] That is $740 for every man, woman, and child. To put it another way, it costs America $25 million every hour for alcohol-related problems. More than 60% of the cost is due to lost employment or reduced productivity, and 13% of the cost is due to medical and treatment costs. Health care costs for alcoholics are about twice those for nonalcoholics.[10]

Alcohol and other drugs are contributing factors to a variety of unintentional injuries and injury deaths. The risk of a motor vehicle crash increases progressively with alcohol consumption and **blood alcohol concentration (BAC)** (see Figure 12.5).

> Compared with drivers who have not consumed alcohol, the risk of a single-vehicle fatal crash for drivers with BAC's between 0.02 and 0.04 percent is estimated to be 1.4 times higher; for those with BAC's between 0.05 and 0.09 percent, 11.1 times higher; for drivers with BAC's between 0.10 and 0.14 percent, 48 times higher; and for those with BAC's at or above 0.15 percent, the risk is estimated to be 380 times higher.[19]

Young drivers are particularly at risk because they are inexperienced drivers and inexperienced drinkers. This combination can be deadly. One study found that 23% of drivers 16 to 20 years old who were involved in fatal motor vehicle crashes, and for whom any alcohol consumption is illegal, had alcohol in their blood.[19]

Despite these grim figures, significant progress has been made in reducing the overall rate of alcohol-related vehicle deaths. In 1987, there were 9.8 deaths per 100,000 people; in 1998 the rate had declined to 5.3 deaths per 100,000 people. The *Healthy People 2010* objective has set a target of 4.8 deaths per 100,000. By 2002, the rate had declined further to 5.2 per 100,000 people. The rate among 15–24-year-olds actually increased between 1998 and 2002 (see Box 12.1). Past success and the promise of future achievement of the target came through public policy changes—raising the minimum legal drinking age, strengthening and enforcing state license revocation laws, and lowering the BAC tolerance levels from 0.10% to 0.08% in some states—stricter law enforcement, and better education for those cited for driving while intoxicated.[20] In October 2000 President Clinton signed a bill that made 0.08% BAC the national standard. States that refused to impose the standard by 2004 would lose millions of dollars of federal highway construction money.[21] By the end of 2004, all 50 states, Puerto Rico, and the District of Columbia had adopted the 0.08% standard.[22]

Alcohol has also been found to increase one's risk for other types of unintentional injuries, such as drowning, falls, fires, and burns. Associations between unintentional injuries and the abuse of other drugs are less well documented, but given a knowledge of the effects of such drugs, one can assume that they increase neither the alertness nor the coordination of users.

Alcohol also contributes to intentional violence in the community. For example, 50% of spouse abuse, 49% of murders, 62% of assaults, 52% of rapes, 38% of child abuse cases, and 20% to 35% of suicides are traceable to alcohol consumption (see Figure 12.1).

"Alcohol is the number 1 rape drug," according to Henry Wechsler of the Harvard University School of Public Health.[23] The incidence of rape on college campuses is estimated at 35 per 1,000 female students, making rape the most common violent crime on American campuses. Yet, less than 5% of these rapes are reported to police. About half of the

blood alcohol concentration (BAC) the percentage of concentration of alcohol in the blood

FIGURE 12.5
The risk of a motor vehicle crash increases progressively with alcohol consumption.

<table>
<tr><td>BOX
12.1</td><td colspan="4">HEALTHY PEOPLE 2010 OBJECTIVES: ADVERSE CONSEQUENCES OF SUBSTANCE USE AND ABUSE</td></tr>
</table>

Objective 26-1:   Reduce deaths caused by alcohol-related motor vehicle crashes.

Target and baseline:

Objective	Reduction in Consequences of Motor Vehicle Crashes	1998 Baseline	2002	2010 Target
		Per 100,000 population		
26-1a	Alcohol-related deaths			
	General population (all ages)	5.9	5.2	4.8
	Selected population group (Persons aged 15–24 years)	11.8	12.4	NA

NA = Not applicable

For Further Thought

The reduction of alcohol-related vehicle deaths is one of the greatest success stories of public health during the 1990s. The 1987 baseline was 9.8 deaths per 100,000 people, and the objective for the year 2000 was 8.5 deaths. By 1998, a level of 5.3 deaths per 100,000 was achieved, and the 2010 target has been set for just 4.8 deaths per 100,000. Similar success has not been achieved for drug-related deaths overall, or for drug abuse–related emergency department visits. What explanation can you offer for these differences?

Source: CDC (2007). *Data2010 . . . The Healthy People 2010 Database—January, 2007 Edition*. Available at http://wonder.cdc.gov.

perpetrators and rape survivors on college campuses were drinking alcohol at the time of the assault. Ninety percent of college women who are raped know their assailants. A new law in Wisconsin was designed to protect women at risk of sexual assault by acquaintances at social gatherings where alcohol is served. A person convicted under the new law can be fined up to $100,000 and sentenced up to 25 years in prison. Wisconsin is the 50th state to enact such a law.[23]

Another community health problem resulting from pathological drinking is fetal alcohol spectrum disorder (FASD). FASD includes diagnoses such as fetal alcohol syndrome (FAS), fetal alcohol effects (FAE), alcohol-related birth defects (ARBD), and alcohol-related neurodevelopmental disorders (ARND). "Every year, about 40,000 babies are born with symptoms of prenatal alcohol exposure," according to a 2003 publication of the Substance Abuse and Mental Health Services Administration.[24] These babies cost society thousands of dollars over their lifetimes. Estimates vary greatly based upon estimated prevalence rates, from a low rate of 0.33 cases of FASD per 1,000 live births to 2.0 cases per 1,000. Costs can be attributable to medical treatment for pre- and postnatal growth defects requiring surgery; services for developmentally disabled children; home health care, special education, social services, training and supervision, and institutional care for affected individuals with mental retardation to age 65 years; and lost productivity. Estimates of the annual cost of FASD in the United States range from $0.5 million to $6 billion. Likewise, estimates for the lifetime costs for a specific individual with FASD range from $1 million to $5 million.[24] Clearly, this is a community health problem for which an ounce of prevention is worth a pound of cure. It is also clear that women of childbearing age who could become pregnant should exercise caution in their alcohol use.

Nicotine

Nicotine is the psychoactive and addictive drug present in tobacco products such as cigarettes, cigars, smokeless or "spit" tobacco (chewing tobacco and snuff), and pipe tobacco. For many years the enforcement of state laws prohibiting the sale of cigarettes and other tobacco products to minors was uneven. In other cases, cigarettes could easily be purchased by youth from vending machines. Thus, until recently many American youths have had ready access to tobacco products, and American tobacco companies made the most of this situation during the 1990s. With their seductive "Joe Camel" advertisements (now retired) and other similar youth-oriented marketing approaches, they made smoking highly attractive to today's youth. In a more recent effort to market cigarettes to children and adolescents, Reynolds Tobacco began selling candy-, fruit-, and liquor-flavored cigarettes. An agreement between Reynolds Tobacco and the attorneys general of 38 states to end the sale of these items was announced October 10, 2006.[25] The **Synar Amendment** is a federal law that requires all states to adopt legislation that prohibits the sale and distribution of tobacco products to people under age 18. States that do not comply with this regulation lose federal dollars for alcohol, tobacco, and other drug prevention and treatment programs.[26]

Synar Amendment a federal law that requires states to set the minimum legal age for purchasing tobacco products at 18 years and requires states to enforce this law

The 30-day prevalence of cigarette smoking among high school seniors, which had declined to 27.8% in 1992 and then rebounded to 36.5% by 1997, reached a new low of 23.2% in 2005. The prevalence of daily smoking among high school seniors also declined in 2003, to 13.6%.[4] While it is true that some of these students are light smokers (less than half a pack a day), studies show that many light smokers become heavy smokers (more than half a pack a day) as they become older. The prevalence of cigarette smoking in young adults (aged 19–28) seems to be related to college attendance. For college students, the 30-day prevalence of daily use of cigarettes was 12.4%; for young adults, it was 19.6%.[4]

The health consequences of tobacco use are familiar to all, even smokers (see Box 12.2). They include increased risks for heart disease, lung cancer, chronic obstructive lung disease, stroke, emphysema, and other conditions. Smoking accounted for an estimated 438,000 premature deaths per year in the United States and 4.8 million premature deaths per year worldwide.[27] The economic costs of tobacco smoking in the United States are estimated at $167 billion, of which about 55% is due to lost productivity and 45% is attributable to medical costs.[27,28] A significant portion of the medical costs attributed to smoking (43%) are paid with government funds, including Medicaid and Medicare.[1] Inasmuch as tobacco use and nicotine addiction increase the cost of these programs, they clearly add to the economic burden on society.

Well-established research findings have demonstrated that one does not have to use tobacco products to be adversely affected. The 1986 Surgeon General's report on the effects of **environmental tobacco smoke (ETS)** or **secondhand smoke** indicated that adults and children who inhale the tobacco smoke of others (passive smoking) are also at increased risk for cardiac and respiratory illnesses.[29,30] These findings resulted in new smoking regulations in many indoor environments. Then, in December 1992, the Environmental Protection Agency (EPA) released the report *Respiratory Health Effects of Passive Smoking: Lung Cancer and Other Disorders.*[31] This report stated that ETS is a human class A carcinogen (the same class that contains asbestos) and that it is responsible for 3,000 lung cancer deaths annually among nonsmoking Americans. Further, it stated that ETS exposure is causally associated with as many as 150,000 to 300,000 cases of lower respiratory infections (such as bronchitis and pneumonia) in infants and young children up to 18 months of age. The EPA study also found that ETS aggravates asthma in children and is a risk factor for new cases of childhood asthma.

environmental tobacco smoke (ETS) (secondhand smoke) tobacco smoke in the ambient air

The use of smokeless (spit) tobacco also carries with it serious health risks, including addiction, periodontal disease, and oral cancer. Approximately 3.7% of 12- to 17-year-old males and 9.7% of 18- to 25-year-old males reported using smokeless tobacco within the past 30 days in 2005.[32] The subgroup of Americans who reported the highest rate of smokeless tobacco use was the American Indians/Alaskan Natives. In 2005, 8.6% of this population aged 12 or older reported using smokeless tobacco in the past 30 days.[32] This habit begins in high school,

TEN GREAT PUBLIC HEALTH ACHIEVEMENTS, 1900–1999: RECOGNITION OF TOBACCO USE AS A HEALTH HAZARD

Less Smoke, More Prevention

During the twentieth century, smoking went from being an accepted norm to being recognized as the Number 1 preventable cause of death and disability in the United States. Although substantial progress has been made and millions of lives have been saved, increased prevention efforts are needed to reduce the impact of tobacco use on public health.

> **SURGEON GENERAL'S WARNING: Smoking Causes Lung Cancer, Heart Disease Emphysema, And May Complicate Pregnancy**

Each year, smoking kills more people than all of the following health hazards combined:

- AIDS
- Alcohol abuse
- Drug abuse
- Motor vehicle crash injuries
- Murders
- Suicides

Per capita consumption of cigarettes has decreased from a high of more than 4,000 cigarettes/year in the early 1960s to a low of 2,261/year in 1998, the lowest level seen since the early 1940s. Some of the changes appear to be associated with notable smoking and health events.

- 1964 Surgeon General's report
- Doubling of federal cigarette taxes
- Master Settlement Agreement
- Banning of tobacco advertising in many venues

During this century, smoking prevalence among adults aged 18 years decreased from approximately 40% in the mid-1960s to 25% in 1999, with the rate for men being approximately five percentage points higher than for women.

Source: Centers for Disease Control and Prevention. Available at http://www.cdc.gov/phtn/tenachievements/tobacco1/to1.htm.

where in 2005, 5.3% of eighth-grade males, 9.7% of tenth-grade, males, and 12.7% of twelfth-grade males reported using smokeless tobacco in the past 30 days.[4]

Over-the-Counter Drugs

over-the-counter (OTC) drugs (nonprescription drugs) drugs (except tobacco and alcohol) that can be legally purchased without a physician's prescription

Over-the-counter (OTC) drugs are those legal drugs, with the exception of tobacco and alcohol, that can be purchased without a physician's prescription. Included in this category are internal analgesics such as aspirin, acetaminophen (Tylenol), and ibuprofen (Advil); cough and cold remedies (Robitussin, Contac); emetics; laxatives; mouthwashes; vitamins; and many others.[33] Thousands of different OTC products are sold by pharmacies, supermarkets, convenience stores, and in vending machines. These products are manufactured and sold to those who self-diagnose and self-medicate their own illnesses.

Over-the-counter drugs are carefully regulated by the **Food and Drug Administration (FDA),** an agency of the Department of Health and Human Services. The FDA ensures the safety and effectiveness of these products when they are used according to their label directions. There is no person or agency that supervises the actual sale or use of these substances.

Naturally, some of these substances are misused and abused. Examples of misuse are not following the dosage directions or using the drugs after their expiration date. A specific example of OTC drug abuse is the taking of laxatives or emetics to lose weight or to avoid gaining weight. Other OTC drugs that are often abused are appetite suppressants (Dexatrim), stimulants (NoDoz), and nasal sprays (Neo-Synephrine). Recently, common cold OTC products that contain pseudoephedrine have been the target of thieves whose intent is to manufacture methamphetamine. This has led to tighter regulation that restricts the amounts that can be sold at one time.[34]

Most OTC drugs provide only symptomatic relief and do not provide a cure. For example, cough and cold remedies relieve the discomfort that accompanies a cold but do not in any way rid a person of the cold virus that is causing these symptoms. Therefore, a real danger of OTC drug misuse and abuse is that symptoms that should be brought to the attention of a physician remain unreported. Another danger is that those who abuse these drugs may become dependent, thus unable to live normally without them. Lastly, abuse of OTC drugs may establish a pattern of dependency that predisposes the abuser to developing dependent relationships with prescription drugs or illicit drugs.

Prescription Drugs

Because all prescription drugs have serious side effects for some people, they can be purchased only with a physician's (or dentist's) written instructions (prescription). Like OTC drugs, prescription drugs are carefully regulated by the FDA. More than 4,000 prescription drugs are listed in each annual edition of the *Physician's Desk Reference.*[35] The written prescription connotes that the prescribed drugs are being taken by the patient under the prescribing physician's supervision. Each prescription includes the patient's name, the amount to be dispensed, and the dosage.

Nonetheless, prescription drugs are also subject to misuse and abuse. Types of misuse include those previously cited for the OTC drugs and also the giving of one person's prescription drug to another. Furthermore, certain prescription drugs such as stimulants (amphetamines), depressants (Valium), and pain relievers such as narcotics (morphine, codeine) have a higher potential for abuse than others. Because prescription drugs are usually stronger or more concentrated than OTC drugs, there is a greater risk of developing dependence or taking an overdose from these drugs. Those who develop dependence may try to obtain duplicate prescriptions from other physicians or steal the drugs from hospital dispensaries or pharmacies.

While the abuse of prescription drugs is a concern, levels of abuse are much lower for these drugs than for alcohol and tobacco. After marijuana, however, this group of drugs, the psychotherapeutics, is the most abused. Nearly 6.3% of people aged 12 and older took one of these addictive drugs without a prescription in 2005. Included in this group of substances are prescription narcotics such as Darvocet, Darvon, Percocet, Percodan, Vicodin (hydrocodone), and OxyContin, among others. Among those aged 18 to 25, the prevalence of nonmedical use of pain relievers in the past month was 4.7%. Most nonmedical users of prescription pain relief drugs get them "free" from friends and relatives.[32]

One serious consequence of the misuse of prescription drugs, in addition to becoming dependent, is the development of drug-resistant strains of pathogens. When patients fail to complete the entire antibiotic treatment (i.e., three days of a ten-day prescription), some of the bacteria survive and multiply, re-infecting the body with drug-resistant organisms. Thus, succeeding treatments are less effective. When this strain of the disease is transmitted to another, the antibiotic treatment fails. New drugs are then needed to treat these patients. As drug misuse continues to occur, bacteria become resistant to multiple drugs. Multidrug-resistant tuberculosis (MDR-TB) is an example. Another example is the growing number of reports of community-associated methicillin-resistant *Staphylococcus aureus* (CA-MRSA) infections. These are bacterial infections of the skin or other organs that are resistant to some antibiotics.[36] The prevalence of MDR-TB and the increase in the incidence of CA-MRSA point both to the dangers of drug misuse and the need to continue to develop new antibiotics for the treatment of bacterial infections.

Food and Drug Administration (FDA) a federal agency in the Department of Health and Human Services charged with assuring the safety and efficacy of all prescription and nonprescription drugs

controlled substances
drugs regulated by the Comprehensive Drug Abuse Control Act of 1970, including all illegal drugs and prescription drugs that are subject to abuse and can produce dependence

Another problem with prescription drug use is that of adverse drug reactions. Researchers estimated that in 1994 there may have been as many as 106,000 deaths in the United States from adverse drug reactions.[37] If this is true, adverse drug reactions would be one of the top ten leading causes of death in the country. Indeed, poisoning has now become the second leading cause of unintentional injury deaths in the United States (see Chapter 17).

Controlled Substances and Illicit (Illegal) Drugs

Controlled substances are those regulated by the **Controlled Substances Act of 1970** (CSA), officially called the **Comprehensive Drug Abuse Control Act of 1970**. Many of the drugs discussed next belong to Schedule I under this Act because they have a high potential for abuse and have no accepted medical uses and, hence, no acceptable standards of safe use. These are considered **illicit (illegal) drugs.** They cannot be cultivated, manufactured, bought, sold, or used within the confines of the law. Well over 100 drugs are listed in this category, including heroin, methaqualone, marijuana (see Figure 12.6), LSD, psilocybin, mescaline, MDMA, and DMT.[38]

Controlled Substances Act of 1970 (Comprehensive Drug Abuse Control Act of 1970)
the central piece of federal drug legislation that regulates illegal drugs and legal drugs that have a high potential for abuse

Other drugs, which do have medical uses, are placed in Schedules II to V of the act, depending upon their potential for abuse and risk of causing dependence. Included in Schedule II is a variety of very powerful compounds that have specific medical uses but have a high risk for potential abuse. Included in this category are many opium derivatives, such as morphine, fentanyl, and methadone. Also included in Schedule II are the stimulants amphetamine and methamphetamine, certain depressants such as amobarbital, pentobarbital, secobarbital and phencyclidine, and several other drugs. Schedule III drugs have medical uses and exhibit a lower risk of potential abuse than Schedule II drugs. Included are less concentrated forms of certain Schedule II drugs and also many of the anabolic steroids. Schedule IV drugs exhibit even less potential for abuse than Schedule III drugs. Included are many milder stimulants and depressants. Schedule V drugs are primarily very dilute concentrations of opium or opiates used in such medicines as cough syrups.[38]

illicit (illegal) drugs
drugs that cannot be legally manufactured, distributed, or sold, and that usually lack recognized medicinal value. Drugs that have been placed under Schedule I of the Controlled Substances Act of 1970

The **Drug Enforcement Administration (DEA),** under the Department of Justice, has the primary responsibility of enforcing the provisions of the Controlled Substances Act. Once a drug is placed in Schedule I of the CSA, it becomes the primary responsibility of the DEA to interdict the trafficking (manufacturing, distribution, and sales) of the substance. The only sources of these drugs are illegal growers and manufacturers. Schedule II to V substances often reach the street illegally, either by illegal production (in clandestine labs) or by diversion of legally manufactured prescription drugs.

Drug Enforcement Administration (DEA)
the federal government's lead agency with the primary responsibility for enforcing the nation's drug laws, including the Controlled Substances Act of 1970

Marijuana

Marijuana is the most abused illicit drug in the United States. "Pot" and the related products, hashish and hash oil, are derived from the hemp plant, *Cannabis sativa*. The products are most commonly used by smoking but can also be ingested. While marijuana abuse has declined, it remains a concern for several reasons. First, it is illegal, and therefore brings the user into contact with those involved in illegal activities. Second, the act of smoking is detrimental to one's health. Third, marijuana smoking often occurs in conjunction with the drinking of alcohol or the use of other drugs. The effects of **polydrug use** (the use of more than one drug at a time) may be more serious than those of single-drug use. Lastly, as is true of all drugs, the adolescent who uses marijuana is delaying the accomplishment of developmental tasks such as attaining an adult self-identity, achieving independence, and developing the interpersonal skills necessary for successful independent living.

marijuana
dried plant parts of the hemp plant, *Cannabis sativa*

In a 2002 survey, the percentage of high school seniors who reported having smoked marijuana at least once in their lives was 44.8%. Also, 21.2% reported having smoked marijuana in the past 30 days.[4] As with many of the other drugs, the prevalence of marijuana use has waxed and waned over the past 30 years. The perceived risk of use is one of the factors that seems to contribute to the level of use. In 1992, when 76.5% of high school seniors felt there was great risk associated with regular marijuana use, the 30-day use prevalence was 11.9%. In 2005, when 53.0% of seniors felt there was great risk associated with regular marijuana use, the 30-day use prevalence was 19.8%.[4] Another measurement of students' attitudes is disapproval rates. National anti-drug-use campaigns directed at youth, aimed at increasing disapproval rates, may be working. Although still lower than their highest levels in the early 1990s, disapproval rates for trying marijuana once or twice edged upward in eighth, tenth, and twelfth graders in 2002.[4] One of the objectives of *Healthy People 2010* is to increase the proportion of adolescents who disapprove of trying marijuana or hashish once or twice (see Box 12.3).

FIGURE 12.6
Marijuana is the nation's most popular illicit drug.

The acute health effects of marijuana use include reduced concentration, slowed reaction time, impaired short-term memory, and impaired judgment. Naturally, these effects can have serious consequences for someone operating a motor vehicle or other machinery or can even result in a medical emergency. The increase in both marijuana use and its potency in the 1990s were reflected in an increase in the number of marijuana-related emergency room episodes, which rose from 15,706 in 1990 to 33,954 in 2004.[39] Marijuana use in combination with other drugs can be especially dangerous because drugs in combination may affect the brain differently. In 2004, marijuana, used alone or with one or more other drugs, was involved in an estimated 215,665 emergency department visits.[39]

polydrug use
concurrent use of
multiple drugs

BOX 12.3   HEALTHY PEOPLE 2010 OBJECTIVES: ADVERSE CONSEQUENCES OF SUBSTANCE USE AND ABUSE

Objective: An increase in adolescents who disapprove of trying marijuana or hashish once or twice.

Target and baseline:

Objective	1998 Baseline	2004	2010 Target
		Percent	
26-16d. Eighth graders	69	76	72
26-16e. Tenth graders	56	60	72
26-16f. Twelfth graders	52	53	72

Target setting method: Better than the best.

Source: Monitoring the Future Study, NIH, National Institute of Drug Abuse (NIDA).

For Further Thought

Attitudes and beliefs are often a key factor influencing drug-taking behavior among adolescents. Studies have shown that when there is high level of disapproval of marijuana use by adolescents, the prevalence of marijuana use declines. Conversely, an increase in marijuana use occurs when there is an apparent decline in those expressing strong disapproval of use. How strong are prevailing feelings of disapproval of marijuana use in your community? Do adolescents in your community feel that it is "OK" to try marijuana once or twice?

Source: CDC (2007). *Data2010 . . . The Healthy People 2010 Database—January, 2007 Edition.* Available at http://wonder.cdc.gov.

**amotivational
syndrome**
a pattern of behavior
characterized by
apathy, loss of
effectiveness, and a
more passive,
introverted
personality

The chronic effects of smoking marijuana include damage to the respiratory system by the smoke itself and, for some, the development of a controverisal condition known as **amotivational syndrome.** Amotivational syndrome has been described as a chronic apathy toward maturation and the achievement of the developmental tasks listed previously (e.g., developing skills for independent living, setting and achieving goals, and developing an adult self-identity). There is also evidence now that long-term marijuana users experience physiological and psychological withdrawal symptoms. While these "unpleasant behavioral symptoms are less obvious than those for heroin or alcohol, they are significant and do perhaps contribute to continued drug use."[40] Further evidence of the dependence-producing nature of marijuana is the number of persons seeking admission to treatment programs. Between 1994 and 2004, the proportion of admissions to treatment programs for marijuana abuse rose 9%. Nearly 16% of those entering drug abuse treatment programs in 2004 were admitted for marijuana abuse; this was more than for any other single drug except alcohol.[41] Finally, one of the chief concerns with marijuana is that those who smoke marijuana are more likely to use other, more addictive drugs. For example, 89% of those who use cocaine first used cigarettes, alcohol, and marijuana.[42]

Narcotics: Opium, Morphine, Heroin, and Others

narcotics
drugs derived from or
chemically related to
opium that reduce
pain and induce
stupor, such as
morphine

Opium and its derivatives, morphine and heroin, come from the oriental poppy plant, *Papaver somniferum.* These **narcotics** numb the senses and reduce pain. As such, they have a high potential for abuse. The narcotic that is most widely abused is heroin, a derivative of morphine. In 2000, about 3.5 million (1.5%) of the 243 million noninstitutionalized people over the age of 12 reported the use of heroin in their lifetime, while 379,000 (0.2%) reported use in the past year.[32] This estimate is low because this survey undoubtedly missed a great many addicts who may be homeless and living in shelters. Use in the past year among high school seniors has increased significantly, from 0.6% in 1992 to 0.8% in 2005.[4]

Opium poppies do not grow in the continental United States. Heroin arrives in the United States from four geographic areas: Southwest Asia, Southeast Asia, Mexico, and South America. While Asia and Mexico have supplied heroin to U.S. markets for many years, South America has only recently become an important source of heroin. While South American heroin predominates in the east, Mexican heroin predominates west of the Mississippi River.[43]

Heroin is the Number 1 narcotic of abuse and is also the illicit drug responsible for more deaths than any other.[1] But, there are many other narcotics that are also abused and some of the heroin deaths could be attributable to fentanyl, a potent synthetic narcotic sometimes mixed with heroin.[43] Prescription narcotics abusers take opiates that are obtained through diversion of compounds intended for legitimate medical use as pain relievers. Examples include natural narcotics such as morphine and codeine, synthetic narcotics such as Demerol and Darvon, and quasi-synthetic narcotics such as OxyContin, Vicodin, Dilaudid, and Percodan. As mentioned earlier, these prescription narcotics are highly addictive and subject to abuse.

tolerance
physiological and
enzygmatic
adjustments that
occur in response to
the chronic presence
of drugs, which are
reflected in the need
for ever-increasing
doses

Narcotics produce euphoria, analgesia, and drowsiness. They reduce anxiety and pain without affecting motor activity the way alcohol and barbiturates do. If use continues, the body makes physiological adjustments to the presence of the drug. This **tolerance** means that larger and larger doses are required to achieve the same euphoria and numbing as the initial dose. While tolerance develops rapidly to the euphoric effects, the depressing effects on respiration may continue to increase with dose level, increasing the risk of a fatal overdose. As the cost of the drug habit becomes higher, the abuser usually attempts to quit. This results in withdrawal symptoms because the body has become physically dependent upon the drug. Heroin addicts have a difficult time changing their lifestyle for several reasons. First there is the addiction itself, both physical and psychological. Often, there are underlying psychosocial problems as well, such as poor self-image, lack of job skills, and absence of supporting family and friends. Addicts usually mistrust official programs set up to help them. They are usually in poor health mentally and physically. Because the duration of action of heroin is only four to five hours, the addict is usually too concerned with finding the next dose or recovering from the previous one to be productive in the community.

The community is affected by more than just the loss of productivity. The addict must obtain money to purchase heroin, and the price of the habit can be very high—as much as $200 per day. The money is usually obtained illegally through burglaries, thefts, robberies, muggings, prostitution (male and female), and selling drugs. If a prostitute can make $50 dollars a trick, he or she needs to turn at least four tricks a day just to maintain the habit. The result is not only a deteriorating community but also epidemics of sexually transmitted diseases, such as gonorrhea, syphilis, chlamydia, herpes, and AIDS. Because most heroin addicts inject the drug, there are also epidemics of bloodborne diseases, such as those caused by HIV and hepatitis viruses. In this way, drug abuse increases the burden on community health resources. Addicts who turn to dealing drugs to support their habit do even more damage, because they increase the availability of the drug and may introduce it to first-time users. There is an additional burden on the criminal justice system when these addicts are arrested, prosecuted, incarcerated, and rehabilitated.

Cocaine and Crack Cocaine

Cocaine is the psychoactive ingredient in the leaves of the coca plant, *Erythoxolyn coca,* which grows in the Andes Mountains of South America. Cocaine is a **stimulant;** that is, it increases the activity of the central nervous system. For centuries, natives of the Andes Mountains have chewed the leaves to improve stamina during work and long treks. In its more purified forms, as a salt (white powder) or dried paste (crack), cocaine is a powerful euphoriant/ stimulant and very addictive.

Cocaine use among high school seniors peaked in 1985, when 6.7% reported use within the past 30 days. By 1992 this figure had dropped to only 1.3%, but by 1999 those reporting use in the past 30 days had doubled to 2.6%.[3,4] The 2005 30-day prevalence rate among high school seniors was 2.3%. Estimates for 2005 indicated that as many as 2.4 million Americans had used cocaine or crack in the past 30 days.[32] Therefore, cocaine remains a serious drug problem in the United States.

Hallucinogens

Hallucinogens are drugs that produce illusions, hallucinations, and other changes in one's perceptions of the environment. These effects are due to the phenomenon known as **synesthesia,** a mixing of the senses. Hallucinogens include both naturally derived drugs like mescaline, from the peyote cactus, and psilocybin and psilocin, from the Psilocybe mushroom; and synthetic drugs, such as lysergic acid diethylamide (LSD). While physical dependence has not been demonstrated with the hallucinogens, tolerance does occur. Though overdose deaths are rare, "bad trips" (unpleasant experiences) do occur, and a few people have experienced permanent visual disturbances. Because there are no legal sources for these drugs, users are always at risk for taking fake, impure, or adulterated drugs.

Stimulants

As previously mentioned, stimulants are drugs that increase the activity level of the central nervous system. Examples include the amphetamines, such as amphetamine itself (bennies), dextroamphetamine (dexies), methamphetamine (meth), and dextromethamphetamine (ice); methylphenidate (Ritalin); and methcathinone (cat). These drugs cause the release of high levels of the neurotransmitter dopamine, which stimulates brain cells. Tolerance builds quickly, so abusers must escalate their doses rapidly. Chronic abusers can develop tremors and

cocaine
the psychoactive ingredient in the leaves of the coca plant, *Erythoxolyn coca*, which, when refined, is a powerful stimulant/euphoriant

stimulant
a drug that increases the activity of the central nervous system

hallucinogens
drugs that produce profound distortions of the senses

synesthesia
impairment of mind characterized by a sensation that senses are mixed

amphetamines
a group of synthetic
drugs that act as
stimulants

methamphetamine
the amphetamine
most widely abused

barbiturates
depressant drugs
based on the structure
of barbituric acid

benzodiazapines
nonbarbiturate
depressant drugs

methaqualone
an illicit depressant
drug

depressants
drugs that slow
central nervous
system activity, for
example, alcohol,
barbiturates,
benzodiazapines

club drugs
a general term for
those illicit drugs,
primarily synthetic,
that are most
commonly
encountered at night
clubs and "raves"
(examples include
MDMA, GHB, GBL,
LSD, PCP, ketamine,
Rohypnol, and
methamphetamine)

confusion, aggressiveness, and paranoia. The long-term effects include permanent brain damage and Parkinson's disease-like symptoms.[44]

Amphetamines are Schedule II prescription drugs that have been widely abused for many years. Increased regulatory efforts in the 1970s probably contributed to the rise in the cocaine trade in the 1980s. When cocaine abuse declined in the late 1980s, there was a resurgence of amphetamine abuse, primarily **methamphetamine,** also known as "crystal," "crank," "speed," "go fast," or just "meth." At first, the clandestine labs that produced methamphetamine, and those abusing the substance, were concentrated primarily in the southwestern states. However, by 1995 production and abuse had spread to the Midwest, and by 1999 methamphetamine abuse had become the fastest growing drug threat in America. In 2005, 3.9% of high school seniors reported abusing amphetamines and 0.9% reported abusing methamphetamine in the past 30 days.[4] In 2005, the DEA seized 2,148 kilograms of methamphetamine and recorded 12,484 clandestine lab incidents, including labs, dumpsters, chemicals and glassware, and equipment (see Figures 12.7 and 12.8).[45,46]

Methylphenidate (Ritalin) is a Schedule II drug used to treat attention-deficit hyperactivity disorder. Though not produced in clandestine labs, the drug is often diverted from its intended use and abused by those for whom it was not prescribed.

Depressants
Barbiturates, benzodiazapines, methaqualone, and other **depressants** slow down the central nervous system. They are attractive to some people because, like alcohol, among the first effects of taking these drugs are the lowering of anxiety and the loss of inhibitions. These effects produce the feeling of a "high," even though these drugs depress the central nervous system. As one continues to use these drugs, tolerance develops, and the user experiences the need for greater and greater doses in order to feel the same effects that the previous dose provided. Strong physical dependence develops, so that abstinence results in severe clinical illness; thus, abusers of these substances must often rely on medical assistance during detoxification and recovery.

Club Drugs and Designer Drugs
"**Club drugs** is a term for a number of illicit drugs, primarily synthetic, that are most commonly encountered at nightclubs and 'raves.'"[47] These drugs include MDMA, ketamine, GHB, GBL, Rohypnol, LSD, PCP, methamphetamine, and others. Because these drugs are illegal, there is no guarantee of their safety or even their identity. Also, these drugs are often taken in combination with alcohol or other drugs. As a result, the number of emergency reports for many of these club drugs quadrupled between 1994 and 1998.[47] MDMA, also known as "Ecstasy," is the most popular of the club drugs. Use of MDMA rose sharply among eighth, tenth, and twelfth graders through 2001 and then declined sharply. Five percent of high school seniors surveyed in 2005 had taken MDMA at least once, 3% in the past year.[4] Long-term effects of MDMA are still under evaluation, but there is evidence that the drug causes brain damage.[47]

Rohypnol (flunitrazepan) is another club drug that is also known as a date-rape drug. This drug, which exhibits all of the characteristics of a depressant, is a legal prescription drug in more than 50 countries. In the United States, the drug is regarded as more dangerous, and thus less medically useful than other sedatives. Thus, it is an illegal (Schedule I) drug.

Designer drugs is a term coined in the 1980s to describe drugs synthesized by amateur chemists in secret laboratories. By constantly changing the design of their drugs, these chemists hoped to stay one step ahead of law enforcement. Examples of designer drugs included MDMA (3,4-methylenedioxy-methamphetamine), synthetic narcotics, and dissociative anesthetics like PCP (angel dust) and ketamine. Under the Controlled Substance Act of 1970, only those drugs that were listed as illegal were illegal, whereas similar, but slightly altered, drugs were not. The Controlled Substances Analogue Act of 1986 was enacted to reduce the flow of designer drugs into the market and make it easier to prosecute those involved in manufacturing and distributing these drugs. Designer and club drugs are still a problem.

Anabolic Drugs

Anabolic drugs are protein-building drugs. Included are the anabolic/androgenic steroids (AS), testosterone, and human growth hormone (HGH). These drugs have legitimate medical uses, such as the rebuilding of muscles after starvation or disease and the treatment of dwarfism. But they are sometimes abused by athletes and body builders as a shortcut to increasing muscle mass, strength, and endurance. Abuse of steroids is accompanied by numerous acute and chronic side effects for men, including acne, gynecomastia (the development of breasts), baldness, reduced fertility, and reduction in testicular size. Side effects for women are masculinizing: development of a male physique, increased body hair, failure to ovulate (menstrual irregularities), and a deepening of the voice. Long-term abuse of anabolic steroids can result in psychological dependence, making the discontinuation of use very difficult.[48]

In the late 1980s, it became apparent that increasing numbers of boys and young men of high school and college age were taking anabolic steroids as a shortcut to muscle building or to maturity (see Figure 12.9). Because of these trends in the abuse of anabolic

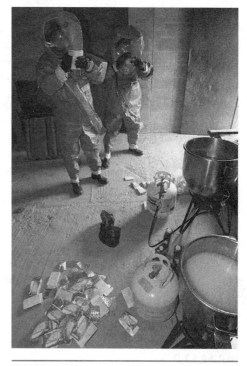

FIGURE 12.7

Dismantling a clandestine methamphetamine lab is hazardous work.

FIGURE 12.8

Total of all clandestine laboratory incidents involving methamphetamine (including labs, dump sites, and chemicals, glassware, or equipment), calendar year 2005.

Source: Drug Enforcement Administration, Department of Justice (2006). "Maps of Methamphetamine Lab Incidents." Available at http://www.usdoj.gov/dea/concern/map_lab_seizures.html.

Rohypnol (flunitrazepan) a depressant in the benzodiazapine group that has achieved notoriety as a date-rape drug

designer drugs drugs synthesized illegally that are similar to, but structurally different from, known controlled substances

anabolic drugs compounds, structurally similar to the male hormone testosterone, that increase protein synthesis and thus muscle building steroids, these drugs were placed in Schedule III of the Controlled Substance Act in 1990. Abuse of steroids increased during the 1990s, but has leveled off recently. As with other drugs discussed earlier, "steroids" sold on the Internet may not be authentic. Purchasing such things online is certainly an example of the phrase "Buyer, beware."

Inhalants

Inhalants are a collection of psychoactive, breathable chemicals. They include paint solvents, motor fuels, cleaners, glues, aerosol sprays, cosmetics, and other types of vapor. Because of their easy availability and low cost, they are often the drug of choice for the young. The primary effect of most of the inhalants is depression. As with alcohol, the user may at first experience a reduction of anxieties and inhibitions, making the user feel high. Continued use may result in hallucinations and loss of consciousness. Many of these chemicals are extremely toxic to the kidneys, liver, and nervous system. The use of inhalants by youth results from boredom and perhaps peer pressure and represents a maladaptation to these conditions.

FIGURE 12.9
Abuse of anabolic drugs carries the risk of serious acute and chronic health problems.

inhalants
breathable substances that produce mind-altering effects

PREVENTION AND CONTROL OF DRUG ABUSE

The prevention and control of alcohol and other drug abuse require a knowledge of the causes of drug-taking behavior, sources of illicit drugs, drug laws, and treatment programs. Also required are community organizing skills, persistence, and cooperation among a vast array of concerned individuals and official and unofficial agencies.

From a community health standpoint, drug abuse tends to be a chronic condition. Thus, the activities of drug abuse and prevention agencies and organizations can be viewed as chronic disease-prevention activities. This approach, involving three different levels of prevention, was first discussed in Chapter 4 and is discussed next in relation to drug abuse prevention and control.

Levels of Prevention

Drug abuse prevention activities can be viewed as primary, secondary, or tertiary depending upon the point of intervention. *Primary prevention* programs are aimed at those who have never used drugs, and their goal is to prevent or forestall the initiation of drug use. Drug education programs that stress primary prevention of drug and alcohol use are most appropriate and successful for children at the elementary school age. In a broader sense, almost any activity that would reduce the likelihood of primary drug use could be considered primary prevention. For example, raising the price of alcohol, increasing cigarette taxes, arresting a neighborhood drug pusher, or destroying a cocaine crop in Bolivia could be considered primary prevention if it forestalled primary drug use in at least some individuals.

Secondary prevention programs are aimed at those who have begun alcohol or other drug use but who have not become chronic abusers and have not suffered significant physical or mental impairment from their drug or alcohol abuse. Alcohol and other drug abuse education programs that stress secondary prevention are often appropriate for people of high school or college age. They can be presented in educational, workplace, or community settings.

Tertiary prevention programs are designed to provide drug abuse treatment and aftercare, including relapse prevention programs. As such, they are usually designed for adults. Tertiary programs for teenagers are far too uncommon. Tertiary prevention programs may receive clients who "turn themselves in" for treatment voluntarily, but more often than not their clients are referred by the courts.

Elements of Prevention

There are four basic elements that play a role in drug abuse prevention and control. These are (1) education, (2) treatment, (3) public policy, and (4) enforcement. The goals of education and treatment are the same: to reduce the demand for drugs. Likewise, setting effective public policy and law enforcement share the same goal: to reduce the supply and availability of drugs in the community.

Education

The purpose of **drug abuse education** is to limit the demand for drugs by providing information about drugs and the dangers of drug abuse, changing attitudes and beliefs about drugs, providing the skills necessary to abstain from drugs, and ultimately changing drug abuse behavior. Education, principally a primary prevention activity, can be school-based or community-based. Examples of school-based drug abuse prevention programs are *Here's Looking at You, 2000* and *Project DARE (Drug Abuse Resistance Education).* For these programs and other school-based programs to be successful, other community members such as parents, teachers, local business people, and others must visibly support the program. Examples of community-based programs are the American Cancer Society's *Great American Smokeout; Race Against Drugs (RAD),* a nationwide program that links drug abuse prevention with motor sports; and the *Reality Check Campaign,* a program to boost awareness of the harmful effects of marijuana smoking among youth.

drug abuse education providing information about drugs and the dangers of drug abuse, changing attitudes and beliefs about drugs, providing the skills necessary to abstain from drugs, and ultimately changing drug abuse behavior

Treatment

The goal of **treatment** is to remove the physical, emotional, and environmental conditions that have contributed to drug dependency. Like education, treatment aims to reduce demand for drugs. It also aims to save money. Consider the money saved on law enforcement, medical costs, and lost productivity when treatment is successful. It is estimated that for every $1 spent on treatment, between $5 and $7 are saved.[49,50] Treatment for drug abuse occurs in a variety of settings and involves a variety of approaches. Treatment may be residential (inpatient) or nonresidential (outpatient). Under managed care, "behavioral health care" guidelines usually limit inpatient care to 28 days, after which the care may continue on an outpatient basis. In drug abuse treatment, what happens after the initial treatment phase is critical. **Aftercare,** the continuing care provided the recovering former drug abuser, often involves peer group or self-help support group meetings, such as those provided by Alcoholics Anonymous (AA) or Narcotics Anonymous (NA). Despite frequent relapses, treatment for drug dependence is viewed as an important component of a community's comprehensive drug abuse prevention and control strategy.

treatment (for drug abuse and dependence) care that removes the physical, emotional, and environmental conditions that have contributed to drug abuse and/or dependence

aftercare the continuing care provided the recovering former drug abuser

Public Policy

Public policy embodies the guiding principles and courses of action pursued by governments to solve practical problems affecting society. Examples include passing drunk-driving laws or zoning ordinances that limit the number of bars in a neighborhood and enacting ordinances that regulate the type and amount of advertising for such legal drugs as alcohol and tobacco. Public policy should guide the budget discussions that ultimately determine how much a community spends for education, treatment, and law enforcement. Further examples of public policy decisions are restrictions of smoking in public buildings, the setting of 0.08% blood alcohol concentration as the point at which driving becomes illegal, and zero tolerance laws for BACs for minors. Setting the level of state excise taxes on alcohol and tobacco is also a public policy decision.

public policy the guiding principles and courses of action pursued by governments to solve practical problems affecting society

Law Enforcement

Law enforcement in drug abuse prevention and control is the application of federal, state, and local laws to arrest, jail, bring to trial, and sentence those who break drug laws or break laws because of drug use. The primary roles of law enforcement in a drug abuse prevention and control program are to (1) control drug use, (2) to control crime, especially crime related to drug use and drug trafficking—the buying, selling, manufacturing, or transporting of illegal drugs—(3) to prevent the establishment of crime organizations, and (4) to protect neighborhoods.[51] Law enforcement is concerned with limiting the supply of drugs in the community by interrupting the source, transit, and distribution of drugs. There are law enforcement agencies at all levels of government. The principal agencies are discussed next.

Governmental Drug Prevention and Control Agencies and Programs

Governmental agencies involved in drug abuse prevention, control, and treatment include a multitude of federal, state, and local agencies. At each of these levels of government, there are numerous offices and programs aimed at reducing either the supply of, or the demand for, drugs.

Federal Agencies and Program

Our nation's anti-drug efforts are headed up by the White House **Office of National Drug Control Policy (ONDCP),** which annually publishes a report detailing the nation's drug control strategy and budget. The 2004 National Drug Control Strategy included three priorities:[52]

1. Stopping drug use before it starts (prevention)
2. Intervening and healing America's drug users (treatment)
3. Disrupting the (drug) market (interdiction)

Progress toward youth goals would be measured from the baseline established by the Monitoring the Future survey for the 2000–2001 school year. Progress toward adult goals would be measured from the baseline of the 2002 National Survey on Drug Use and Health.[52]

Two-Year Goals

- A 10% reduction in current use of illegal drugs by eighth, tenth, and twelfth graders.
- A 10% reduction in current use of illegal drugs by adults aged 18 and older.

Five-Year Goals

- A 25% reduction in current use of illegal drugs by eighth, tenth, and twelfth graders.
- A 25% reduction in current use of illegal drugs by adults aged 18 and older.

According to the National Drug Control Strategy issued by the White House in February 2006, the two-year goal for reducing current illicit drug use by youths was met and exceeded. As of 2005, illicit drug use in this group was down 19%. It remains to be seen whether the five-year reduction goal of 25% will be met. No mention was made of progress toward reaching use reduction goals for adults.[53]

The National Drug Control Strategy budget request for the fiscal year (FY) 2007 was $12.66 billion.[54] Although this may seem like a lot of money, it is considerably less than the figure given in 2001, namely, $18.1 billion.[55] The department scheduled to receive the largest portion of funds in FY 2007 is the Department of Health and Human Services (the National Institute on Drug Abuse and the Substance Abuse and Mental Health Services Administration). The Department of Justice (DOJ) is slated for the second-largest portion. DOJ agencies include the Bureau of Prisons, the Drug Enforcement Administration, the Interagency Crime and Drug Enforcement Agency, and the Office of Justice Programs. Two agencies that will receive significant funding belong in the Department of Homeland Security—the U.S. Coast Guard and Border and

Transportation Security. The remainder of the funding is spread over the Departments of Defense, State, Education, and Veterans Affairs and the Office of National Drug Control Policy.[54]

Department of Health and Human Services
The Department of Health and Human Services (HHS) receives the largest portion of the federal drug budget, more than $3.41 billion in FY 2007. This money is spent on drug prevention education, treatment programs, and research into the causes and physiology of drug abuse. The preponderance of these funds is spent to reduce the demand for drugs. The approach of HHS to the drug problem is broad and includes research, treatment, and educational activities.

The misuse and abuse of tobacco, alcohol, and other drugs are addressed primarily as lifestyle problems, that is, as health promotion issues—like physical fitness and nutrition. As such, HHS recognizes that the problems of drug misuse and abuse are complex—involving inherited, environmental, social, and economic causes. Therefore, the solutions are also viewed as being complex. The typical approach involves the application of the three levels of prevention—primary, secondary, and tertiary. It also recognizes the importance of incorporating the three primary prevention strategies of education, regulation, and automatic protection. These are discussed in greater detail in Chapter 17.

The HHS has published health status, risk reduction, and service and protection objectives on the use of tobacco, alcohol, and other drugs in *Healthy People 2010* (see Boxes 12.1 and 12.2). These objectives set the direction and standards for success of all our national drug control efforts.

The lead agency within HHS is the **Substance Abuse and Mental Health Services Administration (SAMHSA).** Within SAMHSA, there are three centers: the Center for Substance Abuse Prevention (CSAP), the Center for Substance Abuse Treatment (CSAT), and the Center for Mental Health Services (CMHS). In addition to SAMHSA, there are two other important agencies that deal with the problems of alcohol and other drugs: the National Institute on Drug Abuse and the Food and Drug Administration (see Chapter 2 for more information on these agencies).

The **National Institute on Drug Abuse (NIDA)** is the largest institution in the world devoted to drug abuse research. At NIDA, research efforts are aimed at understanding the causes and consequences of drug abuse and at evaluating prevention and treatment programs. Within NIDA are several important divisions and centers, such as the Division of Clinical Research, the Division of Epidemiology and Prevention Research, the Division of Preclinical Research, the Division of Applied Research, the Medications Development Division, and the Addiction Research Center. These agencies conduct research and publish articles on the causes, prevention, and treatment of tobacco, alcohol, and other drug abuse.

Another important agency in HHS is the Food and Drug Administration (FDA). As stated earlier, the FDA is charged with ensuring the safety and efficacy of all prescription and non-prescription drugs. The FDA dictates which drugs reach the market, and how they must be labeled, packaged, and sold. The FDA is more concerned with drug misuse than abuse.

Department of Justice
The second-largest portion of federal spending for drug control, $2.95 billion in FY 2007, goes to the Department of Justice (DOJ).[54] The DOJ addresses the supply side of the drug trade most directly by identifying, arresting, and prosecuting those who break drug laws. It tries to protect the welfare of society by incarcerating the most serious offenders, deterring others from becoming involved in drug trade, and providing a clear picture to all of the cost of drug trade and abuse. Regarding the latter, the DOJ indirectly contributes to reducing the demand for drugs.

The DOJ's budget is large, because in addition to its enforcement responsibilities, the department maintains prisons and prisoners. The DOJ employs not only those who manage

Substance Abuse and Mental Health Services Administration (SAMHSA) the agency within the Department of Health and Human Services that provides leadership in drug abuse prevention and treatment. It houses the Center for Substance Abuse Prevention and the Center for Substance Abuse Treatment.

National Institute on Drug Abuse (NIDA) the federal government's lead agency for drug abuse research, one of the National Institutes of Health the penal system, but also many marshals, attorneys, and judges. The single largest portion of the DOJ's budget goes to the Bureau of Prisons. The DOJ also operates treatment, education, and rehabilitation programs in these prisons.

Within the DOJ are several important drug-fighting agencies. The lead agency in this respect is the Drug Enforcement Agency (DEA), which investigates and assists in the prosecution of drug traffickers and their accomplices in the United States and abroad and seizes the drugs as well as the assets on which they depend. The DEA employs more than 7,000 special agents and support personnel.

Three other important agencies in the DOJ that are involved in the prevention and control of drug abuse are the Federal Bureau of Investigation (FBI), the Office of Justice Programs (OJP), and the **Bureau of Alcohol, Tobacco, Firearms and Explosives (ATF).** The FBI investigates multinational organized-crime networks that control the illegal drug market. The OJP provides "federal leadership in developing the nation's capacity to prevent and control crime, improve the criminal and juvenile justice systems, increase knowledge about crime and related issues, and assist crime victims."[56] For example, the OJP forms partnerships with and provides funds for state and local programs to "control drug abuse and trafficking; reduce and prevent crime and rehabilitate neighborhoods."[56] The ATF was only recently transferred to the DOJ from the Department of the Treasury, where it had been administered since its inception. Part of ATF's mission is to prevent the diversion of taxes (loss of revenue) caused by trafficking in contraband tobacco and alcohol products and to bring those involved in this activity to justice.

Bureau of Alcohol, Tobacco, Firearms, and Explosives (ATF) the federal agency in the Department of Justice that regulates alcohol and tobacco

Department of Homeland Security

Shortly following the terrorist attacks on the World Trade Center and the Pentagon on September 11, 2001, President George W. Bush authorized the establishment of the Department of Homeland Security (DHS). Subsequently, a number of federal agencies involved in drug control activities were transferred into this new department, which is scheduled to receive the third-largest portion of funding from the National Drug Control Budget ($3.30 billion).[54] Those agencies receiving funds are Immigration and Customs Enforcement, Customs and Border Protection, and the United States Coast Guard. In the current environment, in which protection from terrorist acts is DHS's primary concern, the prevention and control of drug trafficking seems somewhat less urgent by comparison. Nonetheless, it is part of the mission of these agencies. For example, Immigration and Customs Enforcement works to prevent the immigration to this country of criminals, including those involved in drug trafficking. Customs and Border Protection, made up of employees from the Department of Agriculture, the Immigration and Naturalization Service, the Border Patrol, and the U.S. Customs Service, works with the Immigration and Customs Enforcement to protect our borders from external threats, including illegal drugs (see Figure 12.10). The United States Coast Guard helps to interdict illegal drug trafficking in our coastal waters.

FIGURE 12.10
Customs agents assist in the arrest and prosecution of those involved in drug trafficking.

Other Federal Agencies

Other federal agencies involved in drug abuse prevention and control are the Departments of State, Defense, Veterans' Affairs, and Education. The State Department, through various diplomatic efforts, including "drug summits," attempts to achieve a reduction in the production and shipment of illicit drugs into this country. The Defense Department assists foreign allies to control the cultivation of illegal drug crops and the production of illegal drugs. Funding slated for the Department of Veterans' Affairs is aimed primarily at the treatment of drug-related health problems of veterans.

The Department of Education (DE) launched a program to support drug-free schools and communities in the late 1980s. The effort was aimed at encouraging schools to adopt clear "no drug use" policies and to provide a message that both communities and schools do not condone or approve of alcohol or drug use by minors. A handbook titled *What Works: Schools Without Drugs* was prepared and distributed to schools and communities.[57] The Department of Education continues to participate in the federal drug prevention effort, although the amount of funding for the DE has declined annually since 2002. The National Drug Control Budget for fiscal year 2007 cut $346.5 million from the Drug Free Schools and Safe Communities Program and $32 million from the alcohol abuse reduction program, but provided a $15 million increase in funding for drug testing in schools.[54]

State and Local Agencies and Programs

While considerable economic resources can be brought to bear on the drug problem at the federal level, it is becoming increasingly clear that to achieve success, the drug war in America must be fought at the local level—in homes, neighborhoods, and schools. State support usually comes in the form of law enforcement expertise in education and mental health, the coordination of local and regional programs, and sometimes funding initiatives. It is usually up to local citizens to put these state initiatives into action or to begin initiatives of their own.

State Agencies

State agencies that address drug abuse prevention and control issues include the offices of the governor, as well as state departments of health, education, mental health, justice, and law enforcement. Sometimes there is an umbrella agency that coordinates the activities of these various offices and departments; other times there is not. To review agencies involved in the prevention and control of drug abuse and drug dependence problems in your state, visit the Web site of the Office of National Drug Control Policy (www.whitehousedrugpolicy.gov/statelocal/index.html) and click on the State and Local button. This button should take you to a page that lists each of the states. By clicking on a state, you can view all the state agencies involved in drug abuse prevention and control. For example, the Minnesota page lists the governor's office, the state drug program coordinator, the state legislative contact, the attorney general, the corrections agency, the judicial agency, the statistical analysis center, the Uniform Crime Reports contact, the state's drug and alcohol agency, a prevention resource center, the Department of Children, Families and Learning (Safe and Drug Free Schools), the Department of Human Services (and the chemical dependency program division), and other agencies.

The role of these state-level agencies is evident from their titles. Some state agencies provide actual services; others provide statistics or other information. Still others provide expertise or serve as a conduit for federal funding aimed at local (city or county) governments.

The role of state government is to promote, protect, and maintain the health and welfare of its citizens. Thus, each state has its own laws regulating the sale of tobacco, alcohol, and prescription drugs. It is the states that issue licenses to doctors, dentists, pharmacists, liquor stores, and taverns. Each state also passes laws and sets the penalties for the manufacture, sale, and possession of illicit drugs such as marijuana. For example, in California, possession of 28.5 grams (one ounce) of marijuana or less is a misdemeanor but not an arrestable offense; it carries a $100 fine. Possession of more than 28.5 grams is also a misdemeanor, punishable by six months in jail and a $500 fine. In Utah, however, possession of less than one ounce of marijuana is a misdemeanor punishable by six months in jail and a $1,000 fine. Possession of more than one pound is a felony punishable by five years in jail and a $5,000 fine.[58]

In some cases, states have passed laws that conflict with federal laws. For example, some states have decriminalized marijuana cultivation and possession for medical use. In Hawaii, patients with a signed statement from their physician affirming that they suffer from a certain medical condition are protected under law. These patients must be on a state-run registry that issues identification cards. They are then permitted to cultivate up to seven marijuana plants (only three mature plants) and to be in possession of no more than one ounce of usable marijuana. These people could still be arrested by the DEA and prosecuted under federal law.

Local Agencies

Agencies of local governments that are involved in drug abuse prevention and control include mayors' offices, police and sheriffs' departments, school corporations, health departments, family services offices, mental health services, prosecutors' offices, the juvenile justice system, judges and courts, drug task forces, and so on. In some communities, there is a community drug task force or coordinating council that includes both government officials and representatives of nongovernmental agencies. Such task forces or councils might include local religious leaders, representatives from local industry (both labor and management), health care providers, and members from local voluntary agencies. The task of these organizations is usually to prioritize problems faced by the community and decide on approaches to solving them. The goal is to develop a coordinated and effective effort to resolve the issue. Sometimes a solution might involve selecting an approach that has been used with success in another community or school system.

Nongovernmental Drug Prevention and Control Agencies and Programs

Many nongovernmental programs and agencies make valuable contributions to the prevention and control of drug abuse in America. Among these are community- and school-based programs, workplace programs, and voluntary agencies.

Community-Based Drug Education Programs

Community-based drug education can occur in a variety of settings, such as child care facilities, public housing, religious institutions, businesses, and health care facilities. Information about the abuse of alcohol, tobacco, and other drugs can be disseminated through television and radio programs, movies, newspapers, and magazines.

Community-based drug education programs are most likely to be successful when they include six key features:[59]

1. A comprehensive strategy
2. An indirect approach to drug abuse prevention
3. The goal of empowering youth
4. A participatory approach
5. A culturally sensitive orientation
6. Highly structured activities

Community-based drug education programs that address broader issues (e.g., coping and learning skills) are most effective, as are those embedded in other existing community activities (see Figure 12.11). Participation can be increased by planning drug education programs around sporting or cultural events. Culturally sensitive programs are crucial for reaching minorities in the community. Use of the appropriate language, reading level, and spokespersons can mean the difference between success or failure of a program.

In the past 30 years a great many drug abuse prevention education programs have been conceived and tested. Some of these

FIGURE 12.11

Use of appropriate language can be the difference between success and failture of a community drug prevention program.

have been scientifically proven to be effective. The Center for Substance Abuse Prevention (CSAP), a branch of the Substance Abuse and Mental Health Services Administration in the U.S. Department of Health and Human Services, has developed a list of effective programs. The list is available online at the CSAP Web site.[60]

An example of a community-based program with a record of success is *Across Ages.*

> Across Ages is a school- and community-based drug prevention program for youth 9 to 13 years, that seeks to strengthen the bonds between adults and youth and provide opportunities for positive community involvement. The unique and highly effective feature of Across Ages is the pairing of older adult mentors (age 55 and above) with young adolescents, specifically youth making the transition to middle school. The program employs mentoring, community service, social competence training, and family activities to build youths' sense of personal responsibility for self and community.[60]

Across Ages has been able to demonstrate success in the following areas: decreased substance use, decrease in tobacco and alcohol use, increased problem-solving ability, increased school attendance, decreased suspensions from school, improved attitude toward adults, and improved attitude toward school and the future.[60] Many other successful community- and school-based drug abuse prevention programs are listed on the CSAP Web site.

School-Based Drug Education Programs

Most health educators believe that a strong, comprehensive school health education program (see Chapter 6)—one that occupies a permanent and prominent place in the school curriculum—is the best defense against all health problems, including drug abuse. However, many schools lack these strong programs, and in their absence, substitute drug education programs developed specifically for school use.

One such program is the Drug Abuse Resistance Education (DARE) program, which began in Los Angeles. In the DARE program, local police enter the classroom to teach grade-school children about drugs (see Figure 12.12). While imparting some knowledge, the program's primary approach is to change attitudes and beliefs about drugs. It is also successful in improving children's images of the police themselves. Unfortunately, while very popular in many communities, DARE programs have been unable to demonstrate any real success in reducing actual drug use.[61]

An example of a program from the CSAP list that has been scientifically proven to be effective is Project ALERT. Project ALERT reduced students' initiation of marijuana use by 30%, decreased current marijuana use by 60%, reduced past-month cigarette use by 20% to 25%, decreased regular and heavy smoking by 33% to 55%, and substantially reduced students' pro-drug-use attitudes and beliefs.[60]

Student assistance programs (SAPs) are school-based programs modeled after employee assistance programs in the workplace. They are aimed at identifying and intervening in cases of drug problems. **Peer counseling programs** are also present in some schools. In these programs, students talk about mutual problems and receive support and perhaps coping skills from peers who have been trained in this intervention activity and do not use drugs.

Workplace-Based Drug Education Programs

In September 1986, concern about widespread drug use in the workplace led then President Ronald Reagan to sign Executive

student assistance programs (SAPs) school-based drug education programs to assist students who have alcohol or other drug problems

peer counseling programs school-based programs in which students discuss alcohol and other drug-related problems with peers

FIGURE 12.12
Drug Abuse Resistance Education (DARE) programs involve police in school drug education.

Order 12564, proclaiming a Drug Free Federal Workplace.[62] The rationale for the order signed in September 1986 was cited in the document itself: the desire and need for the well-being of employees, the loss of productivity caused by drug use, the illegal profits of organized crime, the illegality of the behavior itself, the undermining of public confidence, and the role of the federal government as the largest employer in the nation to set a standard for other employers to follow in these matters. It had also become apparent to all that drug abuse is not just a personal health problem and a law enforcement problem, but that it also is a behavior that affects the safety and productivity of others, especially at work. Studies have shown that substance abusers (1) are less productive, (2) miss more work days, (3) are more likely to injure themselves, and (4) file more workers' compensation claims than their non-substance-abusing counterparts.

The Drug Free Federal Workplace order required federal employees to refrain from using illegal drugs, and it required agency heads to develop plans for achieving drug-free workplaces for employees in their agencies. The order further required the setting up of drug testing programs and procedures and employee assistance programs that would include provisions for rehabilitation.[62] Similar workplace substance abuse programs, which include drug testing, soon spread to the private sector, so that by the mid-1990s, such programs were in place in more than 80% of American companies.[63]

A typical workplace substance abuse prevention program has five facets.[64] The first is a formal written substance abuse policy that reflects the employer's commitment to a drug-free workplace. The second is an employee drug education and awareness program. Third is the supervisor training program. Fourth is the **employee assistance program (EAP)** to help those who need counseling and rehabilitation. The last component is a drug testing program. Large companies are more likely than small companies to have the major components of a drug-free workplace program.

While a substantial part of the problem can be attributed to alcohol consumption, illicit drug use remains a problem in many workplaces. While it is true that the prevalence of illegal drug abuse in the unemployed adult population is twice that of the employed adult population, 70% of all the illegal users are employed.[65] Fortunately, the prevalence of workplace drug use has declined significantly, in part because of the proliferation of workplace drug abuse and prevention programs that include drug testing. In 1987, the first year of workplace drug testing, 18.1% of all tests were positive;[66] by 1998, this figure had dropped below 5%, where it has remained. In 2005, only 4.1% of all workplace drug tests were positive (see Figure 12.13).[67]

Voluntary Health Agencies

Drug prevention and control programs are carried out at the local level with the cooperation and effort of many community members. Some of these programs are of local origin, while others have received national recognition and even endorsement. The people who actually deliver drug abuse prevention programs include teachers, community health educators, social workers, law enforcement officers, and volunteers.

The programs presented vary greatly in their message and approach. Some programs seek to educate or provide knowledge, others seek to change beliefs or attitudes about alcohol or other drug use, while still others seek to alter behavior by providing new behavior skills. Studies have shown that programs incorporating all these approaches are most successful.

A large number of voluntary health agencies have been founded to prevent or control the social and personal consequences of alcohol, tobacco, and other drug abuse. Among these are such agencies as Mothers Against Drunk Driving (MADD), Students Against Destructive Decisions (SADD), Alcoholics Anonymous (AA), Narcotics Anonymous (NA), the American Cancer

employee assistance program (EAP) a workplace drug program designed to assist employees whose work performance is suffering because of a personal problem such as alcohol or other drug problems

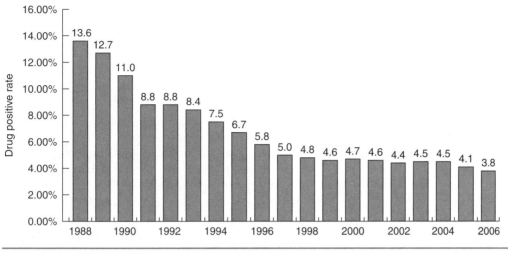

FIGURE 12.13

Drug positivity rates for combined U.S. workforce, 1988 through 2006.

Source: The Quest Diagnostics Drug Testing Index® (2006), from Quest Diagnostics Incorporated. Available at www.questdiagnostics.com. Reprinted with permission.

Society (ACS), and many others. Each of these organizations is active locally, statewide, and nationally.

An important function of community leaders is to encourage parents, school officials, members of law enforcement, businesses, social groups, community health workers, and the media to work together in an effort to reduce the abuse of alcohol, tobacco, and other drugs. Every approach should be used, including seeking favorable legislation and judicial appointments, fairness in advertising, school and community education and treatment, and law enforcement. Only through citizen support and vigilance can there be a reduction in the threat that alcohol and other drugs pose to our community.

CHAPTER SUMMARY

- The abuse of alcohol, tobacco, and other drugs is a major community health problem in the United States.

- Alcohol, tobacco, and other drug abuse affects not only individuals but also communities, where it results in a substantial drain both socially and economically.

- Investigations into the causes of drug experimentation, drug abuse, and drug dependence indicate that both inherited and environmental factors contribute to the problem.

- Rates of tobacco, alcohol, and other drug use rose during the 1990s. After peaking in 1998, use of these drugs began to level off and decline.

- Chronic alcohol and tobacco use results in the loss of billions of dollars and thousands of lives in America each year.

- The misuse and abuse of prescription and nonprescription drugs remains a problem of concern.

- There are four principal elements of drug abuse prevention and control—education, treatment, public policy, and law enforcement.

- Prevention activities can be categorized as primary, secondary, and tertiary prevention.

- There are substantial federal, state, and local efforts to reduce the use, misuse, and abuse of drugs in the United States.

- Federal agencies involved include the Departments of Health and Human Services, Justice, Homeland Security, and many others.

- Efforts at the state level vary from state to state but usually include attempts to coordinate federal and local efforts.

- Drug testing in the workplace reveals a decline in illicit drug use in the workplace since testing began in 1987.

- Alcohol, tobacco, and other drug abuse continues to cause injuries and lost productivity in the American workplace.
- A typical workplace substance abuse prevention program has five components: A written policy, a drug education program, a supervisor training program, an employee assistance program, and a drug testing program.
- A large number of voluntary health agencies are involved in drug abuse prevention and control activities.

REVIEW QUESTIONS

1. What are some personal consequences resulting from the abuse of alcohol and other drugs?
2. What are some community consequences resulting from the abuse of alcohol and other drugs?
3. What are the recent trends in drug use by high school seniors?
4. What do you feel is our most serious drug problem? Why?
5. Explain the differences among drug use, misuse, and abuse.
6. How are physical and psychological dependence different?
7. What are the two sources of risk factors that contribute to substance abuse?
8. Name the four categories of environmental risk factors that contribute to substance abuse and give an example of each.
9. What are the two major types of abused drugs? Give examples of each.
10. Why is alcohol considered the Number 1 problem drug in America?
11. In what forms do Americans consume nicotine, and in what groups of people do we see the heaviest users?
12. What agency regulates over-the-counter and prescription drugs? What two characteristics must a drug have to be approved for sale?
13. How can misuse of prescription drugs become a risk to your health?
14. What is the most commonly abused illicit drug? Why is this drug a concern?
15. What are controlled substances? Give some examples.
16. What are the side effects for both men and women that result from the use of anabolic drugs?
17. What are the four elements of drug prevention and control?
18. What are primary, secondary, and tertiary prevention strategies for the drug problem?
19. Describe the roles of each of the following federal departments in controlling drug abuse: Health and Human Services, Justice, and Homeland Security.
20. What role do state governments play in preventing and controlling drug abuse? Local governments?

SCENARIO: ANALYSIS AND RESPONSE

Please reread the scenario at the beginning of this chapter. How would you respond to the following questions?

1. Re-examine Table 12.2. Which of the personal consequences of drug use were evident in Larissa's story?
2. Re-examine Figure 12.1. Which of the violent acts was mentioned or inferred in the scenario?
3. Which of the factors, discussed in this chapter, that contribute to drug abuse could have contributed to Larissa's drug dependence?
4. Methamphetamine has become a nationwide problem. Figure 12.8 is a map showing the number of incidents involving methamphetamine clandestine laboratories in each state. Which states appear to have the most serious methamphetamine problem? Is methamphetamine a widespread problem in your state? Have you heard about any meth lab busts in your community?
5. Child maltreatment, a serious problem in the United States, is discussed in Chapter 17. Larissa left her baby with her parents. How many grandparents in the United States are forced into raising their children's children? If Larissa had had no parents, what do you think would have happened to her baby?
6. What state or local agencies are available to help Larissa get into and stay in recovery?

21. What is Across Ages? What does it do? What is Project ALERT? What does it do?

22. How would you respond to the statement "Most drug abusers are unemployed"?

23. What are the names of four voluntary agencies and self-help groups involved in the prevention, control, and treatment of alcohol, tobacco, and other drug abuse?

ACTIVITIES

1. Schedule an appointment with the vice president of Student Affairs, the Dean of Students, or the alcohol and drug abuse prevention educator on your campus to find out more about drug (including alcohol) problems. Find out what the greatest concerns are and how the administration is trying to deal with the issues.

2. Make an appointment with the health educator or another employee in your local health department to find out more about the existing alcohol, tobacco, and other drug problems in the community. Collect the same information as noted in the first activity, except find information for the community, not the campus.

3. Find six articles that appeared in your local paper during the past two weeks that deal with drugs. Find two that related to problems at the national or international level, two at the state level, and two at the local level. Summarize each and present your reaction to these articles in a written paper.

4. Conduct a survey of at least 100 students on your campus. Try to get a random sample of people. Interview these people and find out what they think are the major drug problems on your campus and how they might be solved. Feel free to include other questions on your survey. Summarize the results in a two-page paper.

5. Attend a meeting of a community group that is involved in the prevention and control of drug abuse (e.g., local drug task force, AA, a smoking cessation group, MADD, or SADD). In a two-page paper, summarize the meeting and share your reaction to it.

COMMUNITY HEALTH ON THE WEB

The Internet contains a wealth of information about community and public health. Increase your knowledge of some of the topics presented in this chapter by accessing the Jones and Bartlett Publishers Web site at **http://health.jbpub.com/book/communityhealth/6e** and follow the links to complete the following Web activities.

- National Clearinghouse for Alcohol and Drug Information
- MADD
- Office on Smoking and Health

REFERENCES

1. Horgan, C., K. C. Skwara, and G. Strickler (2001). *Substance Abuse: The Nation's Number One Health Problem*. Princeton, NJ: Robert Wood Johnson Foundation.

2. The National Center on Addiction and Substance Abuse at Columbia University (2006). *The Commercial Value of Underage and Pathological Drinking to the Alcohol Industry: A CASA White Paper*. Available at http://www.casacolumbia.org/absolutenm/templates/Home.aspx.

3. Johnston, L. D., P. M. O'Malley, and J. G. Bachman (1993). *Monitoring the Future National Survey Results on Drug Use, 1975–1992. Vol. I: Secondary School Students* (NIH pub. no. 93-3597). Bethesda, MD: National Institute on Drug Abuse.

4. Johnston, L. D., P. M. O'Malley, J. G. Bachman, and J. E. Schulenbert (2006). *Monitoring the Future National Survey Results on Drug Use 1975–2005. Vol. I: Secondary School Students* (NIH pub. no. 06-5883). Rockville, MD: National Institute on Drug Abuse. Available at http://www.monitoringthefuture.org/pubs/.

5. Glantz, M., and R. Pickens (1992). "Vulnerability to Drug Abuse: Introduction and Overview." In M. Glantz and R. Pickens, eds., *Vulnerability to Drug Abuse*. Washington, DC: American Psychological Association.

6. Cotton, N. S. (1979). "The Familial Incidence of Alcoholism: A Review." *Journal of Studies on Alcohol*, 40: 89–116.

7. Cloninger, C. R., M. Bohman, and S. Sigvardsson (1981). "Inheritance of Alcohol Abuse." *Archives of General Psychiatry*, 38: 861–868.

8. Schuckit, M. A., S. C. Risch, and E. O. Gold (1988). "Alcohol Consumption, ACTH Level, and Family History of Alcoholism." *American Journal of Psychiatry*, 145(11): 1391–1395.

9. Tabakoff, B., and P. L. Hoffman (1988). "Genetics and Biological Markers of Risk for Alcoholism." *Public Health Report*, 103(6): 690–698.

10. U.S. Department of Health and Human Services (1990). *Seventh Special Report to the U.S. Congress* (DHHS pub. no. ADM-90-1656). Washington, DC: U.S. Government Printing Office.

11. Zickler, P. (2000). "Evidence Builds That Genes Influence Cigarette Smoking." *NIDA Notes*, 15(2): 1–2.

12. Needle, R., Y. Lavee, S. Su, et al. (1988). "Familial, Interpersonal, and Intrapersonal Correlates of Drug Use: A Longitudinal Comparison of Adolescents in Treatment, Drug-Using Adolescents Not in Treatment, and Non-Drug-Using Adolescents." *International Journal of Addictions*, 239(12): 1211–1240.

13. Meller, W. H., R. Rinehart, R. J. Cadoret, and E. Troughton (1988). "Specific Familial Transmission in Substance Abuse." *International Journal of Addictions*, 23(10): 1029–1039.

14. Shedler, J., and J. Block (1990). "Adolescent Drug Use and Psychological Health: A Longitudinal Inquiry." *American Psychologist*, 45(5): 612–630.

15. Horgan, C., K. C. Skwara, and G. Strickler 2001. *Substance Abuse: The Nation's Number One Health Problem*. Princeton, NJ: Robert Wood Johnson Foundation, 30.

16. Dembo, R., W. R. Blount, J. Schmeidler, and W. Burgos (1986). "Perceived Environmental Drug Use Risk and the Correlates of Early Drug Use or Nonuse Among Inner-City Youths: The Motivated Actor." *International Journal of Addictions*, 21(9–10): 977–1000.

17. Foster, S. E., R. D. Vaughan, W. H. Foster, and J. A. Califano Jr. (2006). "Estimate of the Commercial Value of Underage Drinking and Adult Abusive and Dependent Drinking to the Alcohol Industry." *Archives of Pediatrics and Adolescent Medicine*, 160(5): 473–478.

18. Morse, R. M., and D. K. Flavin (1992). "The Definition of Alcoholism." *JAMA*, 268(8): 1012–1014.

19. National Institute on Alcohol Abuse and Alcoholism (January 1996). "Drinking and Driving." *Alcohol Alert*, 31(362): 1–4.

20. U.S. Department of Health and Human Services, Public Health Service (2000). *Healthy People 2010: Understanding and Improving Health*. Washington, DC: U.S. Government Printing Office.

21. Hunt, T. (4 October, 2000). "Tough Standard Set for Drunken Driving." *USA Today*, 4A.

22. Insurance Institute for Highway Safety, Highway Loss Data Institute (2007). "DUI/DWI Laws as of March 2007." Available at http://www.iihs.org/laws/state_laws/dui.htm.

23. Cole, T. B. (2006). "Rape at U.S. Colleges Often Fueled by Alcohol." *JAMA*, 296(5): 504–505.

24. Lupton, C. (2003). "The Financial Impact of Fetal Alcohol Syndrome." Substance Abuse and Mental Health Services Administration, FASD Center for Excellence. Available at http://fasdcenter.samhsa.gov/publications/cost.cfm?&print=y.

25. Office of New York Attorney General Eliot Spitzer (11 October 2006). "Attorneys General and R. J. Reynolds Reach Historic Settlement to End the Sale of Flavored Cigarettes [Press release]." Available at http://www.oag.state.ny.us/press/2006/oct/oct11a_06.html.

26. Department of Health and Human Services (August 1993). "Substance Abuse Prevention and Treatment Block Grants: Sale or Distribution of Tobacco Products to Individuals Under 18 Years of Age: Proposed Rule." *Federal Register Part II*, 45: 96.

27. American Cancer Society (2006). *Cancer Facts and Figures—2006*. Atlanta, GA: Author.

28. Centers for Disease Control and Prevention (2002). "Annual Smoking-Attributable Mortality, Years of Potential Life Lost, and Economic Costs—United States, 1995–1999." *Morbidity and Mortality Weekly Report*, 51(14): 300–303.

29. U.S. Department of Health and Human Services, Public Health Service, Centers for Disease Control (1986). *The Health Consequence of Involuntary Smoking. A Report of the Surgeon General* (DHHS pub. no. CDC-87-8398). Washington, DC: U.S. Government Printing Office.

30. Byrd, J. C., R. S. Shapiro, and D. L. Schiedermayer (1989). "Passive Smoking: A Review of Medical and Legal Issues." *American Journal of Public Health*, 79(2): 209–215.

31. Environmental Protection Agency (1991). *Respiratory Health Effects of Passive Smoking: Lung Cancer and Other Disorders* (EPA/600/6-90/006F). Washington, DC: Indoor Air Quality Clearinghouse.

32. Department of Health and Human Services, Substance Abuse and Mental Health Services Administration (2006). *Results from the 2005 National Survey on Drug Use and Health: National Findings*. Available at http://www.oas.samhsa.gov/NSDUH/2k5NSDUH/2k5results.htm.

33. Thomson Healthcare. (2006). *2007 PDR for Nonprescription Drugs, Dietary Supplements, and Herbs*, 2nd ed. Montvale, NJ: Thomson Healthcare. Available at http://www.pdr.net.

34. U.S. Department of Justice, Drug Enforcement Administration (2006). "Pseudoephedrine Notice." Office of Diversion Control. Available at http://www.deadiversion.usdoj.gov/pubs/brochures/pseudo/pseudo_notice.pdf.

35. Thomson Healthcare. (2006). *Physicians' Desk Reference*, 61st ed. Montvale, NJ: Thomson Healthcare. Available at http://www.pdr.net.

36. Centers for Disease Control and Prevention (2006). "MRSA (Methicillin-Resistant *Staphylococcus aureus*)." Available at http://www.cdc.gov/ncidod/diseases/submenus/sub_mrsa.htm.

37. Lazarou, J., B. H. Pomeranz, and P. N. Corey (1998). "Incidence of Adverse Drug Reactions in Hospitalized Patients: A Meta-Analysis of Prospective Studies." *JAMA*, 279(15): 1200–1205.

38. Federal Register, Code of Federal Regulations, Food and Drugs, Part 1308. *Schedules of Controlled Substances*, Rev. April 1, 1998. Washington, DC: Author.

39. Substance Abuse and Mental Health Services Administration, Office of Applied Studies (2006). *Drug Abuse Warning Network, 2004: National Estimates of Drug-Related Emergency Department Visits* (DAWN Series D-28, DHHS pub. no. SMA 06-4143). Rockville, MD: Author.

40. Zickler, P. (2000). "Evidence Accumulates That Long-Term Marijuana Users Experience Withdrawal." *NIDA Notes*, 15(1).

41. Substance Abuse and Mental Health Services Administration, Office of Applied Studies (2006). *Treatment Episode Data Sets (TEDS). Highlights—1004. National Admissions to Substance Abuse Treatment Services* (DASIS Series S-31, DHHS pub. no. SMA 06-4140). Rockville, MD: Author.

42. Center for Addiction and Substance Abuse at Columbia University (1994). *Cigarettes, Alcohol, Marijuana: Gateways to Illicit Drug Use*. New York: Author.

43. Department of Justice, National Drug Intelligence Center (October 2006). *National Drug Threat Assessment 2007* (product no. 2006-Q0317-003). Johnstown, PA: Author. Available at http://www.usdoj.gov/ndic/topics/ndtas.htm.

44. Leshner, A. I. (30 July 1999). "The Drug Addiction Treatment Act of 1999. Testimony before the House Subcommittee on Health and Environment." Available at http://165.112.78.61/Testimony/7-30-99Testimony.html.

45. Drug Enforcement Administration, Department of Justice (2006). *Stats and Facts. National Statistics*. Available at: http://www.usdoj.gov/dea/statistics.html.

46. Drug Enforcement Administration, Department of Justice (2006). "Maps of Methamphetamine Lab Incidents." Available at http://www.usdoj.gov/dea/concern/map_lab_seizures.html.

47. Drug Enforcement Administration, Intelligence Division (2000). *An Overview of Club Drugs* (DEA-20005). Washington, DC: Drug Enforcement Agency.

48. National Institute on Drug Abuse (2000). *Anabolic Steroid Abuse* (NIH pub. no. 00-3721). Bethesda, MD: Author.

49. Center for Substance Abuse Prevention, Substance Abuse and Mental Health Services Administration (1997). *A Look at Successful and Cost-Effective State Treatment Programs: Treatment Works Fact Sheet*. Rockville, MD: Author.

50. Yates, B. T. (1999). *Measuring and Improving Cost, Cost-Effectiveness, and Cost-Benefit for Substance Abuse Treatment Programs* (NIH pub. no. 99-4518). Available at http://www.drugabuse.gov/PDF/Costs.pdf.

51. Bureau of Justice Statistics (1992). *Drugs, Crime and the Justice System 1992*. Washington, DC: U.S. Government Printing Office.

52. Office of National Drug Control Policy (March 2004). *2004 National Drug Control Strategy*. Available at http://www.whitehousedrugpolicy.gov/publications/policy/ndcs04/index.html.

53. Office of National Drug Control Policy (February 2006). *National Drug Control Strategy*. Available at http://www.whitehousedrugpolicy.gov/publications/policy/ndcs06/.

54. Office of National Drug Control Policy (February 2006). *National Drug Control Strategy FY 2007 Budget Summary*. Available at http://www.whitehousedrugpolicy.gov/publications/policy/07budget/.

55. Office of National Drug Control Policy (February 2002). *2002 National Drug Control Strategy*. Washington, DC: U.S. Government Printing Office. Available at www.whitehousedrugpolicy.gov/publications/policy/03ndcs/index.html.

56. U.S. Department of Justice, Office of Justice Programs. "About OJP." Available at www.ojp.usdoj.gov/about.htm.

57. U.S. Department of Education (1987). *What Works: Schools without Drugs*. Washington, DC: U.S. Government Printing Office.

58. NORML (National Organization for the Reform of Marijuana Laws). Available at http://www.norml.org/.

59. Brown, M. E. (1993). "Successful Components of Community and School Prevention Programs." *National Prevention Evaluation Report: Research Collection*, 1(1): 4–5.

60. Center for Substance Abuse Prevention (2004). *SAMHSA Model Programs*. Available at http://modelprograms.samhsa.gov/.

61. Lynam, D. R., R. Milich, R. Zimmerman, S. P. Novak, T. K. Logan, C. Martin, C. Leukefeld, and R. Clayton (1999). "Project DARE: No Effects at 10-Year Follow-up." *Journal of Consulting and Clinical Psychology*, 67(4): 590–593.

62. Drug-Free Federal Workplace (Executive Order 12564) (17 September 1986). *Federal Register*, 51(180).

63. American Management Associates (1996). *AMA Survey: Workplace Drug Testing and Drug Abuse Policy*. New York: Author.

64. U.S. Department of Labor (1991). *What Works: Workplaces without Alcohol or Other Drugs* (pub. no. 282-148/54629). Washington, DC: U.S. Government Printing Office.

65. Substance Abuse and Mental Health Services Administration, Office of Applied Studies (1999). *Worker Drug Use and Workplace Policies and Programs: Results from the 1994 and 1997 NHSDA* (DHHS pub. no. SMA 99-3352). Rockville, MD: Author.

66. SmithKline Beecham Clinical Laboratories (29 February 1996). "Drug Detection in the Workplace in 1995 Declines for the Eighth Straight Year [Press release]." Collegeville, PA: Author.

67. Quest Diagnostics (2006). "Drug Testing Index: Amphetamine Use Declined Significantly among U.S. Workers in 2005, According to Quest Diagnostics' Drug Testing Index." Available at http://www.questdiagnostics.com/employersolutions/dti/2006_06/dti_index.html.

UNIT THREE

HEALTH CARE DELIVERY

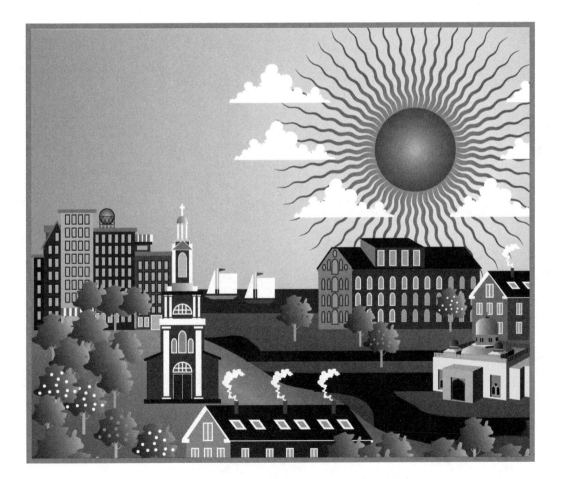

Chapter 13

Health Care System: Structure

Chapter Outline

Chapter Objectives

After studying this chapter, you will be able to:

1 Define the term *health care system*.

2 Trace the history of health care delivery in the United States from colonial times to the present.

3 Discuss and explain the concept of the spectrum of health care delivery.

4 Distinguish between the different kinds of health care, including population-based public health practice, medical practice, long-term practice, and end-of-life practice.

5 List and describe the different levels of medical practice.

6 List and characterize the various groups of health care providers.

7 Explain the differences among allopathic, osteopathic, and nonallopathic providers.

8 Define *complementary* and *alternative medicine*.

9 Explain why there is a need for health care providers.

10 Prepare a list of the different types of facilities in which health care is delivered.

11 Explain the differences among private, public, and voluntary hospitals.

12 Explain the difference between outpatient and ambulatory care facilities.

13 Briefly discuss the options for long-term care.

14 Explain what the Joint Commission does.

SCENARIO

Marcus had had a busy summer. Not only was he working 45 hours a week in order to earn enough money to return to college in the fall, but he was a member of two different softball teams and played in the golf league sponsored by his summer employer. He really enjoyed sports. In fact, one of his softball teams was a traveling team that played a 60-game schedule, traveling as far as 100 miles away to play in some tournaments.

Marcus was an aggressive softball player who enjoyed good competition and was always willing to slide hard into second base to break up a double play. In fact, it was his excessive sliding into the different bases that led to his medical problem. Toward the end of the season, Marcus had realized that the scab on his leg really never got a chance to heal over the summer

because of his sliding, and now it was getting tender and a redness appeared around it. So he decided to go see his physician. After a quick look and a little probing, Dr. Duncan said "Marcus, you have a basic infection. Are you allergic to any antibiotics?" When Marcus said no, Dr. Duncan wrote a prescription and sent him on his way.

Two weeks passed. Marcus had taken all his medication, but his leg didn't look any better. He called Dr. Duncan for another appointment. At the second appointment, Dr. Duncan took another look at the leg and prescribed a second medication. Another two weeks passed and still no change. So at his third visit, Dr. Duncan stated, "I'm not sure what the problem is. I'd like to refer you to a specialist. I think you should see Dr. Kennedy, the dermatologist."

INTRODUCTION

The process by which health care is delivered in the United States is unlike the processes used in other countries of the world. Other developed countries have national health insurance run or organized by the government and paid for, in large part, by general taxes. Also, in these countries almost all citizens are entitled to receive health care services, including routine and basic health care.[1] Health care in the United States is delivered by an array of **providers,** in a variety of settings, under the watchful eye of regulators, and paid for in a variety of ways. Because of this process, many question the notion that the United States has a health care delivery system (see Figure 13.1). That is, "[a]lthough these various individuals and organizations are generally referred to collectively as 'the health care delivery system,' the phrase suggests order, integration, and accountability that do not exist. Communication, collaboration, or systems planning among these various entities is limited and is almost incidental to their operations."[2] Whether or not health care delivery in the United States should be called a "system," there is a process in place in which health care professionals, located in a variety of facilities, provide services to deal with disease and injury for the purpose of promoting, maintaining, and restoring health to the citizens. In this chapter, we will outline the history of health care delivery in the United States, examine the spectrum of health care delivery, and describe the various types of health care providers and the facilities in which health care is delivered.

providers
health care facilities or health professionals that provide health care services

A BRIEF HISTORY OF HEALTH CARE DELIVERY IN THE UNITED STATES

For as long as humankind has been concerned with disease, injury, and health, there has always been a category of health care in which people have tried to help or treat themselves. This category of care is referred to as *self-care* or *self-treatment*. For example, in most American homes, there are usually provisions to deal with minor emergencies, nursing care, and the relief of minor pains or ailments. This type of care continues today. The following discussion of the history of health care in the United States does not include self-care, because it is assumed that most people would engage in some type of self-care prior to seeking professional help. Instead, we will review the development of professional care provided by those trained to do so.

As might be assumed with the birth of a new country, from colonial times through the latter portion of the nineteenth century, health care and medical education in the United States lagged far behind their counterparts in Great Britain and Europe. During this period of time anyone, trained or untrained, could practice medicine. Much of the early health care was provided by family members and neighbors and consisted of home and folk remedies that had been handed down from one generation to another. When a person did receive training as a physician, it was nothing like the rigorous training that a physician goes through today. The early medical education in the colonies was not grounded in science, but rather was experience based.[1] Prior to 1870, medical education was provided primarily through an apprenticeship with a practicing physician who may have been trained in the same way.[3] Consequently, medical care was primitive and considered to be more a trade than a profession.[1] In addition, most of the health care was provided in the patient's home and not in an office or clinic.

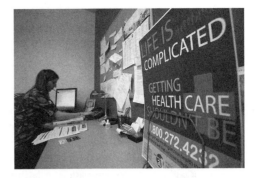

FIGURE 13.1
Do we really have a health care system?

There were some hospitals during these early years, but they were located primarily in large cities and seaports such as New York, Philadelphia, and New Orleans. However, the hospitals were much different from the hospitals of today and served more in a social welfare function than as places to receive health care. They were not very clean, and unhygienic practices prevailed. The forerunner of today's hospital and nursing home was the *almshouse* (also called a *poorhouse*).[1] Almshouses were run by the local government primarily to provide food, shelter, and basic nursing care for indigent people (i.e., the elderly, homeless, orphans, the ill, and the disabled) who could not be cared for by their own families.[1] In addition to almshouses, local government also operated *pesthouses*, which served as a place to isolate people who had contracted an infectious disease such as cholera, smallpox, or typhoid.[1]

In the late-nineteenth century, formal health care gradually moved from the patient's home to the physician's office and into the hospital. The primary reason for this change was the building and staffing of many new hospitals. It was felt that patients could receive better care in a setting designed for patient care, staffed with trained people, and equipped with the latest medical supplies and instruments. In addition, physicians could treat more patients in a central location because of the reduced travel time.

It was also during the latter portion of the nineteenth century that the scientific method began to play a more important role in medical education and health care. Medical procedures backed by scientific findings began to replace "rational hunches," "good ideas," and "home remedies" as the standards for medical care. With the acceptance of the germ theory of disease and the identification of infectious disease agents, there was real hope for the control of communicable diseases, which were the leading health problems of that period.

At the beginning of the twentieth century, although communicable diseases were still the leading causes of death, mortality rates were beginning to decline. Most of the decline can be attributed to improved public health measures. Yet, at the end of World War I, mortality rates spiked not only in the United States but also worldwide because of the 1918–1919 influenza pandemic. This deadliest pandemic in history killed as many as 100 million people. Shortly after the pandemic in the early 1920s, a major shift took place in the United States as chronic diseases moved past communicable diseases as the leading causes of death.

At the same time that chronic diseases were pushing to the top of the list of causes of death, much change was taking place in health care. New medical procedures such as X-ray therapy, specialized surgical procedures, and chemotherapy were developed, group medical practices were started, and new medical equipment and instruments (such as the electrocardiograph to measure heart function) were invented. The training of doctors and nurses also improved and became more specialized. By 1929 the United States was spending about 3.9% of its gross domestic product (GDP) on health care, which means that 3.9% of all goods and services produced by the nation that year were associated with health care.

Even with some of these "new" advances in the practice of medicine, U.S. medicine was still limited pretty much to two parties—patients and physicians. "Diagnosis, treatment, and fees for services were considered confidential between patients and physicians. Medical practice was relatively simple and usually involved long-standing relationships with patients and, often, several generations of families. Physicians collected their own bills, set, and usually adjusted their charges to their estimates of patients' ability to pay. This was the intimate physician-patient relationship the professional held sacred."[4]

By the early 1940s the United States was again at war. World War II affected health care in the United States in a variety of ways. One consequence of the war that would have a lasting impact on health care was employers' use of health insurance to lure workers to their companies. Because of the large number of men and women in the armed services, there was a shortage of workers to fill the jobs back home. Also, because of the need for resources for the war effort, the U.S. government put restrictions on the wages that companies could pay their employees. However, there were no restrictions on the health care insurance that employers could provide for their employees. Thus, companies began using health insurance to recruit and retain workers, and as a result employer-provided health insurance took a foothold at this time.

Also as a result of World War II, huge technical strides were made in the late 1940s and 1950s as medical procedures and processes developed during the war found applications in civilian medicine. However, adequate health facilities to treat long-term diseases were lacking in many areas of the country. The **Hospital Survey and Construction Act of 1946,** better known as the **Hill-Burton Act** (after the authors of the legislation), provided substantial funds for hospital construction. The infusion of federal funds helped to remedy the serious hospital shortage caused by the lack of construction during the Depression and World War II. The Hill-Burton Act was primarily a federal-state partnership. State agencies were given grants to determine the need for hospitals and then were provided with seed money to begin construction of the facilities.[5] However, the major portion of construction dollars came from state and local sources.[6] Through the years, the Hill-Burton Act has been amended several times to help meet health care needs in the United States. Funds have been made available for additional construction, modernization, and replacement of other health care facilities and for comprehensive health planning.

With improved procedures, equipment, and facilities and the increase in noncommunicable diseases, the cost of health care began to rise. As the cost of health care rose, it became too expensive for some people. Concerns were expressed about who should receive health care and who should pay for it. The debate over whether health care is a basic right or a privilege in America began in earnest. By the end of the 1950s, there remained an overall shortage of quality health care in America. There was also a maldistribution of health care services—metropolitan areas were being better served than the less-developed rural areas.

In the 1960s, there was an increased interest in health insurance, and it became common practice for workers and their bargaining agents to negotiate for better health benefits (see Figure 13.2). Undoubtedly, some employers preferred to increase benefits rather than to raise wages. Few then could foresee the escalation in health care costs for Americans that would continue through the early 1990s. Thus, the **third-party payment system** for health care became solidified as the standard method of payment for health care costs in the United States. The third-party payment system gets its name from the fact that the insurer—either government or a private insurance company (third party)—reimburses (pays the bills) to the provider (second party) for the health care given to the patient (first party).[7] (A detailed explanation of the third-party payment system is presented in Chapter 14.) More recently, when some speak

Hospital Survey and Construction Act of 1946 (Hill-Burton Act) federal legislation that provided substantial funds for hospital construction

third-party payment system a health insurance term indicating that bills will be paid by the insurer and not the patient or the health care provider of the third-party payment system, they add a fourth party—the purchaser of the insurance, usually an employer.[8] It should be noted that the government and private insurers pay the medical bills with tax dollars and collected premiums, respectively—not with their own funds.

With the growth of the third-party system of paying for health care, the cost of health care rose even more rapidly than before because patients enjoyed increased access to care without out-of-pocket expenses. However, those without insurance found it increasingly difficult to afford care. When the Democrats regained the White House in the 1960s, they led a federal policy change to increase citizen access to health care, which culminated in 1965 with the authorization of Medicare and Medicaid by Titles XVIII and XIX, respectively, of the Social Security Act. (These programs, which were enacted to help provide care for the elderly, the disabled, and the poor, are also discussed at length in Chapter 14.) Also in the 1960s, the federal government increased funding for medical research and technology to support transplants and life extension.

By the late 1960s and early 1970s, it had become apparent that the Hill-Burton Act had stimulated not only the growth of health care facilities, but also the demand for health care services. With this growth came a continuing rise in health care costs and a need for better planning in health care delivery.

Among the early attempts at planning were the 1964 amendments to the Hill-Burton Act. The amendments called for comprehensive planning on a regional level. Their purpose was to make more efficient use of federal funds by preventing the duplication of facilities. However, they depended on good faith efforts and could not be enforced. It soon became evident that more powerful legislation was needed to control costs and to coordinate and control rapid growth in health care facilities.

FIGURE 13.2
Health benefits have become an important part of the total compensation package for workers.

Another attempt was made to encourage better planning two years later. The Comprehensive Health Planning and Public Service Amendments of 1966 authorized funds for state- and area-wide Comprehensive Health Planning Agencies. These too failed because they had no teeth. Then, in 1974, Public Law 93-641 was passed. This law, known as the National Health Planning and Resources Development Act of 1974, combined several pieces of previous legislation to put teeth into comprehensive planning efforts. There were high hopes and expectations that these pieces of legislation would provide reason and order to the development and modification of health care services.[9] This legislation led to the formation of Health Systems Agencies throughout the entire country. Their purpose was to cut costs by preventing the building of "unnecessary" facilities or the purchase of unnecessary equipment. While some money may have been saved, the Health Systems Agencies were viewed by some as yet another unnecessary government bureaucracy, and when the late President Reagan took office in 1980, he, along with Congress, eliminated this program.

Before leaving our health care discussion of the 1970s, it should be noted that another piece of legislation was passed that did not seem all that important at the time but would have a profound impact on the way health care was delivered later. This legislation was the Health Maintenance Organization (HMO) Act of 1973. This act "provided both loans and grants for the planning, development, and implementation of combined insurance and health care delivery organizations and required that a minimum prescribed array of services be included in the HMO arrangement."[4]

The 1980s brought many changes to the health care industry, the most notable of which was probably the deregulation of health care delivery. In 1981, with Ronald Reagan in the White House, it was announced that the administration would let the competitive market, not governmental regulation, shape health care delivery.[10] Open competition is a philosophy of allowing consumers to regulate delivery by making choices about where and from whom they receive their care. In theory, those who provide good care will get more patients and in turn be able to offer the care at a lower price. In other words, the resulting competition would help squeeze out costly waste and ineffective care.[11]

There are some economists, however, who do not believe that the health care system behaves like a normal market. For example, it is not likely that an ill patient seeking medical care will shop for a less expensive physician. Physicians do not advertise the cost of their services. Also, it is the physician who tells the patient which hospital to go to and when to check in and out, due to the admitting privileges that physicians have. In addition, providers tend to offer more and more services to entice the market to "shop with us," which in effect drives up health care spending. For these reasons, the competitive market approach is of questionable value in lowering health care costs.

The 1980s also saw a proliferation of new medical technology (e.g., MRIs and ultrasound). Along with this new technology have come new health care issues such as medical ethics (e.g., prolonging life and ending life) and more elaborate health insurance programs (e.g., policies that cover specific diseases such as cancer and AIDS, home care, and rehabilitation).

Many of the concerns of the 1980s continued into the 1990s. The 1992 presidential campaign again brought attention to America's problems with health care delivery. Bill Clinton, then governor of Arkansas, based his election campaign strategy on being a new kind of Democrat—one who could take on the nation's domestic ills. He saw health care as one of those ills because the present system failed to cover all, and its spiraling costs threatened to bankrupt the government and cripple American industry.

Shortly after being elected president, Mr. Clinton appointed the first lady, Hillary Rodham Clinton, to head a committee to develop a plan to overcome the shortcomings of the health care system. By the fall of 1993, the committee had completed a plan that the president then presented to a joint session of Congress in front of a national television audience. This detailed plan, referred to informally as the president's Health Security Plan and formally as the **American Health Security Act of 1993,** was over 1,500 pages in length. The plan rested on six major points: (1) providing security (universal coverage), (2) controlling costs, (3) enhancing quality, (4) expanding access to traditionally undeserved areas, (5) reducing bureaucracy, especially paperwork, and (6) reducing fraud and abuse.[12] President Clinton's health care plan was much discussed in Congress in 1994; however, opposition kept it from ever reaching the floor for a vote before Congress adjourned. Although the plan was never approved, the pressures generated by the plan transformed the private health care system in the United States.

In the mid- to late-1990s, rapid changes occurred in the organization and financing of health care. These changes can be summed up in two words—managed care. **Managed care** has many meanings but will be referred to here as health plans "that integrate the financing and delivery of health care services to covered individuals by means of arrangements with selected providers to furnish comprehensive services to members; explicit criteria for the selection of health care providers; significant financial incentives for members to use providers and procedures associated with the plan; and formal programs for quality assurance and utilization review."[13]

With the advent of managed care, the increase of health care costs slowed in the mid-1990s; in fact, the actual growth for several years was almost flat. Even so, both the percentage of the GDP and the dollars spent on health care continued to inch up. In 1996, for the first time in history, the total health care bill for the United States topped $1 trillion

American Health Security Act of 1993
the comprehensive health care reform introduced by then President Clinton, but never enacted

managed care
health plans that integrate the financing and delivery of health care services to individuals who are covered by arrangements with selected providers who furnish comprehensive services to members; explicit criteria for the selection of health care providers; significant financial incentives for members to use providers and procedures that are associated with the plan; and formal programs for quality assurance and utilization review

($1,039 billion, 13.6% of the GDP).[14] In 2006, health care expenditures were approximately $2.16 trillion (16.2% of the GDP).[15] (See Table 13.1 for comparisons to other countries in 2003.)[16] Put another way, almost one-sixth of all the output of the United States in 2006 was spent on health care. Health care is the one segment of the U.S. economy that continues to grow consistently faster than the cost of inflation (see Table 13.2). Ever-newer technology, ever-increasing demands for the best care, growing medical liability, new diagnostic procedures, the lengthening of lifespans, the development of new drugs (e.g., Viagra), and newly identified diseases put great demands on the system.

By the mid- to late 1990s managed care had become the dominant form of health care financing and delivery, but it became apparent that support for it, with some exceptions, was not deep.[17] In addition, it was obvious that the slowdown in health care costs, which was attributed to managed care, would be just a one-time savings if other measures were not taken. President Clinton saw this as an opportunity to again seek health care reform.

This time then President Clinton treaded carefully, offering small but politically popular programs like health care coverage for uninsured children (see the discussion of SCHIP in Chapter 14) and a mandatory minimum hospital stay for childbirth to counter the so-called "drive-by deliveries" created by managed care.[18] So in 1996, through an executive order and with an amendment by way of a second executive order in 1997, President Clinton created the Advisory Commission on Consumer Protection and Quality in the Health Care Industry.[19] Formally, "the Commission was charged to advise the President on changes occurring in the health care system and, where appropriate, to make recommendations on how best to promote and ensure consumer protection and health care quality."[19] Informally, this meant

Table 13.1
Spending on Health Care in Selected Countries: 1960, 1980, and 2003

Country	Health Expenditures as a Percentage of GDP			Per Capita Health Expenditures* ($)		
	1960	1980	2003	1960	1980	2003
Australia	4.1	7.0	—	93	691	2,699
Austria	4.3	7.4	—	77	764	—
Canada	5.4	7.1	9.6	123	783	3,003
Czech Republic	—	—	9.9	—	—	1,298
France	3.8	7.1	10.1	70	711	2,903
Germany	—	8.7	11.1	—	965	2,996
Ireland	3.7	8.4	8.4	43	518	—
Italy	—	—	—	—	—	2,258
Japan	3.0	6.5	5.6	30	580	—
Korea	—	—	—	—	—	1,074
Mexico	—	—	6.2	—	—	583
Netherlands	—	7.5	9.8	—	757	2,976
New Zealand	—	5.9	8.1	—	506	1,886
Poland	—	—	9.6	—	—	—
Portugal	—	5.6	5.9	—	295	1,797
Slovak Republic	—	—	7.7	—	—	777
Spain	1.5	5.4	—	16	365	1,835
Sweden	—	9.1	11.5	—	936	—
Switzerland	4.9	7.4	—	166	1,033	3,781
Turkey	—	3.3	—	—	75	—
United Kingdom	3.9	5.6	—	84	482	—
United States	5.0	8.7	15.0	144	1,055	5,635

GDP, gross domestic product. —, Data not available.
*Per capita health expenditures for each country have been adjusted to U.S. dollars using gross domestic product purchasing power parities for each year.

Source: National Center for Health Statistics (2006). *Health, United States, 2006 with Chartbook on Trends in the Health of Americans.* Hyattsville, MD: Author, 373.

Table 13.2
Consumer Price Index and Average Annual Percentage of Change for All Items and Selected Items: United States, Selected Years 1960–2005

[Data are based on reporting by samples of providers and other retail outlets.]

Year	All Items	Medical Care	Food	Apparel	Housing	Energy
1960	29.6	22.3	30.0	45.7	—	22.4
1970	38.8	34.0	39.2	59.2	36.4	25.5
1980	82.4	74.9	86.8	90.0	81.1	86.0
1990	130.7	162.8	132.4	124.1	128.5	102.1
2000	172.2	260.8	167.8	129.6	169.6	124.6
2005	195.3	323.2	190.7	119.5	195.7	177.1

—, Data not available.

Note: 1982–1984 = 100.

Sources: National Center for Health Statistics (2006). *Health, United States, 2006, with Chartbook on Trends in the Health of Americans*. Hyattsville, MD: Author.

creating a "consumer bill of rights" and conducting a comprehensive review of the quality of health care in the nation.

In November 1997, the commission delivered its interim report to the President, which contained "A Consumer Bill of Rights and Responsibilities" (see Box 13.1). President Clinton endorsed the report and challenged insurance companies and managed care organizations to voluntarily adopt the commission's "bill of rights." Only a handful did so, and President Clinton asked that Congress pass a federal law requiring health plans to adopt such protections.

The final report of the commission was delivered to President Clinton in March 1998. Included, in addition to the "Consumer Bill of Rights and Responsibilities," was a proposed statement of purpose for the health care system, evidence of quality problems within health care, and more than 50 recommendations to advance health care in the United States. The commission felt that the first step in improving health care in the United States was to create a statement of purpose that the president could articulate. The commission proposed "The purpose of the health care system must be to continuously reduce the impact and burden of illness, injury, and disability and to improve the health and functioning of the people of the United States."[19] The quality problems identified by the commission included (1) an unacceptably high rate of medical errors (e.g., medication errors), (2) the extensive overuse of some services (e.g., hysterectomies), (3) the underuse of other services (e.g., use of beta blockers in Medicare patients with myocardial infarctions), and (4) a wide variation in patterns of care across the country.[19] Few of the recommendations of the commission were approved before President Clinton left office in 2001. However, in 2002 both the House and the Senate passed differing versions of the Patients' Bill of Rights,[3] but as of 2007 no compromise had been worked out. "Frustrated by years of congressional inaction, over 40 states have already passed their own version of a 'Patients' Bill of Rights.'"[4]

Not only has no "Patients' Bill of Rights" been passed, but also few changes have occurred in health care in recent years. The lone notable exception was the passage of the Medicare Prescription Drug, Improvement, and Modernization Act of 2003 (MMA). The most visible components of the MMA have been the voluntary outpatient prescription drug benefit for people on Medicare, know as Part D (see the discussion of Medicare Part D in Chapter 14), and health savings accounts (HSAs). HSAs are tax-free savings accounts that can be used to pay for near-term medical expenses incurred by individuals, spouses, and dependents and to save for future longer-term costs.[20] (HSAs are also discussed in greater detail in Chapter 14.)

Even with these recent changes, both consumers and health care providers are in agreement that the American health care delivery system needs to be changed. Recent reports from the Institute on Medicine[2,21,22] claim that "health care today harms too frequently and routinely

BOX 13.1	CONSUMER BILL OF RIGHTS AND RESPONSIBILITIES

I. Information Disclosure

Consumers have the right to receive accurate, easily understood information and to require assistance in making informed health care decisions about their health care plans, professionals, and facilities.

II. Choice of Providers and Plans

Consumers have the right to a choice of health care providers that is sufficient to ensure access to appropriate high-quality health care.

III. Access to Emergency Services

Consumers have the right to emergency health care services when and where the need arises. Health plans should provide payment when the consumer presents to an emergency department with acute symptoms of sufficient severity—including severe pain—such that a "prudent lay person" could reasonably expect the absence of medical attention to result in placing that consumer's health in serious jeopardy, serious impairment to bodily functions, or serious dysfunction of any bodily organ or part.

IV. Participation in Treatment Decisions

Consumers have the right and responsibility to fully participate in all decisions related to their health care. Consumers who are unable to fully participate in treatment decisions have the right to be represented by parents, guardians, family members, or other conservators.

V. Respect and Nondiscrimination

A. Consumers have the right to considerate, respectful care from all members of the health care system at all times and under all circumstances. An environment of mutual respect is essential to maintain a quality health care system.

B. Consumers must not be discriminated against in the delivery of health care services consistent with the benefits covered in their policy or as required by law based on race, ethnicity, nation-ality, religion, sex, age, mental or physical disability, sexual orientation, genetic information, or source of payment.

C. Consumers who are eligible for coverage under the terms and conditions of a health plan or program or as required by law must not be discriminated against in marketing and enrollment practices based on race, ethnicity, nationality, religion, sex, age, mental or physical disability, sexual orientation, genetic information, or source of payment.

VI. Confidentiality of Health Information

Consumers have the right to communicate with health care providers in confidence and to have the confidentiality of their individually identifiable health care information protected. Consumers also have the right to review and copy their own medical records and request amendments to their records.

VII. Complaints and Appeals

All consumers have the right to a fair and efficient process for resolving differences with their health plans, health care providers, and the institutions that serve them, including a rigorous system of internal review and an independent system of external review.

VIII. Consumer Responsibilities

In a health care system that protects consumers' rights, it is reasonable to expect and encourage consumers to assume reasonable responsibilities. Greater individual involvement by consumers in their care increases the likelihood of achieving the best outcomes and helps support a quality improvement, cost-conscious environment.

Source: The President's Advisory Commission on Consumer Protection and Quality in the Health Care Industry (1998). *Quality First: Better Health Care for All Americans.* Washington, DC: U.S. Government Printing Office, A5–A12.

---

fails to deliver its potential benefits."[21] Further, the health care system suffers from lack of coordinated, comprehensive services, resulting in both the wasteful duplication of efforts and unaccountable gaps in care.[21] In its reports, the IOM outlines a number of recommendations for changing health care delivery in the United States. These recommendations, combined with the release of the World Health Organization's report *The World Health Report 2000— Health Systems: Improving Performance*, in which the U.S. health system was ranked 37th out of 191 countries,[23] provide some direction for changing the current system.

Where is health care in the United States headed? No one can accurately predict that. However, a couple of things are certain. The U.S. health care system will continue to change and evolve; technology and the mapped human genome will play a bigger and bigger role in how health care is delivered; and the aging U.S. population, along with increasing health care costs, will mandate that change occur.

THE SPECTRUM OF HEALTH CARE DELIVERY

Because health care in the United States is delivered by an array of providers in a variety of settings, reference is sometimes made to the spectrum of health care delivery (see Table 13.3). The *spectrum of health care delivery* refers to the various types of care. Within this spectrum, four levels of practice have emerged: population-based public health practice, medical practice, long-term practice, and end-of-life practice.

Population-Based Public Health Practice

population-based public health practice incorporates interventions aimed at disease prevention and health promotion, specific protection, and a good share of case findings

Population-based public health practice incorporates interventions aimed at disease prevention and health promotion, specific protection, and a good share of case findings.[24,25] A primary component of population-based public health practice is education. If people are going to behave in a way that will promote their health and the health of their community, they first must know how to do so. Health education not only provides such information but also attempts to empower and motivate people to put this information to use by discontinuing unhealthy behaviors and adopting healthy ones. Though much of public health practice takes place in governmental health agencies, it also takes place in a variety of other settings (such as

Table 13.3
The Spectrum of Health Care Delivery

Level of Practice	Description	Examples of Delivery Settings
Population-based public health practice	Practice aimed at disease prevention and health promotion that shapes a community's overall health; emphasizes education and prevention	Public, community, and school health programs; public health clinics
Medical practice		
Primary care	Clinical preventive services, first-contact treatment services, and ongoing care for commonly encountered medical conditions; emphasizes prevention, early detection, and routine care	Primary care provider offices; public clinics; managed care organizations; community mental health centers
Secondary care	Specialized attention and on-going management for common and less frequently encountered medical conditions, including support services for people with special challenges due to chronic or long-term conditions	
Acute care	Short-term, intense medical care that may require hospitalization	Emergency rooms; urgent/emergent care centers; outpatient/inpatient surgical centers; hospitals
Subacute care	After acute care, need for more nursing intervention	Special subacute units in hospitals (e.g., transitional care units); skilled nursing facilities; home health care
Tertiary care	Subspecialty referral care requiring highly specialized personnel and facilities	Specialty hospitals (e.g., psychiatric, chronic disease) and general hospitals with highly specialized facilities
Long-term practice		
Restorative care	Intermediate follow-up care such as surgical post-operative care	Home health; progressive and extended care facilities; rehabilitation facilities that specialize in therapeutic services; halfway houses
Long-term care	Care for chronic conditions; personal care	Nursing homes; facilities for the mentally retarded or emotionally disturbed; geriatric day care centers
End-of-life practice	Care provided to those who have less than six months to live	Hospice services provided in a variety of settings

Sources: Cambridge Research Institute (1976). *Trends Affecting the U.S. Health Care System.* Washington, DC: U.S. Government Printing Office; U.S. Public Health Service (1994). *For a Healthy Nation: Return on Investments in Public Health.* Washington, DC: Author; Turnock, B. J. (2004). *Public Health: What It Is and How It Works,* 3rd ed. Sudbury, MA: Jones and Bartlett Publishers; Shi, L., and D. A. Singh (2005). *Essentials of the U.S. Health Care System,* Sudbury, MA: Jones and Bartlett Publishers.

voluntary health agencies, social service agencies, schools, businesses and industry, and even in some traditional medical care settings).[24]

Medical Practice

Medical practice means "those services usually provided by or under the supervision of a physician or other traditional health care provider."[24] Such services are offered at several different levels. You may remember that in Chapter 4 we used the terms *primary, secondary,* and *tertiary* as they related to levels of prevention. These terms have a similar meaning here, but they are now applied to health care delivery rather than prevention.

Primary Medical Care

Primary care is "front-line" or "first-contact" care. "The unique characteristic of primary care is the role it plays as a regular or usual source of care for patients and their families."[2] Formally, **primary care** has been defined as "the provision of integrated, accessible health care services by clinicians who are accountable for addressing a large majority of personal health care needs, developing a sustained partnership with patients, and practicing in the context of family and community."[26] Eighty percent of medical care is primary care.[24] Primary care includes routine medical care to treat common illnesses or to detect health problems in their early stages, and thus includes such things as semiannual dental checkups; annual physical exams; health screenings for hypertension, high blood cholesterol, and breast or testicular cancer; and sore throat cultures. Primary care usually is provided in practitioners' offices, clinics, and other outpatient facilities by physicians, nurse practitioners, physician assistants, and an array of other individuals on the primary care team. Primary care is the most difficult for the poor and uninsured to obtain (see Box 13.2).

> **primary care**
> the provision of integrated, accessible health care services by clinicians who are accountable for addressing a large majority of personal health care needs, developing a sustained partnership with patients, and practicing in the context of family and community

The World Health Organization has stated that primary health care rests on the following eight elements:[27]

- Education concerning prevailing health problems and the methods of preventing and controlling them.
- Promotion of food supply and proper nutrition.
- An adequate supply of safe water and basic sanitation.
- Maternal and child health care, including family planning.
- Immunization against the major infectious diseases.
- Prevention and control of locally endemic diseases.
- Appropriate treatment of common diseases and injuries.
- Provision of essential drugs.

In the United States, the supplies of food and clean water are taken for granted. But other elements, such as maternal and child health services, immunizations, and routine dental and medical care, are not available to large segments of our population—primarily for economic reasons.

Secondary Medical Care

Secondary medical care is specialized attention and ongoing management for common and less frequently encountered medical conditions, including support services for people with special challenges due to chronic or long-term conditions.[25] This type of care is usually provided by physicians, ideally upon referral from a primary care source.[24] Secondary medical care can be further divided into acute and subacute care. *Acute care* is short-term, intense medical care for an illness or injury that may require hospitalization. *Subacute care* is a "transitional level of care between acute care and traditional skilled nursing or home care."[28] Patients receiving subacute care "may still have an unstable condition requiring active monitoring and treatment, or they may require technically complex nursing treatments such as wound care, intravenous therapy, blood transfusion, or AIDS care."[1]

> **secondary medical care**
> specialized attention and ongoing management for common and less frequently encountered medical conditions, including support services for people with special challenges due to chronic or long-term conditions

HEALTHY PEOPLE 2010: OBJECTIVES

Objective 1-5: Increase the proportion of persons with a usual primary care provider.

Target: 85%.

Baseline: 77% of the population had a usual primary care provider.

	1996 Baseline	2003 Status	2010 Target
		Percent	
TOTAL	77	78	85
Race and ethnicity			
American Indian or Alaska Native	79	79	85
Asian or Pacific Islander	72	DNC	85
Asian	DNC	71	85
Native Hawaiian and other Pacific Islander	DNC	70	85
Black or African American	74	73	85
White	77	78	85
Hispanic or Latino	64	63	85
Not Hispanic or Latino	78	80	85
Black or African American	74	74	85
White	80	82	85
Gender			
Female	80	81	85
Male	74	74	85
Education level (aged 18 years and older)			
Less than high school	70	68	85
High school graduate	74	74	85
At least some college	74	77	85
Geographic location			
Within MSA	76	77	85
Outside MSA	78	81	85
Disability status			
Persons with activity limitations	84	85	85
Persons without activity limitations	76	77	85

DNC = Data are not collected. DSU = Data are statistically unreliable. MSA = Metropolitan statistical area.

*Data for office hours, prescription medications, and treatments are displayed to further characterize the practices of primary care providers.

For Further Thought

Why is it important that the United States reach the objective previously noted by the year 2010?

Tertiary Medical Care

Tertiary medical care is even more highly specialized and technologically sophisticated medical and surgical care than secondary medical care.[24] It is "care for those with unusual or complex conditions (generally no more than a few percent of the need in any service category)."[24] This care is not usually performed in smaller hospitals; however, it is provided in specialty hospitals, academic health centers, or on specialized floors of general hospitals. Such facilities are equipped and staffed to provide advanced care for people with illnesses such as cancer and heart disease, and procedures such as heart bypass surgery.

Long-Term Practice

Long-term practice can be divided into two subcategories—restorative care and long-term care.

tertiary medical care
specialized and technologically sophisticated medical and surgical care for those with unusual or complex conditions (generally no more than a few percent of the need in any service category)

Restorative Care

Restorative care is the health care provided to patients after surgery or other successful treatment, during remission in cases of an oncogenic (cancerous) disease, or when the progression of an incurable disease has been arrested. This level of care includes follow-up to secondary and tertiary care, rehabilitative care, therapy, and home care (see Figure 13.3). Typical settings for this type of care include both inpatient and outpatient rehabilitation units, nursing homes, halfway houses, and private homes.

Long-Term Care

Long-term care includes the different kinds of help that people with chronic illnesses, disabilities, or other conditions that limit them physically or mentally need. In some situations time-intensive skilled nursing care is needed, while some people just need help with basic daily tasks like bathing, dressing, and preparing meals. This type of care is provided in various settings such as nursing homes, facilities for the mentally and emotionally disturbed, and adult and senior day care centers, but often long-term care is used to help people live at home rather than in institutions.

FIGURE 13.3
Restorative care can follow either secondary or tertiary care.

End-of-Life Practice

The final level of practice in the health care delivery is end-of-life practice. **End-of-life practice** is usually thought of as those health care services provided to individuals shortly before death. The primary form of end-of-life practice is hospice care. **Hospice care** "is a program of palliative and support care services providing physical, psychological, social, and spiritual care for dying persons, their families, and other loved ones by a hospice program or agency."[29] The most common criterion for admission to hospice care is being terminally ill with a life expectancy of less than six months. The first hospice program in the United States was established in 1974.[30] In 2004, there were 2,645 Medicare-certified providers and suppliers of hospice services in the United States, compared with 164 in 1985.[16] Hospice services are available in home and inpatient settings.

TYPES OF HEALTH CARE PROVIDERS

To offer comprehensive health care that includes services at each of the levels just mentioned, a great number of health care workers are needed. In 2005, the number of civilians employed in the health service industry was 14 million. These 14 million represented approximately one of every 10 (9.9%) employed civilians in the United States.[16]

Despite the large number of health care workers, the demand for more is expected to continue to grow. The primary reasons for this growth are the aging U.S. population (by the year 2030, it is estimated that 71.5 million [one in five] people will be 65 years old or older)[16] and the expectation of more demand for long-term health care. Due to the continuing geographic maldistribution of health care workers, the need will be greater in some settings than in others. The settings of greatest need will continue to be the rural and inner-city areas (see Box 13.3).

In 2005, approximately two-fifths (42%) of all health care workers were employed in hospitals, about 13% in nursing and personal facilities, 13% in physicians' offices and clinics, 6% in dentists' offices and clinics, and about 1% in chiropractors' offices and clinics.[16] The remaining 25% practice in a variety of settings, including governmental and nongovernmental

restorative care
care provided after successful treatment or when the progress of a incurable disease has been arrested

long-term care
different kinds of help that people with chronic illnesses, disabilities, or other conditions that limit them physically or mentally need

end-of-life practice
health care services provided to individuals shortly before death

hospice care
a program of palliative and support care services providing physical, psychological, social, and spiritual care for dying persons, their families, and other loved ones by a hospice worker

<table>
<tr><td colspan="2" style="text-align:center">BOX 13.3</td><td colspan="4" style="text-align:center">HEALTHY PEOPLE 2010: OBJECTIVES</td></tr>
</table>

Objective 1-8: In the health professions, allied and associated health profession fields and the nursing field, increase the proportion of all degrees awarded to members of underrepresented racial and ethnic groups.

Target and baseline:

Objective	Increase in Degrees Awarded to Underrepresented Populations	1996–97 Baseline (unless noted)	2004 Status (unless noted)	2010 Target
		Percent		
	Health professions, allied and associated health profession fields (For the baselines, health professions include medicine, dentistry, pharmacy, and public health.)			
1-8a.	American Indian or Alaska Native	0.6	0.5	1.0
1-8b.	Asian or Pacific Islander	16.2	20.3	4.0*
1-8c.	Black or African American	6.7	7.4	13.0
1-8d.	Hispanic or Latino	4.0	5.9	12.0
	Nursing			
1-8e.	American Indian or Alaska Native	0.7 (1995–96)	0.9 (2003)	1.0
1-8f.	Asian or Pacific Islander	3.2 (1995–96)	3.5 (2003)	4.0
1-8g.	Black or African American	6.9 (1995–96)	10.6 (2003)	13.0
1-8h.	Hispanic or Latino	3.4 (1995–96)	5.0 (2003)	12.0
	Medicine			
1-8i.	American Indian or Alaska Native	0.6	0.6	1.0
1-8j.	Asian or Pacific Islander	15.9	20.0	4.0*
1-8k.	Black or African American	7.3	6.5	13.0
1-8l.	Hispanic or Latino	4.6	6.5	12.0
	Dentistry			
1-8m.	American Indian or Alaska Native	0.5	0.3	1.0
1-8n.	Asian or Pacific Islander	19.5	24.7	4.0*
1-8o.	Black or African American	5.1	4.5	13.0
1-8p.	Hispanic or Latino	4.7	6.3	12.0
	Pharmacy			
1-8q.	American Indian or Alaska Native	0.4	0.4	1.0
1-8r.	Asian or Pacific Islander	17.5	22.8	4.0*
1-8s.	Black or African American	5.7	7.5	13.0
1-8t.	Hispanic or Latino	2.8	3.6	12.0

*The Asian or Pacific Islander group has exceeded its target, which represents the minimum target based on this group's estimated proportion of the population.

For Further Thought

Minority and disadvantaged Americans lag behind the general U.S. population on virtually all health status indicators. Furthermore, among the poor, minorities, and the uninsured, access to medical care has been deteriorating. What impact do you think meeting the just noted objectives will have on this community health problem? Please defend your response.

agencies, home health care, and other private practices. As changes have come to the way health care is offered, the proportions of health care workers by setting have also changed, with fewer persons working in hospitals (in 1970, 63% worked in hospitals), and more employed in nursing homes and ambulatory care settings (such as surgical and emergency centers).[16] This trend is expected to continue in the future, with special needs in the area of long-term care workers to meet the needs of the aging baby boom generation.

There are well over 200 different careers in the health care industry. To help simplify the discussion of the different types of health care workers, they have been categorized into six different groups—independent providers, limited care providers, nurses, nonphysician practitioners, allied health care professionals, and public health professionals.

Independent Providers

Independent providers are those health care workers who have the specialized education and legal authority to treat any health problem or disease that an individual has. This group of workers can be further divided into allopathic, osteopathic, and nonallopathic providers.

Allopathic and Osteopathic Providers

Allopathic providers are those who use a system of medical practice in which specific remedies for illnesses, often in the form of drugs or medication, are used to produce effects different from those of diseases. The practitioners who fall into this category are those who are referred to as Doctors of Medicine (MDs). The usual method of practice for MDs includes the taking of a health history, a physical examination—perhaps with special attention to one area of the complaint—and the provision of specific treatment, such as antibiotics for a bacterial infection or a tetanus injection and sutures for a laceration.

Another group of physicians that provides services similar to those of MDs are **osteopathic providers**—Doctors of Osteopathic Medicine (DOs). At one time, MDs and DOs would not have been grouped together because of differences in their formal education, methods, and philosophy of care. While the educational requirements and methods of treatment used by MDs have remained essentially consistent over the years, those of DOs have not. The practice of osteopathy was started in 1874 by Andrew Taylor Still, MD, DO, who was dissatisfied with the effectiveness of nineteenth-century medicine.[31] At that time, the education and training of osteopaths was aimed at a thorough understanding of the musculoskeletal system because, according to osteopathic theory, all health problems, including diseases, could be cured by manipulating this system. During that time, DOs were often referred to as "bone doctors" and were often called upon to set fractured bones. During the twentieth century, osteopathic medicine changed. It is now based on a philosophy of health care that emphasizes the interrelationships of the body's systems in the prevention, diagnosis, and treatment of illness, disease, and injury. The distinctive feature of osteopathic medicine is the recognition of the reciprocal interrelationship between the structure and function of the body. The actual work of DOs and MDs is very similar today. Both types of physicians use all available scientific modalities, including drugs and surgery, in providing care to their patients. Both can also serve as primary care physicians (about one-third of MDs[1] and more than two-thirds of DOs are primary care physicians)[31] or as board-certified specialists. Their differences are most notably the DOs' greater tendency to use more manipulation in treating health problems and the DOs' perception of themselves as being more holistically oriented than MDs. Few if any patients today would be able to tell the difference between the care given by a DO and a MD.

The educational requirements for MD and DO degrees are very similar. Both educational programs generally accept students into their classes after they have completed a bachelor's degree. Medical education takes four years to complete. The first two years include course work in the sciences, while the final two years emphasize clinical experiences and rotations through the specialty areas of medicine. At the end of the second year of medical school and again at the end of the fourth year, medical students take the first two parts of their licensing examination. During the fourth year of medical school, the students apply for entrance into a medical residency program. It is during their residency program that the physicians receive the training to specialize in a particular field of medicine. The residency programs typically range in length from three (such as in family medicine) to five (such as in pathology) years. The first year of a residency is referred to the *internship year,* and the physicians are referred to as **interns** or first-year **residents.** During this year, the interns can only practice medicine

independent providers
health care professionals with the education and legal authority to treat any health problem

allopathic providers
independent providers whose remedies for illnesses produce effects different from those of the disease

osteopathic providers
independent health care providers whose remedies emphasize the interrelationships of the body's systems in prevention, diagnosis, and treatment

intern
a first-year resident

resident
a physician who is training in a specialty

under the guidance of a licensed physician. Upon successful completion of the internship year, the interns are then eligible to sit for the third part of the licensing examination. If they pass the exam, they are then entitled to practice medicine without the supervision of another licensed physician. At this point, almost all interns will complete the remaining years of residency (and are referred to generically as residents) in order to be eligible to sit for the board specialty examinations. Passing this examination will make them "board certified" in their specialty. A list of such medical care specialties and subspecialties is presented in Figure 13.4.

With so many specialties and subspecialties, health care experts are worried that not enough primary care physicians (which includes general practice/family medicine, internal

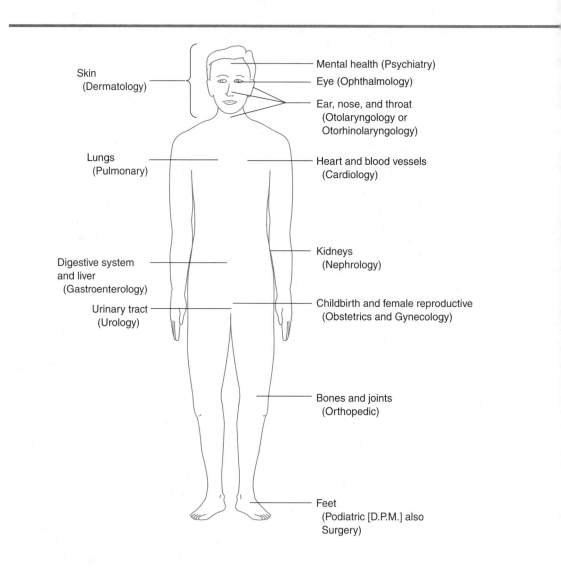

FIGURE 13.4

Listing of medical specialties and subspecialties.

medicine, obstetrics/gynecology, and pediatrics) will be trained. There are some data to support this claim. In 1949, 59% of active doctors of medicine (MDs and DOs) practiced as primary care physicians. This percentage dropped to 43% by 1970 and to approximately 38% by 1990. However, the percentage has remained fairly stable since 1990. In 2004, the figure was 37.4%.[16] This stabilizing effect may in part be because of the managed care movement and its need for primary care practitioners and not specialists.

Nonallopathic Providers

Nonallopathic providers are identified by their nontraditional means of providing health care. Some have referred to much of the care provided by these providers as complementary/

nonallopathic providers independent providers who provide nontraditional forms of health care

Allergy and immunology (immune systems)
Anesthesiology (administer drugs for pain during surgery)
Cardiology (heart and circulatory system)
Colon and rectal surgery
Dermatology (skin)
Dermatopathology
Emergency medicine
Family medicine (general family health)
  Geriatric medicine
  Sports medicine
Internal medicine
  Cardiovascular medicine
  Clinical cardiac electrophysiology
  Critical care medicine
  Diagnostic laboratory immunology
  Endocrinology (diabetes and metabolism)
  Gastroenterology (digestive organs)
  General practice (usually just for adults)
  Geriatric medicine
  Hematology (blood, spleen, and lymph glands)
  Infectious disease
  Medical oncology (cancer)
  Nephrology (kidney)
  Neurology
  Pulmonary disease (lungs)
  Rheumatology (joints, muscle, bones, and tendons)
Nuclear medicine (use radioactive substances to diagnose, research, and treat disease)
Obstetrics and gynecology (female reproductive system, the fetus, and the newborn)
  Gynecologic oncology
  Maternal-fetal medicine
  Reproductive endocrinology
Ophthalmology (eye)
Otolaryngology (ear and throat)
Otorhinolaryngology (ear, nose, and throat)
Pathology
  Blood banking/transfusion medicine
  Cytopathology (tumors)
  Dermatopathology
  Forensic pathology (cause of death)

Hematology
Immunopathology
Medical microbiology
Neuropathology
Pediatric pathology
Radioisotopic pathology
Pediatrics (children)
  Adolescent medicine (adolescents and young adults)
  Diagnostic laboratory immunology
  Neonatal–prenatal medicine (problems of the fetus and newborns)
  Pediatric cardiology
  Pediatric critical care
  Pediatric emergency medicine
  Pediatric endocrinology
  Pediatric gastroenterology
  Pediatric hematology-oncology
  Pediatric infectious disease
  Pediatric nephrology
  Pediatric rheumatology
  Pediatric sports medicine
Physical medicine and rehabilitation
  Sports medicine
Plastic and reconstructive surgery
Preventive medicine
  Public health and general preventive medicine
  Aerospace medicine
  Occupational medicine
Psychiatry
Radiology (radiation to diagnose and treat disease)
  Radiation oncology
  Diagnostic radiology
Surgery
  Colon and rectum surgery
  General vascular surgery
  Hand surgery
  Orthopedic
  Pediatric surgery
  Surgical critical care
  Thoracic surgery (chest area)
Urology (genitals and urinary tract)

FIGURE 13.4
Continued.

alternative medicine (CAM) or complementary/integrative medicine. Included in this group of providers are chiropractors, acupuncturists (see Figure 13.5), naturopaths (those who use natural therapies), herbalists (those who use herbal brews for treating illness), and homeopaths (those who use small doses of herbs, minerals, and even poisons for therapy).

The best known and most often used nonallopathic providers in the United States are **chiropractors.** The underlying premise of the care provided by chiropractors is that all health problems are caused by misalignments of the vertebrae in the spinal column. The chiropractic (done by hand) approach to the treatment is (1) the identification of the misalignment through X-rays, and (2) the realignment of the bones through a series of treatments called "adjustments."

Chiropractors are educated in four-year chiropractic colleges. The Council on Chiropractic Education accredits colleges of chiropractic medicine in the United States. As with allopathic and osteopathic programs, students usually enter chiropractic programs after earning a bachelor's degree. Those who graduate from chiropractic colleges earn a Doctor of Chiropractic (DC) degree. Chiropractors are licensed in all 50 states and must pass either a state licensing examination or an examination given by the National Board of Chiropractic Examiners. Although the educational standards for chiropractors have improved over the years, many people still question their ability to help the ill and injured. However, it should be noted that the American Public Health Association recognizes chiropractors as a professional group, and many insurance companies and Medicare and Medicaid provide reimbursement for chiropractic care.

As noted earlier, much of the care provided by nonallopathic providers is often referred to as **complementary/alternative medicine (CAM)** or *complementary/integrative medicine*. CAM has been defined as "a group of diverse medical and health care systems, practices, and products that are not presently considered to be a part of conventional medicine."[4] When used together with conventional medicine, a therapy is identified as *complementary*. "An example of a complementary therapy is using aromatherapy to help lessen a patient's discomfort following surgery."[32] When a therapy is used in place of a conventional medicine, it is labeled as *alternative*. "An example of an alternative therapy is using a special diet to treat cancer instead of undergoing surgery, radiation, or chemotherapy that has been recommended by a conventional doctor."[32] When mainstream medical therapies are combined with CAM therapies for which there is some high-quality scientific evidence of safety and effectiveness, it is referred to as *integrative medicine*.[32] CAM is one of the fastest growing areas of health care today. Data indicate that about two-thirds of adults in the United States have reported ever using CAM and just over half have reported using it in the past year,[33] although the percentage varies depending on what is considered CAM. The percentage is the highest when the definition of CAM therapy includes prayer specifically for health reasons. Compared with other countries, the United States is at the low end of using alternative forms of healing.[34] Even with its popularity, most CAM is paid for out of pocket by Americans because coverage for CAM by insurance companies is limited and is different depending on the state and insurer.[35] Yet, "insurers say that when traditional medicine is ineffective and an alternative form of therapy, such as acupuncture, for a condition like chronic pain costs less and satisfies the patient, they will pay for it."[4]

FIGURE 13.5
Many people seek out nontraditional means of health care, such as acupuncture.

chiropractor
a nonallopathic, independent health care provider who treats health problems by adjusting the spinal column

complementary/ alternative medicine (CAM)
a group of diverse medical and health care systems, practices, and products that are not presently considered to be a part of conventional medicine

The growth in the American public's interest in CAM therapies is evidenced by the emphasis placed on the research by the U.S. government. In 1992, the National Institutes of Health (NIH) created an Office of Alternative Medicine (OAM) with a budget of $2 million to investigate whether or not the CAM therapies actually work. In 1998, the NIH OAM was elevated to the National Center for Complementary and Alternative Medicine (NCCAM) and its mandate expanded. Its funding also expanded, reaching $122.7 million in fiscal year 2006."[36]

There are literally hundreds of systems, approaches, and techniques that fall within the CAM rubric (see Box 13.4), but the NCCAM classifies them into five general categories.[32] They include:

- Alternative Medical Systems
- Mind-Body Interventions
- Biologically Based Therapies
- Manipulative and Body-Based Methods
- Energy Therapies

BOX 13.4 — **COMPLEMENTARY/ALTERNATIVE MEDICINE APPROACHES**

Alternative Medical Systems
  Acupuncture
  Ayurvedic Medicine (traditional medicine of India— means "Science of Life")
  Faith Healing
  Homeopathic Medicine
  Naturopathic Medicine
  Shamanism
  Traditional Oriental Medicine [includes several techniques and methods such as acupuncture, herbal medicine, oriental massage, and qi gong (a form of energy therapy)]

Mind-Body Interventions
  Bioenergetics
  Biofeedback
  Biorhythms
  Body-Oriented Psychotherapy
  Breathing Techniques
  Color Therapy
  Dance Therapy
  Growth Astrology
  Hypnosis
  Hypnotherapy
  Human Aura
  Martial Arts
  Music Therapy
  Past Life Therapy
  Relaxation Therapy
  Spiritual Healing
  Visualization
  Yoga

Biologically Based Therapy
  Bee Venom
  Colonics
  Copper
  Ginseng
  Macrobiotics
  Microdose Pharmacology
  Natural Food Diets
  Nutritional Therapy
  Shark Cartilage
  Veganism
  Vegetarianism

Manipulative and Body-Based Methods
  Acupressure
  Alexander Technique
  Applied Kinesiology
  Belly Dancing
  Chiropractic Manipulation
  Massage
  Myotherapy
  Osteopathic Manipulation
  Polarity Therapy
  Reflexology
  Rolfing
  Shiatsu
  Trager Work

Energy Therapies
  Bioelectromagnetic-Based Therapies
  qi gong
  Reiki
  Therapeutic Touch

Sources: Levinson, D., and L. Gaccione (1997). *Health and Illness: A Cross-Cultural Encyclopedia.* Santa Barbara, CA: ABC-CLIO; Quander, L. (2001). "Complementary and Alternative Medicine Research on HIV/AIDS." *HIV Impact* (Winter), 10; Sultz, H. A., and K. M. Young (2006). *Health Care USA: Understanding Its Organization and Delivery,* 5th ed. Sudbury, MA: Jones and Bartlett Publishers; National Center for Complementary and Alternative Medicine (2006). *What Is Complementary and Alternative Medicine (CAM)?* Available at http://nccam.nih. gov/health/whatiscam/.

"Although alternative approaches use a wide range of techniques, most share a number of common features. These include:

1. A focus on disease prevention and health maintenance
2. A holistic approach in which the whole person—mind, emotions, and spirit are considered
3. The use of natural processes and materials in healing
4. A focus on the cause of the disease rather than symptoms
5. A consideration of lifestyle and emotional issues
6. A belief that the body has an innate ability to heal itself when it is brought into balance and harmony"[34]

Limited (or Restricted) Care Providers

limited (restricted) care providers health care providers who provide care for a specific part of the body

Much health care is provided by **limited (or restricted) care providers** who have advanced training, usually a doctoral degree, in a health care specialty. Their specialty enables them to provide care for a specific part of the body. This group of providers includes but is not limited to dentists (teeth and oral cavity), optometrists (eyes, specifically refractory errors), podiatrists (feet and ankles), audiologists (hearing), and psychologists (mind).

Nurses

We have categorized nurses into a group of their own because of their unique degree programs, the long-standing tradition of nursing as a profession, and their overall importance in the health care industry. It has been estimated that there are a little over 4 million individuals who work in the nursing profession. These include registered nurses, licensed practical nurses, and ancillary nursing personnel such as nurse's aids.[16] Nurses outnumber physicians, dentists, and every other single group of health care workers in the United States.[16] Even with such numbers, the need for nurses will continue (see Figure 13.6). In 2005, it was reported that there was a 10% shortage of registered nurses that if not addressed in terms of supply and demand would grow to a 27% shortage by the year 2015 and 36% by 2020.[37] The nurse "shortage is driven by a broad set of factors related to recruitment and retention—among them, fewer workers, an aging workforce, and unsatisfying work environments—that have contributed to a different kind of shortage that is more complex, more serious, and expected to last longer than previous shortages."[38]

Training and Education of Nurses

licensed practical nurse (LPN) those prepared in one- to two-year programs to provide nontechnical bedside nursing care under the supervision of physicians or registered nurses

Nurses can be divided into subcategories based on their level of education and type of preparation. The first are those who are prepared as licensed practical nurses. Once they complete their one to two years of education in a vocational, hospital, or associate degree program and pass a licensure examination, these nurses are referred to as **licensed practical nurses (LPNs),** or *licensed vocational nurses* (LVNs) in some states,[39] and are able to work under the supervision of physicians or registered nurses. The duties of LPNs vary depending upon their work setting. In a hospital, LPNs usually perform routine duties and provide nontechnical bedside nursing care. In a nursing home, they may handle a more broad range of duties, including routine and more complex nursing procedures such as treating bedsores, preparing and giving injections, and inserting catheters. In outpatient settings, LPNs may perform a variety of clinical and clerical duties depending on the size and nature of the practice, and in home health care their duties may range from education to routine nursing care to use of technical equipment.[39] Not too many years ago it was thought that LPNs would be phased out and replaced with more qualified nurses, but with the current nursing shortage, employment of LPNs is now expected to grow.

The second group of nurses includes those who have successfully completed a diploma program or an associate degree (ADN) and a state licensing (registration) examination. They are referred to as **registered nurses (RNs).** Diploma programs are offered by hospitals and last about two to three years.[39] ADN programs take about two years to complete and are typically offered by community or junior colleges.

The third group of nurses includes the baccalaureate-prepared nurses who hold the degree of Bachelor of Science in Nursing (BSN). These nurses also must pass a state licensing examination to become RNs. RNs holding BSN degrees are referred to as **professional nurses** and are considered to have been more thoroughly prepared for additional activities involving independent judgment. The total number of licensed RNs in the United States in 2004, regardless of their level of preparation, was approximately 2.9 million. Approximately 58% of these nurses were employed full-time, 25% part-time, and the remaining 17% were not employed in the nursing profession. Of the employed registered nurses, 56% worked in hospitals, 15% in public or community health settings, 11.5% in ambulatory care, 6% in nursing homes/extended care facilities, 2.5% in nursing education, and 8.5% in other areas, including schools, prisons/jails, and insurance companies.[40]

FIGURE 13.6
There is still a need for more nurses.

registered nurse (RN)
an associate- or baccalaureate degree-prepared nurse who has passed the state licensing examination

Advanced Practice Nurses

With advances in technology and the development of new areas of medical specialization, there is a growing need for specialty-prepared advanced practice nurses (APNs). Many professional nurses continue their education and earn master's and doctoral degrees in nursing. The master's degree programs are aimed primarily at specialties such as nurse practitioners (NPs) (e.g., pediatric nurse practitioners and school nurse practitioners), clinical nurse specialists (CNSs), certified registered nurse anesthetists (CRNAs), and certified nurse midwives (CNMs). These APNs are qualified to conduct health assessments, diagnose and treat a range of common acute and chronic illnesses, and manage normal maternity care. Not only do they provide high-quality care in a cost-effective manner, but they are also considered primary care providers in chronically medically underserved inner-city and rural areas. Like other nurses, the demand for APNs is also expected to increase, especially as a greater portion of the population gains access to health care and more of the population becomes enrolled in managed care. In 2004, the number of RNs prepared to practice in at least one advanced practice role was estimated to be 240,461, or 8.3% of the total RN population.[40] The largest portion of these APNs were nurse practitioners (see Figure 13.7).

The relatively few nurses who hold doctorate degrees in nursing are highly sought after as university faculty. Nurses with doctorates teach, conduct research, and otherwise prepare other nurses or hold administrative (leadership) positions in health care institutions.

professional nurse
a registered nurse holding a bachelor of science degree in nursing (BSN)

Nonphysician Practitioners

Nonphysician practitioners (NPPs) (also known as nonphysician clinicians [NPCs] or midlevel providers or physician extenders) constitute a relatively new classification of health care workers. This group is composed of those "clinical professionals who practice in many

nonphysician practitioners
clinical professionals who practice in many of the areas similar to those in which physicians practice, but do not have an MD or DO degree

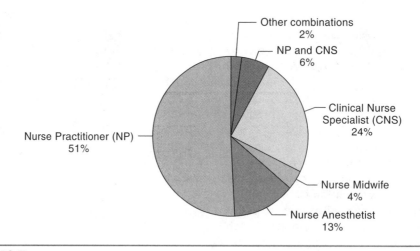

FIGURE 13.7

Registered nurses prepared for advance practice, 2004.

Source: Health Resources and Services Administration, Department of Health and Human Services (2006). *Preliminary Findings: 2004 National Sample Survey of Registered Nurses.* Available at http://www.bhpr.hrsa.gov/healthworkforce/reports/rnpopulation/preliminaryfindings.htm.

of the areas similar to those in which physicians practice, but do not have an MD or a DO degree."[1] NPPs are middle-level health workers with training and skills beyond those of RNs and less than those of physicians.[39] This group typically includes the just discussed nurse practitioners and certified midwives as well as physician assistants (PAs).[1] Because the former two were just presented as part of the section on advanced practice nurses, we will discuss only PAs here.

Physician assistant programs began in response to the shortage of primary care physicians. PAs' academic programs usually last two years and are offered in a variety of formats, including diploma and certificate programs, or as associate, bachelor's, or master's degrees. After completion of the program or degree, PAs must pass a national certifying examination. PAs always work under the direct supervision of a licensed physician (thus the name *physician extenders*). They carry out many of the same duties that are thought of as the responsibilities of physicians, such as taking medical histories, examining patients, ordering and interpreting laboratory tests and X-rays, counseling patients, making preliminary diagnoses, treating minor injuries, and, in most states, prescribing medications.[39]

Allied Health Care Professionals

allied health care professionals
health care workers who provide services that assist, facilitate, and complement the work of physicians and other health care specialists

Allied health describes a large group of health-related professions that fulfill necessary roles in the health care delivery system. These **allied health care professionals** assist, facilitate, and complement the work of physicians, dentists, and other health care specialists. These health care workers provide a variety of services that are essential to patient care. Oftentimes they are responsible for highly technical services and procedures. Allied health care professionals can be categorized into several groups.[4] They include (1) laboratory technologists and technicians (e.g., medical technologists, emergency medical technicians, nuclear medicine technicians, operating room technicians, dental technicians and hygienists, and radiographers [X-ray technicians]); (2) therapeutic science practitioners (e.g., occupational, physical, radiation, and respiratory therapists and speech pathologists); (3) behavioral scientists (e.g., health educators, social workers, and rehabilitation counselors); and (4) support services (e.g., medical record keepers and medical secretaries). The educational backgrounds of allied health workers range from vocational training to master's degrees. Most of these professionals also must pass a state or national licensing examination before they can practice.

The demand for allied health care workers in all of the areas previously noted is expected to continue well into the twenty-first century. The primary reasons for this are the growth of the entire health care industry and the impending arrival of the baby boomers as senior citizens.

Public Health Professionals

A discussion about health care providers would be incomplete without the mention of a group of health workers who provide unique health care services to the community—**public health professionals.** "Public health professionals—in their roles as environmental monitors, inspectors, consumer educators, and health care providers—significantly reduce the number of preventable deaths."[41] They support the delivery of health care by such hands-on providers as public health physicians, dentists,

FIGURE 13.8
Public health professionals make up a key component of the health care system.

nurses, and dieticians who work in public health clinics sponsored by federal, state, local, and voluntary health agencies (see Figure 13.8). Examples of other public health professionals are environmental health workers, public health administrators, epidemiologists, health educators, public health nurses and physicians, biostatisticians, the Surgeon General, and the research scientists at the Centers for Disease Control and Prevention. Public health professionals often make possible the care that is practiced in immunization clinics, nutritional programs for women, infants, and children (WIC), dental health clinics, and sexually transmitted disease clinics. School nurses are also considered public health professionals. Public health services are usually financed by tax dollars and, while available to most taxpayers, serve primarily the economically disadvantaged.

**public health
professional**
a health care worker
who works in a public
health organization

HEALTH CARE FACILITIES AND THEIR ACCREDITATION

Health care is provided in a variety of settings in the United States. The major settings and the accreditation of these facilities are discussed in the sections that follow.

Health Care Facilities

Health care facilities are the physical settings in which health care is actually provided. They include practitioners' private offices, public and private clinics, hospitals, ambulatory care facilities, rehabilitation centers, and continuing care facilities. One other place that many people do not think of as a health care facility is a patient's home. Yet, for a variety of reasons, more and more health care is being provided in this setting.

Practitioner Offices

The setting for much of the preventive and primary care provided in America is the offices of health care practitioners. In 2004, there were over 910,857,000 patient visits to physician offices in the United States.[16] Practitioner offices are privately owned buildings such as physicians' and dentists' offices, where care is provided by the practitioner and his or her staff.

Because it is very expensive to set up a private practice, it is increasingly common to see more than one practitioner sharing both an office and staff. These practices are often referred to as *group practices* to distinguish them from *solo (single practitioner) practices.*

Clinics

When two or more physicians practice as a group, the facility in which they provide medical services is called a *clinic.* Some clinics are small, with just a few providers, while others are very large with many providers, such as the Mayo Clinic in Rochester, Minnesota, or the Cleveland Clinic in Cleveland, Ohio. Some clinics provide care only for individuals with special health needs such as treatment of cancer or diabetes or assistance in family planning; others accept patients with a wide range of problems. A misconception held by many is that clinics are not much different from hospitals. One big difference is that clinics do not have inpatient beds, and hospitals do. Some clinics do have an administrative relationship with inpatient facilities so that if a person needs to be admitted to a hospital, it is a relatively simple process; other clinics may be free-standing, or independent of all other facilities.

Although many of the clinics are run as either for-profit or not-for-profit facilities, some are also funded by tax dollars. These clinics have been created primarily to meet the needs of the **medically indigent**—those lacking the financial ability to pay for their own medical care. Most of these clinics are located in large urban areas or rural areas that are underserved by the private sector. Two examples of this type of clinic are *public health clinics* and *community health centers.* The former are usually a part of a local health department (LHD). The scope of health care services offered by LHDs varies greatly. These services can range from prevention-oriented programs, such as immunizations and well-baby care, to complete personal health services such as those offered at private-sector clinics.[4] Community health centers have been around since the late 1960s, known initially as *neighborhood health centers.* Today, community health centers operate under the auspices of the Bureau of Primary Health Care, which is part of the U.S. Department of Health and Human Services.[1] "Community health centers are recognized as an important 'safety net' for the nation's low-income populations as well as the uninsured populations who have no, or limited access to services from other sources."[4]

medically indigent those lacking the financial ability to pay for their own medical care

Hospitals

Like clinics, hospitals vary in size, mission, and organizational structure. The major purpose of hospitals is to provide secondary and tertiary care.

Hospitals can be categorized in several different ways; one way is by hospital ownership (see Figure 13.9 and Table 13.4). A **private (proprietary or investor-owned) hospital** is one that is owned as a business for the purpose of making a profit. "Most for-profit hospitals belong to one of the large hospital management companies that dominate the for-profit hospital network."[4] Recently, a new type of for-profit hospital has been popping up in the United States: the **specialty hospital.** These are hospitals that provide mainly one type of medicine—usually surgery, either cardiac or orthopedic; most are owned, at least in part, by the physicians who practice in them.[42] A lot of controversy surrounds these hospitals.

FIGURE 13.9
Hospitals are often categorized by ownership.

Table 13.4
Hospitals According to Ownership: United States, 2005

Type	Number
All hospitals	5,756
Federal	226
Nonfederal community hospitals	4,936
Private or proprietary or investor-owned (for-profit)	868
Public (state or local)	1,110
Voluntary (not-for-profit)	2,958
Other (e.g., psychiatric, long-term care, prisons, college infirmaries)	594

Source: American Hospital Association (2006). "Fast Facts on US Hospitals." Available at http://www.aha.org.

Larger general hospitals, who are losing patients and revenue to the specialty hospitals, say that these specialty hospitals are just a "grab for money" by the physicians who own them. Physicians say specialty hospitals allow them to practice medicine the way it should be practiced, without answering to a hospital administrator who is trying to cut corners to make a profit. Currently, specialty hospitals make up about 2% of all hospitals in the United States, with more being planned for construction in the near future.[42]

A second type is a **public hospital.** These hospitals are supported and managed by governmental jurisdictions and are usually found in larger cities. Public hospitals can be operated by agencies at all levels of government. Hospitals operated by the federal government include military hospitals (e.g., Walter Reed Army Hospital and the Bethesda Naval Hospital) and the many hospitals run by the Veterans Administration and Indian Health Service. There are also hospitals that are owned or partially financed by states and local governments. Examples include university hospitals, state mental hospitals, and local city and county hospitals.

Voluntary hospitals make up the third category of hospitals. These are nonprofit hospitals administered by not-for-profit corporations or religious, fraternal, and other charitable community organizations. These hospitals make up about one-half of all hospitals in the United States.[16] Examples of this latter group are the Southern Baptist hospitals, the many Shriners' hospitals, and many community hospitals. In recent years, voluntary hospitals have been expanding their scope of services and many now include wellness centers, stress centers, chemical dependency programs, and a variety of satellite centers.

A second way of classifying hospitals is by dividing them into *teaching* and *nonteaching hospitals.* Teaching hospitals have, as a part of their mission, the responsibility to prepare new health care providers. These hospitals are typically aligned with medical schools, universities, and medical residency programs. However, there are a number of hospitals that are not affiliated with medical schools that provide clinical education for nurses, allied health personnel, and a wide variety of technical specialties.[4]

A third means of categorizing hospitals is by the services offered. **Full-service hospitals,** or general hospitals, are those that offer care at all or most of the levels of care discussed earlier in the chapter. These are the most expensive hospitals to run and are usually found in metropolitan areas. **Limited-service hospitals** offer the specific services needed by the population served, such as emergency, maternity, general surgery, and so on, but they lack much of the sophisticated technology available at full-service hospitals. This type of hospital is more common in rural areas. Many limited-service hospitals were once full-service hospitals but have become limited-service hospitals because of the low volume of patients, a shortage of health care personnel, and financial distress.

private (proprietary) or investor-owned hospitals for-profit hospitals

specialty hospital a hospital that provides mainly one type of medicine, is for-profit, and is owned at least in part by the physicians who practice in it

public hospitals hospitals that are supported and managed by governmental jurisdictions

voluntary hospitals nonprofit hospitals administered by not-for-profit corporations or charitable community organizations

full-service hospitals hospitals that offer services in all or most of the levels of care defined by the spectrum of health care delivery

limited-service hospitals hospitals that offer only the specific services needed by the population served

Outpatient and Ambulatory Care Facilities

In the strictest sense, the term *outpatient care* refers to any care that does not require an overnight stay in a hospital, whereas *inpatient care* is the care provided to those patients who have been admitted to a hospital. Thus, going to a doctor's office for a checkup or having same-day surgery would qualify as outpatient care. Today, care and procedures that once were performed only on an inpatient basis are increasingly being performed in a variety of outpatient settings.[30] In fact, today the majority of all surgical procedures are performed on an outpatient basis.[4] The term given to facilities in which many of these medical procedures are performed is **ambulatory care facilities.** There are many different types of ambulatory care facilities, ranging from hospital-based facilities, generally in various building complexes surrounding the main hospital, to independently owned freestanding facilities that provide a wide, and rapidly expanding, array of services (see Figure 13.10). The growth and movement of services to ambulatory care facilities has resulted from a combination of new medical and diagnostic procedures, technological advances, consumer demand for user-friendly environments, the reimbursement process, and financial mandates from insurance companies and government.[4] The ownership and operation of ambulatory care facilities includes hospitals, hospital systems, physician groups, and for-profit or not-for-profit chains.[4] The types of ambulatory care facilities most often found in communities are primary care centers, urgent/emergent care centers, ambulatory surgery centers, and freestanding service facilities.

Primary care centers present another way to offer primary care in addition to the more traditional physician office mode. Though they may appear to be just another physician's office or group practice, many of these facilities are owned by hospitals and also include laboratory, radiology, and pharmacy services. "In hospital-operated facilities, staff physicians are commonly employees of the owner hospital, or, in the case of a teaching facility, physicians may be jointly compensated through a medical school—affiliated faculty practice group and the hospital."[4] In some parts of the country, depending on licensing procedures, it may be common to see nurse practitioners and physician assistants, under physician supervision, as the primary care practitioners in these facilities.[4]

Some of the most recent additions to ambulatory care facilities offering primary care services are grocery and retail stores. In late 2005 and early 2006, Hy-Vee, a small grocery chain, and retail giants Wal-Mart and Target began offering a limited range of basic tests and treatments in select locations. The facilities are operated by an outside company and are generally staffed by nurses, nurse practitioners, and physician assistants.[43] Experts feel that these facilities have been created to increase foot traffic in the stores rather than as a new revenue stream.[43] Early reports indicate that patients like them for both cost and convenience. Time will tell if they will become common in all parts of the country.

Urgent/emergent care centers have been around in the United States since the early 1970s. They "fill gaps in the delivery system created by the rigidity of private physician appointment and unavailability during nonbusiness hours. The centers also can provide a much more convenient and user friendly alternative to a hospital emergency department during hours when private physicians are not available."[4] Urgent/emergent care centers often provide quicker service with less paperwork, particularly for those with cash or credit cards. These facilities (often not much

ambulatory care facilities
facilities that provide a wide array of outpatient services; these can range from hospital-based facilities to independently owned freestanding facilities

FIGURE 13.10
Ambulatory care facilities provide medical services safely and efficiently without the overhead of a hospital.

larger than a fast-food restaurant) have sometimes been referred to as "Docs in a Box"! These facilities are not appropriate for all emergency cases. A majority of patients with life-threatening conditions are still taken to hospital emergency rooms, where top-of-the-line, advanced life support equipment and emergency physicians are on staff. Although emergency rooms are expensive for hospitals to maintain, they obviously perform a needed service.

Ambulatory surgery centers do not perform major surgery, such as heart transplants, but perform same-day surgeries where a hospital stay following the surgery is not needed. As noted earlier, today the majority of all surgical procedures are performed in these types of facilities.[4] The factors that have promoted the increase in ambulatory surgical procedures as alternatives to inpatient surgery include the development of new, safe, and faster- acting general anesthetics, advances in surgical equipment and materials, development of noninvasive or minimally invasive surgical and nonsurgical procedures, and reduced coverage by insurance companies for hospital stays.

One area of tremendous growth in ambulatory care facilities in recent years has been in the development of freestanding, non-hospital based, specialty facilities. Often, these facilities offer a single service, such as dialysis for individuals with kidney failure, or several similar services, such as those found in a diagnostic imaging center. In this latter example, the services often included are simple radiograph technology (X-rays) and computed tomography (CT) and magnetic resonance imaging (MRI), which are used for viewing the body's anatomical structures in several planes. These technologies are ideal for ambulatory facilities because of their noninvasive nature and profitability.

Even though convenience and cost are often the reason for the development of new ambulatory care facilities, the establishment of a new ambulatory care facility in a community is not always received with enthusiasm. In previously underserved communities, fast-growing communities, or communities with many temporary residents such as resort communities, they have been well received. However, in stable or shrinking communities where there is an adequate number of health providers, the arrival of a new freestanding ambulatory care facility is sometimes viewed as unfriendly competition. In some of these cases the "unfriendly competition" has come from outside for-profit health care companies, but a more recent trend has been physicians breaking away from voluntary (independent or not-for-profit) hospitals where they once performed the procedures in the hospital's outpatient facility to create their own facilities in which to perform the procedures. The primary reasons for this trend are physicians wishing to have control over how the facility is run (i.e., the times and days procedures are scheduled, who is hired to work in the facilities) and to receive a greater share of the profits.

Rehabilitation Centers
Rehabilitation centers are health care facilities in which patients work with health care providers to restore functions lost because of injury, disease, or surgery. These centers are sometimes part of a clinic or hospital but may also be freestanding facilities. Rehabilitation centers may operate on both an ambulatory and an inpatient basis. Those providers who commonly work in a rehabilitation center include physical, occupational, and respiratory therapists as well as exercise physiologists.

rehabilitation center a facility in which restorative care is provided following injury, disease, or surgery

Long-Term Care Options
Not too many years ago, when the topic of long-term care was mentioned, most people thought of nursing homes and state hospitals for the mentally ill and emotionally disabled. Today, however, the term *long-term care* includes not only the traditional institutional residential care, but also special units within these residential facilities (such as for Alzheimer patients), halfway houses, group homes, assisted living facilities, transitional (step-down) care in a hospital, day care facilities for patients of all ages with health problems that require

special care, and personal home health care. Many of these options were discussed in Chapter 9 because elders are the biggest users of long-term care, but other users include those with disabilities or chronic conditions, and those with acute and subacute conditions who are unable to care for themselves.

One area of long-term care that has received special attention in recent years is home health care. The demand for home health care has been driven by the restructuring of the health care delivery system, technological advances that enable people to be treated outside a hospital and to recover more quickly, and the cost containment pressures that have shortened hospital stays.[44] Home health care should not be confused with home care. *Home care* is a more inclusive term and "denotes a range of services provided in the home, including skilled nursing and therapies, personal care, and even social services, such as meals, and home modifications"[45] (see Chapter 9 for a discussion of personal care). **Home health care** involves providing health care via health personnel and medical equipment to individuals and families in their places of residence, for the purpose of promoting, maintaining, or restoring health or to maximize the level of independence while minimizing the effects of disability and illness, including terminal disease. Home health care can be either long term, to help a chronically ill patient avoid institutionalization, or it can be short term to assist a patient following an acute illness and hospitalization until the patient is able to return to independent functioning. Home health care can be provided either through a formal system of paid professional health caregivers (e.g., home health care agency), or through an informal system where the care is provided by family, friends, and neighbors[4] (see Chapter 9 for more on caregivers). Medicare is the largest single payer for home health care, accounting for about one-third of the total annual expenditures.[4]

The need for professional health caregivers will continue into the future because of the "increase in the number of older persons and their expressed desire to remain in their homes for care whenever possible."[4] In 2004, there were 7,519 Medicare-certified home health agencies in the United States. That number is almost three times as many as existed in 1980, but down from the high of 10,807 in 1997.[16] Changes in Medicare reimbursement and regulation beginning in the late 1990s resulted in significant downward shifts in both expenditures and the number of Medicare-certified home health agencies.[4] In addition, the Medicare changes led to some consolidations, mergers, and closures of home health agencies and thus reduced home health expenditures.[46]

Accreditation of Health Care Facilities

One way of determining the quality of a health care facility is to find out if it is accredited by a reputable group. **Accreditation** is the process by which an agency or organization evaluates and recognizes an institution as meeting certain predetermined standards. The predominant organization responsible for accrediting health care facilities is the **Joint Commission**, formerly known as the Joint Commission on Accreditation of Healthcare Organizations (JCAHO). The Joint Commission is an independent, not-for-profit organization that accredits about 15,000 health care organizations in the United States and in many other countries. The health care facilities/organizations that can be accredited by the Joint Commission include ambulatory care organizations, assisted living facilities, behavioral health care organizations, critical access hospitals, clinical laboratories, health care networks, home care organizations, hospitals, long-term care facilities, and office-based surgery practices. To earn and maintain JCAHO accreditation, a facility or organization must complete an application and undergo an on-site survey by a Joint Commission survey team at least every three years.[47] However, laboratories must be surveyed every two years.

When home health care was discussed earlier, mention was made of Medicare-certified home health agencies. To receive Medicare and Medicaid reimbursement, home health agencies must have this certification. Certification is a quality assurance process. Medicare does not directly certify home health agencies, but rather uses approved national accreditation organizations to handle the process. However, prior to allowing an accrediting organization to review home health agencies, the Centers for Medicare and Medicaid Services (CMS) must grant the accrediting organization "deeming authority" to determine if indeed an agency is in compliance with CMS Quality Standards for Suppliers of Durable Medical Equipment, Prosthetics, Orthotics, and Supplies (DMEPOS). If the accrediting organization indicates that all of the Medicare conditions are met or exceeded, the agency is certified. A number of different accrediting organizations have "deeming authority." JCAHO is one, but other examples include the Community Health Accreditation Program (CHAP) and the Accreditation Commission for Health Care, Inc. (ACHC).

CHAPTER SUMMARY

- The concept of a health care system has been and continues to be questioned in the United States. Is it really a system or is treatment provided in an informal, cooperative manner?

- Health care in the United States has evolved from home and folk remedies to the modest services of the independent country doctor who often visited the sick in their homes to a highly complex two trillion dollar-plus industry.

- There are medical specialists and health care facilities for almost every type of illness and health problem.

- The spectrum of health care includes four domains of practice—population-based public health practice, medical practice, long-term practice, and end-of-life practice.

- Within the medical practice domain of health care are the following types of health care providers: independent providers (allopathic, osteopathic, and nonallopathic); limited (restricted) care providers; nurses; nonphysician practitioners; allied health care professionals; and public health professionals.

- Complementary and alternative medicine (CAM) is "a group of diverse medical and health care systems, practices, and products that are not presently considered to be a part of conventional medicine."[4]

- Health care providers perform services in a variety of settings, including practitioners' offices, clinics, hospitals, ambulatory care facilities, rehabilitation centers, and long-term care facilities, including patients' places of residence.

- Ambulatory care facilities range from hospital-based facilities, generally in various building complexes surrounding the main hospital, to independently owned freestanding facilities that provide a wide, and rapidly expanding, array of services.

- Long-term care options include traditional institutional residential care as well as special units within these residential facilities, halfway houses, group homes, assisted living facilities, transitional (step-down) care in a hospital, day care facilities for patients, and personal home health care.

- The predominant organization responsible for accrediting health care facilities is the Joint Commission.

REVIEW QUESTIONS

1. Why have some questioned whether or not the United States really has a health care system?
2. Describe some of the major changes that have taken place in health care delivery over the years.
3. What is meant by third-party payment?
4. Why has the cost of health care in the United States continued to grow faster than the cost of inflation?
5. What is meant by a spectrum of health care?
6. What are the domains of practice noted in the spectrum of health care?
7. Is there a demand for health care workers in the United States today? If so, why?
8. In what type of facility are most health care workers employed?

SCENARIO: ANALYSIS AND RESPONSE

1. Have you ever experienced a situation similar to the one described in the scenario? If so, briefly describe it.

2. If we truly had a "health care system" in this country, how would this scenario be different?

3. If you were Marcus, how would you have handled this situation?

9. What is the difference between independent and limited (restricted) care providers?

10. What are the differences between allopathic and nonallopathic health care providers?

11. Define complementary and alternative medicine and give a few examples of each.

12. What kind of education do limited (restricted) care providers have?

13. What is the difference between LPNs and RNs?

14. What are advanced practice nurses (APNs)?

15. What are nonphysician practitioners?

16. What role do public health professionals play in health care delivery?

17. What are the advantages of ambulatory care facilities?

18. What is meant by a long-term care facility? Give two examples.

19. Why has the number of home health care agencies dropped in recent years?

20. What is the Joint Commission? What does it do?

ACTIVITIES

1. Using Table 13.3 from this chapter, identify two different health care facilities in your community for each of the levels of care. Briefly describe each facility and determine whether each one is private, public, or voluntary.

2. Make an appointment to interview three health care workers in your community who have different types of jobs. Ask them what they like and dislike about their work, what kind of education they needed, whether they are happy with their work, and whether they

would recommend that others seek this line of work. Summarize your findings in a written paper.

3. Obtain a copy of a local newspaper (the Sunday edition is best) and look through the "want ads" for health care worker jobs. In a one-page paper, briefly describe what you have found and summarize the status of health care position openings in your community.

4. Create a list of all the health care providers from whom your family has sought help in the past five years. Group the individuals into the six provider groups outlined in the chapter. When appropriate, identify the providers' specialties and whether they were allopathic, osteopathic, or nonallopathic providers.

5. Make an appointment to interview an administrator in the local (city or county) health department. In the interview, find out what kind of people, by profession, work in the department. Also find out what type(s) of health care services and clinics are offered by the department. Summarize your findings in a two-page paper.

COMMUNITY HEALTH ON THE WEB

The Internet contains a wealth of information about community and public health. Increase your knowledge of some of the topics presented in this chapter by accessing the Jones and Bartlett Publishers Web site at **http://health.jbpub.com/book/communityhealth/6e** and follow the links to complete the following Web activities.

- American Hospital Association
- American Medical Association
- Joint Commission

REFERENCES

1. Shi, L., and D. A. Singh (2005). *Essentials of the US Health Care System*. Sudbury, MA: Jones and Bartlett.

2. Institute of Medicine (2003). *The Future of the Public's Health in the 21st Century*. Washington, DC: National Academy Press.

3. Rothstein, W. G. (1972). *American Physicians in the Nineteenth Century: From Sect to Science*. Baltimore, MD: Johns Hopkins University Press.

4. Sultz, H. A., and K. M. Young (2006). *Health Care USA: Understanding Its Organization and Delivery*, 5th ed. Sudbury, MA: Jones and Bartlett.

5. Cambridge Research Institute (1976). *Trends Affecting the U.S. Health Care System* (DHEW pub. no. HRA 75-14503). Washington, DC: U.S. Government Printing Office, 261.

6. U.S. Department of Health, Education and Welfare, Health Resources Administration (September 1974). "Fact Sheet: The Hill-Burton Program." Washington, DC: U.S. Government Printing Office.

7. Lokkeberg, A. R. (1988). "The Health Care System." In E. T. Anderson and J. M. McFarlane, eds., *Community as Client: Application of the Nursing Process*. Philadelphia: JB Lippincott, 3-14.

8. Centers for Disease Control and Prevention (1995). "Prevention and Managed Care: Opportunities for Managed Care Organizations, Purchasers of Health Care, and Public Health Agencies." *Morbidity and Mortality Weekly Report*, 44(RR-14): 1-12.

9. Koff, S. Z. (1987). *Health Systems Agencies: A Comprehensive Examination of Planning and Process*. New York: Human Services Press.

10. Stockman, D. A. (1981). "Premises for a Medical Marketplace: A Neoconservative's Vision of How to Transform the Health System." *Health Affairs*, 1(1): 5-18.

11. Wessel, D. (7 September 2006). "In Health Care, Consumer Theory Falls Flat." *Wall Street Journal*, A2.

12. White House Domestic Policy Council (1993). *The President's Health Security Plan: The Clinton Blueprint*. New York: Times Books.

13. U.S. Department of Health and Human Services (1996). *Assessing Roles, Responsibilities, and Activities in a Managed Care Environment: A Workbook for Local Health Officials* (AHCPR pub. no. 96-0057). Rockville, MD: Agency for Health Care Policy and Research.

14. MacKay, A. P., L. A. Fingerhut, and C. R. Duran (2000). *Health, United States, 2000, with Adolescent Health Chartbook*. Hyattsville, MD: National Center for Health Statistics.

15. Borger, C., S. Smith, C. Truffer, S. Keehan, A. Sisko, J. Poisal, and M. K. Clemens. (2006). "Health Spending Projections through 2015: Changes in the Horizon." *Health Affairs Web Exclusive*, 25(2): 61-73.

16. National Center for Health Statistics (2006). *Health United States, 2006 with Chartbook on Trends in Health of Americans*. Hyattsville, MD: Author.

17. Zatkin, S. (1997). "A Health Plan's View of Government Regulation." *Health Affairs*, 16(6): 33-35.

18. Dickerson, J. F. (8 December 1997). "Dr. Clinton Scrubs Up." *Time*, 48.

19. President's Advisory Commission on Consumer Protection and Quality in the Health Care Industry (1998). *Quality First: Better Health Care for All Americans*. Washington, DC: U.S. Government Printing Office.

20. The White House (5 April 2006). "Fact Sheet: Health Savings Accounts: Affordable and Accessible Health Care [*Press release*]."

21. Institute of Medicine (2001). *Crossing the Quality Chasm: A New Health System for the 21st Century*. Washington, DC: National Academy Press.

22. Institute of Medicine (2000). *To Err Is Human: Building a Safer Health System*. Washington, DC: National Academy Press.

23. World Health Organization (2000). "World Health Organization Assesses the World's Health Systems." Available at http://www.who.int/whr/2000/en/press_release.htm.

24. Turnock, B. J. (2004). *Public Health: What It Is and How It Works*, 3rd ed. Sudbury, MA: Jones and Bartlett.

25. U.S. Public Health Service (1994). *For a Healthy Nation: Return on Investments in Public Health*. Washington, DC: U.S. Department of Health and Human Services.

26. Donaldson, M., K. D. Yordy, K. N. Lohr, and N. A. Vanselow, eds. (1996). *Primary Care: America's Health in a New Era*. Washington, DC: National Academy Press.

27. Kekki, P. (2003). *Primary Health Care and the Millennium Development Goals: Issues for Discussion*. Available at http://www.who.int/chronic_conditions/primary_health_care/en/mdgs_final.pdf.

28. Slee, V., D. Slee, and H. J. Schmidt (2001). *Slee's Health Care Terms*, 4th ed. St. Paul, MN: Tringa Press.

29. Freid, V. M., K. Prager, A. P. MacKay, and H. Xia (2003). *Health, United States, 2003, with Chartbook on Trends in Health of Americans*. Hyattsville, MD: National Center for Health Statistics.

30. Bernstein, A. B., E. Hing, A. J. Moss, K. F. Allen, A. B. Siller, and R. B. Tiggle (2004). *Health Care in America: Trends in Utilization*. Hyattsville, MD: National Center for Health Statistics.

31. American Osteopathic Association (2006). "What Is a Doctor of Osteopathic Medicine (D.O.)?" Available at http://www.osteopathic.org.

32. National Center for Complementary and Alternative Medicine, National Institutes for Health (2006). "What *Is* Complementary and Alternative Medicine (CAM)?" Available at http://nccam.nih.gov/health/whatiscam/.

33. U.S. Census Bureau (2006). *The 2006 Statistical Abstract: The National Data Book*. Available at http://www.census.gov/compendia/statab/health_nutrition/.

34. Levinson, D., and L. Gaccione (1997). *Health and Illness: A Cross-Cultural Encyclopedia*. Santa Barbara, CA: ABC-CLIO.

35. National Center for Complementary and Alternative Medicine, National Institutes for Health (2006). "Frequently Asked Questions." Available at http://nccam.nih.gov/tools/faq.htm.

36. National Center for Complementary and Alternative Medicine, National Institutes for Health (2006). "NCCAM Funding: Appropriations History." Available at http://nccam.nih.gov/about/appropriations/index.htm.

37. Health Resources and Services Administration, Department of Health and Human Services (2006). "What Is Behind HRSA's Projected Supply, Demand, and Shortage of Registered Nurses?" Available at http://bhpr.hrsa.gov/healthworkforce/reports/behindprojections/4.htm.

38. Hassmiller, S. B., and M. Cozine (2006). "Addressing the Nurse Shortage to Improve the Quality of Patient Care." *Health Affairs*, 25(1): 268-274.

39. Stanfield, P. S., and Y. H. Hui (2002). *Introduction to the Health Professions*, 4th ed. Sudbury, MA: Jones and Bartlett.

40. Health Resources and Services Administration, Department of Health and Human Services (2006). "Preliminary Findings: 2004 National Sample Survey of Registered Nurses." Available at http://www.bhpr.hrsa.gov/healthworkforce/reports/rnpopulation/preliminaryfindings.htm.

41. Health Resources and Services Administration, Department of Health and Human Services (2006). "Public Health." Available at http://.bhpr.hrsa.gov/publichealth/index.htm.

42. Carbonara, P., and J. Caplin (2004). "The Hospital Wars." *Money*, 33(2): 147-148, 151-152.

43. The Associated Press (3 February 2006). "Health Care Hits Retail With In-*Store* Clinics." *The StarPress Newspaper*.

44. Ester, C. L. (2001). "The Uncertain Future of Home Care." In C. Barrington and C. L. Ester, eds., *Health Policy*, 3rd ed. Sudbury, MA: Jones and Bartlett, 102-113.

45. Coleman, B. (2000). *Assuring the Quality of Home Care: The Challenge of Involving the Consumer*. Washington, DC: American Association of Retired People.

46. Levit, K., C. Cowan, H. Lazenby, A. Sensenig, P. McDonnell, J. Stiller, A. Martin, and the Health Accounts Team (2001). "Health Spending in 1998: Signals of Change." In C. Harrington and C. L. Ester, eds., *Health Policy: Crisis and Reform in the U.S. Health Care Delivery System*, 3rd ed. Sudbury, MA: Jones and Bartlett, 254-262.

47. Joint Commission (2007). Facts About the Joint Commission. Available at http://www.jointcommission.org/aboutus/joint_commission_facts.htm.

Health Care System: Function

Chapter Objectives

After studying this chapter you will be able to:

1 Identify the major concerns with the health care system in the United States.

2 Explain fee-for-service and prepaid health plans.

3 Briefly describe the purpose and concept of insurance.

4 Define the term *insurance policy*.

5 Briefly describe the State Children's Health Insurance Program (SCHIP).

6 Explain the insurance policy terms *deductible, co-insurance, co-payment, fixed indemnity, exclusion,* and *pre-existing condition.*

7 Explain what is meant when a company or business is said to be self-insured.

8 List the different types of medical care usually covered in a health insurance policy.

9 Briefly describe Medicare, Medicaid, and Medigap insurance.

10 Briefly explain long-term care health insurance.

11 Define *managed care.*

12 Define the terms *preferred provider organization* (PPO) and *exclusive provider organization* (EPO) and explain how these organizations function.

13 Briefly describe the two main organizational models of health maintenance organizations (HMOs).

14 Explain point-of-service, physician-hospital organizations, and Medicare Advantage.

15 Identify the advantages and disadvantages of managed care.

16 Identify the strengths and weaknesses of national health insurance and the Canadian health care system.

17 Briefly discuss health care reform in the United States.

18 Define *consumer-directed health care.*

19 Explain health savings accounts.

SCENARIO

Greg, a young father, is awakened in the middle of the night by his 8-year-old son, Zack, who has all the typical signs and symptoms of influenza. Greg does not want to disturb his family physician at this time of night, but he does want Zack to receive appropriate medical care. Therefore, he decides to take Zack to the hospital emergency room for treatment. After examining the boy, Dr. Rainey, the attending physician, declares that Zack has the flu. Dr. Rainey then instructs Greg that Zack should drink plenty of clear fluids, take a nonaspirin analgesic for his fever, and get plenty of rest. Dr. Rainey concludes by indicating that the illness should pass in a couple of days. As Greg and Zack leave the hospital, they stop at the business desk to pay the bill. The billing clerk informs Greg that there is no charge. "You have zero deductible health insurance." The amount of the bill was for $743.00.

INTRODUCTION

In Chapter 13, we described the structure of the health care delivery system in the United States, including such concepts as the spectrum of health care delivery and levels of care. We also surveyed the various types of health care providers and the types of facilities in which health care is provided. In this chapter, we will build on that information by explaining how consumers obtain health care services, how these services are paid for, and by whom. We will also discuss three serious issues of concern with our health care delivery system—access, quality, and cost—and examine some current and potential solutions to these issues.

GAINING ACCESS TO AND PAYING FOR HEALTH CARE IN THE UNITED STATES

The services offered by health care providers in the United States are perhaps the best offered anywhere in the world (see Figure 14.1). Unfortunately, the services are not accessible to all Americans because they cannot afford them. Even when services are accessible, racial and ethnic minorities in the United States "often receive a lower quality of care than do their white counterparts, especially for more complicated procedures."[1] For example, black Americans with heart problems are referred less frequently than white Americans for catheterization and bypass grafting. In cases of bone fractures and cancers, black Americans and Americans of Hispanic origin receive prescriptions for pain control less often than whites.[1] To further complicate the health care problem, the cost of services continues to rise. In a nutshell, the major problems with the health care system in the United States can be represented by the cost containment, access, and quality triangle noted by Kissick[2] (see Figure 14.2). In Kissick's equilateral triangle, the equal 60-degree angles represent equal priorities. That is, access is just as important as quality and cost containment and vice versa. However, an expansion of any one of the angles compromises one or both of the other two. For example, if we were interested in increasing the quality of our already good services, it would also increase the costs and decrease access. Or, some feel, if we

FIGURE 14.1

Health care services offered by U.S. providers are perhaps the best in the world, but at what cost?

increase access, costs will go up, and the quality will decrease. Or, if we concentrate on containing costs, both quality of care and access will decrease. With such dilemmas, the United States continues to struggle to find the right combination of policy and accountability to deal with these shortcomings.

Access to Health Care

Even with several different means of gaining access to health care services (see Figure 14.3), access has been and continues to be a major health policy issue in the United States. Health insurance coverage and the generosity of coverage are major determinants of access to health care.[3,4] Although the majority of people (84%) in the United States do have health insurance, approximately 46.6 million Americans were uninsured throughout 2005 (see Box 14.1). Millions more lacked health insurance coverage for shorter periods during that year. The likelihood of being uninsured is greater for younger persons, those with less education, those

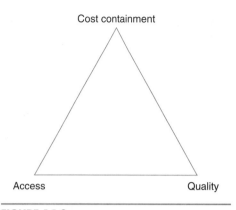

FIGURE 14.2

The cost containment, access, and quality triangle of health care.

Source: Kissick, W. L. (1994). *Medicine's Dilemmas: Infinite Needs Versus Finite Resources.* New Haven, CT: Yale University Press. Used with permission.

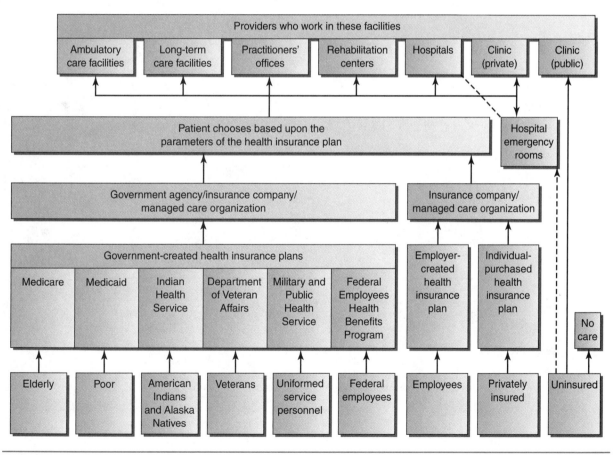

FIGURE 14.3

Means of gaining access to health care.

BOX
14.1   **HEALTHY PEOPLE 2010: OBJECTIVES**

Objective 1-1:   Increase the proportion of persons with health insurance.

Target: 100%.

Baseline: 83% of persons under age 65 years were covered by health insurance in 1997 (age-adjusted to the year 2000 standard population).

Persons Under 65 Years	1997 Baseline	2005 Status
	Percent	
TOTAL	83	84
Race and ethnicity		
American Indian or Alaska Native	62	68
Asian or Pacific Islander	81	DNC
Asian	81	83
Native Hawaiian or other Pacific Islander	80	80
Black or African American	80	82
White	84	84
Hispanic or Latino	66	67
Cuban	79	77
Mexican American	61	64
Puerto Rican	81	84
Not Hispanic or Latino	85	87
Black or African American	80	82
White	86	88
Gender		
Female	84	85
Male	81	82
Family income level		
Poor	66	69
Near poor	69	71
Middle/high income	91	90
Geographic location		
Within MSA	83	84
Outside MSA	80	82
Disability status		
Persons with disabilities	83	86
Persons without disabilities	83	83
Sexual orientation	DNC	DNC
Select populations		
Age groups		
10–24 years	DNA	81
10–14 years	DNA	90
15–19 years	DNA	85
20–24 years	DNA	68

DNA = Data have not been analyzed. DNC = Data are not collected. MSA = Metropolitan statistical area.

Note: Age-adjusted to the year 2000 standard population.

Sources: National Health Interview Survey (NHIS), CDC, NCHS.

For Further Thought

In your opinion, what kinds of things will have to happen by the year 2010 for the previously noted objective to be met? Do you think this objective will be met? Why or why not?

with lower incomes, nonwhites, those who are not U.S. citizens, and males. It also increases based upon where one lives. For the three-year average from 2003 to 2005, some states had fewer than 10% uninsured (Iowa, Hawaii, Minnesota), whereas other states had 18% or more uninsured (Arizona, California, Florida, Louisiana, Montana, Nevada, New Mexico, Oklahoma, Texas).[5] (See Figure 14.4 for reasons why people are uninsured.) Interestingly enough, the uninsured do not lack emergency or urgent care because no one needing such care and willing to go to a hospital emergency room will be turned away. However, the uninsured usually do not have access to primary care (see Box 13.2 in Chapter 13), such as checkups, screenings for chronic illnesses, and prenatal care. Without adequate primary care, many patients eventually find themselves in need of more costly and often less effective medical treatment. The primary factors that limit access to this type of care are total lack of health insurance, inadequate insurance, and poverty. Those who are unable to receive medical care because they cannot afford it are referred to as "medically indigent."[6] The medically indigent in America include people and families with income above the poverty level who are thus ineligible for Medicaid, or government health insurance for the poor, but who are unable to afford health care or health insurance. "Eight out of ten uninsured persons are members of working families. In most of these cases, the worker holds a job that does not offer health insurance. In others, subsidized coverage may be offered, but the employee turns it down because of the cost or because they do not perceive the need for coverage."[3] Those who have a job but are unable to afford health insurance are referred to as the *working poor*. It has been estimated that there are 30 million working poor in the United States.[7] Others may be uninsured because "individual health policies are quite expensive and may be unavailable for those who have a preexisting health problem. Young adults often lose their eligibility under their parent's policy when they turn 19 or graduate from college. Spouses lose coverage under a family policy through separation, divorce, retirement, or upon the death of a policy holder"[3] (see Figure 14.4).

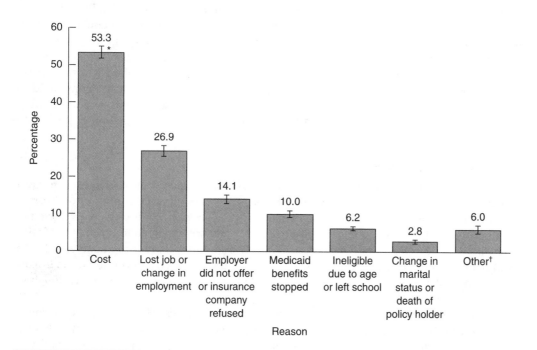

FIGURE 14.4

Reasons for lack of health insurance coverage among uninsured persons aged 65 years or younger: National Health Interview Survey, United States, 2004.

Notes: Based on response to a survey regarding the reasons a household member stopped being covered by health insurance or did not have health insurance. Persons might be counted in more than one category.
*95% confidence interval.
†Includes moved, self-employed, never had coverage, did not want or need coverage, and other unspecified reasons.

Source: Adams, P. F., and P. M. Barnes (2006). "Summary Health Statistics for the U.S. Population: National Health Interview Survey, 2004." *Vital and Health Statistics*, 10(229). Available at http://www.cdc.gov/nchs/data/series/sr_10/sr10_229.pdf.

Even those who have adequate health insurance suffer. Most Americans pay three or four times for health care: "we pay once through taxes, a second time through insurance premiums and co-payments, a third time through supplemental insurance, and a fourth time through the cost of products we buy."[8]

Quality of Health Care

The quality of health care can be measured in a number of ways. For example, the World Health Organization has developed an index of performance based on how efficiently health systems translate expenditure into health as measured by disability-adjusted life expectancy (DALE). (See Chapter 3 for a discussion of DALE.) In the United States, several different groups have developed means for measuring health care quality. The U.S. government, via several agencies of the Department of Health and Human Services—led by the Agency for Healthcare Research and Quality (AHRQ)—collaborates to annually publish the *National Healthcare Quality Report* (NHQR), which was started in 2003. The NHQR is built on 179 measures assembled across four dimensions of quality—effectiveness, patient safety, timeliness, and patient centeredness.[9] Nongovernmental groups are also involved in measuring quality. As was noted in Chapter 13, the accreditation of health care facilities is a means of measuring health care services. The National Committee for Quality Assurance (NCQA) assesses and ranks almost 700 health care plans (i.e., managed care programs, specifically HMOs, POSs, and PPOs) on their clinical performance, patient experience and satisfaction, as well as their NCQA accreditation status.[10] Even though each of these measures of health care quality quantifies *quality* in a different way, the general consensus regarding the quality of health care in the United States is that it is getting better at a modest pace but is not as good as it could be. In fact, in *The World Health Report 2000*, the World Health Organization ranked the United States 37th of 191 countries on its overall health system performance.[11] Schoen and colleagues provide a nice summary of the quality of the U.S. health care system: "The United States has broad opportunities to improve. It can do better, given the level of resources it has committed to health care. There is also much risk in failing to act: Cost and coverage vital signs are moving in the wrong direction. To assure a healthy, productive nation, transformation of the health system is of great urgency."[12]

Paying for Health Care

The health care services in America have not only been labeled the best, but also the most expensive (see Table 13.1 in Chapter 13). Health care expenditures continue to absorb a growing share of the national economy. In 2006, health care expenditures were projected to consume 16.2% of the gross domestic product (GDP) and are expected to reach 20% of GDP by 2015.[13] America spends more per capita annually on health care (approximately $7,129 in 2006) than any other nation.[13] Under the U.S. system, the actual cost of the service is usually not known until after the service has been provided, unless the consumer is bold enough to inquire ahead of time. Most are not.

Payments for the U.S. health care bill come from four sources. The first is the consumers themselves. In 2004 these direct or out-of-pocket payments represented approximately one-sixth (15.1%) of all payments. The remaining portion of health care payments, four-fifths, comes almost entirely from indirect, or third-party, payments. The first source of third-party payments is private insurance companies. Private insurance companies paid 36.1% of the health care bill in 2004. These payments were made from premiums paid to the insurance company by the employees and/or their employers. The second source of third-party payments is public or governmental insurance programs (i.e., Medicare, Medicaid, Veterans Administration, Indian Health Service, or military). These government programs are funded by a combination of taxes and premiums from those insured (as in the case of Part B Medicare coverage). In 2004, 44.4% of the health care bill was paid for by public or governmental insurance programs. Finally, a small percentage of health care bills are paid by other private funds. In 2004, it was 4.4% (see Figure 14.5).[4]

There are two broad divisions of arrangements for paying for and delivering health care—fee-for-service indemnity and prepaid health care. The most traditional system of health care financing is **fee-for-service.** This arrangement is based on the assumption that services are provided in a set of identifiable and individually distinct units such as a doctor's office visit or a specific medical procedure.[14] Under the fee-for-service format, consumers select a provider, receive care (service) from the provider, and incur expenses (a fee) for the care. The provider is then reimbursed for covered services in part by the insurer (private insurance company or the government) and in part by the consumer, who is responsible for the balance unpaid by the insurer. Initially, the providers set the fees and insurers would pay the claim. But more recently, insurers started to limit the amount they would pay for "usual, customary, and reasonable." The biggest drawback of the fee-for-service format is that providers have a greater incentive to provide services, some of which sometimes are nonessential.[14]

Under the fee-for-service format, consumers are obligated to pay their fee at the time the service is rendered. In the past, before health insurance was common, some physicians provided care when needed and worried about payment later. Others often accepted "in kind" payment, such as farm produce or other products or services, as payment in full for a medical service rendered. Today, in order for patients to receive care via fee-for-service, they are often required to demonstrate the ability to pay (to assume financial responsibility for the fee) before the service is rendered. A provider's receptionist may ask, "How do you plan to settle your bill?" In other cases, providers have signs placed around the waiting room that state, "Payment is expected when service is rendered, unless other arrangements have been made prior to the appointment."

A variation of the fee-for-service format that is used in many managed care plans is a *fee schedule*. Instead of using the "usual, customary, and reasonable" amount to reimburse providers, managed care organizations negotiate discounted fees to be paid for specific procedures and services.

fee-for-service
a method of paying for health care in which after the service is rendered, a fee is paid

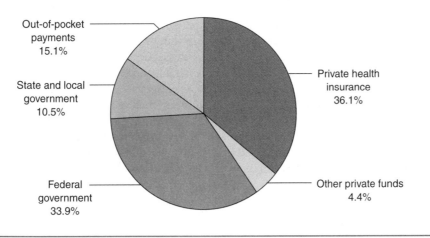

FIGURE 14.5
Personal health care expenditures by source of funds, United States, 2004.

Source: National Center for Health Statistics (2006). *Health United States, 2006 with Chartbook on Trends in Health of Americans*. Hyattsville, MD: Author.

Though prepaid health care has been available in the United States since the late 1920s, it was not until the 1970s that it achieved recognition as a mainstream approach to financing medical costs, with the passage of the Health Maintenance Organization (HMO) Act of 1973. And it was not until the early to mid-1990s, that the managed care movement, or HMOs, became the predominant form of health care coverage. Under **prepaid health care** arrangements, insurers make arrangements with health care providers to provide agreed-upon covered health care services to a given population of consumers for a (usually discounted) set price—the per-person premium fee—over a particular time period. Often the arrangements are set up on a per-member, per-month (PMPM) rate called a *capitated fee*. Thus, this arrangement for reimbursing the providers is referred to as a *capitation system*. The provider receives the capitated fee per enrollee regardless of whether the enrollee uses health care services and regardless of the quality of services provided. The provider is responsible for providing all needed services determined to be medically necessary and covered under the plan.[14] "Thus, under capitation, a portion of the risk is shifted from managed care organization to the provider, and theoretically the providers should become more prudent in providing services cost effectively because they are bearing some of the risk."[14] In addition to the capitated fee, consumers may pay additional fees (co-payments) for office visits and other services used. The insurer organizes the delivery of care by building an infrastructure of providers and implementing the systems to monitor and influence the cost and quality of care.

Of the two broad divisions of arrangements of paying for and delivering health care, prepaid health care arrangements have taken on the label of "managed care." However, both arrangements can include elements of managed care, and not all managed care plans use prepaid health care arrangements. Initially, many managed care plans focused on using their market power to obtain discounts from the providers. However, as they evolve, more organized arrangements are being developed where the providers are asked to assume some of the risk in the plan. Thus, providers are offered incentives for containing costs while maintaining patient satisfaction with the care received.[15]

Third-Party Payment

The process for receiving a third-party payment usually begins when a health care provider or his or her staff requests information about the patient's health insurance plan. They normally request the name of the insuring company (e.g., Blue Cross/Blue Shield), the policy number, and a personal identification number (PIN). This information is usually provided to the insured on a wallet-sized card by the insurer. The provider may then ask the patient to sign an insurance claim form in two places (see Figure 14.6). The first signature indicates that the service has been provided and authorizes the provider to submit patient information with the claim for payment. The second signature instructs the insurance company to make the payment directly to the provider. Upon receiving and reviewing the completed and signed form, the insurance company then issues payments to the provider for services based upon the provisions of the insurance policy. Depending upon the level of reimbursement for the claim, the provider will either consider the bill paid in full or will request payment from the patient in the amount of the difference between the provider's full fee and the portion paid by the insurance company.

HEALTH INSURANCE

Health insurance, like all other types of insurance, is a risk- and cost-spreading process. That is, the cost of one person's injury or illness is shared by all in the group. Each person in the group has a different chance (or risk) of having a problem and thus needing health care. Some members of the group, for example, those who suffer from chronic and/or congenital health

---

prepaid health care
a method of paying for covered health care services on a per-person premium basis for a specific time period prior to the service being rendered (also referred to as capitation)

FIGURE 14.6
Insurance claim form.

problems, will probably need more care while others in the group will need less. The concept of insurance has everyone in the group, no matter what their individual risk, helping to pay for the collective risk of the group. The risk of costly ill health is spread in a reasonably equitable fashion among all persons purchasing insurance, and everyone is protected from having to pay an insurmountable bill for a catastrophic injury or illness.

There are some exceptions to the "equitable fashion." If someone in the group knowingly engages in a behavior that increases his or her risk, such as smoking cigarettes or driving in a reckless manner, that person may have to pay more for the increased risk. In short, the greater the risk (or probability of using the insurance), the more the individual or group has to pay for insurance.

The concept of health insurance is not a new one in this country. Group health and life insurance are considered American inventions of the early twentieth century. In 1911 Montgomery Ward and Company sold health insurance policies based upon the principles still used today in the business. Currently, hundreds of companies in the United States sell health and life insurance policies.

Because of the expense of health care, those without health insurance find it difficult to pay for the care. If people do not have insurance, they are more likely to lack a usual source of primary medical care,[16] use less care, and often suffer adverse consequences due to delayed or postponed care.[17] As noted earlier in the chapter, 46.6 million Americans were without health insurance in 2005. One bright note for some of the uninsured came in 1997 when the 105th Congress enacted the **State Children's Health Insurance Program** (SCHIP; codified as Title XXI of the Social Security Act) as part of the Balanced Budget Act of 1997. SCHIP, which was authorized for 10 years at a cost of about $40 billion, was enacted to extend insurance to a significant portion of the estimated 11.3 million U.S. children without insurance (one in seven, and nearly one-quarter of all uninsured). For low-income and minority children, this proportion is even higher. The figure of 11.3 million was the highest one ever recorded by the Census Bureau, and roughly 3,000 children lose health insurance every day.[18] More than 92% of all uninsured children have working parents, and two-thirds have at least one parent that works full-time and year-round.[18] However, these parents either cannot afford family health care insurance through work, or they are included in those who cannot get family coverage through work at any price.

SCHIP is specifically targeted at low-income children who are ineligible for other insurance coverage, including Medicaid (see the discussion of Medicaid later in this chapter). "Uninsured children pay a heavy price: Study after study shows that they are more likely to report poor health, to see doctors less often (even when they are sick), to go without preventive care, and to turn to emergency rooms when they need treatment. The result is needless illness, learning problems, disabilities, and sometimes even death."[18]

SCHIP is a voluntary grant-in-aid program for states. That is, states can choose to participate or not. If they do, states can provide child health assistance by either expanding Medicaid or by creating a new health assistance program to aid children who are ineligible for Medicaid or are not covered by another form of "creditable coverage." States can also combine the two approaches by using some of their SCHIP funds to expand Medicaid and the rest to provide another form of child health assistance.[19]

At some point during 2005, approximately 6.1 million children were enrolled in SCHIP. However, in that same year the monthly average number of children covered by SCHIP was only 4.2 million.[20] In addition, several states have sought and received approval (waivers) from the U.S. Department of Health and Human Services—the federal agency that administers the SCHIP program—to extend coverage to children not originally covered in the legislation, and to parents of children eligible under either SCHIP or Medicaid.[21] However, even with the SCHIP program, it is estimated that 8.3 million children under the age of 18 in the United States are still uninsured.[22]

As noted earlier, the SCHIP was initially authorized for a 10-year period—until 2007. At the time this edition of *An Introduction to Community Health* was going to press, the 10-year period was ending and Congress was discussing its reauthorization. Proponents of the program were hoping that Congress would not only reauthorize the program but also strengthen

State Children's Health Insurance Program (SCHIP) a title insurance program under the Social Security Act that provides health insurance to uninsured children it by expanding it to cover many of the millions of children still uninsured and to ensure its sustainability into the future.

The Health Insurance Policy

A *policy* is a written agreement between a private insurance company (or the government) and an individual or group of individuals to pay for certain health care costs during a certain time period in return for regular, periodic payments (a set amount of money) called *premiums.* The insurance company benefits in that it anticipates collecting more money in premiums than it has to pay out for services; hence, it anticipates a profit. The insured benefits by not being faced with medical bills he or she cannot pay, because the insurance company is obligated to pay them according to the terms of the contract. The added benefit for those insured as a group is that group premiums are less expensive than premiums for individuals.

The expectations of both insurers and insured are not always met. An insurer occasionally has to pay out more than it collects in premiums. Alternatively, the insured often purchases insurance that is never used.

Although the language of health insurance policies can be confusing, everyone needs to understand several key terms. One of the most important is **deductible.** The deductible is the amount of expenses (money) that the beneficiary (insured) must incur (pay out of pocket) before the insurance company begins to pay for covered services. A common deductible level is $250 per individual policy holder, or a maximum of $1,000 per family. This means that the insured must pay the first $250/$1,000 of medical costs before the insurance company begins paying. The higher the deductible of a policy, the lower the premiums will be.

Usually, but not always, after the deductible has been met, most insurance companies pay a percentage of what they consider the "usual, customary, and reasonable" charge for covered services. The insurer generally pays 80% of the usual, customary, and reasonable costs, and the insured is responsible for paying the remaining 20%. This 20% is referred to as **co-insurance.** If the health care provider charges more than the usual, customary, and reasonable rates, the insured will have to pay both the co-insurance and the difference.[16] A form of co-insurance, often associated with managed care programs, is **co-payment** (or *co-pay* for short). A co-payment is a negotiated set amount a patient pays for certain services—for example, $20 for an office visit and $15 for a prescription. Some insurance policies may have both co-insurance and co-payments included. The greater the proportion of co-insurance paid by the insured, the lower the premiums.

A fourth key term, **fixed indemnity,** refers to the maximum amount an insurer will pay for a certain service. For example, a policy may state that the maximum amount of money paid for orthodontia is $2,000. Depending upon the language of a policy, the fixed indemnity benefit may or may not be subject to the provisions of the deductible or co-insurance clause. Costs above the fixed indemnity amount are the responsibility of the insured.

Another key term related to health insurance is **exclusion.** When an exclusion is written into a policy, it means that a specified health condition is excluded from coverage. That is, the policy does not pay for service to treat the condition. Common exclusions include a pregnancy that began before the health insurance policy went into effect or a chronic disease or condition such as diabetes or hypertension that has been classified as a pre-existing condition. A **pre-existing condition** is a medical condition that had been diagnosed or treated usually within the six months before the date the health insurance policy went into effect. Because of such exclusions, people who have a serious condition or disease are often unable to get health insurance coverage for the condition/disease or in general. Some health insurance policies also exclude a condition/disease for a specified period of time, such as nine months for pregnancy or one year for all other exclusions.

deductible
the amount of expenses that the beneficiary must incur before the insurance company begins to pay for covered services

co-insurance
the portion of the insurance company's approved amounts for covered services that a beneficiary is responsible for paying

co-payment
a negotiated set amount that a patient pays for certain services

fixed indemnity
the maximum amount an insurer will pay for a certain service

exclusion
a health condition written into the health insurance policy indicating what is not covered by the policy

pre-existing condition
a medical condition that had been diagnosed or treated usually within the six months before the date a health insurance policy goes into effect

The rule that a pre-existing condition could be an exclusion "trapped" many people in jobs, because the employees were afraid of losing their health insurance for the condition if they changed employers. To deal with this issue, Congress passed the Health Insurance Portability and Accountability Act of 1996 (PL 104-102, known as HIPAA). This law was created, in part, to ensure that people will not have to wait for health insurance to go into effect when changing jobs. More specifically, a pre-existing condition will be covered without a waiting period when a person joins a new plan if the person has been insured for the previous 12 months. This means that if a person remains insured for 12 months or more, he or she will be able to go from one job to another, and the pre-existing condition will be covered—without additional waiting periods—even if the person has a chronic illness. If a person has a pre-existing condition and it has not been covered the previous 12 months before joining a new plan, the longest that person will have to wait before being covered for that condition is 12 months.

Types of Health Insurance Coverage

As has been noted in the previous discussions, there are a number of different types of services that health insurance policies cover. The more common types of coverage are hospitalization, surgical, regular medical, major medical, dental, and disability. Table 14.1 presents a short overview of each of these coverage types.

Though the types of health insurance coverage remain constant, several trends associated with health insurance plans and the products they offer are emerging. The trends that characterize health insurance plans today are (1) the plans are becoming more complex and are concentrated in a fewer number of companies, (2) there is an increase in the diversity of products, so consumers have many more options in the type of plan they select, (3) there is an increased focus on delivering care through a network of providers rather than independent providers, (4) there is a movement of shifting to financial structures and incentives between purchasers, health plans, and providers and away from the fee-for-service payment, and (5) more health insurance plans are developing clinical infrastructures to manage utilization and to improve the quality of care.[23] Such trends will make understanding health insurance plans more challenging for consumers. These trends will require a greater investment in education and information to help consumers understand how insurance products differ, how best to navigate managed care systems, and what differences exist in structure or performance across the plans.[23]

Table 14.1
Types of Health Insurance Coverage

Dental	Dental procedures.
Disability (income protection)	Income when insured is unable to work because of a health problem.
Hospitalization	Inpatient hospital expenses including room, patient care, supplies, and medications.
Long-term care	An umbrella term for an array of supportive services to help people function in their daily lives. Services may include but are not limited to nursing care, home health care, personal care, rehabilitation, adult day care, case management, social services, assistive technology, and assisted living services. Services may be provided at home or in another place of residence like a nursing home.
Major medical	Large medical expenses usually not covered by regular medical or dental coverage.
Optical (vision)	Nonsurgical procedures to improve vision.
Regular medical	Nonsurgical service provided by health care providers. Often has set amounts (fixed indemnity for certain procedures).
Surgical	Surgeons' fees (for inpatient or outpatient surgery).

The Cost of Health Insurance

Over the years, the cost of health insurance has pretty much mirrored the cost of health care. From the early 1970s through the early 1990s, health care costs and the costs of health care insurance were growing in the neighborhood of 10% to 12% per year.[24] But as the cost of health care slowed in the early to mid-1990s, so did the cost of health insurance. This deceleration in premium growth paralleled the dramatic shift in the health insurance marketplace away from traditional fee-for-service indemnity insurance to managed care. However, the managed care revolution created a one-time-only cost savings, and all the underlying cost drivers, such as an aging population, increased use of prescription drugs, and technology, have again increased costs (see Figure 14.7). The burden of the cost of health insurance for those who are working falls primarily on the employer and, to a lesser extent, on the employee. Most Americans under 65 years of age receive their health insurance through their employer or the employer of their parent or spouse/partner. However, because of the increases in the cost of health insurance, the percentage of employers who offer health benefits to their employees continues to drop (69% offered it in 2000, compared with 61% in 2006).[25] Of those employers who continue to offer health benefits to their employees, most are shifting more of the cost onto their employees by (1) increasing the workers' share of the premium, (2) raising the deductibles that workers must pay, (3) increasing the co-payments for prescription drugs, and (4) increasing the number of items on the exclusion list. A vivid example of the cost of health insurance comes from the automobile industry, where it has been estimated that workers' health insurance adds about $1,500 to the cost of every new car.

In the end, the actual cost of a policy is determined by two major factors—the risk of those in the group and the amount of coverage provided. An increase in either risk or coverage will result in an increase in the cost of the policy.

Self-Insured Organizations

With the high cost of health care today, some employers "(or other group, such as a union or trade association)"[26] that provide health insurance for their employees are deciding to cut their costs by becoming self-insured. With such an arrangement, a **self-insured organization**

self-insured organization one that pays the health care costs of its employees with the premiums collected from the employees and the contributions made by the employer

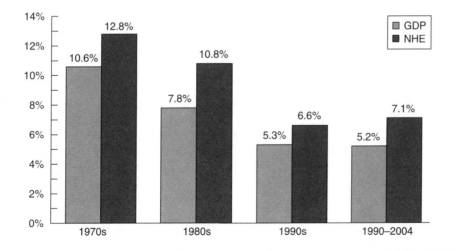

FIGURE 14.7

Average annual growth rates for nominal national health expenditures (NHE) and gross domestic product (GDP) for select time periods.

Source: Centers for Medicare and Medicaid Services, Office of the Actuary (2006). "National Health Expenditure Data." Available at http://www.cms.hhs.gov/NationalHealthExpendData.

pays the health care costs of its employees with the premiums collected from the employees and the contributions made by the employer instead of using a commercial carrier.[26] Self-insured organizations "often use the services of an actuarial firm to set premium rates and a third-party administrator (TPA) to administer benefits, pay claims, and collect data on utilization. Many third-party administrators also provide case management services for potentially extraordinarily expensive cases to help coordinate care and control employee risk of catastrophic expenses."[26] There are several benefits to being self-insured. First, the organization gets to set most of the parameters of the policy—deductibles, co-insurance, fixed indemnities, and exclusions. If the organization wants to exclude some services and include others, it can. For example, if the organization has an older workforce, it may wish to delete obstetrics from the policy but include a number of preventive health services. Second, the organization holds on to the cash reserves in the benefits account instead of sending them to a commercial carrier, and thus gets to accrue interest off of them. Third, the self-insured organizations have been exempt from the *Employee Retirement and Income Security Act of 1974* (ERISA), which mandates minimum benefits under state law.[26] And fourth, generally the administrative costs of self-insured organizations have been less than traditional commercial carriers and, in general, health insurance costs to these groups have risen at a slower rate.[26] For self-insurance to work, there must be a sizable group of employees over which to spread the risk. Larger organizations usually find it more useful than smaller ones. However, if a small workforce is comprised primarily of low-health-risk employees, say for example younger employees, self-insured programs make sense.

HEALTH INSURANCE PROVIDED BY THE GOVERNMENT

Although there are some in the United States who would like to see all health insurance provided by the government—a national health insurance plan—at the present time government health insurance plans are only available to select groups in the United States. The only government health insurance plans—those funded by governments at federal, state, and local levels—that exist today are Medicare, Medicaid, the State Children's Health Insurance Program (SCHIP), Veterans Administration benefits (see Figure 14.8), Indian Health Service, and health care benefits for the uniformed services (military and Public Health Service), federal employees (Federal Employees Health Benefits Program), and prisoners. Our discussion here will be limited to Medicare and Medicaid. These programs were created in 1965 by amendments to the Social Security Act and were implemented for the first time in 1966.

Medicare

Medicare a national health insurance program for people 65 years of age and older, certain younger disabled people, and people with permanent kidney failure

Medicare, which currently covers over 42.5 million people,[4] is a federal health insurance program for people 65 years of age or older, people of any age with permanent kidney failure, and certain disabled people under 65. It is administered by the Centers for Medicare and Medicaid Services (CMS) of the U.S. Department of Health and Human Services (HHS). The Social Security Administration provides information about the program and handles enrollment. Medicare is considered a contributory program, in that employers and employees are required to contribute a percentage of each employee's wages/salaries through Social Security (FICA) tax to the Medicare fund. Medicare has four parts: hospital insurance (Part A), medical insurance (Part B), managed care plans (Part C), and prescription drug plans (Part D).

The Medicare hospital insurance (Part A) portion is mandatory and is provided for those eligible without further cost. Some seniors who are not eligible for premium-free Part A because they or their spouses did not pay into Social Security at all, or paid only a limited amount, may be able to purchase Part A coverage. In 2007, those premiums ranged from $226 to $410 per month.[27] While Medicare Part A has deductible ($992 in 2007) and co-insurance provisions, it helps pay for inpatient care in a hospital and in a skilled nursing facility after a hospital stay, hospice care, and some home health care.[27] Those who are enrolled in Part A of Medicare are automatically enrolled in Part B unless they decline. In 2007, the premium for Part B was $93.50 per month.[27] Most Part A enrollees are also enrolled in Part B and have their premium deducted directly from their Social Security check. Part B of Medicare helps cover physicians' services, outpatient hospital care, and selected other health care services and supplies that are not covered by Part A. Part B also has a deductible ($131 per year in 2007) and co-insurance (80/20 coverage). A recent change to the premiums for Part B was instituted to help reduce the cost of the program to the federal government. The change, which affected about 4% of the enrollees, was to charge enrollees with higher incomes income-related premiums. In 2007, the income-related Part B premiums were $105.80, $124.40, $142.90, or $161.40, depending on the extent to which an individual beneficiary's income exceeded $80,000 (or a married couple's income exceeded $160,000), with the highest premium rates only paid by less than 1% of beneficiaries whose incomes were over $200,000 (or $400,000 for a married couple). A beneficiary who paid the highest income-related premium in 2007 paid $1,936.80 per year in Part B premiums, but was estimated to receive an average of $4,363 in Medicare Part B benefits.[27]

FIGURE 14.8

Insurance provided for veterans is one of several insurance plans paid for by the U.S. government.

Part C of Medicare is the managed care plans of Medicare (see the discussion of managed care later in this chapter). Formally, Part C is called Medicare Advantage (formerly Medicare + Choice) and was added to Medicare as part of the Balanced Budget Act (BBA) of 1997. It was introduced primarily as a means to try to reduce costs compared with the original fee-for-service Medicare plan. Medicare Advantage plans provide all of the coverage provided in Parts A and B and must cover medically necessary services. They generally offer extra benefits; thus, there is no need to purchase a separate supplemental Medigap policy (see the discussion of Medigap later in this chapter), and many include Part D prescription drug coverage. Medicare Advantage plans are not available in all parts of the country.[28]

New to Medicare Advantage plans in 2007 was an option to enroll in a Medicare medical savings account (MSA) (see the discussion of health savings accounts [HSAs] later in this chapter). MSAs combine a high-deductible health plan with a medical savings account that beneficiaries can use to manage their health care costs.[28]

The newest component of Medicare is Part D, the Medicare prescription drug program. The program was introduced as part of the Medicare Prescription Drug, Improvement, and Modernization Act of 2003 and went into effect on January 1, 2006. Part D is optional and run by insurance companies and other private companies approved by Medicare. To use it, those eligible must sign up for it and pay a monthly premium (most range from $20 to $40 per month). The premium varies based upon the plan selected (most states offer approximately 50 different plans). A special provision in Part D—"Extra Help"—offers drug coverage at low cost for qualified people with limited incomes and resources. Although Part D has provided welcome help with the cost of prescription drugs to those who are eligible, the process of using Part D has been hard for many seniors to understand. It is complicated for several reasons. The first is the large number of plans available. The plans vary in drugs covered and costs. For example, one drug may be on the list of drugs covered (called the *formulary*) by one plan but not another. Many plans only cover generic drugs, whereas others cover both generic and brand-name drugs. Most plans have co-payments or co-insurance. And then there is the coverage gap, or what has become known as the *donut hole*. In 2007, all plans (with the exception of the Extra Help plan) had a $265 deductible. Once the deductible was met, the plans covered the cost of drugs (minus co-payment/co-insurance) between $266 and $2,400. Then at $2,401, the enrollees had to pay out of pocket all costs of drugs while in the coverage gap until they had spent $3,850. (This includes yearly deductible, co-payment/co-insurance, and $3,051.25 while in the coverage gap. This does not include the plan's premium.) Once enrollees reached the plan's out-of-pocket limit, the donut hole closed and the enrollees had catastrophic coverage. This means that those covered paid a co-insurance amount (e.g., 5% of the drug cost) or a co-payment (e.g., $2.15 or $3.15 for each prescription) for the rest of the calendar year.[28]

Finally, it should be noted that when health care providers take assignment (are willing to accept Medicare patients) on a Medicare claim, they agree to accept the Medicare-approved amount as payment in full. These providers are paid directly by the Medicare carrier, except for the deductible and co-insurance amounts, which are the patient's responsibility.

Medicare, like private health insurance programs, is affected by the high costs of health care and, therefore, the government is always looking for ways of cutting the costs of the programs. Several different procedures have been put into place. One procedure, added in 1983, that has helped to control the costs is the **prospective pricing system (PPS).** In the PPS, hospitals are paid predetermined amounts of money per procedure for services provided to Medicare patients. The predetermined amounts are based upon over 470 **diagnosis-related groups (DRGs)** rather than the actual cost of the care rendered. Each hospital stay by a Medicare patient is assigned a DRG. "The correct DRG for each patient is decided by considering the patient's major or principal diagnosis; any complications or other problems that might arise; any surgery performed during the hospital stay; and other factors."[29] The amount of money assigned to each DRG is not the same for each hospital. The figure is based on a formula that takes into account the type of service, the type of hospital, the location of the hospital, and the sex and age of the patient. Using this prospective pricing system, hospitals are encouraged to provide services at or below the DRG rate. If the hospital delivers the service below the DRG rate, the hospital can retain the difference. If it is delivered above the DRG rate, the hospital incurs the extra expenses. "However, when a Medicare patient's condition requires an unusually long hospital stay or exceptionally costly care, Medicare makes additional payment to the hospital."[29] Because of DRGs, some have felt that hospitals are quicker to discharge Medicare patients to keep their expenses down. This phenomenon has resulted in an increase in the need for skilled nursing care in homes, in adult day care facilities, and in nursing homes.

In recent years, much discussion has centered around whether there are sufficient funds in Medicare to pay for the health care costs of the 76 million baby boomers when they begin to become eligible in 2011. Most projections about the Medicare program indicate that there is enough money to begin to cover the baby boomers, but as they age Medicare will run out of money unless changes are made. The more difficult questions to answer now are:

When will Medicare run out of money, if no changes are made?

What changes should be made (e.g., decrease benefits, raise eligibility standards, reimburse health care providers less)?

Where should the money come from to build up the program (e.g., increase taxes, increase premiums)?

With the exception of the Medicare Modernization Act of 2003, there has been little agreement in Congress on what to do with Medicare. Both the Democratic and Republican parties agree changes need to be made, but they disagree on what and when changes should be made.

prospective pricing system (PPS) one in which providers are paid predetermined amounts of money per procedure for services provided

diagnosis-related groups (DRGs) a procedure used to classify the health problems of all Medicare patients when they are admitted to a hospital

Medicaid

A second type of government health insurance is **Medicaid,** a health insurance program for the poor. Currently, approximately 45+ million people are covered by Medicaid.[27] Eligibility for enrollment in Medicaid is determined by each state. Many Medicaid recipients are also enrolled in other types of public assistance programs (welfare). Unlike Medicare, there is no age requirement for Medicaid; eligibility requirements are strictly financial. Also, unlike Medicare, Medicaid is a noncontributory program jointly administered through federal and state governments. Both programs cover skilled nursing care but under different conditions.

For many states, the most costly item appearing in the annual state budget is the Medicaid program. Thus, like the federal government, state governments are always looking for ways to reshape their programs to become more efficient. As noted earlier in this chapter, several states have combined their Medicaid program with their State Children's Health Insurance Program (SCHIP) to provide better health care for the poor. In addition, the HHS has provided, on a competitive basis, some states with special grants to develop other plans for extending health care coverage to the uninsured.

Medicaid
a jointly funded federal-state health insurance program for the poor

Problems with Medicare and Medicaid

In theory, both the Medicare and Medicaid programs seem to be sound programs that help provide health care to two segments of the society who would otherwise find it difficult or impossible to obtain health insurance. In practice, there are two recurrent problems with these programs. One problem is that some physicians and hospitals do not accept Medicare and Medicaid patients because of the tedious and time-consuming paperwork, lengthy delays in reimbursement, and insufficient reimbursement. As a result, it is difficult if not impossible for many of those eligible for Medicare and Medicaid to receive health care. The second problem occurs when physicians and hospitals file Medicare and Medicaid paperwork for care or services not rendered or rendered incompletely. This is known as *Medicare/Medicaid fraud.*

Another drawback to these public insurance programs is the lack of coverage for catastrophic illness and long-term care, two situations that could quickly deplete the lifetime savings of an individual or family. People who wish to be protected in these situations must purchase their own catastrophic and long-term care insurance. The late President Ronald Reagan proposed that catastrophic illness insurance should be included with Medicare; in fact, Congress approved it in 1988 for implementation in 1990, but it was repealed in 1989 because the elderly objected to the increased cost.

SUPPLEMENTAL HEALTH INSURANCE

Medigap

As noted earlier, Parts A and B of Medicare have deductibles and co-insurance stipulations. To help cover these out-of-pocket costs and some other services not covered by Medicare, people can purchase supplemental policies from private insurance companies. These policies have come to be known as **Medigap** policies because they cover the "gaps" not covered by Medicare. Federal law mandates national standardization of Medigap policies. Under these standards, insurance companies can offer no more than 12 standardized plans. Prior to 2005, there were only 10 plans (A–J) available. These plans ranged from simple (basic benefits only) to more complex plans with additional benefits. In 2005 two new lower-cost plans (K and L) were offered for the first time.[30] All plans are required to have a core set of benefits referred to as *basic benefits*; however, some of the basic benefits of plans K and L are offered at a reduced level (see Box 14.2). By law, the letters and benefits of the individual plans cannot be changed by the insurance companies. However, they may add names or titles to the letter

Medigap
private health insurance that supplements Medicare benefits

BOX 14.2

OVERVIEW OF MEDIGAP PLANS A THROUGH L

Medigap policies (including Medicare SELECT) can only be sold as standardized plans. This chart gives you a quick look at Medigap Plans A through L and their benefits. This chart doesn't apply if you live in Massachussets, Minnesota, or Wisconsin. If you need more information call your State Insurance Department or State Health Insurance Assistance Program.

A	B	C	D	E	F[a]	G	H	I	J[a]	K	L
Basic benefits[c]	Basic benefits[c]	Basic benefits[c]	Basic benefits[c]	Basic benefits[c]	Basic benefits[c]	Basic benefits[c]	Basic benefits[c]	Basic benefits[c]	Basic benefits[c]	Basic benefits[c]	Basic benefits[c]
		Skilled nursing facility co-insurance	Skilled nursing facility co-insurance	Skilled nursing facility co-insurance	Skilled nursing facility co-insurance	Skilled nursing facility co-insurance	Skilled nursing facility co-insurance	Skilled nursing facility co-insurance	Skilled nursing facility co-insurance	Skilled nursing facility co-insurance (50%)	Skilled nursing facility co-insurance (75%)
	Medicare Part A deductible	Medicare Part A deductible	Medicare Part A deductible	Medicare Part A deductible	Medicare Part A deductible	Medicare Part A deductible	Medicare Part A deductible	Medicare Part A deductible	Medicare Part A deductible	Medicare Part A deductible (50%)	Medicare Part A deductible (50%)
		Medicare Part B deductible			Medicare Part B deductible				Medicare Part B deductible		
					Medicare Part B excess charges (100%)	Medicare Part B excess charges (80%)		Medicare Part B excess charges (100%)	Medicare Part B excess charges (100%)		
		Foreign travel emergency	Foreign travel emergency	Foreign travel emergency	Foreign travel emergency	Foreign travel emergency	Foreign travel emergency	Foreign travel emergency	Foreign travel emergency		
			At-home recovery			At-home recovery		At-home recovery	At-home recovery		
				Preventive care[b]					Preventive care[b]		

Note: As of January 1, 2006, you can't buy Medigap policies covering prescription drugs. If you bought a policy with prescription drug coverage before January 1, 2006, you must decide if you want to keep this coverage.

[a]Medigap Plans F and J also have a high-deductible option.
[b]Medigap policies cover some preventive care that isn't covered by Medicare.
[c]See following table for basic benefits.

Source: Centers for Medicare and Medicaid Services (2006). *2006 Choosing a Medigap Policy: A Guide to Health Insurance for People with Medicare.* Baltimore, MD: Author.

A QUICK LOOK AT THE BASIC BENEFITS FOR MEDIGAP PLANS A THROUGH L

Basic Benefit

What Medigap Plans A through L Paid in 2007
(These amounts can change each year.)

Medicare Part A co-insurance and hospital benefits

Medigap Plans A through L pay
- $238 per day for days 61–90 of a hospital stay
- $476 per day for days 91–150 of a hospital stay (while using your 60 lifetime Medicare-covered days)
- Up to 365 more days for hospital stays during your lifetime after you use all Medicare hospital benefits

Medicare Part B co-insurance or co-payment

Medigap Plans A through J pay all co-insurance and co-payment amounts after you meet the $124 yearly deductible for Medicare Part B.

Medigap Plan K pays 50% of the Medicare Part B co-insurance after you meet the $124 yearly deductible for Medicare Part B. It pays 100% of the co-insurance for Medicare Part B preventive services.

Medigap Plan L pays 75% of the Medicare Part B co-insurance after you meet the $124 yearly deductible for Medicare Part B. It pays 100% of the co-insurance for Medicare Part B preventive services.

Blood

Medigap Plans A through J pay for the first three pints of blood or equal amounts of packed red blood cells per calendar year, unless you or someone else donates blood to replace what you use.

Medigap Plan K pays 50% of the first three pints of blood or equal amounts of packed red blood cells per calendar year, unless you or someone else donates blood to replace what you use.

Medigap Plan L pays 75% of the first three pints of blood or equal amounts of packed red blood cells per calendar year, unless you or someone else donates blood to replace what you use.

Hospice care

Medigap Plan K pays 50% of the hospice cost-sharing for all Medicare Part A Medicare-covered expenses and respite care.

Medigap Plan L pays 75% of the hospice cost-sharing for all Medicare Part A Medicare-covered expenses and respite care.

designations. Companies are not required to offer all the plans. Three states—Minnesota, Massachusetts, and Wisconsin—have exceptions to the 12-plan setup because they had alternative Medigap standardization programs in effect before the federal legislation was enacted. Individuals should contact the state insurance office in these states if interested in these plans.

Two other variances to these Medigap rules should be noted. The first deals with those individuals enrolled in the Medicare Advantage program. Because Medicare Advantage is more comprehensive in coverage than the traditional Medicare program, Medigap policies are not needed. In fact, it is illegal for insurance companies to sell a Medigap policy if they know a person is enrolled in Medicare Advantage.[30] Another variance in Medigap policy deals with Medicare SELECT. *Medicare SELECT* is a type of Medigap policy that is available in some states. This type of policy still provides one of the standardized Medigap plans (A–L), but requires policy holders to use specific hospitals and, in some cases, doctors (except in emergencies) to receive full Medigap benefits.[30]

Other Supplemental Insurance

Medigap is a supplemental insurance program specifically designed for those on Medicare. However, a number of supplemental insurance policies exist for people regardless of their age. Included are specific-disease insurance, hospital indemnity insurance, and long-term care insurance. Specific-disease insurance, though not available in some states, provides benefits for only a single disease (such as cancer) or a group of specific diseases. Many policies are written as fixed-indemnity policies. Hospital indemnity coverage is insurance that pays a fixed amount for each day a person receives inpatient hospital services, and it pays up to a designated number of days. Long-term care insurance, which pays cash amounts for each day of covered nursing home or at-home care, is of great concern to many people, and it is presented next.

Long-Term Care Insurance

With people living longer and the cost of health care on the rise, more and more individuals are considering the purchase of long-term care insurance. It has been estimated that more than 9 million people in the United States received some type of help with their daily activities—either at home or in assisted living facilities, board and care homes, adult foster care homes, nursing homes, and places that provide adult day care in 2006.[31] By 2020, 12 million older Americans will need long-term care.[31] Most will be cared for at home; family and friends are the sole caregivers for 70% of the elderly.[31] Yet, planning for long-term care requires people to think about possible future health care needs and how they will pay for it. Obviously, the cost of long-term care varies based on the level of care, the length of time the care is provided, and where the care is provided. The most costly long-term care is nursing home care. Recent figures show that the average cost of residing in a nursing home was $64,240 per year,[32] and the average length of stay for a person was about 2.4 years.[32] About 10% of the people who enter a nursing home will stay there five years or more.[31] A study by the HHS says that people who reach age 65 will likely have a 40% chance of entering a nursing home.[31] The costs vary by parts of the country, but such costs for long-term care have many people worried about their financial future. This cost is something that can quickly deplete a lifetime of savings. In fact, the majority of Americans who have to pay for long-term care are impoverished within the first few years of making long-term health care payments. Those caring for a spouse find that they quickly exhaust both their spouse's resources and their own. Though the majority of long-term care is paid for by the government (see Figure 14.9), it is only after patients have exhausted many of their assets that Medicaid will begin to cover the costs.

Though long-term care is expensive, not everyone needs to buy long-term care insurance. Those who do not need it are those with low incomes and few assets who could be covered by Medicaid, and the very wealthy who are able to pay the cost of the care out of pocket.

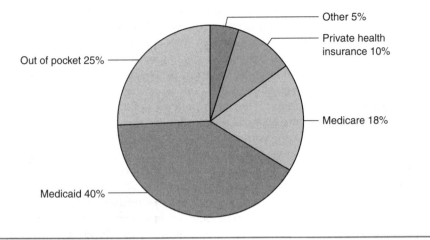

FIGURE 14.9

Who pays for long-term care services?

Source: Center for Medicare and Medicaid Services (2006). "Long-Term Care Expenditures." Available at http://www.cms.hhs.gov.

Those who are most likely to benefit from long-term care insurance are those in between the poor and wealthy, especially older women. About half of women over 65 will spend some time in a nursing home. In addition, about 75% of nursing home residents are women and two-thirds of home care consumers are women. However, there are several reasons why all people should consider purchasing long-term insurance. They include:

- To preserve financial assets
- To prevent the need for family members or friends to provide the care
- To enable people to stay independent in their homes longer
- To make it easier to get into the nursing home or assisted living home of their choice

As with life insurance, the earlier one purchases long-term care insurance the less expensive it is; however, it also may be purchased and never used. Like life insurance, the cost of a policy varies based on the benefits received and the age at which it is purchased.[33] In 2006, the approximate cost of a fairly standard long-term care policy ($150 per day benefit) was $2,732 for a 50-year-old, $3,657 for a 60-year-old, and $7,299 for a 70-year-old.[34]

MANAGED CARE

In 1993, when then President Bill Clinton took office, a comprehensive reform of the U.S. health care system seemed likely. After much debate, the comprehensive reform initiated by the government did not come to pass. Even so, the U.S. health care system did and continues to experience a great deal of change. The change, which has occurred with great speed and controversy, surfaced in the form of managed care. Managed care plans include "a set of techniques used by or on behalf of purchasers of health care benefits to manage health care costs by influencing patient care decision making through case-by-case assessments of the appropriateness of care prior to its provision."[35] The transition to managed care in the United States was largely driven by a desire by employers, insurance companies, and the public to control soaring health care costs. In fact, the goal of managed care is to control costs by controlling health care utilization.[14] Although the exact number of individuals enrolled in managed care programs is constantly changing, it has been estimated that at the end of 2005, almost 176 million Americans[36]—about three-fifths of the total population—belonged to some form of a managed health care plan. These numbers cover not only workers who received their health care coverage from employers, but also some individuals who were covered by Medicare and Medicaid.

Managed health care plans are offered by managed care organizations (MCOs). MCOs function like insurance companies. "They offer policies, collect premiums, and bear financial risk."[36] That is, MCOs take on the financial responsibility if the costs of the services exceed the revenue from the premiums. Approximately 17% to 20% of the premiums are used to manage the risk and to cover administrative expenses, while the remainder is spent on health care services.[14] These organizations have agreements with certain doctors, hospitals, and other health care providers to give a range of services to plan members at reduced cost. MCOs have been structured in a variety of ways and are similar to the other health care organizations with which we are familiar (such as hospitals). Some are structured as nonprofit organizations, while others are for-profit and owned by a group of investors. "Regardless of their structure, their goals, however, are similar: to control costs through improved efficiency and coordination, to reduce unnecessary or inappropriate utilization, to increase access to preventive care, and to maintain or improve quality of care."[37]

The managed health care plans offered by these organizations vary and are always evolving as managed care practices mature. The plans also differ, both in cost and ease of receiving needed services. Although no plan pays for all the costs associated with medical care, some plans cover more than others. Common features in managed care arrangements include (1) provider panels—specific physicians and other providers are selected to care for plan members; (2) limited choice—members must use the providers affiliated with the plan or pay an additional amount; (3) gatekeeping—members must obtain a referral from a case manager for specialty care or inpatient services; (4) risk sharing—providers bear some of the health plan's financial risk through capitation and withholds; and (5) **quality management and utilization review**—the plan monitors provider practice patterns and medical outcomes to identify deviations from quality and efficiency standards.[26]

> **quality management and utilization review** the analysis of provided health care for its appropriateness by someone other than the patient and provider

Types of Managed Care

As noted earlier, there are several different types of managed care arrangements, and because of the increasing cost of health care and the demands of consumers for better health care service these arrangements continue to be adapted and developed. "Until about 1988, the various types of MCOs were quite distinct. Since then, the differences between traditional forms of health insurance and managed care have narrowed considerably."[14] The following are the most commonly available arrangements.

Preferred Provider Organizations

> **preferred provider organization (PPO)** an organization that buys fixed-rate health services from providers and sells them to consumers

The **preferred provider organization (PPO)** is a form of managed care closest to a fee-for-service plan. A PPO differs from the traditional fee-for-service plan in that the fee has been fixed (at a discounted rate) through a negotiation process between a health care provider (e.g., physicians, dentists, hospitals, etc.) and the PPO, and the provider agrees to accept this discounted rate as payment in full. It works in the following manner: A PPO approaches a provider, such as a group dental practice, and contracts with the dentists to provide dental services to all those covered by the PPO's insurance plan at a fixed (discount) rate. To the extent that the PPO succeeds in obtaining favorable prices, it can offer lower premiums, co-insurance, and co-payments, and hence can attract more patients to enroll in its insurance plan. In addition to the PPO doctors making referrals, plan members can refer themselves to other doctors, including ones outside the plan. However, if they do choose to go outside the plan, they will have to meet the deductible and pay higher co-insurance. In addition, they may have to pay the difference between what the provider charges and what the plan pays. PPOs also control costs by requiring (1) preauthorization for hospital admissions (excluding emergencies), and (2) second opinions for major procedures such as surgery.[26] Advantages for the providers are that they (1) do not share in any financial risk as a condition of participation,[26] (2) are reimbursed on a fee-for-service basis to which they are accustomed,[26] (3) are assured a certain volume of patients, and (4) are assured that the patients will pay promptly (via the PPO). PPOs are the most common form of managed care, with about 108 million people enrolled in 2005.[36] Much of the increase in enrollment in PPOs was the result of people leaving HMOs (see the discussion of HMOs later in this chapter) because of increased costs and the restrictions in the choice of providers.

Exclusive Provider Organizations

Exclusive provider organizations (EPOs) are like PPOs except that they have stronger financial incentives for enrolled members to use the exclusive (only) provider. Stronger financial incentives usually mean no deductible, co-insurance, or co-payments. If the members were to go outside the plan to another provider, they would be responsible for a larger percentage of the bill. Typically, the number of providers (physicians, dentists, hospitals, etc.) is much smaller in an EPO, which strengthens the ability of the organization to receive a greater discount because the providers are guaranteed a larger share of patients. Because of such arrangements, a business or corporation is able to create a more stringent utilization and monitoring program with an EPO.

exclusive provider organization (EPO) like a PPO but with fewer providers and stronger financial incentives

Health Maintenance Organizations

Health maintenance organizations (HMOs) are the oldest form of managed care. In 2005, almost 68 million people were enrolled in HMOs, but this number was down from a high of about 80 million in 1999.[36] As noted earlier, many of those leaving HMOs switched to PPOs. In an HMO, the insurance coverage and the delivery of medical care are combined into a single organization. The organization hires (through salaries or contracts) an individual doctor or groups of doctors to provide care and either builds its own hospital or contracts for the services of a hospital within the community. The organization then enrolls members, usually, but not always, through the workplace. Members (or their employers or the government [in the case of HMOs for Medicare and Medicaid]) make regular payments in advance on a fixed contract fee to the HMO. This contract may also include a deductible and co-payment when service is provided. In return, the HMO is contractually obligated to provide the members with a comprehensive range of outpatient and inpatient services that are spelled out in the contract for a specific time period.

health maintenance organizations (HMOs) groups that supply prepaid comprehensive health care with an emphasis on prevention

When members enroll in an HMO, they are given a list (network) of specific physicians/providers from which to select their primary care doctor (usually a family physician, internist, obstetrician-gynecologist, or pediatrician) and other health care providers. The primary care doctor (which some have referred to as the gatekeeper) serves as the member's regular doctor and coordinates the member's care, which means the member must contact his or her primary care doctor to be referred to a specialist. In many plans, care by a specialist is only paid for if the member is referred by the primary care doctor, thus the term *gatekeeper*. Also, if patients receive care outside the network, they must pay for all the costs, except in cases of emergency when physically not near a member of the network.

How do HMOs make a profit? An HMO's focus of care is different from that of a traditional fee-for-service provider. In an HMO, ill and injured patients become a "cost." An HMO does not make money on the ill but on keeping people healthy. The less the providers of an HMO see a patient, the lower the costs and the more profitable the organization. Therefore, most HMOs emphasize health promotion activities and primary and secondary care.

There are two main organizational models of HMOs—staff models and individual practice models—and each type has spawned several hybrids. These hybrids are referred to **mixed model HMOs** and make up almost 40% of the HMOs.[38]

Staff Model

In **staff model HMOs,** the health care providers are employed (usually salaried) by the HMO and practice in common facilities paid for by the HMO. Staff model HMOs employ providers in all common specialties to provide services to their members. Special contracts are established with subspecialties for infrequently needed services. These providers are expected to follow the practice and procedures determined by the HMO. With the exception of the special contracts, the providers work only for the HMO, and thus do not have their own private practices. In most instances, the HMO contracts with a hospital for inpatient services. Nationwide, the number of staff model HMOs has been declining.

Independent Practice Association Model

Under the **independent practice association (IPA) model,** community-based providers, individual practices, or group practices contract with an HMO to provide covered services for members according to the practices and procedures of the IPA model HMO. With this model, providers are free to contract with other HMOs and to maintain fee-for-service patients. The IPA model is the most common form of HMO in the United States, constituting just over 40% of the HMOs.[38] Two variations of the IPA HMO are the group and network models. A **group model HMO** contracts with a multispecialty group practice instead of individual practitioners, whereas a **network model HMO** contracts with more than one medical group practice.[26]

Point-of-Service Option

One of the major objections to HMOs is that the patients cannot freely select their provider. They are restricted to those with whom the HMO has contracted. Some HMOs have solved this problem with the **point-of-service (POS) option,** which allows for a more liberal policy of enabling patients to select providers. With this option, members may choose a provider from within or outside the HMO network. Patients who obtain services outside the network generally must pay a higher deductible and co-insurance. POS plans are among the fastest-growing type of managed care plans.

Physician-Hospital Organizations

In some parts of the country, there has been an emergence of a health care network characterized by a consolidation and integration of the management and delivery of services. One such arrangement is the **physician-hospital organization (PHO).** PHOs are agreements between physicians and hospitals to form units to negotiate with insurers as MCOs. In some PHOs, groups of physicians enter into agreements with hospitals in which both parties negotiate as a single MCO with insurance companies on behalf of all community providers. Other PHOs have been formed when a hospital buys the private or group practices of physicians. Under this arrangement, these physicians become employees of the hospital or hospital's system.

Medicare Advantage

As noted earlier, in some parts of the country Medicare recipients may have an HMO option available to them through the Medicare Advantage plan. In such plans, the Medicare recipient receives all Medicare-covered services from the HMO. In addition, the HMO may charge the beneficiary a premium (in addition to the Medicare Part B premium) to cover co-insurance and deductibles of Medicare and may include items and services not covered by Medicare. If this is the case, Medigap coverage cannot be purchased. In other cases, beneficiaries may receive other services not covered by Medicare at no charge or at a much lower cost than might be expected. In 2005, approximately 14% of the people in Medicare were covered by managed care plans.[36]

Medicaid and Managed Care

As has been noted throughout this chapter, managed care plans are also available for those covered by Medicaid. The rationale for offering such plans is to improve access to care by the establishment of contracted provider networks, as well as by promoting greater accountability for quality and costs. Each state in the United States offers such a plan, and depending on the state requirements, enrollment may or may not be voluntary. If it is mandatory, then the state is required to offer a choice of managed care plans and make efforts to inform beneficiaries about their choices.[26] In 2005, approximately 61% of the people covered by Medicaid were enrolled in managed care plans.[36]

Advantages and Disadvantages of Managed Care

Like all forms of health care delivery before it, managed care has its advantages and disadvantages. "The best features of managed care provide public benefits beyond those available in the fee-for-service system: comprehensive benefits, evidence-based high-quality care, well-documented services provided through integrated delivery systems, and accountability for quality improvement."[39] However, many Americans are still worried about health care and the way it is delivered. Because approximately 60% of people in the United States receive their health care through managed plans, concerns about the health care system in the United States are in large part a reflection of the concerns about managed care. A 2006 poll revealed that 54% of Americans were dissatisfied with the overall quality of their health care. In addition, the poll found that (1) an overwhelming 80% were dissatisfied with the total cost of health care in the United States, (2) one in four had trouble paying for health care in the past year, and (3) 28% said that someone in their family delayed care in the past year because of the cost.[40]

Some have said that the term "managed care" is a misnomer; it should really be called "managed cost." Because Americans had become accustomed to a fee-for-service delivery system in which insurance companies paid almost every medical bill without question, they are now unsatisfied when MCOs question or refuse certain bills and medical procedures. The forms of cost control that have caused the most concern include (1) authorizing only certain practitioners who are under contract to provide services to an enrolled population, (2) reviewing treatment decisions (i.e., utilization review), (3) closely monitoring high-cost cases (i.e., utilization management), (4) reducing the number of days of inpatient hospital stays (e.g., childbirth), and (5) increasing the use of less expensive alternatives to hospitalization (e.g., outpatient surgery and home health care).[37]

As MCOs continue to grow and as Medicare and Medicaid enroll more individuals into managed care plans, the question of quality of care and the criteria and processes used to monitor and report it are being more closely examined.[26] As noted earlier, the organization in the United States that is most influential in regard to the quality of managed care is the National Committee on Quality Assurance (NCQA). The NCQA is an independent, nonprofit organization whose mission is to improve health care quality everywhere. It evaluates health care in four different ways: (1) through accreditation (a rigorous on-site review of key clinical and administrative processes); (2) through certification (a rigorous review of certain functions—for example, credentialing or utilization management—that health plans or employers have delegated to another organization); (3) through the Health Plan Effectiveness Data and Information Set (HEDIS—a tool used to measure performance in key areas like immunization, mammography screening rates), and members' satisfaction with their care in areas such as claims processing, customer service, and getting needed care quickly; and (4) through physician recognition programs that identify

physician-hospital organization (PHO) various agreements between physicians and hospitals to form units to negotiate with insurers as MCOs

physicians who provide quality care in areas such as diabetes and heart/stroke care.[10] Although participation in the accreditation and certification programs is voluntary, 684 plans were renewed by NCQA in 2006.[10] The data generated from these evaluations are available at NCQA's Web site. Many employers use the data as a way of selecting the best managed care program for their employees.

OTHER ARRANGEMENTS FOR DELIVERING HEALTH CARE

Because the majority of people in the United States receive their health care through a managed care plan or a fee-for-service plan, the majority of this chapter and Chapter 13 focused on those plans. However, there are other ways of delivering health care. A few of the more highly visible arrangements are discussed next.

National Health Insurance

National health insurance, or national health care, suggests a system in which the federal government assumes the responsibility for the health care costs of the entire population. In such a system, the costs are paid for with tax dollars. Presently among all the developed countries of the world, there is only one that does not have a national health care plan for its citizens: the United States.

The national health care systems of the developed countries of the world fall into two basic models. The first is a national health service model with universal coverage and a general tax-financed government ownership of the facilities and doctors as public employees. Countries using this model include the United Kingdom, Spain, Italy, Greece, and Portugal. The second is a social insurance model that provides universal coverage under social security, financed by various ways including taxes or contributions paid by employers and employees. In Canada, contributions are made to a government entity. In France and Germany, contributions go to nonprofit funds with national negotiation on fees. Japan also has a compulsory system that relies heavily on employer-based coverage.

When one considers the level of satisfaction with health care, the better access to health care services, the lower health care costs, and the superior health status indicators in these other countries, one must ask why the United States has not adopted such a program. It is not because the United States has not considered such a plan—in fact, there have been six failed attempts at addressing the issue over the past 70 years. The first came when President Roosevelt tried to include it as part of the New Deal. President Harry Truman presented a proposal to Congress on two different occasions, only to have it defeated twice. Other unsuccessful attempts at national health care legislation were made during the Kennedy and Nixon administrations and the last attempt came in the form of President Clinton's Health Security Act of 1993, which never reached the congressional floor.

Though the push for national health insurance has not been successful, many states have tried to move ahead and offer such a program for their citizens. Several of these plans are discussed later in the chapter.

Canadian Health Care System

Because of the proximity of the United States to Canada and due to the similarities of the two countries and their cultures, we present the following information on the national health plan of Canada.

Canada has provided its legal residents with some form of health insurance coverage since 1957. Its current system, in place since 1984 (see Figure 14.10) and outlined in the Canadian Health Act (CHA), is a predominantly publicly financed, privately delivered health care system that is best described as an interlocking set of 10 provincial and three territorial health insurance plans. Known to the Canadians as "Medicare," the system provides access to universal, comprehensive coverage for medically necessary hospital, inpatient, and outpatient physician services. Each provincial and territorial authority must ensure that all residents have access to care regardless of cost, that necessary hospital and physician services are available, that residents have continuous coverage as they travel from one province to another and abroad, and that the provincial programs are run as nonprofit organizations (see Box 14.3).[41]

Health care in Canada is financed through a combination of public funding coming from provincial, federal, and corporate taxes and private funds. With the collected tax dollars, the Canadian federal government provides block grants to the provinces and territories for the health and social programs; this is referred to as the Canada Health Transfer. Some provinces and territories use ancillary funding methods to help support health care, including sales taxes, payroll levies, and lottery (also known as video gambling machines) proceeds, and three provinces (Alberta, British Columbia, and Ontario) utilize health care premiums to help cover costs. Thus, provinces can generate other revenue to help support health care, but they cannot impose user fees or extra billing without loss of federal support.[41]

As noted earlier, the Canadian health care system is not a national health service model of health care. It is a fee-for-service system whereby the government is the single third-party payer. Canadian residents get to select their physicians, who are independent physicians working for themselves—not the government. Providers must accept the provincial plan reimbursement as payment in full if the province is to receive the maximum federal support. In addition, there are no maximum limits on the amount of care provided as long as it is deemed medically necessary. However, not all necessary medical services are covered in the plan. For

FIGURE 14.10
The United States health care system has often been compared to the Canadian health care system.

The five Canada Health Act principles provide for:

Public administration: The provincial and territorial plans must be administered and operated on a nonprofit basis by a public authority accountable to the provincial or territorial government.

Comprehensiveness: The provincial and territorial plans must insure all medically necessary services provided by hospitals, medical practitioners and dentists working within a hospital setting.

Universality: The provincial and territorial plans must entitle all insured persons to health insurance coverage on uniform terms and conditions.

Accessibility: The provincial and territorial plans must provide all insured persons reasonable access to medically necessary hospital and physician services without financial or other barriers.

Portability: The provincial and territorial plans must cover all insured persons when they move to another province or territory within Canada and when they travel abroad. The provinces and territories have some limits on coverage for services provided outside Canada, and may require prior approval for nonemergency services delivered outside their jurisdiction.

Source: Health Canada (2006). "About Health Canada." Available at http://www.hc-sc.gc.ca/ahc-asc/index_e.html.

example, pharmaceuticals needed on an outpatient basis and optometric services are not included. In such cases, these services can be provided at provincial and territorial discretion, on their own terms and conditions, and vary from one province or territory to another. In provinces and territories where they are not covered, people may carry private insurance to cover them.[41]

Compared with the American health care system, the Canadian system has several major strengths. One is that no Canadian is without health insurance. There is equity across income groups. The poor are treated as well as the rich. Canadians regard health care as a basic right, and they value their health system highly. They identify strongly with their health system for several reasons. First, it exemplifies many of the shared values of their society. In addition to equity, it also exemplifies fairness, compassion, and respect for fundamental dignity of all. Second, the administrative costs of the Canadian system are under control. The Canadian system is administered for about one-third the cost of the United States system. Third, the Canadian system is less expensive to run overall. In 2003, the per capita expenditure on health care in Canada was $3,003 compared with $5,635 in the United States. These health care costs amount to 9.9% of the Canadian GDP versus 15.0% in the United States.[4] The controls inherent in the single-payer (the government) approach to health care are recognized as a major contributor to Canada's recent cost containment success. Fourth, the Canadian system places emphasis on prevention and primary care. Though managed care has improved prevention and primary care in the United States for those with health insurance, it cannot match the prevention and primary care afforded through universal access to health care in Canada. One prime example of better prevention and primary care in Canada is the availability of prenatal care for all women (refer to Chapter 7). This is reflected in the lower infant mortality rate in Canada versus that of the United States.

Although the Canadian system sounds good, it is not without its disadvantages. The ever-increasing cost of health care, as in the United States, has also affected the Canadian system. Therefore, the Canadian system has also been going through reform in an effort to become more efficient and cost-effective. Even with such change, the major complaint with the Canadian system remains the same: the long wait lists for procedures associated with the use of high-technology equipment and specialized physicians. The Canadian system does not limit care for life-threatening conditions but does have a tight supply for things such as scanners and MRI equipment. This tight supply has created waiting lists for certain types of care (procedures) in some provinces. Those critical of the Canadian system argue that the availability of innovative technologies conflicts with the quality-of-care concerns. Those Canadians who can afford it have gotten around this limitation by coming to the United States to get needed care.

Even with the many benefits of the Canadian system, the likelihood of a Canadian-type system in the United States is very small. The political and economic barriers are too great. Politically, there are too many people who benefit from not having such a program. Economically, it has been estimated that the implementation of a Canadian-type system in the United States would be prohibitive. In addition, due to the size difference between the two countries—Canada has a population that is about the same size as the state of California—it would be difficult for the national government to be sensitive to regional and local differences and needs. As has been the case with the United States' Medicaid program, it is difficult to provide consistent and equitable administration of the program when the national government delegates authority to state or local agents.

State Plans

Although the push for a national health care plan has not been successful, several states—including Florida, Hawaii, Massachusetts, Minnesota, Oregon, and Vermont—have moved ahead and passed major health care reform packages aimed at providing increased access to health insurance and basic health services to all or most of their residents. Most other states are considering or actively involved in change. Of all the reform movements, the two that attracted the most publicity were Oregon and Massachusetts.

The Oregon Health Plan

Whereas the Canadian plan addresses access first and cost second, the Oregon plan addressed the problem of cost primarily, with the expected result of greater access. Oregon, like all other states, has a finite number of dollars to spend on health care and a significant number of people who lack access because, while they lack health insurance, they do not meet the eligibility for Medicaid, do not work for an employer who provides health insurance, or cannot afford it. Unlike other states, Oregon has attempted to come to grips with the question of whether to spend $250,000 dollars to try to save a prematurely born infant with little hope of a normal life or to spend the same amount to provide maternal and child health services for 400 families.

Beginning in 1989, several pieces of legislation were passed in the Oregon state legislature that set into motion a series of public and private health insurance reforms. Known as the Oregon Health Plan (OHP), these reforms had an initial goal of providing universal access to affordable, quality health care for all Oregonians. More specifically, the plan reformed Medicaid by extending eligibility to all residents with incomes under the federal poverty level, by providing options to small businesses (fewer than 25 employees) to offer health insurance to their employees, and by creating a high-risk insurance pool coordinated by state government. The cornerstone of the plan was the idea that benefit packages should be built on a list of health care services priorities. The initial list comprised 709 line items. Each line consisted of a health condition and its associated treatment. This list was created and prioritized by a state commission after 18 months of statewide hearings and community meetings featuring public input and expert testimony and a random-sample survey. The list was subdivided into 17 categories (priorities). Category 1 has the highest priority. Categories 1 to 9 are considered essential components, 10 to 13 very important, and 14 to 17 valuable to individuals but not certain to improve the health status of the population. It should be noted that the categories were not absolutely discrete. Some items conceptually belonged in one category but have special characteristics that led the commission to place them in another (see Box 14.4).

With the list in place, the state legislature then had to determine how many of the 709 services it could fund with the finite dollars available. They determined that there were enough state dollars available to fund items 1 through 587. Thus, items 588 to 709, or 121 services, would not be funded by state money.

Those who opposed this process did so primarily because they said it rationed health care: A person who needed a health service below item 587 on the list would not get it without being able to pay for it. Thus, the plan rationed care, as even the plan's developers will agree. However, the plan's proponents say that the previous system rationed care based on ability to pay; at least now it is rationed through a policy developed with input from those who help pay for and receive the care—the citizens of the state.

The reason the plan's development received so much publicity was that it needed federal approval. Because Medicaid is a jointly funded federal-state program, approval must be given by the federal Centers for Medicare and Medicaid Services to those states who in changing their program take away services once offered to Medicaid recipients. Obviously, some of the 121 services and procedures that were no longer offered were once available to those on Medicaid. Thus, the need for the waiver.

The waiver was not easily obtained. The state of Oregon applied for the waiver in 1991. This waiver was finally approved in 1993. By any measure, the OHP has been a success. The plan has made health coverage available to (1) almost everyone below the federal poverty level, (2) people who have been turned down or offered limited coverage by insurers because of health status, (3) employees of small businesses and their dependents, and (4) individuals ineligible for group coverage.

BOX 14.4	CATEGORIES OF SERVICES USED IN THE PRIORITIZATION PROCESS AND EXAMPLES OF CONDITION-TREATMENT (CT) PAIRS

Category	Description
"Essential" services	
1. Acute fatal	• Treatment prevents death with full recovery Example: Appendectomy for appendicitis
2. Maternity care	• Maternity and most newborn care Example: Obstetrical care for pregnancy
3. Acute fatal	• Treatment prevents death without full recovery Example: Medical therapy for acute bacterial meningitis
4. Preventive care for children	• Example: Immunizations
5. Chronic fatal	• Treatment improves life span and quality of life Example: Medical therapy for asthma
6. Reproductive services	• Excludes maternity/infertility services Example: Contraceptive management
7. Comfort care	• Palliative therapy for conditions in which death is imminent Example: Hospice care
8. Preventive dental care	• Adults and children Example: Cleaning and fluoride applications
9. Proven effective preventive care for adults	• Example: Mammograms
"Very important" services	
10. Acute nonfatal	• Treatment causes return to previous health state Example: Medical therapy for vaginitis
11. Chronic nonfatal	• One-time treatment improves quality of life Example: Hip replacement
12. Acute nonfatal	• Treatment without return to previous health state Example: Arthroscopic repair of internal knee derangement
13. Chronic nonfatal	• Repetitive treatment improves quality of life Example: Medical therapy for chronic sinusitis
Services that are "valuable to certain individuals"	
14. Acute nonfatal	• Treatment expedites recovery of self-limiting conditions. Example: Medical therapy for diaper rash
15. Infertility services	• Example: In-vitro fertilization
16. Less effective preventive care for adults	• Example: Screening of nonpregnant adults for diabetes
17. Fatal or nonfatal	• Treatment causes minimal or no improvement in quality of life Example: Medical therapy for viral warts

Source: Oregon waiver application (August 1991). Congress of the United States, Office of Technology Assessment (May 1992). *Summary: Evaluation of the Oregon Medicaid Proposal* (pub. no. OTA-H-532). Washington, DC: U.S. Government Printing Office, 6.

Yet even with the success, the Oregon officials still recognize there is work to be done. Some of the state's population remains uninsured, including a small number who are uninsured by choice—generally young, healthy, unmarried males. The state continues to look for ways to cover those people who are uninsured not by choice but because of circumstance. Also, because of the ever-changing technology and increasing cost of health care, the list of covered services needs to be revised periodically. As of April 2006, the list included 710 services, of which 530 were covered.[42]

Finally, when the initial development of the OHP began back in the late 1980s, fee-for-service was the predominant means of delivering care. As the plan evolved, so did managed care. The planners recognized the benefits of such changes and blended those into the plan. Today, most OHP Medicaid clients receive their care through prepaid health plans and a primary care practitioner who is a member of a plan. Others have a primary care case manager.

Massachusetts Health Care Plan

On April 12, 2006, then-Governor Mitt Romney signed into law the Massachusetts health care reform plan. This plan, which was implemented on July 1, 2007, gained considerable publicity because it was the first in the nation that "combined the concept of individual responsibility through an individual mandate on the purchase of health insurance with government subsidies to ensure affordability."[43]

As with any new plan, there are many details involved, but the key components of the program include (1) participation by both individuals and employers, (2) the Commonwealth Health Insurance Connector, (3) government-funded subsidies to low-income individuals to assist with the purchase of health insurance, and (4) an expansion of those covered by Medicaid. The program requires "everyone to purchase health insurance and would impose financial penalties of up to 50% of the cost of a health insurance plan on those who do not via income tax filings. It also includes a requirement that employers with more than 10 employees provide health insurance coverage or pay a 'Fair Share' contribution of up to $295 annually per employee."[43] At the heart of the plan is the Commonwealth Health Insurance Connector, which is designed to "'connect' individuals to insurance by offering affordable, quality insurance products."[43] As such, the Connector will have policies for individuals, small businesses, and a special low-cost plan for those aged 19 to 26 years. These plans will not have deductibles and will be offered through managed care organizations. The plan also provides sliding-scale subsidies to low-income individuals (up to 300% of the federal poverty level) to assist with the purchase of health insurance. People with incomes less than 100% of the poverty level will not be required to pay any premium.[43] Finally, the Medicaid expansion portion of the plan will raise its caps for eligibility, which will make many more children eligible for the program.

The plan is not without its critics. Some think it will drive up the cost of health care, whereas others feel that many small businesses that now offer health insurance to their employees will eliminate it because it is less expensive to pay the annual $295 "fair share" contribution than provide health care coverage. Because this program is the first of its kind in the United States, a lot of eyes will be watching to see how it turns out. Only time will tell.

HEALTH CARE REFORM IN THE UNITED STATES

As noted earlier, there have been at least six major attempts in the last 70 years to make major reforms to the U.S. health care system—all failed. The reform that has taken place in recent years has been with specific smaller portions of the health care system—for example, President Clinton's creation of the SCHIP program. During President George W. Bush's term in office, the reform came in the form of the Medicare Prescription Drug Improvement and Modernization Act of 2003 (PL 108-173). The portions of this act that gained the greatest publicity—those dealing with prescription drugs—were discussed earlier in this chapter. However, another significant portion of this act that has not been discussed is the portion dealing with tax-preferred health savings accounts (HSAs) that are linked to high-deductible health plans (HDHPs). HSAs are an expanded version of medical savings accounts (MSAs), which were created in 1996 by a congressional pilot project.[44] HSAs are part of a handful of reform strategies that are referred to as *consumer-directed health care* "that seek to marshal the power of consumers making cost-conscious choices to constrain rising U.S. health care spending."[45] Simply stated, HSAs require individuals to use their own money (or money set aside by their employers for their use) to pay for medical expenses until a fairly substantial deductible is met (in 2007, the deductible was $1,100 for individuals and $2,200 for families—thus the term *high-deductible health plans*).[46] At that point, traditional health insurance coverage begins. As of January 2007, approximately 5 million Americans were enrolled in an HSA.[47]

HSAs are considered a form of consumer-directed health care because, theoretically, people using their own money for health care will be more aware of the process and will be more likely to shop around for care—saving money for both themselves and their employers. HSAs are comparable to 401(k) plans or other retirement accounts. Money is placed in an HSA and grows tax-free while in the account. In 2007, the maximum amount that could be set aside was $2,850 for an individual or $5,650 for families, or the amount of the deductible of the health insurance policy, whichever was lower. People aged 55 and older can make additional "catch-up" contributions until they enroll in Medicare. Money can be withdrawn from the account without penalty to pay for care before the deductible is met and for things not covered under the health insurance policy after the deductible is met. Money can be withdrawn and pay for anything (nonhealth expenses) after 65 years of age, but the person must pay income tax on it. The advantages of such a plan are reduced premiums and, it is hoped, more prudent use of health care dollars—which should be good for both employers and employees. In addition, HSAs are portable from one employer to another. The major disadvantage for consumers is that they might have to pay more out of pocket for health care, and therefore might skip needed care. At the present, HSAs seem best suited for the healthy and wealthy. It will be some time before it is known whether this type of reform will have a major impact on health care delivery in the United States.

Another reform instituted by President Bush was an executive order he signed in August 2006 to make the health care system more transparent so that Americans will be empowered to find better value and better care. This too is a strategy to move toward a more consumer-directed health care system. The premise behind this executive order is that Americans will become better consumers of health care "if they know their options in advance, know the quality of doctors and hospitals in their area, and know what the procedures will cost."[48] Specifically, the

> Executive Order directs federal agencies that administer or sponsor federal health insurance programs to: (1) Increase Transparency In Pricing. The Executive Order directs Federal agencies to share with beneficiaries information about prices paid to health care providers for procedures, (2) Increase Transparency In Quality. The Executive Order directs Federal agencies to share with beneficiaries information on the quality of services provided by doctors, hospitals, and other health care providers, (3) Encourage Adoption Of Health Information Technology (IT) Standards. The Executive Order directs Federal agencies to use improved health IT systems to facilitate the rapid exchange of health information, and (4) Provide Options That Promote Quality And Efficiency In Health Care. The Executive Order directs Federal agencies to develop and identify approaches that facilitate high quality and efficient care.[48]

At the time this book went to press, the details of this order were still being worked out. As noted, this executive order only applies to those providers associated with federal health insurance programs. It will be interesting to see if the concept trickles down to the private plans in the United States.

Also, when this edition of this book was going to press, President Bush had just outlined several proposals in his State of the Union address to make basic, private health insurance available and affordable for more Americans. The primary component of his proposals was to revise the U.S. tax code to allow for a standard deduction for health insurance. His proposals received mixed responses and promised much debate.

Even with the changes carried out by the Bush administration, there are still many issues facing the U.S. health care system. Some of the more current issues facing health care delivery in the United States include but are not limited to the following:

- The continuing cost of all areas of health care
- The continued health care disparities among minorities and low-income Americans
- The cost of prescription drugs and the fact that the same drugs are less expensive in Canada

- The high cost of malpractice insurance for health care providers, causing some to drop their specialties (e.g., obstetrics) or stop practicing altogether
- The number of medical errors that continue to occur
- The concerns over the privacy of medical information, especially with the use of electronic data sources
- The complexity of navigating the health care delivery system in general and managed care specifically
- The burden on the employer of providing health care insurance
- The ethical issues that arise with the use and availability of new knowledge (e.g., human genome) and technology (e.g., telemedicine)

With so many issues facing health care delivery, it is not a question of whether there will be a major health care reform but of when and in what form. At the heart of reform is access to care at an affordable price. In a series of recent reports, the Institute of Medicine (IOM) has put forth substantial and compelling evidence on the harmful effects of being uninsured.[49-54] The IOM has recommended five principles to assist policy makers as they consider health insurance reform.[52] The principles are supported by clinical, epidemiological, and economic research. The principles are as follows:

1. "Health care coverage should be *universal.*" That is, everyone in the United States should have health insurance. The IOM is not alone regarding this principle—support for a universal system is coming from others, too. The Democratic party, with its most vocal voice being Senator Edward Kennedy, has long pushed for such a program. And in 2006, 56% of Americans said that they preferred a universal system that would provide coverage to everyone under a government program, as opposed to the current employer-based program.[40] However, that support dropped significantly if the universal system would mean a limited choice of doctors or longer waits for nonemergency treatment.[40]
2. "Health care coverage should be *continuous.*" That is, there should never be gaps in coverage, such as when changing employers or when adult children are no longer covered on their parents' policy. Continuous care leads to improved health.
3. "Health care coverage should be *affordable to individuals and families.*" The primary reason given by those who are uninsured for being uninsured is the cost.[55] In fact, six in ten people surveyed in a recent poll say they are worried about being able to afford health insurance in the future.[40]
4. "The health insurance strategy should be *affordable and sustainable for society.*" How much are people willing to spend on health care? It was reported earlier that the United States spends more per capita (approximately \$7,129 in 2006),[13] more total money (approximately \$2.169 trillion in 2006),[13] and more of its gross domestic product (estimated at 16.2% in 2006) on health care than any other country in the world. Is society willing to spend more?
5. "Health insurance should *enhance health and well-being* by promoting access to high-quality care that is effective, efficient, safe, timely, patient-centered, and equitable." In other words, the reform of health care should result in very good health care that is as free as possible from errors, without disparities among groups, and is responsive to the ones being served.

Finally, the IOM's Committee on the Consequences of Uninsurance "calls on the federal government to take action to achieve universal health insurance and to establish an explicit schedule to reach this goal by 2010."[54] Watching health care reform in the United States should be interesting!

Chapter Summary

- The major issues of concern with the health care system in the United States can be summed up by the cost containment, access, and quality triangle.

- Some of the barriers to access to health care in the United States are the lack of health insurance, inadequate insurance, and poverty.

- The two major means by which health care is delivered in the United States are fee-for-service and prepaid health plans.

- Most health care in the United States is paid for via third-party payment.

- The State Children's Health Insurance Program (SCHIP) is for many children who were previously uninsured.

- Key health insurance terms include *deductible, co-insurance, co-payment, fixed indemnity, exclusion,* and *pre-existing condition.*

- The two largest government-administered health insurance programs in the United States are Medicare and Medicaid.

- Two major supplemental insurance programs in the United States are Medigap and long-term care insurance.

- A majority of Americans today are covered by some form of managed care.

- The more common forms of managed care include health maintenance organizations (HMOs), preferred provider organizations (PPOs), exclusive provider organizations (EPOs), point-of-service (POS) options, and physician-hospital organizations (PHOs).

- The United States is the only developed country in the world without national health insurance.

- Alternative ways to provide health care are offered by Canada and selected states in the United States.

- Health savings accounts are the most recent reform in health care.

- Health care reform must take place in the United States.

Review Questions

1. What are three major problems facing the health care system in the United States?

2. Explain the terms *fee-for-service* and *prepaid health care.*

3. How is the quality of health care services measured?

4. Upon what basic concept is insurance based?

5. What is a State Children's Health Insurance Program (SCHIP)?

6. Explain the following insurance policy provisions: (a) a $200 deductible, (b) 20/80 co-insurance, (c) a $4,500 fixed indemnity for a basic surgical procedure, (d) an exclusion of the pre-existing condition of lung cancer, and (e) a $10 co-payment.

7. What is the difference between Medicare and Medicaid? What relationship does Medigap insurance have to Medicare? What is Medicare Part D?

8. Briefly explain the differences among health maintenance organizations (HMOs), preferred provider organizations (PPOs), and exclusive provider organizations (EPOs).

9. Why might a company want to enter into an agreement with a preferred provider organization?

10. Distinguish between the following two main models of health maintenance organizations—staff (group) and independent practice association.

11. What are the point-of-service option and physician-hospital organizations? Medicare Advantage?

SCENARIO: ANALYSIS AND RESPONSE

1. Reread the scenario. In your opinion, did Greg make the right decision in taking his son Zack to the emergency room? Why or why not?

2. What other actions could Greg have taken? What would you have done?

3. What impact do you think a zero deductible health insurance policy has on the health care system? What do you see as the advantages and disadvantages of such a policy? Explain your answer.

4. Do you think all people in the United States should have zero deductible health insurance? Why or why not?

5. How does managed care affect the type of behavior exhibited by Greg?

6. If we had national health insurance, how would this scenario differ?

7. Under the Oregon Health Plan, how would this scenario differ?

12. What are the advantages and disadvantages of managed care?

13. In what ways is the American health care system better than the Canadian system? In what ways is the Canadian system better than that of the United States?

14. Why were the Oregon Health Plan and the Massachusetts Health Care Plan considered to be so innovative?

15. Should the United States have universal health insurance?

16. What is meant by the term *consumer-directed health care*?

17. Define and explain health savings accounts.

ACTIVITIES

1. Obtain a copy of the student health insurance policy available at your school. After reading the policy, summarize in writing what you have read. In your summary, indicate whether it is a fee-for-service or managed care plan, provide the premium costs, and list specifics about the deductible, co-insurance, co-payment, fixed indemnity, and any exclusions.

2. Contact the office in your community that handles the Medicaid insurance program. Find out who is qualified for coverage in your state and the process that one must go through to get registered for such coverage. Also, ask about whom to see if your state has an SCHIP, and if so who qualifies for it.

3. Visit an HMO in your area and find the answers to the following: (a) What type of HMO is it? (b) How does one enroll? (c) What does it cost? (d) What services are provided? and (e) Why should someone get his or her health care from an HMO instead of the more traditional private-practice physician?

4. Write a two-page position paper on one of the following topics: (a) The United States federal government should provide universal health insurance, (b) Health care is a right, or (c) Health care is a privilege.

COMMUNITY HEALTH ON THE WEB

The Internet contains a wealth of information about community and public health. Increase your knowledge of some of the topics presented in this chapter by accessing the Jones and Bartlett Publishers Web site at **http://health .jbpub.com/book/communityhealth/6e** and follow the links to complete the following Web activities.

- Medicare and Medicaid
- Canadian Health Care System
- Health Savings Accounts

REFERENCES

1. Alliance for Health Reform (November 2006). *Racial and Ethnic Disparities in Health Care*. Washington, DC: Author.

2. Kissick, W. L. (1994). *Medicine's Dilemmas: Infinite Needs Versus Finite Resources*. New Haven, CT: Yale University Press.

3. Institute of Medicine (2004). *Insuring America's Health: Principles and Recommendations*. Available at http://www.iom.edu/Object.File/Master/17/732/0.pdf.

4. National Center for Health Statistics (2006). *Health United States, 2006 with Chartbook on Trends in Health of Americans*. Hyattsville, MD: Author.

5. DeNavas-Walt, C., B. D. Protor, and C. H. Lee (2006). *Income, Poverty, and Health Insurance Coverage in the United States: 2005* (Current Population Reports no. P60-231). Washington, DC: U.S. Government Printing Office.

6. Slee, V., D. Slee, and H. J. Schmidt (2001). *Slee's Health Care Terms*, 4th ed. St. Paul, MN: Tringa Press.

7. Institute of Medicine (2002). *Care without Coverage: Too Little, Too Late*. Washington, DC: National Academies Press.

8. Clark, N. (2002). *A Letter from the Dean: Spring/Summer 2002*. Ann Arbor, MI: University of Michigan, School of Public Health.

9. U.S. Department of Health and Human Services, Agency for Healthcare Research and Quality (2005). *2005 National Healthcare Quality Report* (AHRQ pub. no. 06-0018). Rockville, MD: Agency for Healthcare Research and Quality.

10. National Committee for Quality Assurance (2006). *The State of Health Care Quality*. Available at http://www.ncqa.org.

11. World Health Organization (2000). *The World Health Report 2000*. Available at http://www.who.int/en.

12. Schoen, C., K. Davis, S. K. H. How, and S. C. Schoenbaum (2006). "U.S. Health System Performance: A National Scorecard." *Health Affairs Web Exclusive*, 25: w457–w475.

13. Borger, C., S. Smith, C. Truffer, S. Keehan, A. Sisko, J, Poisal, and M. K. Clemens (2006). "Health Spending Projections through 2015: Changes in the Horizon." *Health Affairs Web Exclusive*, 25(2): 61–73.

14. Shi, L., and D. A. Singh (2005). *Essentials of the US Health Care System*. Sudbury, MA: Jones and Bartlett.

15. Donaldson, M., K. D. Yordy, K. N. Lohr, and N. A. Vanselow, eds. (1996). *Primary Care: America's Health in a New Era*. Washington, DC: National Academy Press.

16. U.S. Department of Health and Human Services (2000). *Healthy People 2010: Understanding and Improving Health*, 2 vols. Sudbury, MA: Jones and Bartlett.

17. Rowland, D., J. Feder, and P. Keenan (1998). "Uninsured in America: The Causes and Consequences." In S. H. Alterman, U. Reinhardt, and A. E. Shields, eds., *The Future U.S. Health Care System: Who Will Care for the Poor and Uninsured?* Chicago: Health Administration Press.

18. Dorn, S., M. Teitelbaum, and C. Cortez (1998). *An Advocate's Tool Kit for the State Children's Health Insurance Program*. Washington, DC: Children's Defense Fund.

19. Rosenbaum, S., K. Johnson, C. Sonosky, A. Markus, and C. DeGraw (1998). "The Children's Hour: The State Children's Health Insurance Program." *Health Affairs*, 17(1): 75–89.

20. Centers for Medicare and Medicaid Services (2006). "National SCHIP Policy." Available at http://www.cms.hhs.gov/NationalSCHIPPolicy/.

21. Centers for Medicare and Medicaid Services (2006). "2005 CMS Statistics, Table 11." Available at http://www.cms.hhs.gov/Medicare MedicaidStatSupp/06_CMSStatistics.asp#TopOfPage.

22. Kaiser Family Foundation (2006). *The Uninsured: A Primer*. Available at http://www.kff.org/uninsured/upload/7451.pdf.

23. The President's Advisory Commission on Consumer Protection and Quality in the Health Care Industry (1998). *Quality First: Better Health Care for All Americans*. Washington, DC: U.S. Government Printing Office.

24. Centers for Medicare and Medicaid Services (2006). "National Health Expenditure Data." Available at http://www.cms.hhs.gov/NationalHealthExpendData.

25. Kaiser Family Foundation (2006). *Employer Health Benefits: 2006 Summary of Findings*. Available at http://www.kff.org/insurance/7527/index.cfm.

26. Sultz, H. A., and K. M. Young (2004). *Health Care USA: Understanding Its Organization and Delivery*, 5th ed. Sudbury, MA: Jones and Bartlett.

27. Centers for Medicare and Medicaid Services (2006). "Medicare." Available at http://www.cms.hhs.gov.

28. Centers for Medicare and Medicaid Services (2006). *Medicare and You: 2007* (CMS pub. no. 10050). Baltimore, MD: Author.

29. U.S. Department of Health and Human Services (1989). *Your Hospital Stay Under Medicare's Prospective Payment System* (HHS pub. no. HCFA 02163). Washington, DC: U.S. Government Printing Office.

30. Centers for Medicare and Medicaid Services (2006). *2006 Choosing a Medigap Policy: A Guide to Health Insurance for People with Medicare*. Baltimore, MD: Author.

31. Centers for Medicare and Medicaid Services (2006). "Long-Term Care." Available at http://www.medicare.gov/LongTermCare/Static/Home.asp.

32. AARP (2006). *Who Pays for Long-Term Care Services?* Available at https://aarpltc.metlife.com/aarp/ltc3leftNav.do.

33. Elias, R. (2006). *Financing Long-Term Care 101*. Available at http://www.kaiseredu.org/tutorials/longtermcare/longtermcare.html.

34. Basler, B. (2006). "Pursuing Peace of Mind: Long-Term Care Insurance Provides Security for a Rainy Day. But Can You Afford It?" *AARP Bulletin*, 47(11), 10–11.

35. Halverson, P. K., A. D. Kaluzny, C. P. McLaughlin, et al., eds. (1998). *Managed Care and Public Health*. Gaithersburg, MD: Aspen Publishers.

36. Managed Care On Line (2004). *Managed Care Fact Sheets*. Available at http://www.mcareol.com.

37. Institute of Medicine (1997). *Managing Managed Care: Quality Improvement in Behavioral Health*. Washington, DC: National Academy Press.

38. Kaiser Family Foundation (2006). *Trends and Indications in Changing Health Care Marketplace: 2004 Update*. Available at http://www.kff.org/insurance.

39. Zatkin, S. (1997). "A Health Plan's View of Government Regulation." *Health Affairs*, 16(6): 33–35.

40. ABC News/Kaiser Family Foundation/USA Today (2006). *Health Care in America 2006 Survey*. Available at http://www.kff.org/kaiser-polls/upload/7572.pdf.

41. Health Canada (2006). "About Health Canada." Available at http://www.hc-sc.gc.ca/ahc-asc/index_e.html.

42. Oregon Department of Human Services (2006). "The Prioritized List—An Overview." Available at http://www.oregon.gov/DHS/healthplan/priorlist/main.shtml.

43. Kaiser Family Foundation (2006). *Massachusetts Health Care Reform Plan* (pub. no. 7494). Available at http://www.kff.org/.

44. Minicozzi, A. (2006). "Medical Saving Accounts: What Story Do the Data Tell?" *Health Affairs*, 25(1), 256–267.

45. Alliance for Health Reform (November 2006). *HSAs and High Deductible Health Plans: A Primer*. Washington, DC: Author.

46. U.S. Department of the Treasury (2006). "2007 HSA Indexed Amounts." Available at http://www.ustreas.gov/offices/public-affairs/hsa/07IndexedAmounts.html.

47. PR Web (2006). "Health Savings Accounts Even More Attractive Thanks to Congress." Available at http://www.prweb.com/releases/2006/12/prweb490029.htm.

48. The White House (2006). "Health Care Transparency: Empowering Consumers to Save on Quality Care." Available at http://whitehouse.gov/infocus/healthcare.

49. Institute of Medicine (2001). *Coverage Matters: Insurance and Health Care*. Washington, DC: National Academy Press.

50. Institute of Medicine (2002). *Care without Coverage: Too Little, Too Late*. Washington, DC: National Academy Press.

51. Institute of Medicine (2002). *Health Insurance Is a Family Matter*. Washington, DC: National Academy Press.

52. Institute of Medicine (2003). *A Shared Destiny: Community Effects of Uninsurance*. Washington, DC: National Academy Press.

53. Institute of Medicine (2003). *Hidden Cost, Values Lost: Uninsurance in America*. Washington, DC: National Academy Press.

54. Institute of Medicine (2004). *Insuring America's Health: Principles and Recommendations*. Washington, DC: National Academy Press.

55. Adams, P. F., and P. M. Barnes (2006). "Summary Health Statistics for the U.S. Population: National Health Interview Survey, 2004." *Vital and Health Statistics*, 10(229). Available at http://www.cdc.gov/nchs/data/series/sr_10/sr10_229.pdf.

U N I T
FOUR

ENVIRONMENTAL HEALTH AND SAFETY

Chapter 15

Environmental Concerns: Wastes and Pollution

Chapter Objectives

After studying this chapter you will be able to:

1 Explain how human activities affect the environment through the production of wastes and residues.

2 Name the primary sources of solid waste.

3 Explain the four approaches to solid waste management.

4 Define *hazardous waste*.

5 Explain the difference between sanitary and secured landfills.

6 Identify five approaches to hazardous waste management.

7 Explain what is meant by the term *Superfund*.

8 Explain the Air Quality Index (AQI).

9 Describe acid rain, the ozone layer, global warming, and photochemical smog.

10 Identify the major indoor air pollutants.

11 Explain the difference in point source and non-point source pollution.

12 Identify the different types of water pollutants and their consequences.

13 Describe the purpose of wastewater and drinking water treatment.

14 Identify and describe two important pieces of federal legislation that protect our nation's water.

15 Name the primary sources of radiation.

16 Identify the pros and cons of nuclear power.

17 Explain the difference between sound and noise.

18 Identify approaches to reduce problems associated with noise pollution.

Tom and Mary recently accepted jobs as teachers in the Blackford School Corporation. When they moved to the Blackford community, they purchased a modest home on five acres of land outside the city. They had only been living in their new home two months when they noticed that their water was beginning to taste "different." The source of their water was a well on their own property. A testing of the water by the local health department sanitarian revealed that their water was con-taminated with lead and perhaps other chemicals. The sanitarian recommended that Tom and Mary drink bottled water until the well water could be tested further. After some investigation, county officials determined that Mary and Tom's 15-year-old home had been built close to a former landfill that had been closed about 20 years earlier. Tom and Mary were now faced with an expensive, unforeseen, and long-term problem, not to mention the devaluation of their property.

INTRODUCTION

environment
all the external conditions, circumstances, and influences surrounding and affecting the growth and development of an organism or community of organisms

As humans, we are part of the environment in which we live, and our health is affected by its quality. As population growth, industrialization, and urbanization intensify, human activities often result in pollution and other alterations of the environment that negatively affect our health. The goal of this chapter is to introduce you to various environmental issues that can affect human health and the quality of life in your community.

The **environment** is defined as all the external conditions, circumstances, and influences surrounding and affecting the growth and development of an organism or a community of organisms. In order to fully understand environmental concerns that threaten our health, we must understand how we interact with our environment. The study of how living things interact with each other and their environment is called *ecology*, and the zone of the earth where life is found is known as the *biosphere*.

NATURAL ENVIRONMENTAL HAZARDS

natural hazard
an event of nature that increases the probability of disease, injury, or death of humans

Although the purpose of this chapter is to point out environmental hazards associated with human activities, it is important to recognize the existence and influence of **natural hazards** in the environment that damage or destroy wildlife habitats, kill or harm humans, and damage property. These physical hazards are caused by forces either internal to the earth's surface or on the surface itself. Natural hazards resulting from internal forces include earthquakes, tsunamis, and volcanoes. Those on the surface include avalanches, winds, dust storms, floods, wildfires, droughts, hurricanes, and tornadoes.

Natural environmental hazards can result in serious physical and psychological health consequences for humans. For example, after the 2004 Asian tsunami, the primary health concerns were not only the diseases associated with contaminated water and food but also exposure to insects, high temperatures, and other environmental risks associated with the loss of shelter.[1] Meanwhile, the loss of loved ones left many survivors feeling sad and depressed. Volcanic eruptions are another example of natural environmental hazards that can result in human injury and illness. Large quantities of ash are released into the atmosphere, where they can remain for long periods of time before falling to earth. Acute respiratory symptoms commonly reported by people during and after ash falls include nasal irritation and discharge (runny noses), throat irritation and sore throat, coughing, and uncomfortable breathing. People with pre-existing conditions can develop severe bronchitis, shortness of breath, wheezing, and coughing.[2] Natural hazards and their effects on human health are discussed further in Chapter 16.

In addition to natural disasters, humans can alter, pollute, and destroy their environment through individual and community activities. The resulting environmental degradation has negative consequences for human health. This chapter focuses on the human activities that result in the production of waste and pollution that can negatively affect individual as well as community health.

RESIDUES AND WASTES FROM HUMAN ACTIVITIES

As people participate in their daily activities, they continually produce **residues and wastes.** On any typical day, a person in the United States might generate the following types of residues and wastes:

> **residues and wastes**
> unwanted by-products of human activities

1. Human body wastes: urine and feces (wastewater)
2. Excess materials and foods: trash and garbage
3. Yard wastes: grass clippings and tree branches
4. Construction and manufacturing wastes: scrap wood and metal, contaminated water, solvents, excess heat, and noise
5. Agricultural wastes: animal dung, runoff from feedlot operations, crop residues, and animal carcasses
6. Transportation wastes: carbon monoxide, gaseous pollutants, and used motor oil
7. Energy production wastes: mining wastes, electrical power (combustion of coal) wastes, and nuclear power (radioactive) wastes
8. Defense wastes: weapons production (radioactive) wastes

A healthy environment, one relatively free of pollution, supports healthy communities (see Figure 15.1). Residues and wastes from human activities can adversely affect the

FIGURE 15.1
A healthy environment supports a healthy community.

FIGURE 15.2
Urbanization has led to overcrowding and pollution.

urbanization
tthe process by which cities develop and grow as people from the countryside migrate to cities in search of better jobs and living conditions

environment by damaging wildlife habitats, undermining food production, contaminating sources of water, altering climate, and threatening human health.

Factors contributing to an ever-increasing number of environmental hazards are (1) urbanization, (2) industrialization, (3) human population growth, and (4) the production and use of disposable products and containers. **Urbanization,** the process in which people come together to live in cities, often results in people living in overcrowded conditions and inadequate space for the proper disposal of wastes, making waste management more difficult (see Figure 15.2). Industrialization results in the increased generation of industrial waste, the production of new types of wastes, and the increased production and use of convenient, disposable products (see Table 15.1). Urbanization, industrialization, the production of new and disposable products, and population growth all affect our environment and our health because we live in more crowded and polluted conditions.

While it is unrealistic to expect communities to produce a pollution-free environment, it is possible to work toward minimizing the level of pollution. As the dominant species on this planet, our very survival depends upon our recognition of the deleterious effects our activities have on the rest of the biosphere and our taking responsibility (individually and collectively) for minimizing these effects. If the environment is to remain relatively stable, the frequency and severity of environmental hazards stemming from human activities must be reduced.

TYPES OF WASTES AND POLLUTION

Unwanted items or substances that result from human activities or processes are wastes. Disposal of waste products often results in pollution of the natural resources on which our health and lives depend—air, land, and water.

The types of wastes and pollution we discuss include solid wastes, hazardous wastes, air pollution, water pollution, radiation, and noise pollution. While some types of wastes may merely lower the aesthetic value of the environment, others constitute either an immediate or long-term threat to human health and well-being.

Table 15.1
Reusable versus Throwaway Consumer Goods

Reusable Goods	Throwaway Goods
Milk bottles	Cardboard cartons and plastic jugs
Returnable soft drink bottles	Aluminum cans and plastic bottles
Cloth diapers	Disposable diapers
Garbage cans	Trash bags
Lunch boxes	Paper bags
Cloth napkins	Paper napkins
Refillable pens	Disposable pens
Handkerchiefs	Facial tissues
Cloth towels or rags	Paper towels
Ceramic or plastic dishes	Paper plates

Solid Waste

Household trash, grass clippings, tree trimmings, manure, excess stone generated from mining, and steel scraps from automobile plants are all examples of **solid waste.** With only 4.6% of the world's population, the United States produces 33% of the world's solid waste.[3] Management of solid waste is absolutely crucial for maintaining a healthy living environment. Imagine if trash collection in your community were to be interrupted for merely two weeks. What would be the consequences of this interruption? The resulting accumulation of garbage and other solid waste would produce undesirable odors and attract vermin such as rats, flies, and other disease reservoirs and vectors. Improperly managed solid wastes can be a focal point where hosts, prey, parasites, food, and disease agents and vectors combine to produce a human-made environmental health hazard. Thus, the necessity of proper solid waste management, storage, and disposal is clear.

> **solid waste**
> solid refuse from households, agriculture, and businesses

In addition to causing negative effects on health, solid waste production has led to a major community problem—where to store it. Many communities have used up all available space to bury their solid waste and must look for a neighboring community willing to accept it (see Figure 15.3).

Sources of Solid Waste

Most solid waste can be traced to four major sources: mining and gas and oil production; agriculture; industry; and municipalities (domestic sources) (see Figure 15.4). Mining activities generate about 38% of total solid waste production. Mining wastes include waste generated during the extraction, beneficiation (crushing, grinding, washing, filtration, sorting, sizing, and drying), and processing of minerals. Agricultural waste, such as crop residues, manure, and vegetation trimmings, makes up about 51% of the solid waste total. Agricultural waste from animals is a very big problem in rural areas and causes significant air and water pollution if not properly controlled.

Industrial waste, 8% of the total solid waste generation, includes paper, wood chips, and chemicals. Some industrial waste can be classified as hazardous waste because it is either chemically reactive, toxic, corrosive, or flammable.

FIGURE 15.3
Solid waste is becoming such a problem in some areas that it is shipped elsewhere.

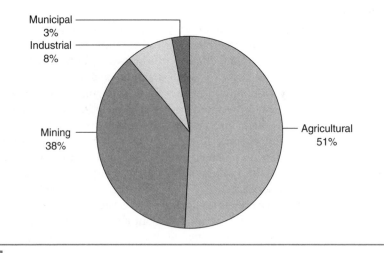

FIGURE 15.4

Contribution of various waste sources generated in the United States.

Source: Elmhurst College Virtual Chembook. "Solid Waste." Available at
http://www.elmhurst.edu/~chm/vchembook/316solidwaste.html.

**municipal solid
waste (MSW)**
waste generated by
individual households,
businesses, and
institutions located
within municipalities

Household and municipal waste makes up the smallest portion (about 3%) of all solid
waste generated each year, although it receives considerable attention because it is visible to
all of us, is malodorous, and is considered a threat to human health. Called **municipal solid
waste (MSW),** and commonly known as *trash* or *garbage,* this type of waste includes all
waste (except wastewater and sewage) generated by households, businesses, and institutions
(e.g., universities, schools, and colleges) located within municipalities. Paper makes up the
largest portion of MSW (34%); yard trimmings, food scraps, and plastics each contribute more
than 10% to the total MSW generation (see Figure 15.5).[4]

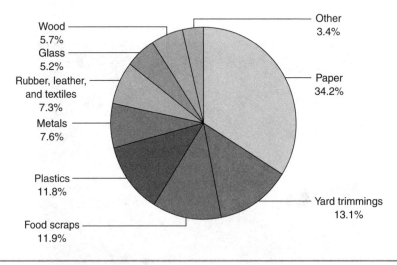

FIGURE 15.5

Types and percentages of municipal solid waste generated (before recycling) in the United States in 2005.

Source: U.S. Environmental Protection Agency (2005). *Municipal Solid Waste in the United States: 2005 Facts and Figures.*
Available at http://www.epa.gov/msw/pubs/ex-sum05.pdf.

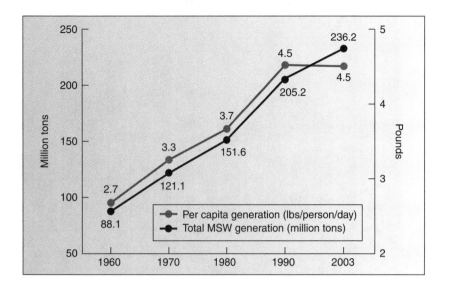

FIGURE 15.6

This line graph indicates the rate by which per capita generation of waste (in pounds per person per day) and total waste generation (in million tons) have increased from 1960 to 2003. In 1960, the per capita generation of waste was 2.7 pounds per person per day, and total waste generation was 88.1 million tons. In 1970, the per capita generation of waste was 3.3 pounds per person per day, and total waste generation was 121.1 million tons. In 1980, the per capita generation of waste of 3.7 pounds per person per day, and total waste generation was 151.6 million tons. In 1990, the per capita generation of waste was 4.5 pounds per person per day, and total waste generation was 205.2 million tons. In 2003, the per capita generation of waste was 4.5 pounds per person per day, and total waste generation was 236.2 million tons.

Source: U.S. Environmental Protection Agency (2005). "Municipal Solid Waste: Basic Facts." Available at http://www.epa.gov.epaoswer/non-hw/muncpl/facts.htm.

So how much waste do you actually produce? In 2003, every one of us produced on average 4.5 pounds of MSW per day. In 1960 a person generated 2.6 pounds of waste per day (see Figure 15.6),[5] which means that the volume of produced waste is growing faster than the U.S. population. The United States is the second-biggest producer of MSW among the countries surveyed by the Organization of Economic Cooperation and Development, with an annual generation of 1,631 pounds per person (see Figure 15.7).[6] To decrease our growing production of waste, we need to lower our consumption, reuse and recycle existing products and materials, and compost our organic waste. These practices will save land from being used for landfills, prevent potential environmental pollution, and protect human health.

The heterogeneous makeup of MSW precludes efficient disposal. There are nine major categories—paper, yard waste, food scraps, rubber and textiles, wood, metals, glass, plastics, and other (see Figure 15.5).[5] Forty years ago, food wastes were the primary component in MSW, but garbage disposals in homes and the preprocessing of foods have reduced that greatly. Today, paper and paper products make up 35.7% of the total. Much of it is packaging. The last and smallest source of solid waste is utilities. The primary solid waste of utilities is cinders from the burning of coal.

Solid Waste Management

In the past, **solid waste management** involved only the collection, transportation, storage, and disposal of waste by incineration or in a landfill. Today, however, it also includes source reduction, reuse of products, recycling, and composting. Normally, municipal sanitary districts or private disposal companies manage the collection, transportation, and disposal of

solid waste management
the collection, transportation, and disposal of solid waste

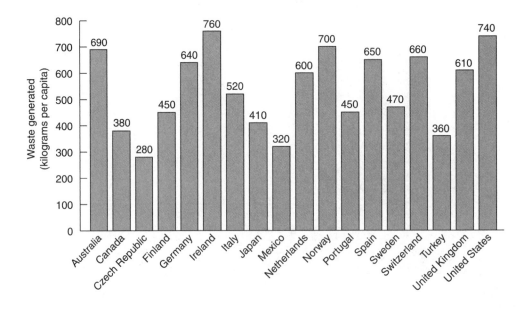

FIGURE 15.7

Municipal solid waste generation in developed countries. (*Note*: 1 kilogram = 2.2 pounds.)

Source: Organization for Economic Cooperation and Development (2005). *OECD in Figures: Statistics on the Member Countries.* Paris: OECD Publishing. Available at http://www.oecd.org/document/62/0,2340,en_2825_495628_2345918_1_1_1_1,00.html.

> **source reduction**
> a waste management approach involving the reduction or elimination of the use of materials that produce an accumulation of solid waste

solid waste so that it does not pollute air or water and causes minimal impact on the land. The degree to which source reduction, reuse, recycling, and composting occur varies from community to community.

Collection

Approximately 80% of the money spent on waste management is spent on the collection process. Faced with ever-increasing amounts of waste, greater efficiency is needed in collecting the wastes so that more money can be spent on environmentally sound disposal. Traditionally, crews of three people and a large truck have collected municipal wastes at the curb or alley. However, experience has shown that crew size, truck size, and special-feature trucks—such as those that can be operated by a single person or those with different storage compartments for separating the trash—can improve efficiency and reduce cost (see Figure 15.8). Moreover, the collection and transportation of trash through pipelines hydraulically and/or pneumatically (the method used at Disney World) can make collection even more efficient and out of sight.

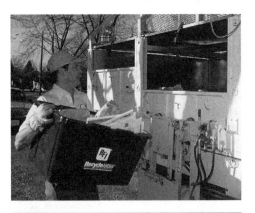

FIGURE 15.8

Household waste picked up at the curbside with a segregated-container recycling truck.

Source Reduction

The ultimate approach to solid waste reduction is to limit its creation in the first place through **source reduction.** This can be achieved by avoiding the use of nonreusable products, such as paper towels and disposable diapers, and by reducing the amount of packaging associated with groceries and carryout foods such as hamburgers and pizzas.

Recycling

Recycling is the collecting, sorting, and processing of materials that would otherwise be considered waste into raw materials that can be used to manufacture new products (see Figure 15.9).[7] This process conserves natural resources, energy, and sanitary landfill space and reduces water pollution and greenhouse gas emissions. Recycling is an important way to divert items, such as paper, glass, plastic, and metals, from the waste stream. These and other materials may be recycled through curbside programs, drop-off centers, buy-back programs, and deposit systems.

In an effort to encourage recycling, the federal government has set a goal of recycling 35% of MSW by 2005 and 38% by 2010 (see Box 15.1).[8] Recycling, including composting, diverted 72 million tons (about 31%) of the generated MSW away from disposal in 2003, an increase from 15 million tons in 1980 and 34 million tons in 1990 (see Figure 15.10).[4,5] The rate of recycling varies depending on the materials. In 2003, U.S. residents recycled about 93% of batteries, 48% of paper and paperboard, and 56% of yard trimmings, but much less plastic and glass (see Figure 15.11).[9] Although there has been great improvement, the recycling rate in the United States is far below the rates of Japan and some European countries.[4,7]

Although the benefits of recycling have been established, the success and practicality of recycling depend on a community's resources and structure. A community must consider the costs of such programs and the availability of markets that would use the recovered materials. However, recycling has grown significantly in the United States. Twenty years ago, only one curbside recycling program existed in the United States, but by 1998, 9,000 curbside programs and 12,000 recyclable drop-off centers were operating across the nation.[10] For recycling to work, everyone has to participate—the government, industry, organizations, institutions, small businesses, and people at home, including you. You and your community can make recycling a part of your daily routine.

One form of recycling, **composting,** can be done at home, since it doesn't require special knowledge or equipment. In composting, yard waste is recycled through a natural process of aerobic biodegradation during which microorganisms convert organic plant and animal matter into compost that can be used as a mulch or fertilizer. Composting can be done by individuals or on a community-wide basis. Yard trimmings and food waste together make up 56%

FIGURE 15.9
Recycling involves collecting, sorting, and processing of materials to manufacture new products that prevent waste, pollution, and use of virgin natural resources.

recycling
the collecting, sorting, and processing of materials that would otherwise be considered waste into raw materials for manufacturing new products, and the subsequent use of those new products

composting
the natural, aerobic biodegradation of organic plant and animal matter to compost

---

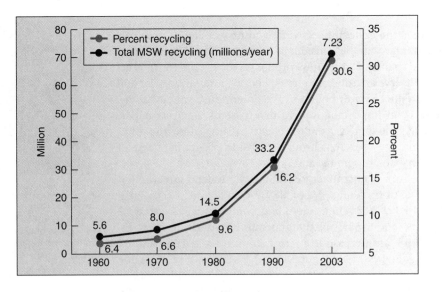

FIGURE 15.10

Changes in materials recycling in the United States between 1960 and 2003.

Source: U.S. Environmental Protection Agency (2005). "Municipal Solid Waste: Basic Facts." Available at http://www.epa.gov/epaoswer/non-hw/muncpl/facts.htm.

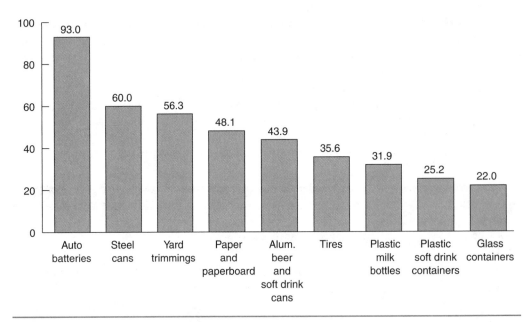

FIGURE 15.11

Recycling rates of selected materials (percentage).

Source: U.S. Environmental Protection Agency (2005). "Municipal Solid Waste: Basic Facts." Available at http://www.epa.gov/epaoswer/non-hw/muncpl/facts.htm.

of MSW in the United States (see Figure 15.11). That's a lot of waste that could become useful and environmentally beneficial! Composting (and use of its final product, compost) keeps organic wastes out of landfills, provides nutrients to the soil, increases beneficial soil organisms, suppresses certain plant diseases, protects soils from erosion, and reduces the need for fertilizers and pesticides that would otherwise pollute our water sources.[11]

Disposal

Waste that cannot be prevented or recycled can be incinerated (combusted) or placed in a sanitary landfill in compliance with environmental regulations.

Sanitary Landfills

Currently, most municipalities dispose of their wastes in **sanitary landfills,** sites judged suitable for inground disposal of solid waste. However, many of these municipal landfills are filling up, and available land suitable for new landfill sites near cities is quickly disappearing. Disposal of MSW on unsuitable land can result in the contamination of groundwater (water found in the ground), which may be the community's only source of drinking water.

The passage of the **Resource Conservation and Recovery Act of 1976 (RCRA,** pronounced Rick-Rah) provided legislation that phased out open dumps and replaced them with sanitary landfills. Only state-of-the-art landfills have been permitted to operate since 1997.[3] These are to be located at sites that can geographically and geologically support them—sites with natural clay soils. If clay soil cannot be found, a clay or double plastic lining must be constructed to prevent **leachates,** that is, liquids created when water mixes with wastes and drains from beneath a landfill. Leachates may contain various conventional and toxic substances that can pollute groundwater. Thus, liners are used to prevent leachates from contaminating water sources. Sanitary landfills are not to be located over sand or gravel deposits that would allow leachates to reach groundwater. In sanitary landfills, all refuse is spread and compacted in thin layers by bulldozers. At the end of each day, unlike an open dump, refuse is covered with a layer of soil. This process continues until the landfill is full, at which time a final layer of soil, about two feet thick, is placed on the top (see Figure 15.12). When this process is strictly followed, sanitary landfills provide little refuge for rodents and insects.

Sanitary landfills are not without problems. The production of leachates and contamination of groundwater can still occur if the clay seal breaks or if the landfill is located improperly. Contaminated groundwater has been detected at 86% of older landfills.[3] Some local governments have enacted legislation that requires sanitary landfills to be lined or double-lined with plastic liners. Another concern is the possibility of explosions and fires caused by the accumulation of dangerous amounts of methane gas created by the anaerobic decomposition of refuse. Although some communities have systems in place to harness the methane gas and use it as an energy source, only a small minority of landfills operating today collect gases. Landfills are responsible for 36% of all methane emissions in the United States.[12]

Today, about 56% of all municipal waste goes into landfills. However, the number of existing landfills in the United States declined from approximately 8,000 in 1988 to fewer than 1,767 in 2002.[4] There are even fewer today. This means that (1) it will be more costly to use existing landfills in the future because of supply and demand, (2) new sites for landfills will be needed, and (3) an alternative means of waste disposal must be developed.

Combustion (Incineration)

Combustion (incineration), or the burning of wastes, is the second major method of refuse disposal. The passage of the Clean Air Act of 1970 severely restricted the rights of individuals and municipalities to burn refuse because most could not comply with the strict emission standards. In 2001, only about 15% of all municipal waste was combusted, and 97 of the nearly

sanitary landfills waste disposal sites on land suited for this purpose and upon which waste is spread in thin layers, compacted, and covered with a fresh layer of clay or plastic foam each day

Resource Conservation and Recovery Act of 1976 (RCRA) the federal law that sets forth guidelines for the proper handling and disposal of hazardous wastes

leachates liquids created when water mixes with wastes and removes soluble constituents from them by percolation

combustion (incineration) the burning of solid wastes

FIGURE 15.12

A state-of-the-art sanitary landfill.

Source: Miller, G. T. (2002). *Living in the Environment: Principles, Connections, and Solutions* (with InfoTrac), 12th ed. Pacific Grove, CA: Brooks/Cole, Thomson Learning. Reprinted with permission of Brooks/Cole, a division of Thomson Learning: www.thomsonrights.com.

200 municipal combustors were energy recovery plants.[4] That is, they are able to convert some of the heat generated from the incineration process into steam and electricity.

Incineration reduces the weight of solid waste by 75% and the volume of solid waste by as much as 90%. Although incineration might seem to be the ultimate solution to the solid waste disposal problem, it is not without its serious drawbacks. First of all, large commercial incinerators are expensive, with start-up costs approaching a quarter of a billion dollars. Additionally, combustion of MSW produces nitrogen oxides, sulfur dioxide, and trace amounts of toxic pollutants such as mercury compounds and dioxins. The emission of these pollutants into the air varies based on the composition of the waste. For example, combustion of MSW containing batteries and tires produces toxic materials that can be released into the air. Consequently, scrubbers and filters are used to reduce toxic air pollutants from MSW power plants, although they do not eliminate them entirely. Furthermore, the remaining ash may be toxic, particularly when plastics have been incinerated. Regular testing of these facilities ensures that residual ash is nonhazardous before being landfilled. Sometimes the residual ash is used for beneficial purposes such as landfill cover or road construction. Another concern is that at least 10% of the volume (25% of the weight) of the original waste remains to be dealt

---

BOX 15.2	TIPS FOR REDUCING SOLID WASTE

Reduce

1. Reduce the amount of unnecessary packaging.
2. Adopt practices that reduce waste toxicity.

Reuse

3. Consider reusable products.
4. Maintain and repair durable products.
5. Reuse bags, containers, and other items.
6. Borrow, rent, or share items used infrequently.
7. Sell or donate goods instead of throwing them out.

Recycle

8. Choose recyclable products and containers and recycle them.

9. Select products made from recycled materials.
10. Compost yard trimmings and some food scraps.

Respond

11. Educate others on source reduction and recycling practices. Make your preferences known to manufacturers, merchants, and community leaders.
12. Be creative—find new ways to reduce waste quantity and toxicity.

Source: U.S. Environmental Protection Agency (1998). *The Consumer's Handbook for Reducing Solid Waste.* Available at http://www.epa.gov/epaanswer/non-hw/reduce/catbook .the12/htm.

---

with. Most of this ash enters landfills, but because of its toxicity poses a threat to local groundwater. Also, it now appears that future restrictions on items placed in landfills may prohibit the disposal of this ash.

Solid waste management has come a long way in the past 30 years. Today, most people know what is and what is not environmentally sound waste management, and the necessary technology to ensure appropriate disposal of waste is available. One question still remains: When will protecting the environment become a high enough priority for most Americans to act and insist upon wise waste management? Tips for more environmentally sound behaviors are plentiful (see Box 15.2).

Hazardous Waste

Hazardous waste is waste with properties that make it dangerous or potentially harmful to human health or the environment. The reason for classifying these wastes separately under the "hazardous" category is that their uncontrolled disposal would create dangerous conditions for humans and the environment. Thus, the identification and properly managed disposal of these materials is required to protect human and environmental health (see Box 15.3).

To be classified and regulated as hazardous, waste must first be identified as solid waste, that is, garbage, refuse, sludge, or other discarded material. This includes not only solids but also semisolids, liquids, and contained gaseous materials. Second, this waste must be specifically designated (listed) as hazardous by the U.S. **Environmental Protection Agency (EPA).** Designated hazardous wastes can be found among the by-products of manufacturing and industrial processes (e.g., solvents that have been used in cleaning or degreasing operations), discarded commercial products (e.g., cleaning fluids), and the by-products of petroleum refining operations and pesticide manufacturing. Furthermore, waste that is not specifically listed as hazardous, but which is ignitable, corrosive, reactive, or toxic, must be managed according to RCRA requirements.

The RCRA of 1976 was the first comprehensive law to address the collection and disposal of wastes. This law, and its 1984 amendments, banned all open dumping of waste, encouraged source reduction and recycling, and promoted the safe disposal of municipal waste. RCRA also established a system for controlling hazardous waste from the time it is generated until its disposal (called *cradle-to-grave regulation*) and mandated strict controls over the treatment, storage, and disposal of hazardous waste.

hazardous waste
a solid waste or combination of solid wastes that is dangerous to human health or the environment

Environmental Protection Agency (EPA)
the federal agency primarily responsible for setting, maintaining, and enforcing environmental standards

ELECTRONIC WASTE

As we become more dependent on electronic products to make our lives more convenient, we also generate a vast amount of electronic waste (e-waste) as we dispose of used and obsolete products (see Figure 15.13). In 1998, over 20 million computers became obsolete, and only 13% were reused or recycled. Electronic waste makes up about 1% to 4% of total municipal solid waste production. The European Union estimates that electronic and electrical equipment waste is growing three times faster than municipal solid waste.[13]

Why Is e-Waste Hazardous?

Color computer monitors and televisions have cathode ray tubes that contain, on average, four pounds of lead, as well as other toxic heavy metals, such as chromium, cadmium, mercury, beryllium, nickel, and zinc, and brominated flame retardants used in plastic. These toxic substances require special handling at the end of their lives. When electronics are not properly disposed of or recycled, these toxic materials can be released into the environment through landfill leachate or incinerator ash—both potential pathways to pollution that can negatively affect nearby communities and the health of community members.

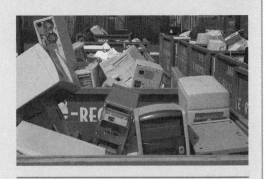

FIGURE 15.13

Electronic waste. As production and use of electronic equipment increases, proper disposal of obsolete equipment through reuse and recycling is necessary to prevent environmental pollution by hazardous substances.

What Should I Do with Used and Obsolete Electronic Products?

Individual users of computer monitors and televisions should check with the local municipal solid waste facility to dispose of these wastes properly. Local facilities may recycle these products, thus promoting the safe management of hazardous components and supporting the recovery and reuse of recyclable materials. Another option is recycling used electronic products by donating them for reuse by others. This extends the life of the products, keeps them out of the waste stream for a longer period of time, and prevents unnecessary e-waste pollution. Donating your used electronics for reuse can benefit schools, nonprofit organizations, and lower-income families who would otherwise be unable to obtain such equipment.

Can I Find Environmentally Friendly Products?

When purchasing new equipment, ask your retailer or supplier about electronics that have environmentally preferable attributes and determine whether the manufacturer offers take-back options. *Buying green* involves purchasing new equipment that has been designed with environmentally preferable attributes. Look for electronics that

- Contain fewer toxic constituents
- Use recycled materials in the new product
- Are energy efficient (look for the Energy Star label)
- Are designed for easy upgrading or disassembly
- Use minimal packaging
- Offer leasing or take-back options
- Have been recognized by independent certification groups (such as TCO or Blue Angel) as environmentally preferable

Where Can I Donate Electronic Products?

- Your municipal solids waste disposal facility may have information
- Reuse Development Organization: www.redo.org
- Students Recycling Use Technology: www. strut.org
- Goodwill Industries: www.goodwill.org

Where Can I Recycle Electronic Products?

- Electronic Industries Alliance (Consumer Education Initiative): www.eiae.org
- International Association of Electronic Recyclers: www.iaer.org/search

Source: U.S. Environmental Protection Agency (2006). "Municipal Solid Waste: eCycling." Available at http://www.epa.gov/epaoswer/hazwaste/recycle/ecycling/index.htm.

It is the responsibility of the EPA to implement the legislation created by RCRA. There are now more than 400 substances that are considered hazardous wastes in the United States. The EPA list includes neither radioactive wastes, which are controlled by the Nuclear Regulatory Commission, nor biomedical wastes, which are regulated by the individual states.

Today, Americans are faced with the dual problem of appropriately disposing of new hazardous waste while working to correct the errors of mishandling of hazardous waste in the past. There are untold numbers of hazardous waste sites that are "polluted" from past actions—legal and illegal—that must be cleaned up. Meanwhile, the production of hazardous wastes continues at a record pace. The United States alone produces almost 300 million metric tons of hazardous industrial waste annually. That is more than 1 ton of waste for every person living in the country. This figure does not include any wastes that are discarded improperly or illegally.

Hazardous Waste Management

The EPA Office of Solid Waste has the responsibility to oversee the management of hazardous waste, including its treatment, storage, and disposal. Some states may add more stringent requirements to management of hazardous wastes. A total of 214 million tons of hazardous waste was generated by the United States in 1995. There are about 15 methods of hazardous waste management overseen and regulated by the EPA.[14] The most commonly used method is deep well or underground injection, which is used for disposal of about 34% of hazardous waste.[14] Deep well injection consists of pumping hazardous waste by way of lined wells, far below the groundwater aquifer, into the layers of permeable rock, typically at a depth of 1,700 to more than 10,000 feet below the surface. The construction of such wells is restricted to sites where impermeable rock overlays the disposal site, thus preventing the movement of toxic contaminants to groundwater and surface water supplies. Most of these wells are found in the states of Texas and Florida.[15]

Other disposal methods of hazardous waste include special landfills (4%) and incineration (3%); all other methods, including treatment and recovery, accounted for the remaining 59% of the hazardous waste disposal in 2003.[14] The principles of these two methods were discussed in the section on MSW disposal. The regulation of these methods for hazardous waste disposal is stricter, however, because of the risk that hazardous wastes pose to the environment and human health.

Because of the difficulties encountered in hazardous waste disposal, source reduction is the best solution to the problem of hazardous waste. Increased public concern and the high cost of disposal have led hazardous waste producers to invest in technological research to reduce the amount of waste produced. Unfortunately, this approach is limited because there are still few incentives for source reduction.

Hazardous Waste Cleanup

Managing present and future hazardous wastes is one issue; dealing with the inappropriate past disposal of hazardous wastes is another.

Leaking underground storage tanks, abandoned mine lands, brownfields, and abandoned hazardous waste sites all present serious threats to human health and the environment (see Box 15.4). An underground storage tank (UST) system includes the tank, underground connected piping, and any containment system that stores either petroleum or certain hazardous substances. As of March 31, 2002, 422,573 releases of hazardous substances caused by leaks, spills, and overfills had been reported from UST systems.[16] Gasoline leaking from service stations is one of the most common sources of groundwater pollution. Just 1.5 cups of leaking hazardous chemicals can contaminate more than one million gallons of groundwater. Because approximately one-half of the population of the United States relies on groundwater as their source of drinking water, groundwater pollution is a serious concern. Many municipal and private wells have had to be shut down as a result of contamination caused by leaky UST systems. Additionally, fumes and vapors can travel beneath the ground and collect in areas such as basements, utility vaults, and parking garages, where they can pose a serious threat of explosion, fire, asphyxiation, or other adverse health effects. Cleaning up petroleum releases in the subsurface is difficult and expensive; therefore, the best prevention of groundwater contamination is appropriate management and maintenance of the UST systems to prevent releases.

The primary participant in the cleanup of hazardous waste in America has been the federal government. In 1980 Congress passed the **Comprehensive Environmental Response, Compensation, and Liability Act (CERCLA)** in response to the public's demand to clean up leaking dump sites. This law, known as *Superfund,* created a tax on the chemical and petrochemical industries to clean up abandoned hazardous waste sites that might endanger human health and the environment. CERCLA established the following:

1. A national priority list (NPL) of hazardous waste sites to be cleaned up
2. The principle that the government would make responsible parties pay for those cleanups whenever possible
3. Funds to support the identification and cleanup of the sites

Comprehensive Environmental Response, Compensation, and Liability Act (CERCLA) the federal law (known as the Superfund) created to clean up abandoned hazardous waste sites

The EPA was responsible for creating the NPL in cooperation with the individual states. These sites were placed on the list in order of priority based upon the threat to public health or the environment. Once on the NPL, sites were eligible for Superfund dollars that could be used for removing and destroying wastes and for the temporary or permanent relocation of residents affected by the harzardous waste dumps. The Superfund did not provide compensation to victims for health-related problems.

Since the inception of this program, 45,826 contaminated sites have been placed in the database from which the individual states and the U.S. EPA select the sites for the NPL and cleanup. The first NPL in 1983 contained 406 sites. Through the end of 2004, the EPA had listed a total of 1,529 sites and deleted 292 sites from the NPL because of the completion of the cleanup process.[16] Between 1993 and 2005, the Superfund provided $15,219,000,000 for cleanup of the NPL sites, an average of about $1.17 billion per year.[17] Another problem is the more than 450,000 abandoned industrial plants and commercial worksites, most of which are contaminated. Examples include empty factories, abandoned junkyards, and old gas stations.[3] These so-called **brownfields** are properties where expansion, redevelopment, or reuse may be complicated by the presence or potential presence of a hazardous substance, pollutant, or

brownfields property where reuse is complicated by the presence of hazardous substances from prior use

---

BOX 15.5   **HEALTHY PEOPLE 2010: OBJECTIVE**

Objective 8-12:   Minimize the risks to human health and the environment posed by hazardous sites.

Target: 98% of sites on the following lists:

8-12a.   National Priority List sites
8-12b.   Resource Conservation and Recovery Act facilities
8-12c.   Leaking underground storage facilities
8-12d.   Brownfield properties

Baseline: 1,200 National Priority List sites; 2,475 Resource Conservation and Recovery Act facilities; 370,000 leaking underground storage facilities; 1,500 brownfield properties in 1998.

For Further Thought

Do you feel it is the responsibility of the party who created a hazardous waste site to pay for the cleanup, even though at the time the site was created it was not illegal to dispose of the waste in such a manner? Why or why not?

---

contaminant. Examples include abandoned industrial plants and commercial worksites, empty factories, and abandoned junk yards. It is estimated that there are more than 450,000 brownfields in the United States that are unsightly, take up space, prevent land development, and can pose a threat to human health. Cleaning up and reinvesting in these properties takes development pressures off undeveloped, open land, increases local tax bases, facilitates job growth, and both improves and protects the environment and human health. One of the *Healthy People 2010* objectives addresses the cleanup of these hazardous waste sites. Its aim is to "Minimize the risks to human health and the environment posed by hazardous sites" (see Box 15.5).[18]

Air Pollution

Until a few hundred years ago, air pollution could be attributed almost entirely to natural causes—dust and sand storms, forest fires, volcanic eruptions, and the gases escaping from deep within the earth or given off by decaying organic matter. While these forms of air pollution still exist today, waste products created by a modern industrialized civilization constitute a greater threat to air quality and our health. Air pollution can cause burning of the eyes and nose, itchy and irritated throat, as well as trouble with breathing. Some chemicals found in polluted air cause cancer, birth defects, brain and nerve damage, and long-term injury to the lungs and breathing passages. Air pollution can also damage the environment and property and can cause haze and reduced visibility. About 141 million tons of pollutants are emitted into the atmosphere in the United States each year.[19]

Contaminants of Outdoor Air

Air pollution is the contamination of the air by substances in amounts great enough to interfere with the comfort, safety, or health of humans and other living organisms. These contaminants occur as gases, liquids, or solids. The most prevalent sources of air pollution in the United States are (1) transportation, including privately owned motor vehicles; (2) electric power plants fueled by oil and coal; and (3) industry, primarily mills and refineries. In addition to these major sources, there are many smaller sources, such as wood and coal burning stoves, fireplaces, drycleaning facilities, and incinerators.

air pollution
contamination of the air that interferes with the comfort, safety, and health of living organisms

Under the Clean Air Act, the EPA sets limits on how much of a pollutant can be in the air anywhere in the United States. The air pollutants of greatest concern in the United States are called **criteria pollutants.** These are sulfur dioxide, carbon monoxide, nitrogen oxides, ground-level ozone, respirable particulate matter, and lead (see Table 15.2). The EPA has established national standards for allowable concentration levels of each of these six pollutants in the ambient (outdoor) air and closely monitors their levels because they are considered harmful to public health. These standards are known as the **National Ambient Air Quality Standards (NAAQSs).** Ground-level ozone and airborne particles pose the greatest threat to human health in the United States.

Widespread concern about the possible ill effects of these criteria pollutants has led to efforts to reduce their concentrations in ambient air. Between 1990 and 2005, the United States substantially reduced the ambient air concentrations of all six of the criteria pollutants, namely, lead by 96%, particulate matter by 25%, ozone by 12%, sulfur dioxide by 48%, carbon monoxide by 60%, and nitrogen oxides by 25%.[19] Nonetheless, in 2005, approximately 122 million people in the United States lived in counties with pollution levels above the NAAQSs (see Box 15.6).[19] Most of these people are exposed to unacceptable levels of ozone. The *Healthy People 2010* objective for the reduction of the levels of criteria pollutants in the ambient air requires that no U.S. residents be exposed to harmful levels of these pollutants (see Box 15.7).[18]

Special Concerns with Outdoor Air

Pollution of the outdoor air has resulted in a number of specific problems for the United States and the world, including acid rain, global warming, destruction of the ozone layer, and photochemical smog. Acid rain and global warming currently have minimal effects on human health and are discussed below briefly. Destruction of the ozone layer and photochemical smog directly affect human health and are discussed in some detail.

Acid Rain

Acid deposition, often referred to as **acid rain** (also acid snow, acid dew, acid drizzle, acid fog, and acid sleet), may occur both within and downwind of areas that produce emissions that contain sulfur dioxide (SO_2) and oxides of nitrogen (NO_2 and NO_3). These emissions result from the burning of fossil fuels—oil, coal, and natural gas—and then react in the atmosphere, combining with water vapor to form sulfuric and nitric acids, which fall to the earth as acid rain. The primary problems associated with acid rain are the acidification of

Table 15.2
Criteria Pollutants

Pollutants (Designation)	Form(s)	Major Sources (in order of percentage of contribution)
Carbon monoxide (CO)	Gas	Transportation, industrial processes, other solid waste, stationary fuel combustion
Lead (Pb)	Metal or aerosol	Transportation, industrial processes, stationary fuel combustion, solid waste
Nitrogen dioxide (NO_2)	Gas	Stationary fuel combustion, transportation, industrial processes, solid waste
Ground-level ozone (O_3)	Gas	Transportation, industrial processes, solid waste, stationary fuel combustion
Particulate matter	Solid or liquid	Industrial processes, stationary fuel combustion, transportation, solid waste
Sulfur dioxide (SO_2)	Gas	Stationary fuel combustion, industrial processes, transportation, other wastes

BOX 15.6   WHAT'S THE COLOR OF YOUR AIR QUALITY TODAY?

How do you know whether the quality of air today is good for your health or for the health of sensitive individuals in your community? Do you know people with asthma? They might react differently to air pollutants than a healthy and young person. To make it easier for all of us to understand daily air quality and what it means for your health, the EPA calculates the **Air Quality Index (AQI)** for five criteria air pollutants regulated by the Clean Air Act. The index tells you how clean or polluted your air is, and what associated health effects might be of concern for you or sensitive people in your community.

The value of the AQI on a particular day can range from 0 (good air quality) to 500 (hazardous air quality). AQI values below 100 are generally thought of as satisfactory, whereas values above 100 are considered to be unhealthy—at first for certain sensitive groups of people. Weather channels and Web sites might use a color-coded AQI for easier understanding (see Figure 15.14). Based on these indices, the cities can declare "action days" when the AQI gets into the unhealthy range. In many cities, action days are called when the AQI is forecast to be Unhealthy (Code Red). In this case, everyone should reduce exposure to air pollution, and especially the members of the sensitive population for the particular pollutant, such as people with asthma or lung disease, and children.

Let's find out the air quality in your town today:

1. Go to www.weather.com, click the tab Stay Healthy, and follow the link Air Quality and Pollution.
2. In the drop-down menu, select the state of interest; a list of cities in your state will be displayed, with color-coded air quality forecasts. Review this information and answer the following questions.
3. Alternatively, you can visit http://airnow.gov/ and follow the link Local Forecast and Conditions. Select your state and review the air quality for today and tomorrow. Answer the following questions.

Questions

1. Which principal pollutants are listed for your town today?
2. What is the Air Quality Index for those pollutants in your area today?
3. Based on your research, summarize the air quality in your area. Is it healthy to enjoy the outdoors or should you or a segment of the population limit outdoor exposure today? Why?
4. Is there an action day declared today for your area?
5. Consider the season right now and explain whether the air quality in your area is at its best or worst. What time of the year would you expect the air quality to be the best and the worst?

Air Quality Index Levels of Health Concern	Numerical Value	Meaning
Good (green)	0–50	Air quality is considered satisfactory, and air pollution poses little or no risk.
Moderate (yellow)	51–100	Air quality is acceptable; however, for some pollutants there may be a moderate health concern for a very small number of people who are unusually sensitive to air pollution.
Unhealthy for Sensitive Groups (orange)	101–150	Members of sensitive groups may experience health effects. The general public is not likely to be affected.
Unhealthy (red)	151–200	Everyone may begin to experience health effects; members of sensitive groups may experience more serious health effects.
Very Unhealthy (purple)	201–300	Health alert: everyone may experience more serious health effects.
Hazardous (maroon)	> 300	Health warnings of emergency conditions. The entire population is more likely to be affected.

Air Quality Index (AQI) an index that indicates the level of pollution in the air and the associated health risk

FIGURE 15.14
Color codes for various Air Quality Indices.

Source: AIRNow. "Air Quality Index (AQI): A Guide to Air Quality and Your Health." Available at http://airnow.gov/index.cfm?action=static.aqi.

HEALTHY PEOPLE 2010: OBJECTIVE

Objective 8-1: Reduce the proportion of persons exposed to air that does not meet the U.S. Environmental Protection Agency's health-based standards for harmful air pollutants.

Target and baseline:

Objective	Reduction in Air Pollutants	1997 Baseline	2004	2010 Target
		Percent		
8-1a.	Ozone*	43	39	0
8-1b.	Particulate matter	12	10	0
8-1c.	Carbon monoxide	19	7	0
8-1d.	Nitrogen dioxide	5	0	0
8-1e.	Sulfur dioxide	2	1	0
8-1f.	Lead	< 1	0	0
		Number		
8-1g.	Total number of people	119,803,000	115,149,000	0

*The targets of zero percent for ozone and particulate matter are set for 2012 and 2018, respectively.

Note: For the purpose of this objective, EPA is counting persons living in nonattainment areas only. Data for population groups currently are not analyzed.

Target setting method: Consistent with the Clean Air Act (Public Law 101-549).

Source: Aerometric Information Retrieval System (AIRS), EPA, OAR. Office of Air and Radiation. Available at http://wonder.cdc.gov/.

For Further Thought

Have you or any members of your family done anything during the past year to help reduce air pollution?

---

global warming
the gradual increase in the earth's surface temperature

surface water, which results in the death of certain aquatic species, damage to vegetation, primarily at higher elevations, and erosion of monuments and buildings (see Figure 15.15). Although acidic air pollutants can contribute to respiratory problems in humans, acid deposition itself is not considered a health hazard.

Global Warming

greenhouse gases
atmosphere gases, principally carbon dioxide, CFCs, methane, and nitrous oxide, that are transparent to visible light but absorb infrared radiation

Global warming is the gradual increase in the earth's surface temperature. One of the conditions that seems to be contributing to global warming is the increase in levels of **greenhouse gases**—namely, carbon dioxide, **chlorofluorocarbons (CFCs)**, methane, and nitrous oxide—which are transparent to visible light but absorb infrared radiation. These gases permit the passage of sunlight to the earth's surface. However, when some of this energy is re-radiated as infrared radiation (heat) back to the atmosphere, it is absorbed by these gases, causing air temperature to rise. Whether or not global warming is occurring at present is a matter of debate. Records show that the average global temperature has gradually increased 0.5–1.0°F since the late nineteenth century. Scientists do not agree on the significance of this increase. If global warming is occurring and if it continues to occur, a number of serious complications can be expected. A few degrees increase in the earth's surface temperature would adversely affect our environment, including the quality of our air, our water, and our health. The George W. Bush administration, which has acknowledged that human activities are probably changing the climate, refused to pursue a policy to reduce emissions of carbon dioxide and other greenhouse gases and refused to force U.S. industries to report their carbon dioxide emissions.[3]

chlorofluoro-carbons (CFCs)
a family of chemical agents used in industry for such items as propellants, refrigeration, solvent cleaning, and insulation

Destruction of the Ozone Layer

Although ground-level ozone (O_3) is considered a criteria pollutant, stratospheric ozone provides a great benefit to life on earth. This stratospheric **ozone layer** filters out 99% of the sun's harmful ultraviolet radiation (see Figure 15.16).[20] Without this protective filter, ultraviolet radiation would reach the earth's surface at dangerously high levels, causing increased rates of skin cancers and eye problems. Further, there would be an increase in the rate of mutations (genetic changes) and perhaps the disruption of the oceanic food chain.

The primary cause of the depletion of the ozone layer is the presence of CFCs in the atmosphere. CFCs are solely a product of the chemical industry; they do not occur naturally in the environment. CFCs are used as propellants in aerosol cans, in the freon of air conditioners and refrigerators, and for blowing plastic foams. Because CFCs are implicated in both ozone depletion and global warming, considerable attention has been placed on controlling their production and release. The United States banned CFC production and sale in this country in 1996 as a result of the international agreement signed in Montreal in 1987. The ozone layer is being depleted faster than originally believed. In fact, scientific evidence suggests that the rate of ozone depletion over the last decade is more than twice what was previously projected. Thinning of the ozone layer has been

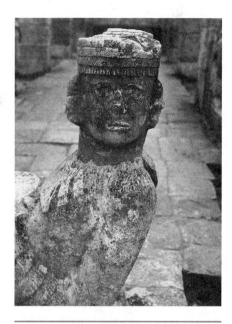

FIGURE 15.15

Acid rain defaces our art and our architecture and is hazardous to the environment.

ozone layer
ozone gas (O_3) found in the stratosphere

FIGURE 15.16

Regions of the atmosphere.

Source: Nadakavukaren, A. (1990). *Man and Environment: A Health Perspective,* 3rd ed. Long Grove, IL: Waveland Press, Inc. Reprinted by permission of Waveland Press, Inc. All rights reserved.

found over the polar regions and in the northern mid-latitudes. Presently, a hole exists in the ozone layer in the Southern Hemisphere, and it is anticipated that one will appear shortly in the Northern Hemisphere. Ozone levels over the Northern Hemisphere are 13% to 14% lower now than they were in the 1970s. The EPA estimates that 1% depletion of the ozone layer would lead to a 2% increase in ultraviolet radiation and that this, in turn, would lead to a 4% increase in the rate of skin cancer cases. Occurrences of cataracts (vision loss) are also expected to increase.[20]

Photochemical Smog

photochemical smog
a secondary air pollutant created when primary and other secondary pollutants react with oxygen and sunlight

Photochemical smog, also called ground-level ozone, is not emitted directly into the air but is created by chemical reactions between nitrogen oxides (NO_x) and volatile organic compounds (VOCs) in the presence of sunlight. The resulting photochemical smog, seen in the air as a brownish haze, is detrimental to human health and to the well-being of other living things.

Major sources of NO_x and VOC emissions are industrial facilities, electric utilities, motor vehicle exhaust, gasoline vapors, and chemical solvents. Peak concentrations of ground-level ozone typically develop during hot, dry, stagnant summertime conditions; concentrations are lower during cloudy, cool, rainy, and windy days. The length of the ozone season differs from one area to another, with southern and southwestern states experiencing the longest ozone season. Anyone who spends time outdoors in the summer may be affected by unhealthy levels of ground-level ozone, particularly children, outdoor workers, and people exercising outdoors.

Breathing ozone can result in a variety of health problems even at low levels, including chest pain, coughing, throat irritation, congestion, bronchitis, emphysema, asthma, and reduced lung function. Repeated exposure to ground-level ozone may permanently scar lung tissue. Even healthy people can experience breathing problems if exposed to ozone at high enough levels.

Many urban and suburban areas throughout the United States have levels of ground-level ozone that exceed the levels set in the NAAQSs. Between 1980 and 2003, ozone levels declined 21%. In spite of this improvement, ozone continues to be a persistent air pollution problem, affecting many areas across the country and harming millions of people. The EPA has designated 474 counties in 31 states as areas that do not meet the national standard for ozone, called nonattainment areas.[21] Thirty-nine percent of Americans (115,149,000 people) are still exposed to ozone levels that are too high (see Box 15.7).

thermal inversion
a condition that occurs when warm air traps cooler air at the surface of the earth

The extent or quantity of photochemical smog, as well as other air pollutants, can be amplified by physical geography. For example, the cities of Denver, Los Angeles, Phoenix, and Salt Lake City have nearby mountains that restrict lateral air movement. Furthermore, this trapped air mass may also be subject to another phenomenon referred to as a **thermal inversion.** Normally, the air surrounding the earth's surface is heated by the sun and rises to mix with the cooler air above it. However, in cases of thermal inversion, a layer of warm air settles above the cooler air at the surface, preventing cooler air from rising. When the cooler air is trapped, it accumulates pollutants. If the thermal inversion continues, the pollutants can reach dangerously high levels (see Figure 15.17).[20]

Just as with other types of pollution, the best way to reduce photochemical smog is to reduce (or eliminate) emissions from the internal combustion engines of motor vehicles. Such a reduction can be achieved through more carpooling, better use of mass transit systems, and the development and use of electric and solar energy sources for motor vehicles.

Protection of Outdoor Air through Regulation

Clean Air Act (CAA)
the federal law that provided the government with authority to address interstate air pollution

Steady deterioration of air quality in the 1950s and 1960s led to the nation's first serious attempt to regulate air pollution, the **Clean Air Act (CAA)** of 1963.[20] The CAA provided the federal government with the authority to address interstate air pollution problems. The CAA

Solar radiation

Cooler air

Cool air

Pollution rises
and disperses

Warm air

(a) Normal pattern

Solar radiation

Cool air

Warm inversion layer

Pollution trapped

Cool air

(b) Thermal inversion

FIGURE 15.17
A thermal inversion.

Source: Chiras, D. D. (2002). *Environmental Science: Creating a Sustainable Future,* 6th ed. Sudbury, MA: Jones and Bartlett
Publishers.

was amended several times in the late 1960s, but much of the regulation was based upon
voluntary compliance.

The 1970 amendments to the CAA provided the first comprehensive approach to dealing
with air pollution nationwide. Three significant components of these amendments were the
development of the NAAQSs, tougher emission standards for automobiles, and *State
Implementation Plans (SIPs)*. The SIPs required each state to submit to the EPA its plan for
achieving and maintaining air quality standards.

The CAA was amended again in 1977, empowering the EPA to regulate air quality.
Specifically, the EPA was authorized to levy fines against those who violated the standards.[3]
The CAA was amended again in 1990 to include (1) mandates to reduce urban smog, sulfur

dioxide, and nitrogen oxides, (2) tighter controls on auto emissions, including a guarantee that auto emission controls will last 100,000 miles, (3) more efficient power plants, and (4) a total ban on the production of CFCs for use in the United States by the year 1996.[20]

Indoor Air

It was once believed that the comfortable confines of the indoors were protected from the ills of air pollution. However, it is now known that indoor air pollution can be a greater threat to human health than outdoor air pollution. Unlike outdoor air pollutants, which are regulated and can be dispersed by the wind, indoor air pollutants can be trapped and concentrated to dangerous levels. This buildup of undesirable gases and airborne particles inside a building is called **indoor air pollution.** Poor indoor air quality combined with the fact that Americans spend 80% to 90% of their time indoors presents a potentially significant health concern.[22]

Indoor Air Pollutants

Indoor air pollution can arise from a number of sources (see Figure 15.18). **Asbestos** is a naturally occurring mineral fiber that was commonly used as an insulation and fireproofing material. It was often used in older buildings to insulate pipes, walls, and ceilings; as a component of floor and ceiling tiles; and sprayed in structures for fireproofing. It is harmless if intact and left alone, but, when disturbed, the airborne fibers can cause serious health problems. **Biogenic pollutants** are airborne materials of biological origin such as living and nonliving

indoor air pollution
the buildup of undesirable gases and particles in the air inside a building

asbestos
a naturally occurring mineral fiber that has been identified as a Class A carcinogen by the Environmental Protection Agency

biogenic pollutants
airborne biological organisms or their particles or gases or other toxic materials that can produce illness

combustion by-products
gases and particulates generated by burning

radon
a naturally occurring, colorless, odorless, radioactive gas formed during the radioactive decay of uranium-238

secondhand smoke
environmental tobacco smoke (ETS)—tobacco smoke in the environment that can be inhaled by nonsmokers

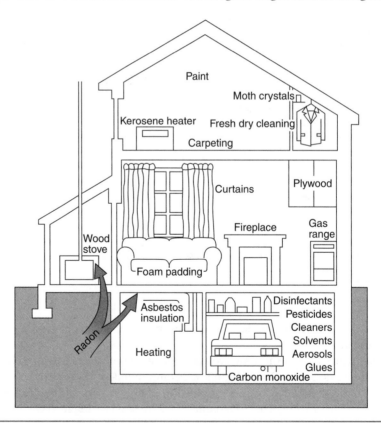

FIGURE 15.18

Air pollution sources in the home.

Source: U.S. Environmental Protection Agency (1991).

fungi and their toxins, bacteria, viruses, molds, pollens, insect parts and wastes, and animal dander. They normally enter the human body by being inhaled. These contaminants can trigger allergic reactions, including asthma; cause infectious illnesses, such as influenza and measles; or release disease-producing toxins. Symptoms of health problems include sneezing, watery eyes, coughing, shortness of breath, dizziness, lethargy, fever, and even digestive problems. Children, elderly people, and people with breathing problems, allergies, or lung diseases are particularly susceptible to airborne biogenic pollutants. You can minimize exposure to these pollutants by controlling the relative humidity level in a home or office; a relative humidity of 30% to 50% is generally recommended for homes. To reduce airborne biogenic pollutants in your home, clean up standing water, remove any wet or water-damaged materials from around your home, and, if you suspect a problem, have your home inspected by someone knowledgeable about indoor air pollution problems.

mainstream smoke
tobacco smoke inhaled and exhaled by the smoker

Combustion by-products include gases (e.g., CO, NO_2, and SO_2) and particulates (e.g., ash and soot). The major sources of these items are fireplaces, wood stoves, kerosene heaters, gas ranges and engines, candles, incense, secondhand tobacco smoke, and improperly maintained gas furnaces. Prolonged exposure to these substances can cause serious illness and possibly death.

sidestream smoke
tobacco smoke that comes off the end of burning tobacco products

Radon is the Number 1 cause of lung cancer among nonsmokers and the second leading cause of lung cancer overall. This radioactive gas, which cannot be seen, smelled, or tasted, is responsible for about 21,000 lung cancer deaths every year.[23] It is a naturally occurring gas that seeps into a home from surrounding soil, rocks, and water and through openings such as cracks, drains, and sump pumps. However, exposure to radon is preventable, and you can do something about it. Every home and office building should be tested for radon, and homeowners can administer this inexpensive and easy test. Increasing the proportion of persons who live in homes that have been tested for radon is one of the *Healthy People 2010* objectives (see Box 15.8).

passive smoking
the inhalation of environmental tobacco smoke by nonsmokers

Environmental tobacco smoke (ETS), also known as **secondhand smoke,** includes both **mainstream smoke** (the smoke inhaled and exhaled by the smoker) and **sidestream smoke** (the smoke that comes off the end of a burning tobacco product). The inhalation of ETS by nonsmokers is referred to as **passive smoking.** There are hundreds of toxic agents and more than forty **carcinogens** (cancer-causing agents) in secondhand smoke. A few of

carcinogens
agents, usually chemicals, that cause cancer

BOX **15.8**   **HEALTHY PEOPLE 2010: OBJECTIVES**

Objective 8-18:   Increase the proportion of persons who live in homes tested for radon concentrations.

Target: 20%.

Baseline: 17% of the population lived in homes in 1998 that had been tested for radon (age adjusted to the year 2000 standard population).

Target setting method: Better than the best.

For Further Thought

Have you tested your house for radon? What was the reading? What is the potential radon level in your area? Go to the EPA Map of Radon Zones and search for the map of your state, where you can identify the potential by county.

Source: National Health Interview Survey (NHIS), CDC, NCHS.

these harmful agents are CO, NO$_2$, CO$_2$, hydrogen cyanide, formaldehyde, nicotine, and suspended particles.[24] The health effects of ETS will be discussed in Chapter 16.

Volatile organic compounds (VOCs) are compounds that exist as vapors over the normal range of air pressures and temperatures. The health effects of these chemicals vary with their concentration and the length of exposure. Acute symptoms include irritation of the eyes and respiratory tract, headaches, dizziness, and memory impairment. Some of these chemicals are either known or suspected carcinogens. In any one building, one might find hundreds of different VOCs. Sources of VOCs include construction materials (e.g., insulation and paint), structural components (e.g., vinyl tile and sheet rock), furnishings (e.g., drapes and upholstery fabric), cleansers and solvents (e.g., liquid detergent and furniture polish), personal care products (e.g., deodorant and eyeliner pencils), insecticides/pesticides, electrical equipment (e.g., computers and VCRs), and combustion of wood and kerosene.[25] **Formaldehyde,** a pungent water-soluble gas, is one of the most ubiquitous VOCs. It is a widely used chemical that can be found in hundreds of products. Exposure occurs when it evaporates from wood products such as plywood and particle board, in which it is a component of the glue that binds these products together. Formaldehyde can also be found in products such as grocery bags, wallpaper, carpet, insulation, wall paneling, and wallboard.[25] Exposure to formaldehyde can cause watery eyes, burning in the eyes and throat, and difficulty in breathing. It can precipitate asthma attacks in susceptible people. Formaldehyde may also be a carcinogen. So, how can you protect your family and yourself? If you are building or renovating a residence, use exterior-grade products that emit less formaldehyde. Increase ventilation in your home, use a dehumidifier and air conditioning to control humidity, and keep temperature at moderate levels in your home to reduce formaldehyde emissions.

Protection of Indoor Air

The energy crisis of the 1970s led to a conservation movement that included reducing the ventilation rate. The accepted rate was reduced from 20 cubic feet per minute to 5 feet per minute as a cost savings and energy savings measure. This reduced ventilation resulted in the creation of "tight buildings," known as "sick buildings," as reports of illness traced to such buildings increased.[9] **Sick building syndrome** refers to a situation in which the air quality in a building produces nonspecific signs and symptoms of ill health in the building occupants. Electronic controls and more efficient filtration, heating, and cooling systems have enabled the ventilation rate of 20 cubic feet per minute to be reinstated.

Even though indoor air pollution may be more harmful to human health than outdoor air pollution, measures to monitor and correct indoor air pollution have been limited. The U.S. government has not yet established a framework for the development of indoor air policies as it has for outdoor air. It has, however, pursued voluntary industry standards. For example, there are safety codes for kerosene space heaters, an "action guideline" for radon, and smoking restrictions for commercial airlines. There also has been federal guidance on the handling of asbestos in schools and a prohibition on new uses of asbestos. In the absence of a federal indoor clean air act, some states and municipalities have developed their own. In an attempt to protect workers and citizens from heart disease, cancer, and respiratory illness, and to reduce forced inhalation through passive smoking, many U.S. counties and states, as well as countries around the world, have banned or are in the process of outlawing smoking in workplaces, sometimes including bars, restaurants, and casinos. In some cases, even outdoor smoking has been banned within a certain distance of public and state-owned building entrances, exits, and air intakes in many cities.

In the absence of any comprehensive policy, individuals are encouraged to take steps to reduce or eliminate sources of indoor air pollution and improve air quality. These may include:[12]

volatile organic compounds (VOCs) compounds that exist as vapors over the normal range of air pressures and temperatures

formaldehyde (CH$_2$O) a water-soluble gas used in aqueous solutions in hundreds of consumer products

sick building syndrome a term to describe a situation in which the air quality in a building produces generalized signs and symptoms of ill health in the building's occupants

1. Selecting safer household products, such as "pump" dispensers instead of spray dispensers
2. Venting dryers outdoors instead of indoors to keep indoor humidity low and therefore discourage mold growth
3. Avoiding products containing formaldehyde
4. Having loose asbestos fibers removed, if found
5. Limiting or prohibiting indoor smoking
6. Maintaining heating, air conditioning, and ventilation systems in good working condition
7. Testing buildings for radon

Water and Its Pollution

Water is necessary for life as we know it. We are dependent on availability of clean water for our health and a good quality of life. In many regions of the world, such as parts of Asia and Africa, water is in scarce supply. Whereas the scarcity of water limits development and challenges health, the lack of basic **sanitation** has immediate and dire health consequences. Consumption of polluted water can result in outbreaks of such waterborne diseases as typhoid fever, cholera, and other gastrointestinal diseases. Such diseases are responsible for 1.8 million deaths every year. Most of those affected are children in developing countries.[26] In 2002, about 42% of the world's population had no access to basic sanitation, and 17% had no access to a supply of clean drinking water.[27]

Here in the United States, 100% of the population has both a clean water supply and sanitation; it is the highest reported rate for any world region.[28] Nonetheless, 419 waterborne disease outbreaks linked to drinking water were reported in the United States between 1980 and 1998, resulting in 511,000 cases of illness.[29]

Pollution of drinking water sources is caused by wastes produced by humans and their daily activities, including sewage. Thus, both the prevention of water pollution and treatment of polluted water are essential community activities.

Sources of Water

We acquire water for our domestic, industrial, and agricultural needs either from surface water or groundwater. Water in streams, rivers, lakes, and reservoirs is called **surface water.** The water that infiltrates into the soil is referred to as *subsurface* or **groundwater.** Groundwater that is not absorbed by the roots of vegetation moves slowly downward until it reaches the zone of soil completely saturated with water, referred to as an *aquifer*. **Aquifers** are porous, water-saturated layers of underground bedrock, sand, and gravel that can yield an economically significant amount of water.[3]

The earth's supply of freshwater available for our use is limited. Only 0.003% of the earth's water is available for use by humans, and much of this is hard to reach and too costly to be of practical value.[20] Thus, the continual contamination of our groundwater through the improper disposal of human waste, trash, and solid and hazardous waste should be of paramount concern to everyone.

Sources of Water Pollution

Water pollution includes any physical or chemical change in water that can harm living organisms or make it unfit for other uses, such as drinking, domestic use, recreation, fishing, industry, agriculture, or transportation.[3] The sources of water pollution (see Figure 15.19) fall into two categories—point sources and nonpoint sources.[3] **Point source pollution** refers to a single identifiable source that discharges pollutants into the water, such as a pipe, ditch, or culvert. Examples of such pollutants might include release of pollutants from a factory or sewage treatment plant. Point sources of pollution are relatively easy to identify, control, and treat.

sanitation the promotion of hygiene and prevention of disease by maintenance of clean conditions through hygienic disposal or recycling of waste material, such as human fecal waste

surface water precipitation that does not infiltrate the ground or return to the atmosphere by evaporation; the water in streams, rivers, and lakes

groundwater water located under the surface of the ground

aquifer an underground soil formation that is saturated with water and available for human use by pumping

water pollution any physical or chemical change in water that can harm living organisms or make it unfit for other uses

point source pollution pollution that can be traced to a single identifiable source

FIGURE 15.19

Sources of groundwater contamination.

Source: U.S. Environmental Protection Agency.

Nonpoint source pollution includes all pollution that occurs through the runoff, seepage, or falling of pollutants into the water. Examples include the runoff of water from cities, highways, and farms due to rain events (called *stormwater runoff*), seepage of leachates from landfills, and acid rain. Nonpoint source pollution is a greater problem than point source pollution because it is often difficult to track the actual source of pollution and, therefore, to control it.

Types of Water Pollutants

As one might guess, the types and numbers of water pollutants are almost endless. The two types of pollutants of primary concern to community health are biological and chemical pollutants. These are briefly described here, but are discussed in more detail in Chapter 16.

Biological Pollutants

Biological pollutants include pathogens such as parasites, bacteria, viruses, and other undesirable living microorganisms. These pathogens enter the water mainly through human and other animal wastes that were disposed of improperly or without being treated before their disposal. Sources of such contamination include **runoff** from animal farms that contains manure; failed septic systems that leach untreated or only partially treated human fecal waste to groundwater and surface water; combined sewer overflow that discharges a mix of untreated stormwater and human sewage to rivers or streams; and stormwater runoff from our cities, highways, and towns that carries animal and human fecal waste left on land surfaces (see Figure 15.20). These biological wastes spread viruses, bacteria, and parasites into rivers, lakes, reservoirs, and drinking water supplies, where they can cause human illness. For example,

nonpoint source pollution
all pollution that occurs through the runoff, seepage, or falling of pollutants into the water

runoff
water that flows over land surfaces (including paved surfaces), typically from precipitation

people can become ill by drinking water from a groundwater well contaminated with fecal waste from a septic system or from ingesting water while swimming in a lake or reservoir contaminated by runoff from surrounding cities or farms. Although many sanitary districts across the United States are implementing new plans to capture and treat urban stormwater runoff from their streets, it is not yet a common practice. Because of increased urbanization and the growing proportion of land that is covered by impervious concrete, rainwater cannot infiltrate the land surface and is therefore collected by storm and sewer lines and often dumped into rivers without any treatment.

Chemical Pollutants

Nonbiological pollutants include inorganic chemicals such as lead, copper, and arsenic; organic chemicals; and radioactive pollutants. Among the organic chemicals are industrial solvents such as trichloroethylene (TCE); pesticides such as dichlorodiphenyltrichloroethane (DDT) and Atrazine, a commonly used herbicide applied to crops in the spring; and the insulating chemicals used in transformers and electrical capacitors, such as the polychlorinated biphenyls (PCBs) and dioxin (TCDD), a substance that is a by-product of the incineration of paper products and chlorinated plastics.

FIGURE 15.20

A warning sign showing a possible contamination of water sources by overflowing sewage has become a common sight in cities and towns across the United States.

Historically, governmental regulation of chemical pollutants has targeted those chemicals discharged by industries and municipal sewage treatment facilities. These pollutants, present in high concentrations and known to be detrimental to human health, are relatively easy to identify. Within the past decade, however, two new types of pollutants have been detected in our waterways and are raising health concerns. These are endocrine-disrupting chemicals (EDCs) and pharmaceuticals and personal care products (PPCPs). Endocrine disruptors include pesticides, commercial chemicals, and environmental contaminants that can disrupt, imitate, or block the body's normal hormonal activity, causing developmental or reproductive problems. Evidence for this has been found in certain species of fish and wildlife. Thus far, the relationship between EDCs and human diseases of the endocrine system is poorly understood and remains scientifically controversial.[30] Currently, the EPA Endocrine Disruption Screening Program is evaluating about 87,000 chemicals to try to determine whether they pose a risk to the human endocrine system.

PPCPs are synthetic chemicals found in everyday consumer health care products and cosmetics. These products include prescription and over-the-counter drugs; cosmetics, including soaps and shampoos; fragrances; sunscreens; diagnostic agents; biopharmaceuticals; and many others. PPCPs have been detected in water supplies around the world, and their effects on human health are the subject of scientific investigations. How do PPCPs get into our water sources? They are flushed down our toilets and washed down our drains and transported to our wastewater treatment plants, where they are discharged, mostly unchanged, into our rivers and streams. The risks posed by PPCPs to humans, aquatic life, and wildlife are essentially unknown. The exception is the increase in resistance of some pathogenic bacteria to antibiotics.[31]

While the EPA and other researchers are working to assess the effects of EDCs and PPCPs, there are no governmental regulations or guidance for the disposal of pharmaceuticals meant for personal use. Because it is important to take some personal action to reduce their presence in our environment, we should dispose of unused or unwanted medication in an environmentally sound manner. Disposal into the domestic sewage system is the *least* desirable option. Two better alternatives are (1) contacting a local pharmacy to see if it takes expired or unwanted medicines, or (2) turning them in to a local hazardous waste collector. If neither of these options is available, disposal in household trash is a better alternative than disposal in the sewage system.[31]

Water quality in the United States has deteriorated in many communities. This deterioration can be attributed to four causes:[32]

1. Population growth—an increase in the number of people generating waste
2. Widespread and ever-increasing chemical manufacture and usage, particularly synthetic organic chemicals
3. Reckless land-use practices that result in runoff of pollutants into waterways
4. Gross mismanagement and irresponsible disposal of hazardous wastes

As the public's knowledge of the endangerment of water quality in the United States grows, so will the number of strategies and the public will to protect it.

Strategies to Ensure Safe Water
Strategies used to ensure safe water in the United States today include proper drinking water and wastewater treatment, pollution prevention, and water quality regulation.

Treatment of Water for Domestic Use
Water in the United States is used for various purposes. In 2002, the greatest use was for thermoelectric power (48%), followed by agriculture, including aquaculture and livestock (36%), public and domestic water supply (11%), and industrial and mining use (6%).[33] Domestic water use in the United States includes water for drinking, cooking, washing dishes and laundry, bathing, flushing toilets, and outdoor use (such as watering lawns and gardens and washing cars). Most people are surprised to learn how much water we use in our homes. Americans use 80 to 100 gallons of water each day, just by flushing the toilet, showering, washing laundry, and other domestic uses.[34]

Whereas many rural residents in the United States obtain their water from untreated private wells (groundwater), urban residents obtain their water from municipal water treatment plants. About two-thirds of the municipalities use surface water, while one-third use groundwater.

Virtually all surface water is polluted and needs to be treated before it can be safely consumed. The steps in surface water treatment vary from plant to plant, but the following four steps are almost always included:

1. *Coagulation and flocculation:* A chemical such as Alum (aluminum sulfate) is added to the water to cause suspended solids to attract one another and form larger particles (floc).
2. *Sedimentation:* The water is permitted to stand so that the large particles (flocs) will settle out.
3. *Filtration:* The water passes through filters (often carbon and sand filters) in order to remove any solids and dissolved chemicals remaining after sedimentation; these are absorbed or retained by the filter media.
4. *Disinfection:* Chlorine is added or sometimes ozone is applied to the water to kill viruses, bacteria, algae, and fungi. Disinfection is sometimes accompanied by fluoridation, which helps prevent dental decay.

The responsibility of municipal water treatment plants is to provide water that is chemically and bacteriologically safe for human consumption. It is also desirable that the water be aesthetically pleasing in regard to taste, odor, color, and clarity. Above all, the municipal water supply must be reliable. Reliability in regard to both quantity and quality has always been regarded as nonnegotiable in planning a treatment facility.

The treated water, now safe to drink, is pumped to community water storage tanks and then to the distribution system, through which it reaches homes. The integrity of this distribution system is not always reliable. There can be breaks in the pipes, sometimes in the vicinity of sewer lines that also may be leaking. Therefore, a residual level of chlorine to kill bacteria must remain in the water until it reaches the tap. This is insurance against contamination during distribution.

The quality of drinking water supplied by municipalities is regulated by the EPA. Each municipality must monitor the water it serves to its customers and report on its quality to the EPA as well as to the public. Your water supplier provides an annual report about the quality of your tap water, its sources, and the processes used to treat it in a consumer confidence report (see Box 15.9).

Wastewater Treatment

Wastewater is the substance that remains after humans have used water for domestic or commercial purposes. Such water, also sometimes referred to as *liquid waste* or *sewage,* consists of about 99.9% water and 0.1% suspended and dissolved solids. The solids consist of human feces, soap, paper, garbage grindings (food parts), and a variety of other items that are put into wastewater systems from homes, schools, commercial buildings, hotels/motels, hospitals, industrial plants, and other facilities connected to the sanitary sewer system. Many municipalities also treat stormwater that has become contaminated by contact with surfaces such as roadways; this water is collected by a system of storm sewers.

wastewater
the aqueous mixture that remains after water has been used or contaminated by humans

The primary purpose of wastewater treatment is to improve the quality of wastewater to the point that it might be released into a body of water without seriously disrupting the aquatic environment, causing health problems in humans in the form of waterborne disease, or causing nuisance conditions.

BOX 15.9 — WHAT IS THE QUALITY OF TAP WATER IN YOUR TOWN OR CITY?

The Consumer Confidence Rule requires public water suppliers to provide consumer confidence reports (CCRs), also known as water quality reports, to their customers. The CCR summarizes information about the sources of drinking water (i.e., rivers, lakes, reservoirs, or aquifers), lists any contaminants detected, provides educational information, and ensures compliance with regulations. To learn about the quality of your municipal tap water, go to the EPA Web site (www.epa.gov) and search for safe water maps.

1. Click on your state and select the city or town of your residence. You will find a link to the water supplier serving that town. The organization of the links will vary for each city. Research the link, make sure you are on the Web page of your town's water supplier, and search the site for the water quality report or consumer confidence report (CCR). This will usually be a PDF (portable document file).

2. Open the water quality report, read it (print it, if necessary), and answer the following questions:

   a. What is the source of drinking water for your town?

   b. Which contaminants were detected in your drinking water system?

   c. What are the sources of these contaminants and what are the consequences of exposure to them?

   d. Did these contaminants exceed the federally allowable level (the maximum contaminant level, or MCL)?

   e. What other contaminants are listed on the report and why?

   f. What are the current concerns and activities of the water utility that provides you with drinking water?

   g. Based on your research, do you consider the water to be safe to drink? Explain your answer.

   h. Is there anything else you would like to see in this report?

Municipal Wastewater Treatment

There are four stages of wastewater treatment: preliminary, primary, secondary, and tertiary. Most municipalities and many large companies have wastewater treatment plants that incorporate at least primary and secondary treatment processes (see Figure 15.21). Upon delivery of wastewater to the treatment facility through a conveyance system, raw sewage passes through preliminary treatment processes that remove larger solids, such as toilet paper, trash, twigs, sand, and small gravel.

Primary Treatment

sludge
a semiliquid mixture of solid waste that includes bacteria, viruses, organic matter, toxic metals, synthetic organic chemicals, and solid chemicals

Primary treatment of wastewater is a physical/mechanical process that uses sedimentation to separate liquid, solids, and oil and grease. This occurs in a sedimentation tank, also called a *clarifier*, where wastewater is in a quiescent condition for about two to four hours. Here, heavier solid particles settle to the bottom, forming a layer referred to as **sludge.** Sludge is a gooey, semisolid mixture that includes bacteria, viruses, organic matter, toxic metals, synthetic organic chemicals, and solids.[3] Above the sludge remains most of the wastewater, including many bacteria and chemicals. On top of the water layer is a layer of oils and fats, also called *scum*. The layers of sludge and scum are removed, and the clarified wastewater enters the secondary stage of treatment.

Secondary Treatment

Secondary treatment consists of biological and physical treatment processes. For the biological process to occur, aerobic bacteria are added and mixed with clarified wastewater to break down the organic waste; this mixture then flows to aeration tanks. Here oxygen is continuously added to support aerobic decomposition of organic waste into carbon dioxide, water, and minerals. When this biological process is completed (after about 6 to 10 hours), the wastewater is sent to sedimentation tanks, where solids and flocks of bacteria are separated from the treated liquid portion of wastewater in quiescent conditions. After this process, many treatment plants discharge treated wastewater to surface water bodies. However, this effluent must comply with federal regulation and not impair the water quality of receiving streams and rivers. Today many wastewater plants perform additional treatment processes.

Tertiary Treatment (Advanced Sewage Treatment)

The third level of treatment usually involves filtration through sand and carbon filters. During this process, many remaining dissolved pollutants are removed.

Finally, whether wastewater is discharged after secondary or tertiary treatment, it is recommended that the wastewater be disinfected. The least expensive way of disinfecting is to chlorinate. After chlorination is completed, chlorine is removed from the water through a process called *dechlorination* to prevent poisoning of aquatic life in streams or rivers downstream of the discharge point. Some municipalities use ozone or ultraviolet radiation for disinfection because these disinfectants do not harm aquatic species downstream and discharged wastewater does not need to be dechlorinated chemically. About half the wastewater treatment plants in the United States disinfect discharged water with chlorine. The treated wastewater discharged to water bodies should not negatively affect aquatic life present in those ecosystems. Discharges of treated wastewater are regulated by the EPA.

FIGURE 15.21
A wastewater treatment facility.

Septic Systems

Septic systems are the means by which those who live in unsewered areas dispose of sewage. Presently, approximately 25% of all Americans live in unsewered areas.[3]

A septic system consists of two major components—a septic tank and a buried sand filter or absorption field (see Figure 15.22). The **septic tank,** which is a watertight concrete or fiberglass tank, is buried in the ground some distance from the house and is connected to it by a pipe. The system works in the following way. Sewage leaves the home via the toilets or drains and goes through the pipe to the septic tank. In the septic tank, the wastewater is retained in quiescent conditions for one to two days, during which separation of heavier solids and lighter scum from liquid wastewater occurs in the process called *sedimentation.* Sludge accumulates at the bottom of the tank. Because the septic tank is airtight, anaerobic conditions occur and part of the sludge will be partially decomposed by anaerobic microorganisms. The liquid portion of wastewater is then carried by a pipe to an absorption field.

The **absorption field** consists of a system of trenches (dugout channels) where perforated pipes are surrounded by gravel. As wastewater trickles through the gravel, films of aerobic microorganisms develop and feed on this liquid wastewater, causing decomposition of organic waste. This treated wastewater then infiltrates through the soil profile into the groundwater. As you can imagine, if this system does not operate correctly, it can be a potential source of fecal contamination of groundwater and surface water that can endanger human

septic tank
a watertight concrete or fiberglass tank that holds sewage; one of two main parts of a septic system

absorption field
the element of a septic system in which the liquid portion of waste is distributed

FIGURE 15.22
A septic system consists of a septic tank and an absorption field. This system is commonly used to treat domestic wastewater in suburban and rural areas.

health. Therefore, the system must be (1) located in appropriate soil, (2) properly constructed and inspected prior to being buried, and (3) maintained regularly. Septic tanks need to be pumped out every three to five years to remove sludge and thus prevent overflow, sewage backup to the house, or failure of the absorption field. Absorption fields must be constructed in soils suitable for carrying out the infiltration of treated wastewater. Soils that are not sufficiently permeable will cause wastewater to build up on the surface above the septic system, resulting in unsanitary conditions and contaminated runoff that could pollute rivers and streams. Additionally, absorption fields must be placed well above the groundwater level to avoid its contamination. Clearly, regular maintenance of the septic system is absolutely crucial for its optimal performance. Failure to properly maintain the system can result in fecal contamination of both land and water sources. Septic systems cannot be installed without a permit. Local health departments are responsible for issuing permits, inspecting the systems, and enforcing state and local regulations regarding them.

Protection of Water Quality through Regulation

Surface water and drinking water are regulated by two different regulations. Growing public concern over the pollution of surface water sources, such as rivers, lakes, estuaries, coastal waters, and wetlands, led to enactment of the Federal Water Pollution Control Act Amendments of 1972 and 1977, when this law became commonly known as the **Clean Water Act (CWA).** The goal of the CWA is to restore and maintain the chemical, physical, and biological integrity of the waters in the United States so that they can support "the protection and propagation of fish, shellfish, and wildlife and recreation in and on the water." In other words, the goal is to return the quality of surface waters to swimmable and fishable status. To achieve this goal, the EPA employs various regulatory and nonregulatory programs to reduce direct pollutant discharges into waterways by industrial and wastewater treatment facilities. In addition, the agency attempts to manage polluted runoff by implementing nonregulatory programs.

In the early years of the CWA's implementation, the agency's efforts focused on regulating discharges from traditional point source facilities, such as municipal sewage plants and industrial facilities. The CWA made it unlawful for any person to discharge any pollutant from a point source into navigable waters without a permit. Not much attention was paid to nonpoint source pollution from urban, agricultural, and stormwater runoff. However, since the late 1980s, the EPA has significantly increased its efforts to address polluted nonpoint source runoff and implemented either voluntary or regulatory programs to curb this problem. In its efforts to reduce and manage water pollution, the EPA considers land use and sources of pollution within the entire **watershed** rather than controlling and regulating only individual pollution sources or contaminants. The watershed approach places emphasis on protecting healthy waters and restoring impaired ones to protect not only human but also environmental health.

The quality of drinking water is of the utmost importance to the health of millions of people in communities around the United States and the world. Drinking water that is not properly treated, disinfected, and distributed in a clean and well-maintained distribution system may pose health risks to entire communities. Although it is easy to take the quality of tap water for granted, there are many threats to drinking water through pollution. Therefore, the quality of our drinking water is regulated by the **Safe Drinking Water Act (SDWA)** and its amendments. The SDWA implements many actions to protect drinking water and its sources (rivers, lakes, reservoirs, springs, and groundwater). Under the SDWA, the EPA sets national standards to limit the levels of contaminants in drinking water and oversees the states, localities, and water suppliers who implement those standards. The national standard for each contaminant is set at the level of the contaminant that is allowed in drinking water in order to protect public health, also called the maximum contaminant level (MCL). Currently, 87 MCLs

Clean Water Act (CWA) the federal law aimed at ensuring that all rivers are swimmable and fishable and that limit the discharge of pollutants in U.S. waters to zero

watershed the area of land from which all of the water that is under it or drains from it goes into the same place and drains in one point; for example, the Mississippi River watershed drains and collects all the water from the land extending from east of the Rocky Mountains to the Appalachian Mountains and from the upper Midwest all the way south to the Gulf of Mexico

Safe Drinking Water Act (SDWA) the federal law that regulates the safety of public drinking water are implemented and enforced for both naturally occurring and human-made contaminants that may be found in drinking water and its sources.[35] Although this number seems insignificant compared with the vast number of chemicals found in drinking water, development of a standard for just one such pollutant takes years of scientific research and discussion. The SDWA requires the EPA to go through a long and intensive process to identify new contaminants that may require regulation in the future. The EPA must periodically release a list of unregulated contaminants—the Contaminant Candidate List—to prioritize research and data collection that would help determine whether it should regulate a specific contaminant.[36]

Environmentalists and others would like to see the provisions of the SDWA strengthened and more vigorously enforced. But Congress is under pressure by water-polluting industries. Lobbyists for these industries, which include mining and timber industries, point to the high administrative and enforcement costs of this act and the cost burden it places on municipal and privately owned water supply systems as reasons not to strengthen the provisions. They also question the benefits of strengthening the act. How many cases of waterborne illness actually would be prevented by passage and enforcement of stricter regulations?

Radiation

Radiation is the energy released when atoms are split or naturally decay from a less stable to a more stable form. This released energy can break chemical bonds among molecules in living cells and tissues. The body may be able to repair this tissue damage, if it is mild, but if the damage is too severe or widespread it cannot be repaired and is manifest in radiation burns or radiation sickness or both. Radiation sickness includes nausea, weakness, hair loss, skin burns, diminished organ function, premature aging, or even death. The amount of radiation and the duration of exposure affect the severity of the injury or illness. (Cancer patients who receive radiation treatments often experience some of the acute effects of radiation, if the dose they receive is high enough.)

Another consequence of chronic radiation exposure is cancer, an uncontrolled growth of cells. (Cancer is discussed in Chapter 4.) Radiation can also cause mutations—changes in the cells' genetic material (DNA). If these are reproductive cells, the changes can be teratogenic (damaging to a fetus or future generation).

Although radiation provides us with certain benefits—in medical use, for example—its misuse or mishandling can have catastrophic consequences, as in the case of the nuclear power plant accident in Chernobyl in 1986. Therefore, a thorough knowledge of the sources, properties, and proper use of radiation, as well as proper methods of its disposal, is necessary to protect human health and the environment.

Sources of Radiation
We are exposed to low levels of radiation daily from both natural and human-made sources (see Figure 15.23).

Naturally Occurring Radiation
Naturally occurring radiation comes from three sources. That which comes to the earth from outer space and the sun is referred to as **cosmic radiation. Terrestrial radiation** comes from radioactive minerals that are within the earth—soil and rocks. Therefore, people who live near these substances (which include traces of uranium), or who live or work in buildings made of brick and stone that contain radioactive materials, have greater exposure. Radon gas is the biggest contributor to terrestrial radiation. The third source of naturally occurring radiation is **internal radiation**—that is, radiation internal to the human body. Exposure to such radiation occurs as a result of ingesting food or drugs and inhaling air that contains radioactive atoms.

radiation
energy released when atoms are split or naturally decay from a less stable to a more stable form

cosmic radiation
radiation that comes from outer space and the sun

terrestrial radiation
radiation that comes from radioactive minerals within the earth

internal radiation
radiation in the human body that occurs as a result of ingesting food and inhaling air containing radioactive particles

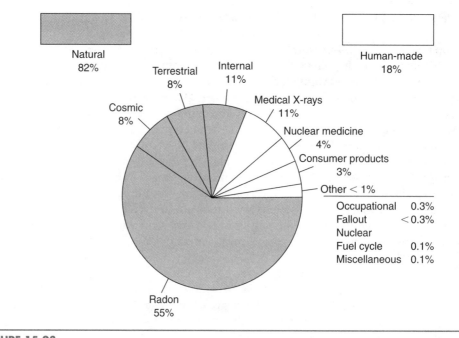

FIGURE 15.23

Sources of ionizing radiation.

Source: National Council on Radiation Protection and Measurements. NCRP Report no. 93. Reprinted with permission.

Individual behavior plays a definite role in the amount of exposure a person receives. For example, those who work or sunbathe outside, especially at higher elevations, increase their exposure to cosmic radiation. Similarly, miners and bricklayers are at greater risk for terrestrial exposure. Those who drink from contaminated wells may be at greater risk of exposure to internal radiation as well.

Human-Made Radiation

Sources of human-made radiation include the radiation used in medical and dental procedures such as X-rays, nuclear medicine diagnoses, and radiation therapy. Other sources of human-made radiation are nuclear power plants, certain consumer products (such as smoke detectors), X-rays for security checks, tobacco, television and computer screens, and nuclear weapons.

Do the benefits derived from the use of radiation outweigh the risks? Most would agree that the use of radiation for medical purposes is justified. However, there is less agreement about the cost/benefit question in the case of nuclear power plants, which currently provide about 7% of our energy.[37]

There is a continually growing demand for energy in this country. The United States and Canada make up only 5% of the world's population but consume 25% of the available energy.[37] America's access to oil is not unlimited, and much of our coal contains sulfur, which contributes to acid deposition. There are advantages as well as dangers to nuclear energy. For example, nuclear power plants do not produce carbon dioxide, and they reduce our reliance on foreign oil reserves. However, these facilities produce large volumes of radioactive waste, pose significant environmental and human health risks when failure occurs, and are costly to build, run, and decommission at the end of their expected life.

Currently, there are 103 nuclear power plants in 31 states. It has been more than twenty years since there has been a serious nuclear accident in this country, and there is stirring interest in maintaining these nuclear power plants and in building new ones. Many analysts feel nuclear power is a technology whose time has passed. It is too centralized and too vulnerable to terrorist attacks. The George W. Bush administration argues that nuclear power is an option we should keep open in case we need it. One concern with nuclear power is how to dispose of high-level radioactive waste because of the limited availability of storage and disposal sites. At this time no country has a permanent storage solution for these wastes. In the United States the area of Yucca Mountain in Nevada, located 90 miles northwest of Las Vegas, was chosen as a new site for high-level nuclear waste disposal.[38] The site was considered to be suitable for storage because it is unpopulated and very dry, and radioactive waste deposited there would be unlikely to cause groundwater contamination. However, the site has experienced seismic activity since its selection, which has been a concern. The Yucca Mountain site has become controversial, and lawsuits have been filed in federal court. Meanwhile, the transportation of radioactive waste to the site has also been controversial, because nobody wants trucks hauling nuclear waste passing near them. As controversies surrounding the safe disposal of high-level nuclear waste continue and the Yucca Mountain site continues to experience construction delays,[38] the U.S. Department of Energy seems unable to resolve these issues.[39] Thus, the outlook for building any new nuclear power plants in the immediate future in the United States appears dim.

Noise Pollution

Of all environmental pollution, the type that receives the least attention in this country is **noise pollution,** or excessive or unwanted sound. However, noise pollution can contribute to hearing loss, stress, and emotional problems; it can interrupt concentration and cause unintentional injuries.

What Is Noise and How Is It Measured?

Sound is heard when energy from vibrations, traveling through air, liquid, or solid media as pressure waves, is received by the ear. Unwanted, unpleasant sound is referred to as *noise.*[3] However, what constitutes unwanted sound is a matter of subjective judgment. What is considered a reasonable amount of sound to teenagers often is noise to their parents. In this regard, noise is measured by an annoyance factor. Yet, there are ways to scientifically measure and quantify noise (sound).

Amplitude refers to the sound volume; that is, its loudness or intensity. Amplitude is measured and expressed as **decibels (dB).** The decibel scale, which is logarithmic in nature, ranges from 0 dB, the threshold of hearing, to 180 dB, the sound of a rocket engine.[3] Thus, a sound measured at 10 dB is 10 times louder than 0 dB, and 20 dB is 100 times louder than 0 dB.

Three standardized weightings—A, B, and C—are used. Currently, federal regulations require the use of the A network when measuring sound in environmental and occupational settings. Thus, the preferred notation using this network is dBA instead of dB. Most sound-level meters are calculated using dBA. Table 15.3 lists some commonly encountered sounds and their dBA levels.

Approaches to Noise Abatement

Because serious hearing problems can arise from noise pollution, communities need to take the necessary steps to control unwanted sound. To date, the most common means of dealing with noise pollution have been policy (legislation), educational programs, and environment changes.

noise pollution
excessive sound;
unwanted sound

amplitude
the loudness or
intensity of sound,
measured in decibels

decibels (dB)
a measure of sound
amplitude

Table 15.3
Commonly Encountered Sounds and Their Decibel (dBA) Levels

			Effects		
Sound Intensity Factor	**Sound Level (dBA)**	**Sources**	**Perceived Loudness**	**Damage to Hearing**	**Community Reaction to Outdoor Noise**
1,000,000,000,000,000,000	180	Rocket engine		Tramatic injury	
100,000,000,000,000,000	170				
10,000,000,000,000,000	160				
1,000,000,000,000,000	150	Jet plane at takeoff	Painful	Injurious range; irreversible damage	
100,000,000,000,000	140				
10,000,000,000,000	130	Maximum recorded rock music			
1,000,000,000,000	120	Thunderclap; textile loom; auto horn, 3.3 ft (1 m) away	Uncomfortably loud	Danger zone; progressive loss of hearing	
100,000,000,000	110	Riveter; jet flyover at 985 ft (300 m)			
10,000,000,000	100	Newpaper press			
1,000,000,000	90	Motorcycle, 26 ft (8 m) away; food blender	Very loud		Vigorous action
100,000,000	80	Diesel truck, 50 mph (80 km/hr), 50 ft (15 m) away; garbage disposal		Damage begins after long exposure	Threats
10,000,000	70	Vacuum cleaner			Widespread complaints
1,000,000	60	Ordinary conversation; air-conditioning unit, 20 ft (6 m) away	Moderately loud		Occasional complaints
100,000	50	Light traffic noise, 100 ft (30 m) away			
10,000	40	Average living room; bedroom	Quiet		No action
1,000	30	Library; soft whisper			
100	20	Broadcasting studio	Very quiet		
10	10	Rustling leaf			
1	0	Threshold of hearing	Barely audible		

Source: Jonathan Turk and Amos Turk (1987). *Physical Science with Environmental and Other Practices,* 3rd ed. Philadelphia: Saunders College Publishing. Reproduced by permission Brooks/Cole, a division of Thomson Learning: www.thomsonrights.com.

Policy

The development of a federal policy for noise control has lagged behind that for other environmental problems—probably because by its very nature, noise is a local problem. However, in 1972, Congress passed the Noise Control Act (NCA). This act was aimed at regulating noise emissions from new consumer products. In 1978, Congress amended the NCA to include the Quiet Communities Act. This set of amendments authorized the EPA to assist local and state governments in developing noise reduction programs that would meet their specific needs. Through the amendments, federal dollars were provided to help local governments put their programs into action. Most people still view noise as a nuisance and not as a health problem. Until noise pollution becomes recognized as detrimental to health, it will continue to be overlooked and underfunded.

Educational Programs

Another approach to noise control is education. The goal in this approach is to alter the behavior of those generating the noise, thereby reducing noise at the source. So far, little measurable progress has been achieved through noise education programs, and no model noise education program has been widely accepted.

Environmental Changes

Noise abatement can be achieved through environmental modification. This modification can be made at the source of the noise, to the path it travels, or to the exposed parties. An example of reducing noise at its source is the common practice of placing a computer printer in a padded compartment. An example of altering the path on which noise travels can be seen in the large dirt mound placed at the beginning of the airport runway to absorb the jet engine sound from surrounding areas. Ways to protect against damaging effects of noise pollution include wearing ear protection in the form of earplugs or headsets, as is often practiced in manufacturing facilities.

CHAPTER SUMMARY

- The environment consists of all the external conditions, circumstances, and influences surrounding and affecting the growth and development of an organism or community of organisms.

- There are both natural and human-made hazards that threaten habitats, climates, and ultimately the health of both individuals and their communities.

- Residues and wastes from human activities have been increasing rapidly because of urbanization, industrialization, population growth, and reliance on disposable products and containers (especially in the United States).

- Types of wastes and pollution include solid wastes, hazardous wastes, air pollution, water pollution, radiation, and noise pollution.

- Widespread recognition of the growing problem of environmental pollution officially occurred in 1970, with the celebration of the first Earth Day and the establishment of the Environmental Protection Agency (EPA).

- A number of significant pieces of federal legislation have been passed to protect our land, air, and water from further contamination, including the Resource Conservation and Recovery Act; the Comprehensive Environmental Response, Compensation, and Liability Act; the Clean Air Act; the Clean Water Act; and the Safe Drinking Water Act.

- Progress has been made in cleaning up our air, water, and even abandoned hazardous waste sites. However, there is still a great deal of work to do.

- Greater effort is needed by communities and individuals to increase the levels of recycling, source reduction, and resource conservation if we are to leave a healthy environment to future generations.

REVIEW QUESTIONS

1. What are the primary sources of solid waste? Why are municipal wastes such a problem?

2. What piece of federal legislation deals with cradle-to-grave regulation of solid hazardous waste?

3. Define the following terms—*sanitary landfill, combustion, recycling,* and *source reduction.* Provide one advantage and one disadvantage for each process.

4. Define the term *hazardous waste* and give several examples.

5. The Superfund was part of what legislation? What is the Superfund used for?

6. What is the Number 1 source of air pollution?

7. In what forms can air pollutants be found?

8. What are the six criteria air pollutants?

9. What is the Air Quality Index (AQI)?

10. Outline the process and conditions that result in acid rain.

11. How does the greenhouse effect result in global warming?

12. Why is ozone depletion occurring?

13. What relationship is there between photochemical smog and thermal inversion?

14. Why was the Clean Air Act so important to the United States?

15. Name six indoor air pollutants.

16. What is meant by *sick building syndrome*?

17. What makes water so important to life?

18. What is the difference between point source and non-point source pollution?

19. How does the Clean Water Act and its amendments help to protect the water supply?

20. What is the Safe Drinking Water Act?

21. What is the purpose of municipal wastewater treatment?

22. What is a septic system?

23. What is radiation?

24. What types of human behavior increase exposure to radiation?

25. What types of radiation are dangerous to humans? Why?

26. How have humans benefited from radiation?

27. What is noise?

28. What are decibels? What do they measure?

29. What level of government passes the most noise ordinances?

ACTIVITIES

1. In order for all of us to be better stewards of our environment, we need to be aware of how our community handles various important environmental issues. Find the answers to the following questions about your community and state:

   How does your community dispose of solid waste?

   How far do you live from a secured landfill? What is the closest community to it?

   Where does your community get its water? If you personally get your water from a well, when was the last time the water was evaluated?

   Where is the closest nuclear power plant to your home? What are you supposed to do in case of an accident?

   Does your state/community have a clean indoor air act? If it does, briefly describe it.

   Does your community have a noise ordinance? If so, briefly describe it.

   What is the most recent piece of legislation your community has enacted to protect the environment? Do you agree with it? Why or why not?

2. Write a one-page paper describing either your support for or opposition to (a) nuclear power plants or (b) strengthening the Safe Drinking Water Act.

3. In a one-page paper, identify what you feel to be the Number 1 waste or pollution problem faced by the United States and then detail your rationale for feeling this way.

4. For two weeks, watch a television weather program that mentions the Air Quality Index (AQI). During that two-week period, chart the AQI in a graph form and identify the major pollutant for each day.

5. During the next week, create a list of at least 10 things you could have done to conserve the water you use.

COMMUNITY HEALTH ON THE WEB

The Internet contains a wealth of information about community and public health. Increase your knowledge of some of the topics presented in this chapter by accessing the Jones and Bartlett Publishers Web site at **http://health.jbpub.com/book/communityhealth/ 6e** and follow the links to complete the following Web activities.

- Environmental Protection Agency
- The Health Effects Institute
- Headquarters Solid Waste and Emergency Response

SCENARIO: ANALYSIS AND RESPONSE

As you know from reading this chapter, the problem Mary and Tom face is not so uncommon. The National Priority List (NPL) associated with the Superfund legislation has over 1,300 known hazardous waste sites that still need to be cleaned up.

1. Knowing what you now know about polluted water, what could Mary and Tom have done before purchasing their house to try to ensure against such a problem?

2. If you were confronted with the problem that Mary and Tom now face, how would you handle it?

3. Would you continue to live in the home, or would you move?

4. If you planned to sell the house, would you tell the realtor or prospective buyers about the problem?

5. Is it fair that Mary and Tom are faced with this problem? Name five things you could do to help prevent such a problem in the future.

REFERENCES

1. Centers for Disease Control and Prevention (2004). "Health Effects of Tsunamis." Available at http://www.bt.cdc.gov/disasters/tsunamis/healtheff.asp.

2. Blong, R. J. (1984). *Volcanic Hazards: A Sourcebook on the Effects of Eruptions.* Australia: Academic Press, 83–91.

3. Miller, G. T. (2004). *Living in the Environment: Principles, Connections, and Solutions,* 13th ed. Pacific Grove, CA: Brooks/Cole-Thomson Learning.

4. U.S. Environmental Protection Agency (October 2006). *Municipal Solid Waste in the United States: 2005 Facts and Figures* (EPA530-S-06-001). Washington, DC: Author. Available at http://www.epa.gov/msw/pubs/ex-sum05.pdf.

5. U.S. Environmental Protection Agency (2007). "Municipal Solid Waste: Basic Facts." Available at http://www.epa.gov/msw/facts.htm.

6. Organization for Economic Cooperation and Development (2005). *OECD in Figures: Statistics on the Member Countries.* Paris: OECD Publishing. Available at http://www.oecd.org/document/62/0,2340,en_2825_495628_2345918_1_1_1_1,00.html.

7. U.S. Environmental Protection Agency (2004). "Municipal Solid Waste: Recycling." Available at http://www.epa.gov/epaoswer/non-hw/muncpl/recycle.htm.

8. U.S. Environmental Protection Agency (2004). "MSW Programs." Available at http://www.epa.gov/epaoswer/non-hw/muncpl/programs.htm.

9. U.S. Environmental Protection Agency (2003). *Municipal Solid Waste Generation, Recycling, and Disposal in the United States: Facts and Figures for 2003* (EPA530-F-05-003). Washington, DC: Author. Available at http://www.epa.gov/epaoswer/non-hw/muncpl/msw99.htm.

10. U.S. Environmental Protection Agency (2006). "Municipal Solid Waste: Recycling." Available at http://www.epa.gov/epaoswer/non-hw/muncpl/recycle.htm.

11. U.S. Environmental Protection Agency (2006). "Municipal Solid Waste: Reduce, Reuse, Recycle." http://www.epa.gov/epaoswer/non-hw/muncpl/reduce.htm.

12. U.S. Environmental Protection Agency (1996). "Standards of Performance for New Stationary Sources and Guidelines for Control of Existing Sources: Municipal Solid Waste Landfills." Final rule and guideline, *Federal Register,* March 12, 1996.

13. U.S. Environmental Protection Agency (2006). "Municipal Solid Waste: eCycling." Available at http://www.epa.gov/epaoswer/hazwaste/recycle/ecycling/index.htm.

14. U.S. Environmental Protection Agency (2003). *National Analysis: The National Biennial RCRA Hazardous Waste Report, Based on 2003 Data* (EPA530-R-03-007). Washington, DC: Author. Available at http://www.epa.gov/epaoswer/hazwaste/data/br03/national03.pdf.

15. U.S. Environmental Protection Agency (2006). "Underground Injection Control Program: Deep Wells (Class I)." Available at http://www.epa.gov/safewater/uic/classi.html.

16. U.S. Environmental Protection Agency (September 2005). *FY 2004 Superfund Annual Report* (EPA-540-R-05-001). Washington, DC: Author. Available at http://www.epa.gov/superfund/action/process/fy2004.htm.

17. U.S. Environmental Protection Agency (2006). "Superfund: Superfund Appropriation History." Available at http://www.epa.gov/superfund/action/process/budgethistory.htm.

18. U.S. Department of Health and Human Services (2000). *Healthy People 2010: Understanding and Improving Health,* 2nd ed. Washington, DC: U.S. Government Printing Office.

19. U.S. Environmental Protection Agency (2006). "Air Trends: Basic Information." Available at http://www.epa.gov/air/airtrends/sixpoll.html.

20. Chiras, D. D. (2002). *Environmental Science: Creating a Sustainable Future,* 6th ed. Sudbury, MA: Jones and Bartlett.

21. U.S. Environmental Protection Agency (2006). "Air Trends: National Trends in Ozone Levels." Available at http://www.epa.gov/air/airtrends/ozone.html.

22. Moeller, D. W. (1997). *Environmental Health.* Cambridge, MA: Harvard University Press, 93.

23. U.S. Environmental Protection Agency (2006). "Radon: Health Risks." Available at http://www.epa.gov/radon/healthrisks.html.

24. National Institute for Occupational Safety and Health (1991). *Environmental Tobacco Smoke in the Workplace: Lung Cancer and Other Health Effects* (HHS pub. no. NIOSH 91-108). Cincinnati, OH: Author.

25. Spengler, J. D. (1991). "Sources and Concentration of Indoor Air Pollution." In J. M. Samet and J. D. Spengler, eds., *Indoor Air Pollution: A Health Perspective.* Baltimore, MD: Johns Hopkins University Press, 33–67.

26. World Health Organization (2004). *The Sanitation Challenge: Turning Commitment into Reality.* Geneva: Author. Available at http://www.who.int/water_sanitation_health/hygiene/envsan/sanitchallenge/en/.

27. World Health Organization and UNICEF (2005). *Water for Life: Making It Happen.* Geneva: WHO/UNICEF Joint Monitoring Programme for Water Supply and Sanitation. Available at http://www.who.int/water_sanitation_health/monitoring/jmp2005/en/index.html.

28. World Health Organization and UNICEF (2000). *Global Water Supply and Sanitation Assessment 2000 Report.* Geneva: WHO/UNICEF Joint Monitoring Programme for Water Supply and Sanitation. Available at http://www.who.int/water_sanitation_health/monitoring/globalassess/en/index.html.

29. U.S. Environmental Protection Agency (September 2005). *Providing Safe Drinking Water in America: 2003 National Public Water Systems Compliance Report* (EPA-305R-05-002). Washington, DC: Author. Available at http://www.epa.gov/compliance/resources/reports/accomplishments/sdwa/sdwacom2003.pdf.

30. U.S. Environmental Protection Agency (2006). "The Endocrine Disruption Screening Program." Available at http://www.epa.gov/scipoly/oscpendo/pubs/edspoverview/primer.htm#3.

31. U.S. Environmental Protection Agency (2006). "Pharmaceuticals and Personal Care Products as Environmental Pollutants." Available at http://www.epa.gov/esd/chemistry/pharma/.

32. Steward, J. C. (1990). *Drinking Water Hazards: How to Know If There Are Toxic Chemicals in Your Water and What to Do If There Are.* Hiram, OH: Envirographics.

33. U.S. Geological Survey (2004). *Estimated Use of Water in the United States in 2000* (USGS Circular 1268). Denver, CO: Author. Available at http://pubs.usgs.gov/circ/2004/circ1268/.

34. U.S. Geological Survey (2005). "Water Q & A: Water Use at Home." Available at http://ga.water.usgs.gov/edu/qahome.html.

35. U.S. Environmental Protection Agency (2006). "Groundwater and Drinking Water: List of Drinking Water Contaminants and Their Maximum Contaminant Levels." Available at http://www.epa.gov/safewater/mcl.html#mcls.

36. U.S. Environmental Protection Agency (2004). "Drinking Water Contaminant Candidate List." Available at http://www.epa.gov/OGWDW/ccl/cclfs.html.

37. Cunningham, W. P., M. A. Cunningham, and B. W. Saigo (2005). *Environmental Science: A Global Concern,* 8th ed. New York: McGraw-Hill.

38. Las Vegas Review-Journal. (2006). "Yucca Mountain: Nuclear Waste in Nevada." Available at http://www.reviewjournal.com/news/yuccamtn/.

39. U.S. Department of Energy (2006). "Civilian Radioactive Waste Management: Yucca Mountain Repository." Available at http://www.ocrwm.doe.gov/ym_repository/index.shtml.

Chapter 16

The Impact of Environment on Human Health

Chapter Outline

Chapter Objectives

After studying this chapter you will be able to:

1 Define the terms *environmental health* and *environmental hazard.*

2 Explain the relationship between environmental sanitation and the prevention of waterborne disease outbreaks.

3 Explain the meaning of waterborne, foodborne, and vectorborne diseases and give an example of each.

4 Define the term *vector* and give examples.

5 Define *pest, pesticides, target organism,* and *persistent* and *nonpersistent pesticides.*

6 Explain the benefits and risks of using pesticides.

7 Define *environmental tobacco smoke, mainstream smoke, sidestream smoke,* and *passive smoking.*

8 Describe the legislation in place to deal with environmental tobacco smoke.

9 Describe the sources of lead in the environment and the progress made in reducing lead levels in the United States.

10 Define *ionizing radiation* and give examples.

11 Explain the dangers of radon gas.

12 Explain how human activities have increased the risk of skin cancer by altering the environment.

13 Explain the relationship between psychological hazards and loss of health and give an example.

14 Describe the state of population growth in the world.

15 Interpret the relationships among population growth, the environment, and human health.

16 Outline some solutions to population growth.

17 Define *natural disaster* and describe two agencies involved in disaster preparedness, response, and recovery.

SCENARIO

Pam and Gary were numb when their physician told them that the laboratory tests indicated that Gary had prostate cancer. Numb, yes—shocked, no, for Gary had served in Vietnam with the 151st Airborne Infantry Rangers in 1968–1969. During that time, his entire unit had been exposed to the herbicide Agent Orange, the defoliant used in Vietnam and Laos to eliminate enemy hiding places by destroying their crops. Agent Orange, composed of an equal mixture of 2,4-D (2,4-dichlorophenoxyacetic acid) and 2,4,5-T (2,4,5-trichlorophenoxyacetic acid), was named for the bright orange stripes on the steel drums in which it was contained. Later it was found that the 2,4,5-T was contaminated with an extremely toxic compound known as dioxin. Gary was aware that a number of other men in his unit had been diagnosed with cancer in the past couple of years, but he thought that somehow maybe the dreaded disease might have passed him by. Prior to the diagnosis Gary had suffered from rashes, and his skin always seemed dry.

INTRODUCTION

Environmental health is the study and management of environmental conditions that affect the health and well-being of humans. **Environmental hazards** are those factors or conditions in the environment that increase the risk of human injury, disease, or death. Regardless of whether the environment contributes a little or a lot to disease, all environment-induced disease is highly preventable.[1] Both individuals and communities can contribute to the elimination of environmental health risks. Individuals can protect their own health and the health of those around them by making wise choices the products they purchase, how they dispose of their waste, and their everyday behavior toward the environment, as well as their personal health behavior. Examples of personal choices are selecting environmentally friendly products (i.e., made from recycled or recyclable materials), not littering, picking up after your dog, disposing of expired medicine properly rather than flushing it down the toilet, properly disposing of household hazardous waste in community facilities rather than leaving them in trash cans or dumping them elsewhere outdoors, and recycling batteries that can be a source of hazardous waste. Communities can limit their exposure to environmental hazards by:

environmental health the study and management of environmental conditions that affect the health and well-being of humans

environmental hazards factors or conditions in the environment that increase the risk of human injury, disease, or death

- Supporting and using community recycling programs
- Protecting the quality of local water sources by reducing or properly managing use of fertilizers
- Keeping the community clean to avoid accumulation of trash
- Supporting local wastewater facilities in implementation of new plans for the treatment of stormwater
- Adopting environmentally sound practices in the production, transport, storage, and disposal of solid and hazardous waste
- Supporting environmentally and ecologically sustainable development in their communities

Environmental hazards can be biological, chemical, physical, psychological, or sociological. Some events, such as natural disasters or terrorist acts, can result in several types of environmental hazards. For example, Hurricane Katrina caused physical hazards (high winds, high precipitation, breach of the levees protecting the communities, infrastructure damage, and disruption of energy and water supplies), followed by biological and chemical hazards (floodwaters contaminated by sewage, oil drums washed inland from the shore, and propagation of insects in the stagnant water), and finally psychological and social hazards (such as fear and loss of homes and business and the witnessing of hardship and death).

Biological Hazards and Human Health

Biological hazards are living organisms (and viruses), or their products, that increase the risk of disease or death in humans. These may be animals (venomous snakes) or plants (toxic mushrooms), but they are usually viruses or microbes such as pathogenic bacteria and parasites. Because the immediate source of many biological hazards is humans themselves, the improper handling of human waste and wastewater can jeopardize the health of the community.

Environmental sanitation is the practice of establishing and maintaining healthy and hygienic conditions in the environment. The mismanagement of wastewater or solid waste can result in epidemics of **waterborne diseases,** illnesses and diseases transmitted through chemical or fecal contamination of drinking water. Environmental sanitation also includes protecting communities from unsafe food. The improper handling, storage, and service of food can result in outbreaks of **foodborne diseases.** Likewise, the overflow of wastewater into open fields and ditches or the mismanagement of solid waste near human habitation can result in outbreaks of **vectorborne diseases,** diseases transmitted by insects.

Waterborne Diseases

Waterborne diseases occur when water contaminated with a disease agent is consumed by a susceptible person. Waterborne disease agents include viruses, bacteria, parasites, and chemicals. Waterborne viral agents and the diseases they cause include poliomyelitis virus (polio) and hepatitis A virus (hepatitis). Waterborne bacteria and the diseases they cause include *Escherichia coli, Legionella* spp., *Salmonella typhi* (typhoid fever), *Shigella* spp. (shigellosis or bacillary dysentery), and *Vibrio cholerae* (cholera). Waterborne parasites include *Entamoeba histolytica* (amebiasis or amebic dysentery), *Giardia lamblia* (giardiasis), and *Cryptosporidium parvum* (cryptosporidiosis). Each of these diseases can be serious, and two in particular—typhoid fever and cholera—have killed thousands of people in single epidemics (see Table 16.1).

One of the earliest carefully documented cholera epidemics was the one that began in London, England, in 1849. This epidemic occurred before the discoveries of Louis Pasteur, during a period of time when most people thought that diseases were caused by malodorous vapors (miasmas) or, perhaps, by spirits. Dr. John Snow believed that water drawn from a particular city well was contaminated. After interviewing many sick and well people, he had the handle removed from the Broad Street pump; the cholera epidemic subsided. This event was so remarkable that the site has been preserved in modern-day London (see Figure 1.8).

biological hazards
living organisms (and viruses) or their products that increase the risk of disease or death in humans

environmental sanitation
the practice of establishing and maintaining healthy or hygienic conditions in the environment

waterborne disease
a disease transmitted through contamination of drinking water (for example, typhoid fever)

foodborne disease
a disease transmitted through the contamination of food (for example, salmonellosis)

vectorborne disease
a communicable disease transmitted by insects or other arthropods (for example, St. Louis encephalitis)

Table 16.1
Waterborne Biological Hazards

Hazard	Agent	Disease
Viruses	Poliomyelitis virus	Polio
	Hepatitis A virus	Infectious hepatitis
Bacteria	*Vibrio cholerae*	Cholera
	Salmonella typhi	Typhoid fever
	Shigella spp.	Bacillary dysentery
	Leptospira spp.	Leptospirosis
Protozoans (parasites)	*Entamoeba histolytica*	Amebic dysentery
	Giardia lamblia	Giardiasis
	Cryptosporidium parvum	Cryptosporidiosis

Source: Heymann, D. L., ed. (2004). *Control of Communicable Diseases Manual,* 18th ed. Washington, DC: American Public Health Association.

A **waterborne disease outbreak (WBDO)** is an event in which at least two persons experience a similar illness after ingestion of drinking water or after exposure to water used for recreational purposes *and* epidemiological evidence implicates water as the probable source of the illness.[2] In the case of chemical poisoning, a single case is considered an outbreak. WBDOs can be associated with drinking water, recreational water, or occupational water exposure. In recent years, the leading causes of WBDOs (in cases in which the cause was identified) have been bacteria and parasites.[2-4] During 2003-2004, 36 WBDOs were associated with drinking water, and a total of 62 were associated with recreational water.[5,6] Overall, the number of outbreaks associated with drinking water has declined and the number of outbreaks associated with recreational water has increased since the 1970s (see Figure 16.1). The specific cause—microbe or chemical—of waterborne diseases associated with drinking water was determined

> **waterborne disease outbreak (WBDO)**
> a disease in which at least two persons experience a similar illness after the ingestion of drinking water or after exposure to water used for recreational purposes and epidemiological evidence implicates water as the probable source of the illness

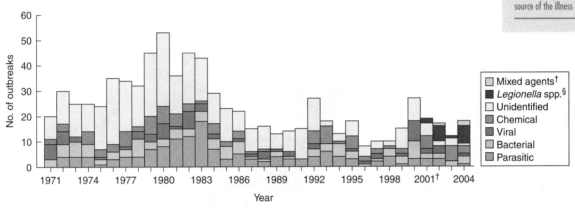

(a)

†Beginning in 2003, mixed agents of more than one etiologic agent type were included in the surveillance system. However, the first observation is a previously unreported outbreak in 2002.

§Beginning in 2001, Legionnaires' disease was added to the surveillance system, and *Legionella* spp. were classified separately in this figure.

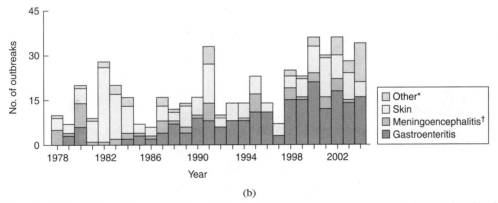

(b)

*Includes keratitis, conjunctivitis, otitis, bronchitis, meningitis, hepatitis, leptospirosis, Pontiac fever, acute respiratory illness, and combined illnesses.

†Also includes data from report of ameba infections.

FIGURE 16.1

(a) Historical trends of number of waterborne disease outbreaks (n = 803) associated with drinking water, by year and etiologic agent—United States, 1971-2004. (b) Historical trends of number of waterborne disease outbreaks (n = 508) associated with recreational water, by year and illness—United States, 1978-2004.

Sources: Centers for Disease Control and Prevention (2004). "Surveillance for Waterborne-Disease Outbreaks Associated with Drinking Water—United States, 2001-2002." *MMWR, 53*(SS08): 23-45. Centers for Disease Control and Prevention (2004). "Surveillance for Waterborne-Disease Outbreaks Associated with Recreational Water—United States, 2001-2002." *MMWR,* 53: 1-22.

in 71% of outbreaks, a significant improvement from the 1999–2000 reporting period, when the cause was determined in only 56.4% of the outbreaks. Where the cause was determined, bacteria of the genus *Legionella* were most often the cause of illness, followed by chemicals or toxins, other bacteria, viruses, and parasites (see Figure 16.2). Bacteria were also the leading cause of outbreaks associated with recreational waters in 2003–2004, constituting 32.3% of those outbreaks in which the causative agent was identified, followed by parasites (24.2%), viruses (9.7%), and chemicals/toxins (4.8%). In 29% of the outbreaks an agent could not be identified (see Figure 16.2).

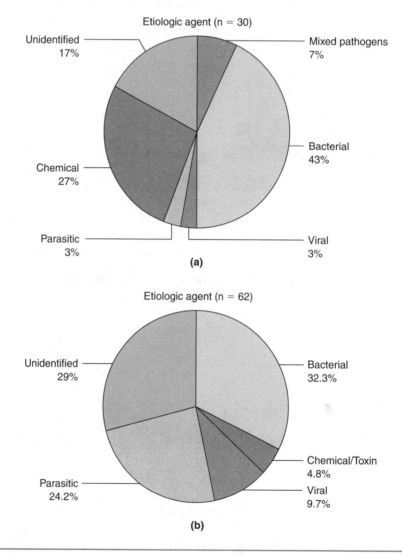

FIGURE 16.2

(a) Waterborne disease outbreaks associated with drinking water, by etiologic agent: United States, 2003–2004.
(b) Waterborne disease outbreaks of gastroenteritis associated with recreational water, by etiologic agent: United States, 2003–2005.

Waterborne disease outbreaks can be traced to individual wells or to a municipal water supply. During 2003–2004, only 42% of WBDOs associated with drinking water were associated with water regulated by water utilities.[6] Nonetheless, outbreaks associated with municipal water systems can become quite large. The largest WBDO ever reported in the United States occurred in Milwaukee, Wisconsin, in 1993. In that outbreak, 403,000 people became ill and 4,400 were hospitalized. The disease agent was identified as the parasite *Cryptosporidium parvum*. This outbreak occurred because of a breakdown in the city's water treatment plant.[4] (Refer to Chapter 15 for a summary of municipal water treatment.)

Waterborne disease outbreaks resulting from excessive levels of fluoride, copper, and nitrates can also occur. In one outbreak during 1993–1994, nitrate poisoning was associated with miscarriages (see Box 16.1).[4] In 2003–2004, eight outbreaks of chemical poisoning affecting 27 people were reported in the United States.[2]

Public health laws that set standards for water and wastewater treatment facilities and plumbing are a community's first line of defense against such epidemics. Although WBDOs occur from time to time in the United States, they occur much less frequently than in countries with developing economies, where access to safe drinking water and sanitation is limited or nonexistent. In 2005, the World Health Organization and the United Nations reported that 1.1 billion people lacked access to safe drinking water, and about 2.4 billion people lacked access to basic sanitation.[5]

One of the most significant achievements in public health during the last century occurred not by removing harmful elements from community drinking water, but by adding something to it. Fluoridation of community drinking water is a major factor responsible for the decline in dental caries (tooth decay) in the United States since 1950 (see Box 16.2). At first, caries reduction rates of 50% to 70% were reported. More recently, the reduction among adolescents has averaged 25%. Because fluoride has appeared in other products, such as toothpaste and mouthwashes, the difference in rates of caries between those who receive fluoridated water and those who do not has declined. By 1992, 144 million people were receiving fluoridated water, at an average cost of 31 cents per person per year. The savings from prevention of dental caries attributable to fluoridation was estimated for the period 1979–1989 at $39 billion (1990 dollars), a savings per person that in some communities reached $53 per person per year.[6]

BOX 16.1   NITRATE POISONING IN INDIANA TRACED TO A LEAKING HOG FARM WASTE PIT

Two episodes of nitrate poisoning, associated with eight miscarriages, were reported in Indiana in the mid-1990s. In the first episode, three women who lived within a mile of each other reported a total of six miscarriages during 1993 and 1994. All three women drank water from private wells on their premises and all three wells tapped the same aquifer, which was probably contaminated by a leaking waste pit on a nearby hog farm. The well water had high nitrate-nitrogen levels, 2 to 3 times the EPA's maximum contaminant level (MCL). No other toxic substances were found in the water. All three women delivered full-term babies after changing to nitrate-free drinking water. During that same period, five women who lived in the same geographical area and who had wells with nitrate levels below the EPA's MCL had five normal pregnancies.[4]

Many states and local communities are being confronted by the establishment of large-scale hog operations in areas that were once occupied by family farms. State regulations, originally passed to protect the family farmer, often shield these large-scale hog operations from stricter regulation. The waste pits on these large hog farms sometimes contaminate nearby water supplies. Is your state or local community experiencing such a problem? What community approaches might be effective in correcting this problem?

From Toothless Grins to Pearly Whites

At the beginning of the twentieth century, tooth decay was rampant, and because no effective preventive measures existed, tooth extraction was routine. Now, thanks to water fluoridation, combined with other dental health advances, adults in the United States are retaining most of their teeth thoughout their lifetime.

In 1901, soon after establishing his dental practice in Colorado Springs, Colorado, Dr. Frederick S. McKay noted an ususual permanent brown stain on the teeth of many of his patients. He concluded that something in the public water supply was probably responsible. McKay also observed that teeth affected by this condition seemed to be less susceptible to dental caries.

In 1931, Dr. H. Trendley Dean, a U.S. Public Health Service Dental Officer, conducted pioneering research into the relationship between fluoride and dental carries. His research laid the groundwork for community water fluoridation in the United States.

In 1945, Grand Rapids, Michigan, became the first city in the world to fluoridate its drinking water. The caries rate among Grand Rapids children born after fluoride was added to the water supply dropped 60%. This finding revolutionized dental care and resulted in tooth decay being preventable for most people.

Water fluoridation is relatively inexpensive in the United States. The benefits of fluoridation are available, on average, for little more than $0.50 per person per year, and even less in large communities.

The documented effectiveness of community water fluoridation in preventing dental caries prompted rapid adoption of this public health measure in cities throughout the United States. In the 1960s, the U.S. Public Health Service provided funding, technical expertise, and leadership to promote and establish fluoridation programs throughout the nation. The federal government continues to promote water fluoridation worldwide.

Foodborne Diseases

One way in which humans interact with their environment is by ingesting bits of it. The act of eating is, in effect, a way of bringing biological hazards into intimate contact with the tissues that line the intestinal tract. "More than 200 known diseases are transmitted through food. In these cases, food is the vehicle; and the agents can be viruses, bacteria, parasite's toxins, metals, and prions."[7] Symptoms of foodborne illness range from mild to severe, and organs involved can include stomach and intestines, liver, kidneys, and brain and nervous system. Foodborne diseases cause between 6 and 81 million cases of illness and up to 9,000 deaths each year in the United States.[7] A majority of these cases are never reported to the Centers for Disease Control and Prevention (CDC).

foodborne disease outbreak (FBDO) the occurrence of two or more cases of a similar illness resulting from the ingestion of food

The CDC defines a **foodborne disease outbreak (FBDO)** as the occurrence of two or more cases of a similar illness resulting from the ingestion of food.[8] During the five-year period 1993-1997, 2,751 FBDOs were reported, which resulted in illness in 86,058 persons. Only 32% of the outbreaks had a known etiology, which accounted for 50,788 illnesses.[9] In outbreaks for which the causative agent was established, bacterial pathogens caused 75% of the outbreaks and 86% of the cases. *Salmonella* serotype enteritidis accounted for the largest number of outbreaks, cases, and deaths, but *E. coli* O157:H7 was also responsible for multistate outbreaks that were associated with consumption of undercooked or raw ground beef. One of the food safety objectives of *Healthy People 2010* is to reduce outbreaks of infections caused by key foodborne bacteria by half (see Box 16.3). Chemicals were the cause of 17% of outbreaks (1% of cases) in which the cause was determined, viruses for 6% of outbreaks (8% of cases), and parasites for 2% of outbreaks (5% of cases) (see Figure 16.3).[9]

The leading factors that were found to contribute to FBDOs during 1993-1997 were improper holding temperatures and inadequate cooking of food.[8] Other factors that often contribute to FBDOs are poor personal hygiene of preparers, contaminated equipment, and obtaining food from an unsafe source (such as shellfish from polluted waters).

HEALTHY PEOPLE 2010 OBJECTIVE: REDUCE OUTBREAKS OF INFECTIONS CAUSED BY KEY FOODBORNE BACTERIA

Objective 10-2:   Reduce outbreaks of infections caused by key foodborne bacteria.

Target and baseline:

Objective	Reduction in Infections Caused by Foodborne Bacteria	Number of Outbreaks per Year		
		1997 Baseline	2002	2010 Target
10-2a.	*Escherichia coli* O157:H7	22	38	11
10-2b.	*Salmonella* serotype Enteritidis	44	20	22

Target setting method: 50% improvement.

Sources: Foodborne Disease Outbreak Surveillance System, CDC, NCID; wonder.CDC.gov/data2010/focus.htm.

For Further Thought

Outbreaks of *E. coli* O157:H7 have been associated with undercooked ground beef. How do you make sure that you are protecting yourself and your guests when you cook hamburgers at home?

The leading vehicle for the transmission of FBDOs during 1993-1997 was fish, followed by salad and beef, but it is important to remember that almost any food can serve as a vehicle of transmission for a foodborne disease agent. For example, transmission of *E. coli* was first associated with contaminated ground beef but has also occurred through unpasteurized fruit juices, lettuce, and contaminated drinking water. In late August and early September 2006, an *E. coli* O157:H7 outbreak infected 199 people and caused three deaths in the United States.[10] This outbreak was traced to a single fresh spinach packing facility. However, the vehicle of infection for more than half of the cases is unknown. In some outbreaks, multiple foods are incriminated. Delicatessens, cafeterias, and restaurants are reported nearly twice as often as homes as places where the contaminated food is eaten. Also, more cases occur in the summer months than during any other season.[9] More and more of our foods are imported. Currently, 38% of the fruits, 12% of the vegetables, and 9% of the meats and poultry Americans consume each year are imported. Foodborne illness has been increasingly related to imported foods.[11]

To protect the public from foodborne diseases requires the coordinated efforts of federal, state, and local health agencies. At the federal level, the CDC, under its Emerging Infections Program, has established the Foodborne Diseases Active Surveillance Network (FoodNet) to provide better data on foodborne diseases. FoodNet tracks nine foodborne diseases in eight catchment areas with a combined surveillance population of 29.5 million people.[12] The CDC coordinates these surveillance activities with officials from the U.S. Department of Agriculture's Food Safety and Inspection Service, the Food and Drug Administration's Center for Food Safety and Applied Nutrition, and with the respective state epidemiologists.

A recent report analyzed the success rate for investigating and reporting FBDOs in FoodNet catchment areas during 1998-1999. The results were disappointing. In 71% of the outbreaks, no confirmed etiology (cause) was found, and in 46% of the outbreaks, no suspected food

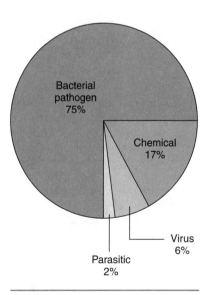

FIGURE 16.3

Foodborne disease outbreaks with known etiology by cause: United States, 1993-1997.

Source: Centers for Disease Control and Prevention (2000). "Surveillance for Foodborne-Disease Outbreaks—United States, 1993-1997." *MMWR,* 49.

was identified. This study illustrates the difficulty of epidemiological and disease control work in the absence of adequate resources.[13]

Enforcing state regulations at the local level are **sanitarians,** also known as registered environmental health specialists. Hired by local health departments, these sanitarians inspect restaurants and other food-serving establishments (such as hospitals, nursing homes, churches, and schools), temporary and seasonal points of food service (such as those at fairs and festivals), and retail food outlets (grocery stores and supermarkets) to ensure that environmental conditions favorable to the growth and development of pathogens do not exist.

By enforcing food safety laws, public health officials protect the health of the community by reducing the incidence of FBDOs. Nevertheless, it is important to recognize that consumers can reduce their risk for foodborne illness by following safe food-handling recommendations and avoiding consumption of unpasteurized milk and milk products, raw or undercooked oysters, raw or undercooked eggs, raw or undercooked ground beef, and undercooked poultry. In fact, safer and healthier foods has been one of the ten greatest achievements in public health in the twentieth century (see Box 16.4).[14] Guidelines for preventing foodborne disease transmission at home are simple and straightforward (see Box 16.5).

Vectorborne Diseases

Standing water, including runoff water from overflowing septic systems or overloaded sewer systems, and improperly handled solid waste are more than unsavory sights. They provide a habitat for, and support the proliferation of, disease vectors. As discussed in Chapter 4, a **vector** is a living organism, usually an insect or other arthropod, that transmits microscopic disease agents to susceptible hosts. Examples of vectors and the diseases they transmit include mosquitoes (malaria, filariasis, and arthropodborne viruses—arboviruses), fleas (murine typhus

sanitarians
environmental workers responsible for the inspection of restaurants, retail food outlets, public housing, and other sites to ensure compliance with public health codes

vector
a living organism, usually an insect or other arthropod, that can transmit a communicable disease agent to a susceptible host (for example, a mosquito or tick)

BOX 16.4 TEN GREAT PUBLIC HEALTH ACHIEVEMENTS, 1900–1999: SAFER AND HEALTHIER FOODS

Food for Thought

Early in the twentieth century, contaminated food, milk, and water were responsible for many foodborne diseases, including typhoid fever, tuberculosis, botulism, and scarlet fever. In the first half of the century, scientific discoveries and public health policies, such as food fortification programs, led to large reductions in diseases caused by nutritional deficiency. More recently, the focus of many public health nutrition programs shifted to the prevention and control of chronic disease, such as cardiovascular disease and obesity, through nutrition.

After the characteristics and sources of foodborne diseases were identified, public health professionals began advocating control of those diseases through technology and safer food-handling procedures, including:

- Hand washing
- Better sanitation
- Refrigeration
- Pasteurization
- Pesticide application
- Reduction of foodborne pathogens
- Better animal care and feeding
- Safer food processing

Prompt refrigeration inhibits bacterial growth, thus reducing the risk for disease.

One notable discovery that reduced disease was the process invented by Louis Pasteur—pasteurization.

New foodborne pathogens have emerged in the United States during the past 20 years as a result of changes in agricultural practices and in food-processing operations and the globalization of the food supply. Seemingly healthy food animals can be reservoirs for human pathogens.

Pesticides have played an important role in increasing crop yields, decreasing food costs, and enhancing the appearance of food. However, without proper controls, the residues of some pesticides remaining on foods also create potential health risks.

BOX 16.5

GUIDELINES FOR PREVENTING FOODBORNE ILLNESSES

To prevent foodborne illness, use the following strategy.

Clean: Wash hands and surfaces often

- Wash your hands with warm water and soap for at least 20 seconds before and after handling food and after using the bathroom, changing diapers, and handling pets.
- Wash your cutting boards, dishes, utensils, and counter tops with hot soapy water after preparing each food item and before you go on to the next food.
- Use paper towels to clean up kitchen surfaces. If you use cloth towels, wash them often in the hot cycle of your washing machine.
- Rinse fresh fruits and vegetables under running tap water, including those with skins and rinds that are not eaten.
- Rub firm-skin fruits and vegetables under running tap water or scrub with a clean vegetable brush while rinsing with running tap water.

Separate: Don't cross-contaminate!

- Separate raw meat, poultry, seafood, and eggs from other foods in your grocery shopping cart, grocery bags, and in your refrigerator.
- Use one cutting board for fresh produce and a separate one for raw meat, poultry, and seafood.
- Never place cooked food on a plate that previously held raw meat, poultry, seafood, or eggs.

Cook to proper temperature

- Use a food thermometer to measure the internal temperature and make sure that the food is cooked to a safe internal temperature (e.g., roasts and steaks to a minimum of 145°F, poultry to a minimum of 165°F in the innermost part of the thigh and wing and the thickest part of the breast). Cook ground meat to at least 160°F.
- Cook eggs until the yolk and white are firm, not runny. Don't use recipes in which eggs remain raw or only partially cooked.
- Cook fish to 145°F or until the flesh is opaque and separates easily with a fork.
- When cooking in a microwave oven, make sure there are no cold spots in food where bacteria can survive. For best results, cover food, stir, and rotate for even cooking.
- Bring sauces, soups, and gravy to a boil when reheating. Heat leftovers thoroughly to 165°F.

Chill: Refrigerate promptly

- Refrigerate foods quickly and as soon as you get them home from the store because cold temperatures slow the growth of harmful bacteria. Keeping a constant refrigerator temperature of 40°F or below is one of the most effective ways to reduce the risk of foodborne illness.
- Never let raw meat, poultry, eggs, cooked food, or cut fresh fruits or vegetables sit at room temperature more than two hours before putting them in the refrigerator or freezer.
- Never defrost food at room temperature. Food must be kept at a safe temperature during thawing, which you can achieve by defrosting your food in the refrigerator, in cold water, and in the microwave.
- Always marinate food in the refrigerator.
- Divide large amounts of leftovers into shallow containers for quicker cooling in the refrigerator.
- Use or discard refrigerated food on a regular basis.

Source: Partnership for Food Safety Education (2006). "Safe Food Handling." Available at http://www.fightbac.org/content/view/6/11/.

---

and plague), lice (epidemic typhus), and ticks (Rocky Mountain spotted fever and Lyme disease) (see Table 16.2).

Mosquito larvae require standing water in which to complete their development. The improper handling of wastewater or inadequate drainage of rainwater provides an ideal habitat for mosquitoes and increases the risk for a **vectorborne disease outbreak (VBDO).** Of particular concern in this regard is the northern house mosquito, *Culex pipiens* (see Figure 16.4). *Culex pipiens* is the most important vector of St. Louis encephalitis (SLE) in the eastern United States. In California, the SLE virus is transmitted by another mosquito species, *Culex tarsalis,* which proliferates in mismanaged irrigation water. SLE is a disease to which the elderly are particularly susceptible. Those at greatest risk live in unscreened houses without air conditioning.

Culex pipiens also transmits West Nile virus (WNV), which causes West Nile fever, West Nile encephalitis, and West Nile meningitis—severe diseases that affect the nervous system.

vectorborne disease outbreak (VBDO) the occurrence of two or more cases of a vectorborne disease

Table 16.2
Vectorborne Biological Hazards

Hazard	Agent	Vector	Disease
Virus	SLE virus	Mosquito	St. Louis encephalitis
	LaCrosse	Mosquito	LaCrosse encephalitis
Rickettsiae	*Rickettsia typhi*	Flea	Murine typhus
	Rickettsia rickettsii	Tick	Rocky Mountain spotted fever
	Ehrlichia chaffeensis	Tick	Ehrlichiosis
Bacteria	*Yersinia pestis*	Flea	Bubonic plague
	Borrelia burgdorferi	Tick	Lyme disease
Protozoa	*Plasmodium* spp.	Mosquito	Malaria
Nematodes	*Wuchereria bancrofti*	Mosquito	Filariasis (elephantiasis)

Source: Chin, J., ed. (2000). *Control of Communicable Diseases Manual,* 17th ed. Washington, DC: American Public Health Association.

Encephalitis refers to an inflammation of the brain; *meningitis* is an inflammation of the membrane surrounding the brain and spinal cord. West Nile virus first appeared in New York in 1999, where it caused 62 human cases of disease, including 7 deaths.[15] An excellent example of the global nature of emerging infectious diseases, WNV had caused outbreaks of encephalitis in Algeria (1994), Romania (1996-1997), the Democratic Republic of the Congo (1998), and Russia (1999) before arriving in the United States.[16] Once established, WNV spread rapidly in the United States (see Figure 16.5). This story underscores the importance of both proper environmental sanitation and active surveillance for vectorborne diseases.

Another species of mosquito that thrives on environmental mismanagement in the north-central and eastern United States is the eastern tree hole mosquito, *Aedes triseriatus*. While the natural habitat for this mosquito is tree holes, it flourishes in water held in discarded automobile and truck tires. It is estimated there are two billion used tires discarded in various places in the United States today, and two million more discarded tires are added to the environment each year. In the eastern United States, *Aedes triseriatus* is the vector for LaCrosse encephalitis, an arbovirus that produces a serious and sometimes fatal disease in children.

Improperly discarded vehicle tires are also the favored habitat of another vector, the Asian tiger mosquito, *Aedes albopictus*. Since 1985, when this species was first discovered in the United States (in Houston, Texas), it has been reported in 866 counties in 26 states.[17] The tiger mosquito arrived in the United States in used tires imported from Japan. *Aedes albopictus* has been called a "super vector" because it can transmit about 10 diseases to humans, including the viruses that cause LaCrosse encephalitis and dengue fever. Larvae of the Asian tiger mosquito can develop in water held in almost any artificial container, including discarded cups and plastic wrap. So far, two pathogenic arboviruses have been isolated from *Ae. albopictus* in the United States—the eastern equine encephalomyelitis virus and the Cache Valley virus.

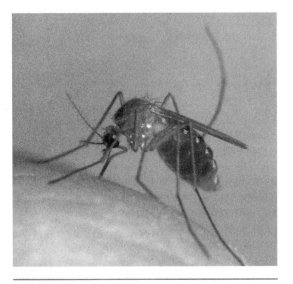

FIGURE 16.4

The northern house mosquito (*Culex pipiens*) is the most important vector of St. Louis encephalitis and West Nile virus in the eastern United States.

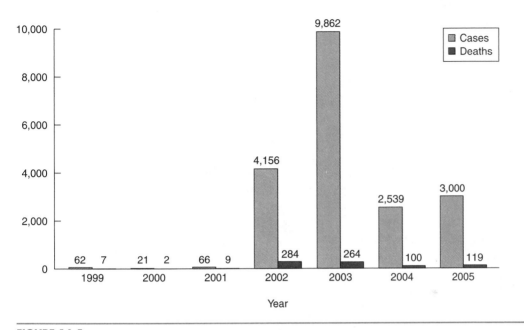

FIGURE 16.5

West Nile virus activity in the United States from 1999 to 2005.

Source: Centers for Disease Control and Prevention (2006). "West Nile Virus: Statistics, Surveillance, and Control." Available at http://www.cdc.gov/ncidod/dvbid/westnile/surv&controlCaseCount99_detailed.htm.

In 1998, yet another Asian species of mosquito, *Aedes japonicus,* was detected in the United States. While no human cases of disease have been traced to *Ae. japonicus* in the United States thus far, the species has been shown to be a good vector of West Nile virus under laboratory conditions.[18]

In summary, the cases of diseases carried by mosquitoes stress the importance of prevention at the community level through actions such as mosquito control and promotion of personal protection against mosquito bites.

Improper management of solid waste—such as occurs at open dumps, ill-managed landfills, and urban slums—fosters the expansion of rat and mouse populations. These rodents are hosts for fleas, which transmit murine typhus, a rickettsial disease characterized by headache, fever, and rash. If the rodent population should decline rapidly because of disease or a successful rodent control program, these fleas could come into contact with humans and spread the disease directly to them. Diseases of animals that are transmissible to humans, such as murine typhus, are referred to as *zoonoses.*

Seemingly harmless interactions with the environment can have unintended consequences. For example, white-tailed deer were decimated throughout much of the Midwest and eastern United States during the nineteenth century. As they declined in numbers, their predators and parasites vanished too. Reintroduced in the 1930s and protected from hunting by strict regulations, white-tailed deer populations became well established. Modern farming practices, which result in field after field of corn, soybeans, or other nutritious crops interspersed with wooded areas, resulted in deer populations large enough to reach pest status in some parts of the Midwest. As deer populations have increased, so have populations of the blacklegged tick, *Ixodes scapularis.* Sometimes called the deer tick, *I. scapularis* is the vector of **Lyme disease** caused by the bacterial spirochete *Borrelia burgdorferi* (see Figure 4.5). Lyme disease is currently the most commonly reported vectorborne disease in the United

Lyme disease
a systemic, bacterial, tickborne disease with symptoms that include dermatologic, arthritic, neurologic, and cardiac abnormalities

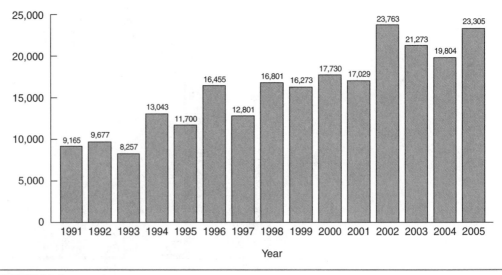

FIGURE 16.6

Number of reported cases of Lyme disease in the United States from 1991 to 2005.

Sources: Centers for Disease Control and Prevention (2004). "Lyme Disease—United States 2001–2002." *MMWR*, 53(17): 365–369; and Centers for Disease Control and Prevention (2006). "Vector-borne Infectious Diseases—Lyme Disease." Available at http://www.cdc.gov/ncidod/dvbid/lyme/ld_UpClimbLymeDis.htm.

States, and its incidence has been increasing almost every year (see Figure 16.6). The states with the highest incidences of Lyme disease in 2005 were Delaware, Connecticut, New Jersey, Massachusetts, Pennsylvania, New York, and Wisconsin.[19] Since there is no vaccine available for Lyme disease, and community tick control is virtually nonexistent, personal protection is the best defense. Avoid entering tick-infested areas when possible; these are usually wooded and bushy areas with high grass and a lot of leaf litter. If this is not possible, dress appropriately—wear long pants and tuck them into your socks and wear a long-sleeved shirt, tucked into your pants. Apply tick repellents and carry out tick checks after leaving these areas, carefully removing any ticks found with a pair of tweezers. May, June, and July are the months of highest risk for Lyme disease; it is during these months that the nymphal stage of the black-legged tick is most active.

There are also several measures you and your community can take to control ticks around your home and in your community. Employ landscaping techniques that reduce leaf litter and tall grass and establish a litter-free (and tick-free) border around the perimeter of your yard. If you have a lawn, keep it short and, if you apply acaricides to your property, be sure to do so in accordance with the instructions on the label. Finally, deer are an essential host for adult blacklegged ticks; consider ways to discourage deer from entering your community.

CHEMICAL HAZARDS AND HUMAN HEALTH

chemical hazards
hazards caused by
the mismanagement
of chemicals

Chemical hazards are those that result from the mismanagement of chemicals. Not all people react to chemicals in the same way; some people are especially susceptible, whereas others are not. One fact is clear: Children are much more vulnerable to chemical assaults than adults. Although chemicals have provided modern society with innumerable benefits, they can have a deleterious impact on human health when mismanaged. This section examines three common sources of chemical exposure that could negatively affect health, namely, pesticides, environmental tobacco smoke, and lead.

Pesticides

The term **pest** refers to any organism (plant, animal, or microbe) that has an adverse effect on human interests. Some common examples are weeds in your vegetable garden, termites in your house, and mold on your shower curtain. **Pesticides** are natural or synthetic chemicals that have been developed and manufactured for the purpose of killing pests. In the United States, there are more than 25,000 different pesticide products that contain more than 600 pest-killing chemicals.[20] It has been estimated that without the use of chemical insecticides, American agricultural production would decrease by 30%. Because of this, it seems certain that pesticides will be present in our environment for the foreseeable future.

While chemical companies market pesticides to control a particular pest, most of them in fact kill a wide range of organisms. The pest organism against which the pesticide is applied is referred to as the **target pest** or **target organism** (see Table 16.3). All other organisms in the environment that may also be affected are called **nontarget organisms.** For example, most weed killers will not only kill the weeds but also (nontarget) flowers and ornamental plant vegetation. Similarly, it is not uncommon for domestic animals to be poisoned and killed by rodenticides (rat poison). Overexposure to these chemicals can have adverse effects on human health.

The two most widely used types of pesticides are **herbicides** (pesticides that kill plants) and **insecticides** (pesticides that kill insects). It is also from these two types of pesticides that most human pesticide poisonings occur. The two groups at highest risk for pesticide poisoning are young children and the workers who apply the pesticides. Many of these persons live on farms or are engaged in farm work. Poisonings occur when the pesticides are consumed orally, inhaled, or when they come in contact with the skin. The majority of children poisoned by pesticides consume them orally. These are frequently unintentional poisonings that occur when pesticides are left within reach of children. Most adult poisonings occur because of careless practice. Examples include eating food without washing hands after handling pesticides, mouth-siphoning to transfer pesticides from one container to another, applying pesticides while one's skin is exposed, or spilling the pesticide on one's body.

In agricultural settings, poisonings can occur when agricultural workers misuse pesticides. For example, illiterate workers or those who do not read English may enter sprayed fields too soon because of the inability to read product directions or posted warning signs. Their employers may even tell them to enter the field too soon, and the workers' children may be with them.

In addition to occupational exposure, we are exposed to low concentrations of pesticides daily because of their presence in our air, water, soil, and food products. The effects of exposure to pesticides depend on the pesticide type, dose, route and duration of exposure, and the

Table 16.3
Types of Pesticides

Type of Agent	Target Pest to Be Destroyed
Acaricides/miticides	Ticks/mites
Bactericides	Bacteria
Fungicides	Fungi, molds
Herbicides	Weeds, plants
Insecticides	Insects
Larvicides/grubicides	Insect larvae
Molluscicides	Snails, slugs
Nematocides	Worms
Rodenticides	Rats, mice

pest
any organism—a multicelled animal or plant, or a microbe—that has an adverse effect on human interests

pesticides
synthetic chemicals developed and manufactured for the purpose of killing pests

target organism (target pest)
the organism (or pest) for which a pesticide is applied

nontarget organisms
all other susceptible organisms in the environment, for which a pesticide was not intended

herbicide
a pesticide that kills plants

insecticide
a pesticide that kills insects

characteristics of the person exposed. Exposures may be acute (single, high-level exposure) or chronic (repeated exposure over an extended period of time). Allowable pesticide concentrations in drinking water are regulated under the Safe Drinking Water Act (see Chapter 15 for more details on this regulation). Some signals of poisoning are headaches, weakness, rashes, fatigue, and dizziness. More serious effects include cancer, mutations, birth defects, respiratory problems, convulsions, coma, and death.

A great deal of money and effort have been spent looking for the "ideal" pesticide for various purposes. The ideal pesticide has been characterized by Enger and Smith as one that would (1) be inexpensive, (2) kill only the target organism, (3) break down rapidly, and (4) break down into harmless materials.[21] Developing the ideal pesticide is an illusive goal, but a number of safe, effective, and useful pesticides have been developed. Pesticide development, like pharmaceutical (drug) development, is expensive because it requires years of research and testing.

Among the first modern pesticides developed were insecticides known as *chlorinated hydrocarbons*. The most famous example of this group is dichloro-diphenyl-trichloroethane (DDT). DDT and its relatives are very stable chemical compounds; that is, they are persistent in the environment. On the one hand, this was helpful because one did not have to make repeated treatments. It has been said that DDT has saved more lives than any other chemical developed by man by killing such disease vectors as lice, mosquitoes, and flies. On the other hand, its persistence meant that the chemical remained in the environment and even accumulated in organisms such as fish and birds that fed on the insects. Therefore, its use was eventually banned in the United States because of this problem. Another problem with DDT is the fact that it is a broad-spectrum insecticide—it kills any and all insects with which it comes into contact.

Beginning in the 1960s, a new generation of pesticides arrived on the market called organophosphates. These pesticides were less persistent, breaking down into harmless products within weeks. The best-known organophosphate pesticide is Malathion, a relatively safe and widely used insecticide. In the 1970s, even less-persistent chemicals were developed, the carbamates. These chemicals break down in days or hours. The best example is carbaryl, which is still in use today. While today's pesticides are much safer for the environment, they are still not species-specific, and some have even a higher acute toxicity to humans and other mammals than DDT.

While there is no doubt that pesticides have provided significant benefits to society, they can be dangerous if used or stored improperly. The victims are often children. In 1998 alone, 73,260 children were involved in common household pesticide-related poisonings or exposures in the United States.[2] An Environmental Protection Agency (EPA) survey revealed that 47% of all households with children under the age of 5 had at least one pesticide stored in an unlocked cabinet less than four feet off the ground (i.e., within the reach of children).[22]

The immediate solutions to the problems of pesticide poisoning and environmental quality are better education about the safe storage and proper application of pesticides, better regulation of pesticides, and better compliance by the homeowner to ensure that the products are used in accordance with instructions on the label. One of the *Healthy People 2010* objectives is to reduce pesticide exposures that result in visits to a health care facility (see Box 16.6).

Environmental Tobacco Smoke

Approximately 24.9% (60.5 million) of adult Americans 12 years of age or older were current cigarette smokers in 2005.[23] As a result, many nonsmokers are exposed to environmental tobacco smoke. As noted in Chapter 15, *environmental tobacco smoke (ETS),* also known as *secondhand smoke*, includes both sidestream smoke and mainstream smoke. The process of inhaling ETS is referred to as *passive smoking*. Secondhand smoke involuntarily inhaled by nonsmokers from other people's cigarettes is classified as a known human (group A) carcinogen and causes approximately 3,000 lung cancer deaths annually in U.S. nonsmokers.[24]

The association between ETS and adverse health effects has been demonstrated in a number of different epidemiological studies.[25-27] These studies provide evidence that adults exposed to ETS have an increased relative risk of lung cancer and possibly heart disease.[25] In addition, the studies show that about 50% of all American children 5 years of age and under have been exposed to ETS from prenatal maternal smoking and/or sidestream smoke from household members after their birth (see Figure 16.7). Such exposure has been shown to increase the risk of adverse prenatal consequences and postnatal health conditions in infants. Specifically, this exposure has been associated with intrauterine growth retardation, low birth weight, preterm delivery, respiratory tract infections, and behavioral and cognitive abnormalities.[27] Furthermore, young children are especially susceptible to secondhand smoke and are likely to suffer from coughing, wheezing, phlegm production, breathlessness, and an increased risk of developing asthma.

The Surgeon General's report states that there is no risk-free level of secondhand smoke exposure and that even brief exposures can be harmful to children. A large body of evidence indicates that ETS is detrimental to human health and can cause or exacerbate a wide range of adverse health effects, including cancer, respiratory infections, and asthma. It is known that tobacco smoke contains about 4,000 substances, many of which have carcinogenic and mutagenic properties. The obvious solution to eliminate the increased health risks associated with ETS is to eliminate exposure to ETS. Though many people do their best to avoid ETS, it is not always possible. In fact, many individuals who report no exposure to ETS have low concentrations of cotinine (a metabolite of nicotine) in their urine, indicating they have indeed been exposed.[27] Such evidence led the EPA to issue a report in 1993 classifying ETS as a known human carcinogen. ETS is responsible for approximately 3,400 lung cancer deaths per year in nonsmoking adults, 22,700 to 69,600 deaths from heart disease in people who are not current smokers, and 150,000 to 300,000 lower respiratory tract infections in American children younger than 18 months of age.[24,28-30]

Educational programs have been helpful in getting nonsmokers and smokers alike to understand the hazard of ETS. As a result, many nonsmokers attempt to avoid ETS, and many smokers have become more courteous about asking those around them for permission to smoke. At the same time, there are many smokers who believe that smoking whenever and

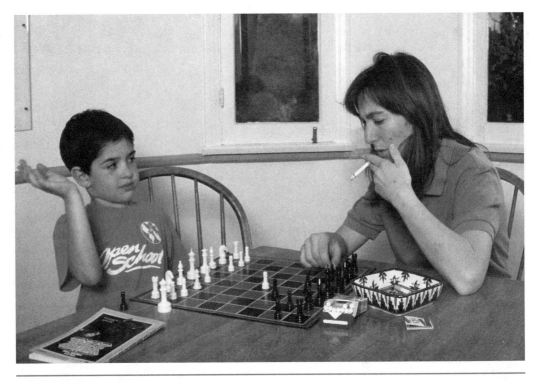

FIGURE 16.7
Too many children are exposed to significant levels of environmental tobacco smoke.

wherever they wish is a right, not a privilege. It is these smokers who necessitate regulations against smoking in certain areas. Such regulations can originate at any level of government. For example, a federal regulation now prohibits smoking on all domestic air flights. Forty-nine states and the District of Columbia have some restriction on smoking in public places; Wyoming has none. Of the 49 states with regulations, 48 restrict smoking in government workplaces and 38 have extended those limitations to private workplaces. "Sixteen states, the District of Columbia, and Puerto Rico have met the American Lung Association's *Smokefree Air 2010 Challenge*, by approving legislation to prohibit smoking in most public places and workplaces, including all restaurants and bars."[31] California has one of the strictest standards; it prohibits smoking in virtually any place of employment (see Box 16.7). Many communities throughout the United States have adopted local ordinances, which regulate smoking in public places when state laws do not. The EPA ruling on ETS as a carcinogen has had a ripple effect across the country, resulting in an increase in the number of smoke-free public places. In addition, many employers are now creating policies (administrative laws) that restrict or prohibit smoking in the workplace, on workplace grounds, and/or in company-owned vehicles.

Regulating smoking behavior, even though it makes perfectly good health sense, can cause hard feelings and much anger between smokers and nonsmokers. If regulation is going to be adopted, it should be jointly developed by representatives of all those affected. Voluntary regulation often works best.

Lead

lead
a naturally occurring mineral element found throughout the environment and used in large quantities for industrial products

Lead is a naturally occurring mineral element that is found throughout the environment and is used in a variety of industrial products, including electric batteries, pipe, solder, paint and

BOX 16.7

PROTECT INDOOR AIR: NO SMOKING IN BARS AND TAVERNS

In California, under existing law, smoking of tobacco products in an enclosed space at a place of employment is prohibited, with certain exceptions. Among the exceptions are bars, taverns, and gaming clubs. These exceptions were suspended on January 1, 1998, "unless and until Occupational Safety and Health Standards Board or Environmental Protection Agency adopts standards for reducing permissible employee exposure to environmental tobacco smoke to an exposure level that will prevent anything other than insignificantly harmful effects to exposed persons."*

This law means that waitresses, waiters, bartenders, and others who are employed in bars, taverns, and gaming clubs do not have to breathe environmental tobacco smoke for an eight-hour shift. Instead, they can work in a smoke-free environment like most other workers. Does your state protect workers employed in bars, taverns, and gaming clubs?

*AB 297, Gaming clubs: bars and taverns: smoking. Available at http://www.sen.ca.gov/htbin/ca-billpage?AB/297/gopher_root2:[bill.current.ab.from0200.ab0297].

plastic pigments, and leaded gasoline. Because of its past widespread use, lead can be found in soil, household dust, drinking water, air, paint, old painted toys and furniture, and foods and liquids stored in lead crystal or lead-based porcelain. However, lead can adversely affect human health and is chronic in nature. The health problems include anemia, birth defects, bone damage, depression of neurological and psychological functions, kidney damage, learning disabilities, miscarriages, and sterility.[32]

Humans are exposed to lead primarily by ingestion and inhalation. Those who are at greatest risk of lead poisoning are young children who may inadvertently ingest lead, adults whose jobs bring them in contact with lead, and people of all ages who live in homes with water pipes made of or soldered with lead.

Lead poisoning is the most significant and prevalent disease of environmental origin among American children.[33] The CDC estimates that approximately 310,000 children aged 1 to 5 years residing in the United States have blood lead levels (BLLs) that exceed the recommended level of 10 micrograms of lead per deciliter of blood during the 1999 to 2002 survey period.[34] Although this situation is not satisfactory and continuous effort is needed to reduce the exposure of children to lead, findings indicate that BLLs continue to decline in the U.S. population. The major source of lead exposure for these children is dust and chips of lead paint in their homes (see Figure 16.8). It is estimated that there are approximately 24 million housing units in the United States that still contain dangerous levels of lead-based paint and that more than 4 million of these dwellings are homes to children.[34] Children are much more susceptible to the effects of lead than adults. It is estimated that as much as 50% of the lead ingested by young children is absorbed, compared with only 10% in adults.

The federal government banned lead-based paints for use in housing in 1978 and completed the elimination of lead from gasoline in 1995. As a result of these actions, there has been significant improvement in the BLLs of the nation's children. However, there is room for further improvement. One of the *Healthy People 2010* objectives is to eliminate elevated BLLs in children (see Box 16.8).[35]

Occupational exposure to lead is the major source of lead intake for adults. Lead is smelted for industrial use in larger quantities than

FIGURE 16.8

Lead poisoning from paint dust continues to be a problem in the United States.

BOX
16.8

Healthy People 2010 Objective: Eliminate Elevated Blood Lead Levels in Children

Objective 8-11:   Reduce elevated blood levels in children aged 1 to 5 years.

Target: 0%.

Baseline: 4.4% of children aged 1 to 6 years had blood lead levels exceeding 10 μg/dL during 1991–1994.

Target setting method: Total elimination.

	Baseline Year	Baseline	2002	2004	Target 2010
	1991–94	4.4%	2/1.6%	3/1.5%	0%
Race and ethnicity					
American Indian or Alaska Native only	1991–94	4/DSU	2/DSU	3/DSU	0%
Asian or Pacific Islander only	1991–94	4/DSA	2/DNC	3/DNC	0%
Asian only	1991–94	DNC	2/DSU	3/DSU	0%
Native Hawaiian and other Pacific Islander only	1991–94	DNC	2/DSU	3/DSU	0%
Black or African American only	1991–94	4/11.5%	2/DNA	3/DNA	0%
White only	1991–94	4/2.6%	2/DNA	3/DNA	0%
Two or more races	1991–94	DNC	2/DSU	3/DSU	0%
American Indian or Alaska Native; White	1991–94	DNC	2/DSU	3/DSU	0%
Black or African America; White	1991–94	DNC	2/DSU	3/DSU	0%
Hispanic or Latino	1991–94	DSU	2/DSU	3/DSU	0%
Mexican American	1991–94	4.0%	2/DSU	3/DSU	0%
Not Hispanic or Latino	1991–94	4.2%	2/DNA	3/DNA	0%
Black or African American only, not Hisp/Latino	1991–94	4/11.2%	2/3.1%	3/3.4%	0%
White only, not Hispanic or Latino	1991–94	4/2.3%	2/DSU	3/1.2%	0%
Gender					
Female	1991–94	3.3%	2/1.5%	3/1.7%	0%
Male	1991–94	5.5%	2/1.7%	3/1.3%	0%
Family income level					
Low	1991–94	a/8.0%	2/1.7%	3/1.8%	0%
Medium	1991–94	1.9%	2/DSU	3/DSU	0%
High	1991–94	DSU	2/DSU	3/DSU	0%
Geographic location					
Population 1 million or more	1991–94	5.4%	2/DNA	3/DNA	0%
Population less than 1 million	1991–94	3.3%	2/DNA	3/DNA	0%

Note: Data may include revisions and may differ from those shown previously. Any displayed age-adjusted data are adjusted to the 2000 standard population.
——— = Data are not available.
BSL = Baseline data available for this year. See Baseline column.
DNA = Data have not been analyzed.
DNC = Data for specific population are not collected.
DSU = Data do not meet the criteria for statistical reliability, data quality, or confidentiality.
NA = Not applicable.
a/Baseline has been revised.
b/Target has been revised.
c/New baseline. Objective was previously developmental.
1/Metropolitan Statistical Area, Consolidated Metropolitan Statistical Area.
2/1999–2002 data.
3/1999–2004 data.
4/Respondents were asked to select one race category; selection of more than one race category was not an option.
5/Respondents were asked to select one or more races and identify one race as best representing their race.

Source: Centers for Disease Control and Prevention (2007). *Healthy People 2010: Data2010.* Available at http://wonder.cdc.gov/.

For Further Thought

While significant progress has been made in reducing BLLs in children through the reformulation of gasoline, it may be more difficult to find and treat the remaining 4.4% of children whose blood levels exceed the target level. Explain how this target could be achieved and what strategies you would employ in your community to eliminate children's exposure to lead.

any other heavy toxic metal. Though lead has many industrial uses, the most notable is in storage batteries. Lead exposure in the workplace often occurs through inhalation.

People of all age groups are exposed to lead if they consume water from lead pipes or pipes connected with lead solder. Lead pipes and solder can become corroded. The exposed lead dissolves in the flowing water that delivers it to the tap. The EPA has estimated that about 40 million Americans who live in homes built before 1930 are drinking water containing more than the legally permissible level of lead (15 parts per billion). Around 1930, copper replaced lead as the metal of choice for water pipes. Federal laws now restrict the use of lead in pipe (no more than 8% lead in brass fittings) and solder (no more than 0.2% lead) in the installation and repair of public water systems. Some local governments have banned lead plumbing components altogether in drinking water systems.

It should also be noted that some well water used for drinking has been contaminated with lead by the inappropriate disposal of lead-containing materials such as old automobile batteries or solvents containing lead. Prior to passage of the laws governing the disposal of toxic substances, it was very common for the toxic substance to end up in dumps or landfills where it could leak into the groundwater.

The solution to preventing lead poisoning includes several strategies—education, regulation, and prudent behavior. Educational efforts to inform people of the dangers of lead in paint have been in effect for a number of years, and for the most part they seem to have been well received, even though there is still an unacceptable number of children being poisoned in this manner. The efforts to educate parents need to continue. National, state, and local laws have been useful in abating the lead poisoning problem. On the national level, the Lead-Based Paint Poisoning Prevention Act of 1971 initiated a national effort to identify children with lead poisoning and to abate the sources in the environment. Passage of the Resource Conservation and Recovery Act (RCRA) in 1976 and the Comprehensive Environmental Response, Compensation, and Liability Act (CERCLA) in 1980 helped to regulate the disposal of lead-based products. Also at the federal level, the Lead Contamination Control Act of 1988 contributed to controlling lead poisoning. This act authorized the CDC to provide grants to state and local agencies for comprehensive programs to (1) screen infants and children for elevated BLLs, (2) ensure referral for medical and environmental intervention for infants and children who have been lead poisoned, and (3) provide education to parents and children about childhood lead poisoning.[36]

While significant progress has been made by the United States to reduce BLLs in children, such is not the case elsewhere in the world. The prevalence of elevated BLLs in Chinese children 1 to 6 years of age has been estimated at 38%, and that for Russian school-aged children at 58%. Thus, it is not unusual to find elevated BLLS in children adopted from these countries as well as other Asian and eastern European countries.[37]

The CDC has begun collaborating with other countries to eliminate childhood lead poisoning worldwide. So far, collaboration efforts are under way with Mexico, China, and India.[38]

PHYSICAL HAZARDS AND HUMAN HEALTH

A number of physical hazards in the environment can negatively affect human health. These include high temperature, equipment and environmental design, and radiation. Two of the most pervasive physical hazards involve radiation from radon gas and ultraviolet light. As discussed in Chapter 15, *radiation* is the energy released when atoms are split or created by natural decay from less stable to more stable forms. The energy, which can be thought of as either waves or particles, can damage the cells that make up living tissue. This damage occurs by a process called *ionization,* the removal of electrons from atoms in the molecules that are part of the living tissue. These molecular changes can result in biochemical lesions that can cause a mutation or cell death. On the skin, these can appear as burns, but the damage also can be internal. If the damage is severe enough, the organism will die.

Radon Contamination

Radon gas in indoor air is the second leading cause of lung cancer in the United States after cigarette smoking. The National Academy of Sciences estimated that 15,000 to 22,000 Americans die every year from radon-related lung cancer.[39] So what is radon gas and where does it come from? **Radon** (radon-222) is a colorless, tasteless, odorless gas that is generated in rock and soil. It is formed during an intermediate step in the radioactive decay process of uranium-238, a natural element that is found in most soil and rock but is more common in some places than in others. Radon gas has the ability to travel miles underground and rise to the earth's surface far away from any source of uranium. When it escapes the earth's crust outdoors, it quickly disperses harmlessly in the atmosphere. However, if it seeps into buildings occupied by humans, it can become a health hazard. It enters buildings through cracks in the foundation walls and floors, joints, openings around sump pump drains, loose-fitting pipes, and porous building materials, where it can then build up to harmful levels.[20] Such harmful levels are most likely to occur in unventilated lower levels of homes and buildings.

Radon becomes attached to dust particles or is present in aerosols that are then inhaled and may be deposited on lung tissues. Environmental tobacco smoke can also pick up radon decay products from the air and make them available for inhalation. This exposes the tissue to ionizing radiation, thereby substantially increasing the risk of lung cancer. Radon is also found in drinking water in homes where the water source of a private well is located in areas with soil containing high radium levels. Some radon can also be ingested with drinking water, but a more serious concern is that radon escapes from water as it is agitated during showers, or when washing dishes or clothes, and can be inhaled. Radon inhaled from water accounts for 90% of the lung cancers traced to the water supply. Overall, radon from domestic water generally contributes less than 1% of the total radon in indoor air in most housing.[39]

Like all other health problems related to environmental hazards, excessive exposure to radon can be prevented. In 1988, the U.S. EPA and the U.S. Surgeon General recommended that all homes below the third floor be tested for radon (see Box 16.9). If levels of radon in a

> **radon**
> a colorless, tasteless, odorless gas formed by the radioactive decay of uranium-238

BOX 16.9

HOW MUCH RADON IS PRESENT IN YOUR GEOGRAPHIC AREA?

The EPA created a map of radon zones to determine radon potential in 3,141 counties in the United States. The map was developed based on indoor radon measurements, local geology, aerial radioactivity, soil permeability, and foundation type. Based on this information, radon potential (highest, moderate, and low) was assigned to U.S. counties. To learn about the situation in your area, visit the EPA Web site and click on "Radon."

1. Locate a map of the radon zones.
2. Select your state and find the county where you live.
3. What is the radon potential in your county of residence?
4. Reflect upon this finding. What does it mean to you and your health?
5. If you found that the potential for the occurrence of radon in your area was moderate or highest, how would you proceed to protect the health of residents in your community?
6. If you found out that your area had the lowest potential for radon, you should still test your home for its occurrence in indoor air and make an informed decision about your next steps.
   a. How can you measure radon in your home?
   b. You can find additional information and guidelines on how to proceed in your situation in "The Citizen's Guide to Radon" on the EPA Web site (click on "Publications").

Source: U.S. Environmental Protection Agency (2006). "Map of radon zones." Available at http://www.epa.gov/iaq/radon/zonemap.html.

FIGURE 16.9

Radon levels in groundwater, soil, air, and indoor and outdoor air can vary dramatically.

home are excessive, steps need to be taken to prevent its entry into the home. Radon levels can be tested by using an easy-to-use, relatively inexpensive test (about $25–$250 per test). "Do it yourself" kits are available in most communities and are sometimes sold in hardware stores. Local health department personnel can usually help you locate one. Once the test has been administered, the kit is returned to the manufacturer for analysis. The average radon level in homes in the United States is 1.5 pCi/L of air (see Figure 16.9). If a home has a reading higher than 4 pCi/L, steps should be taken to reduce the level. Such steps would include filling all cracks in the foundation and walls of a basement or crawl space; creating a barrier between the earth and home, by such means as pouring a concrete floor over a dirt-floor crawl space; and digging a new well if the radon is coming in with the water supply. Some of these steps can be expensive. Most homes with high radon levels can be fixed for $800 to $2,000.[40]

Ultraviolet Radiation

Another source of ionizing radiation is the sun, yet millions of Americans think nothing of exposing (and overexposing) themselves to this form of radiation. Many actually seek it out in the mistaken belief that a tan body is a healthy body (see Figure 16.10). Sunshine comprises energy in many wavelengths, including visible light, heat, and **ultraviolet (UV) radiation.** UV radiation includes energy at wavelengths between 0 and 400 nanometers (nm). UV radiation between 290 and 330 nm, called UV-B, causes most of the harm to humans. In recent years, with the destruction of the ozone layer, the quantity of UV-B radiation reaching the earth has been increasing.[20]

Epidemiological studies have found an association between UV-B, or ionizing, radiation and skin cancer. For example, there is more skin cancer in those living closer to the equator

ultraviolet (UV) radiation
radiation energy with wavelengths 0–400 nm

FIGURE 16.10
Skin cancer is the prevalent type of cancer in the United States.

if they are not protected by darker skin. Also, most skin cancer appears on the exposed body parts (i.e., arms, legs, head, and neck).

Each year over 1,000,000 new cases of skin cancer are reported in the United States, and, in recent years, the incidence rate of skin cancer has been increasing about 3% per year.[20] The vast majority of these cases are the highly curable *basal cell* and *squamous cell carcinomas*. This is the most common form of cancer. The most serious and least common skin cancer is *malignant melanoma*. More than 55,000 new cases of this cancer are diagnosed every year in the United States, and each year about 7,900 patients die of melanoma. This type of skin cancer is the most dangerous because of its ability to grow and spread quickly. However, like the other skin cancers, melanoma is curable if discovered and treated early.[28]

Prevention of and Solutions to UV Radiation Exposure

Solutions for dealing with this physical hazard are simple. The first is for people to reduce their risk of exposure, and the second is to seek early treatment if cancer is suspected. One can reduce the risk of exposure by staying out of the sun or by covering the skin with clothing or commercial sunscreens. Sunscreens work by absorbing, reflecting, or scattering ultraviolet light, thereby reducing the amount that reaches the skin. To reduce your exposure to UV radiation, you can also find out the UV index for a specific day through the weather forecast on the Internet, or visit the EPA Web site called Sunwise.[41] The UV index is reported on a scale of 1 (low danger) to 11 (extreme danger) (see Figure 16.11). The EPA also issues UV Alerts, which are warnings when the level of solar radiation in your area is predicted to be unusually high. Obtaining information about the strength of UV radiation is the most important step in protecting your health. You can find the specific UV index for any day of the year on the EPA Web site (www.epa.gov/sunwise/uvindex.html) or on the Web site of weather.com by following the links "Stay Healthy" and "Skin Protection."

The second way to protect your health is through early diagnosis and prompt treatment. The key to discovering whether treatment is warranted is to practice monthly skin self-examination. Basal and squamous cell carcinomas often appear as a pale, waxlike, peely nodule or a red, scaly, sharply outlined patch. A physician should check either of these abnormalities, or the sudden change in a mole's appearance. Melanomas often start as small mole-like growths. The simple ABCD rule from the American Cancer Society outlines warning signs of melanoma.[28]

A is for *asymmetry* (half of the mole does not match the other half).

B is for *border irregularity* (the edges are ragged, notched, or blurred).

C is for *color* (the pigmentation is not uniform).

D is for *diameter* greater than 6 millimeters (any sudden or progressive change in size should be of concern).

Although not perceived as harmful, UV radiation can be quite damaging to human health. Because the level of UV radiation in the environment cannot be regulated the way other environmental hazards can, personal protection is the only way to prevent overexposure. As a

11+	**11+: Extreme risk of harm from unprotected sun exposure** • Take all precautions. Unprotected skin can burn in minutes. • Apply sunscreen with an SPF of at least 15 liberally every 2 hours. • Try to avoid sun exposure between 10 A.M. and 4 P.M. • Beachgoers—know that white sand and other bright surfaces reflect UV and will increase UV exposure. • Seek shade, cover up, wear a hat and sunglasses, and use sunscreen.
10	
9	**8–10: Very high risk of harm from unprotected sun exposure** • Take extra precautions. Liberally apply sunscreen with an SPF of at least 15. Unprotected skin will be damaged and can burn quickly. • Minimize sun exposure between 10 A.M. and 4 P.M. Seek shade, cover up, wear a hat and sunglasses, and use sunscreen.
8	
7	**6–7: High risk of harm from unprotected sun exposure** • Apply sunscreen with an SPF of at least 15. • Wear a wide-brimmed hat and sunglasses to protect your eyes. • Protection against sunburn is needed. • Reduce time in the sun between 10 A.M. and 4 P.M. • Cover up, wear a hat and sunglasses, and use sunscreen.
6	
5	**3–5: Moderate risk of harm from unprotected sun exposure** • Take precautions, such as covering up, if you will be outside. • Stay in shade near midday when the sun is strongest. • If your shadow is taller than you are (in the early morning and late afternoon, your UV exposure is likely to be low. • If your shadow is shorter than you are (around midday), you are being exposed to high levels of UV radiation. Seek shade and protect your skin and eyes.
4	
3	**2 or less: Low danger/risk from unprotected sun exposure** • Wear sunglasses or goggles on bright days. In winter, reflection off snow can nearly double UV strength. • If you burn easily, cover up and use sunscreen with an SPF of at least 15. • Protect areas that could be exposed to UV rays by the sun's reflection, including under the chin and nose.
<2	

FIGURE 16.11
UV index scale.

Source: U.S. Environmental Protection Agency (2006). "Sunwise Program." Available at http://www.epa.gov/sunwise/uviscale.html.

college-educated member of your community, you can demonstrate your knowledge of the dangers of UV radiation and serve as a role model by exercising personal protection options.

PSYCHOLOGICAL HAZARDS AND HUMAN HEALTH

Psychological hazards can be just as important as biological, chemical, and physical hazards in the determination of human health. However, the precise effects of psychological hazards on human populations are difficult to quantify. Among the health problems associated with psychological hazards are hypochondriasis, depression, hysteria, and stress. (For more information on the effects of stress on health, refer to Chapter 11.)

An important psychological hazard today is international terrorism. Indeed, it has been stated that the primary purpose of terrorist acts, aside from the casualties that usually occur, is

FIGURE 16.12

The September 11, 2001, terrorist attacks on the World Trade Center resulted in fear, stress, and hysteria among some of those who witnessed these events at close range. Others developed post-traumatic stress disorder one to two months after the attack.

to produce a psychological state of fear, stress, and hysteria. Many Americans experienced one or more of these psychological conditions in the aftermath of the World Trade Center (WTC) attack that occurred in New York City on September 11, 2001 (see Figure 16.12).

This terrorist attack was unique because it *did* cause a large number of deaths (2,726) and because it caused an unprecedented environmental assault on Lower Manhattan and resulted in substantial physical and mental health problems in survivors of collapsed or damaged buildings.[42] According to the World Trade Center Health Registry survey, the survivors caught in the dust cloud were two to five times more likely to report physical or mental health problems after September 11 than those who were not. Based on the registry data survey, 64% of building survivors witnessed three or more potentially psychological traumatizing events on September 11, and 11% screened positive for probable serious psychological distress. Also, 15% of adults directly affected by the attacks—such as persons who were in the complex and who were injured, those who lost possessions, a job, a friend, or a relative in this event, or those who were part of the rescue effort—had probable post-traumatic stress disorder (PTSD), compared with only 7.4% of all New York City residents.[42]

A study of Manhattan residents found that 20% of those living near the WTC had symptoms consistent with PTSD five to eight weeks after the attack. Clearly, psychological hazards are an important community health concern, especially during a disaster. In the case of the September 11 terrorist attacks, the full psychological impact on survivors and witnesses of this event is not completely known and continues to be investigated.

SOCIOLOGICAL HAZARDS AND HUMAN HEALTH

Living around other people can create a number of sociological hazards that can affect human health. It is known that noise, overcrowding, traffic jams, isolation, lack of privacy, and crowds can influence human health. As in the case of psychological hazards, the exact impact of these hazards on human health is unknown.

Although sociological hazards alone can create health problems, it is more likely for them to be found in combination with other environmental hazards. For example, the loud music created by a band could very well be harmless in a rural area, but it could create a serious problem in a crowded housing project in the middle of a city. In order to demonstrate the impact of sociological problems on human health, we will discuss population growth.

Population Growth

A population is defined as a group of individuals of the same species occupying a given area.[43] In this section, we focus on human population growth and its impact on human health.

The Principles

The growth of a population can be attributed to three factors—its birth rate, its death rate, and migration. However, because we are discussing the human population on our entire planet,

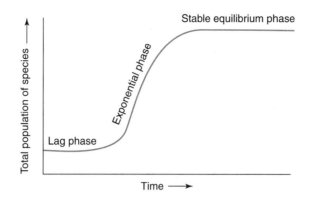

FIGURE 16.13
A theoretical population curve—an S-curve.

lag phase
the initial phase of the population growth S-curve when growth is slow

exponential phase
the middle phase of the population growth S-curve when the birth rate is greater than the death rate

zero population growth (ZPG)
when the birth and death rates for a given population are equal

equilibrium phase
the last phase of the population growth S-curve when the birth and death rates are equal

migration is not a factor. Population growth can be illustrated by an S-curve (see Figure 16.13). Such a curve consists of three phases: the lag phase, the exponential phase, and the stable equilibrium phase. During the **lag phase,** the growth is slow because there are relatively few reproducing individuals and there is little difference between the death rate and the birth rate. The **exponential phase** is characterized by a birth rate that is greater than the death rate, caused by more than one generation producing offspring. When the birth rate and death rate are equal, we have **zero population growth,** or a stable **equilibrium phase.** Prior to movement into the stable equilibrium phase, a J-curve is formed (see Figure 16.14). When a population grows in a J-curve pattern, the environment will eventually put it into an equilibrium

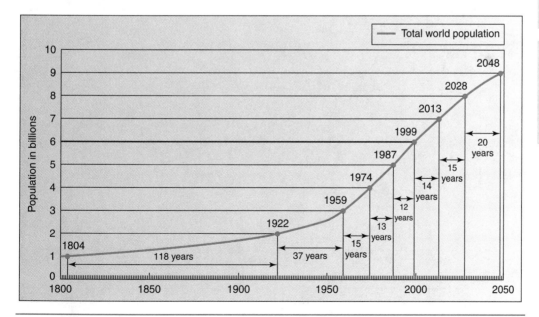

FIGURE 16.14
World population growth in historical perspective between 1750 and 2050, a typical J-shaped curve.
Source: United Nations (1995) and the U.S. Bureau of the Census, International Data Base.

carrying capacity
the maximum
population size that
can be supported by
available resources
(air, water, shelter, etc.)

phase because the resources (food, water, shelter, etc.) to support such growth are limited and thus will not allow the population to grow any further. The maximum population size that can be supported by available resources (air, water, shelter, etc.) is referred to as the **carrying capacity** of the environment.[20]

The Facts

In examining human population growth, one could say its growth followed the J-curve pattern through most of the twentieth century. The world's 6 billionth human inhabitant was born during the first half of 1999. But during the past three decades, the rate of world population growth began to decline because of worldwide efforts to curb the growth and therefore protect the population from disaster due to the declining availability of the natural resources that are needed to support it. Currently, projections are that the number of years required for the population to add one billion more people will increase (see Figure 16.14). While the world population growth rate will continue to decline (see Figure 16.15), the world population will continue to grow during the twenty-first century although somewhat more slowly.[43] At this rate, the U.S. Census Bureau projects that world population will reach 9.4 billion by the year 2050.

About 80% of the world's population lives in the world's less developed countries (LDCs), and virtually all of the world's population increase between now and 2050 will occur in these countries.[44] The largest percentage of growth during the next 45 years (2005–2050) is expected to occur in sub-Saharan Africa. Only one-third the size of China in 1950, sub-Saharan Africa was one-half the size of China in 2002, and is projected to surpass China in size by 2050.[44] By 2050, only the United States, among the more developed countries (MDCs), will

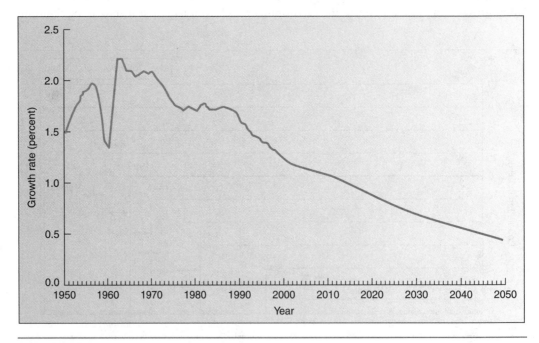

FIGURE 16.15

World population growth rate between 1950 and 2050.

Source: United States Department of Commerce, Bureau of the Census (2006). Available at www.census.gov/ipc/www/img/worldgr.gif.

remain on the list of the top 10 most populous countries; this will be due, in large part, to immigration. Whereas the growth rate remains high for the LDCs as a whole, the growth rate for the MDCs has fallen quite low. In many MDCs, fertility rates are below replacement levels (the level at which children born would just replace those persons lost to mortality).[44]

The Issues

While exponential world population growth is no longer occurring in absolute terms, world population growth continues to be substantial, and it is at a rate that is unsustainable if we wish to maintain the quality of life and health we enjoy today. The ramifications of overpopulation include the prospects of global warming, acid rain, bulging landfills, depletion of the ozone layer, increasing crime rates, increasing vulnerability to epidemics and pandemics, smog, exhaustion and contamination of soils and groundwater, degradation of arable land, and growing international tensions. Between 1990 and 2000, about 610 million hectares were degraded.[45] Also, there will be a dwindling of natural resources for energy, housing, and living space—especially in large cities. Since 1950, the urban population has more than tripled. It is estimated that three-fourths of the current population growth is urban. In 1975, there were only five megacities (cities of more than 10 million residents) in the world; now there are 19. By 2015, there will be 23 megacities, with only two of them in the United States.[45] Such fast growth and large density of humans in one area results in environmental pollution and degradation that negatively affects the health of every one of us.

The Solutions

Most experts agree that the world population is approaching the maximum sustainable limit. However, no one knows what the ultimate population size will be, what the ultimate carrying capacity of the earth is, and how many people it can support. There are some encouraging signs. The world population growth rate was over 2% just 30 years ago; it is now just 1.2%.[44] Although there are still great concerns with the population growth rates in parts of the Middle East and Africa, some developing countries have succeeded in slowing growth. For example, the average number of children born to a Mexican woman has plunged from 7 to just 2.5 in the past 30 years.[46]

The so-called humane means of limiting population growth include (1) various methods of conception control such as the oral contraceptive pill, physical or chemical barrier methods, or sterilization (tubal ligation and vasectomy); (2) birth control methods such as intrauterine devices, legalized abortion, and morning-after pills; and (3) social policies such as financial incentives and societal disincentives for having children, as is the practice in China's one-child family program. While some of these methods are unacceptable to certain people, all are proactive solutions to the mounting population problem. The alternative is to allow exponential population growth to continue until it declines naturally, by way of famine, epidemic diseases, and perhaps warfare. Nature's way will require a good deal more environmental deterioration, social disintegration, poverty, and human suffering. The choice is still ours.

NATURAL DISASTERS AND HUMAN HEALTH

In Chapter 15, we outlined some natural and human-made site and location situations that can be hazardous to humans. To further explain the hazards to human health that site and location may bring, we have chosen to discuss natural disasters.

Natural disasters include those geophysical and meteorological events (disaster agents) that greatly exceed normal human expectations in terms of magnitude or frequency and cause significant injury to individuals and damage to their property. Human health can be adversely affected by a disaster even before it occurs. Knowledge of an impending disaster can cause stress. Such stress can produce serious health problems in those who are unable to control their reaction to the situation. During the event, health can again be affected because of the physical damage causing both injuries and deaths. After a natural disaster, because of the remaining biological, sociological, psychological, and physical conditions, a variety of needs may exist. The primary needs of people after a natural disaster usually include food, clean water, shelter, health care, and clothing. The availability and quality of these items can dictate the impact of the disaster on human health.

A recent example of a natural disaster is Hurricane Katrina, which ravaged the city of New Orleans and coastal and inland areas of Louisiana and Mississippi in August 2005. The sixth-strongest Atlantic hurricane ever recorded, Katrina was also one of the deadliest, and certainly the costliest, forcing the evacuation of more than 1,500,000 people.[47]

Storm surges, violent winds, heavy rains, and flooding are to be expected with any hurricane. But with Katrina, the disaster was magnified because most of New Orleans lies below the level of the surrounding bodies of water. The storm surge damaged the levies that protect the city; once these were breached, 80% of New Orleans was flooded, some areas by as much as three meters of water. There was extensive damage to buildings, roads, and bridges. Utilities, including communication systems, food distribution, and health care were disrupted. Power outages prevented the operation of 200 sewage treatment plants throughout the disaster area, causing untreated sewage to overflow into streets and houses. Damage to oil and gas platforms meant that floodwaters were contaminated with oil as well as sewage.[47] These environmental conditions increased the risk of waterborne and vectorborne disease outbreaks. Three weeks after Katrina made landfall, about 1,000 cases of gastrointestinal (diarrheal) disease and 160 cases of dermatological diseases related to arthropod bites and wound infections were reported among evacuees.[48] Those who were evacuated found shelters crowded, unsanitary, and unsafe. Many of the shelters had insufficient food, drinking water, and medicine.

Finally, when floodwaters were pumped out of the inundated areas, a hazardous sludge remained on the land and in buildings and homes. This sludge, and the mold that grew inside damp buildings, caused respiratory problems for people returning to their homes and for recovery workers. Furthermore, 51 cases of carbon monoxide poisoning occurred in the area because some residents used portable generators and other gasoline-powered appliances for electrical power and cleanup. Finally, mental health issues, although not fully known at this time, may well be among the most serious long-term consequences of Katrina.

The response to and recovery of the communities affected by hurricane Katrina was led by the **Federal Emergency Management Agency (FEMA)**. FEMA, currently an agency within the U.S. Department of Homeland Security, leads efforts to prepare communities around the United States for all hazards and manages federal response and recovery efforts following any national incident, such as earthquake, fire, floods, tornado, landslide, tsunami, wildfires, and winter storms, as well as terrorism. FEMA also initiates proactive mitigation activities, trains first responders, and manages the National Flood Insurance Program.[49]

Federal Emergency Management Agency (FEMA) the nation's official emergency response agency

While the origins of FEMA can be traced back nearly 200 years, it was then President Jimmy Carter who signed the executive order in 1979 merging many of the separate disaster-related responsibilities into one agency. In March 2003, FEMA was placed in the Department of Homeland Security, where it is part of the Emergency Preparedness and Response Directorate. Today, FEMA has 2,600 regular employees supplemented by nearly 4,000 stand-by disaster assistant employees (see Figure 16.16).[49] The FEMA Web site (www.fema.gov) provides links to a vast array of information, reports, and publications that can help individuals and communities prepare for emergencies. Often FEMA works in partnership with other organizations that are part of the nation's emergency management system, including state and local emergency management agencies, 27 other federal agencies, and the American Red Cross.

In the United States, the American Red Cross (ARC), a humanitarian organization led by volunteers and guided by its Congressional Charter and the Fundamental Principles of the International Red Cross Movement, provides relief to victims of disaster and helps people prevent, prepare for, and respond to emergencies."[50] (See Chapter 2 for further discussion of the ARC.)[50]

The ARC works to prevent and alleviate human suffering wherever it may be found, with the purpose of protecting life and health while ensuring respect for human beings. The organization is responsible for giving aid to members of the U.S. Armed Forces and to disaster victims in the United States and abroad while staying neutral and impartial. In the history of the ARC, the natural disaster with the highest death toll in the United States was the hurricane that struck Galveston, Texas, in 1900; 6,000 people were killed. Hurricane Katrina was the most expensive single natural disaster in the organization's history and required the largest mobilization of Red Cross workers.[50]

Each year the ARC responds to more than 67,000 emergencies—from small emergencies such as apartment fires to large ones such as earthquakes and floods.[50] About 85% of all persons trained in disaster relief activities are ARC volunteers.

Natural disasters can occur at any place and at any time. Although a variety of federal and state agencies and organizations have as all or part of their mission to respond to such disasters, recent experiences with disasters should have taught us that local communities, especially those located in high-risk areas, need to prepare too. Only through careful planning and preparation can communities hope to minimize loss of human health and life if a disaster should occur.

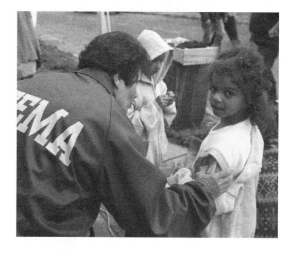

FIGURE 16.16
The mission of the Federal Emergency Response Agency (FEMA) is to lead America to prepare for, prevent, respond to, and recover from disasters with a vision of "A Nation Prepared."

CHAPTER SUMMARY

- Environmental health is the study and management of environmental conditions that affect our health and well-being.

- The environmental factors and conditions that can affect human health are numerous, and many remain to be identified.

- Environmental hazards can be classified as biological, chemical, physical, psychological, social, or natural hazards.

- We come into contact with biological and chemical hazards through the water we drink, the food we eat, and the air we breathe.

- The way communities manage their environment can influence the level of vector populations and, hence, the incidence of vectorborne diseases.

- Chemical hazards include pesticides, environmental tobacco smoke, and lead.

- Radon and ultraviolet radiation are invisible physical hazards that have serious health consequences such as lung cancer and skin cancer.

- Psychological hazards can affect the health of community members.

- Worldwide population growth constitutes a potential sociological hazard for all.

- Natural disasters are unpredictable hazards that can profoundly disrupt community health services and put citizens at risk.

- The Federal Emergency Management Agency (FEMA) and the American Red Cross (ARC) are two agencies that help communities prepare for, prevent, respond to, and recover from disasters.

REVIEW QUESTIONS

1. Define the following terms—*environmental health, environmental hazard,* and *environmental sanitation.*

2. Explain the differences between waterborne, foodborne, and vectorborne diseases and give an example of each.

3. What are chemical hazards and how are they detrimental to human health?

4. What is a pest? What are pesticides?

5. In what ways do pesticides pose a threat to human health?

6. How would you describe the ideal pesticide?

7. What does the term *persistence* mean with regard to pesticides? Give an example of a persistent and a non-persistent pesticide.

8. Explain the differences among environmental tobacco smoke, sidestream smoke, and mainstream smoke.

9. What is passive smoking?

10. To date, how has environmental tobacco smoke been regulated?

11. Who is at the highest risk for lead poisoning?

12. What are the most common ways to get lead poisoning?

13. What can be done to reduce the number of lead poisoning cases?

14. How is radon formed?

15. Why is radon such a concern?

16. How does ultraviolet radiation pose a health risk?

17. Why do you think there are so many cases of skin cancer each year in the United States?

18. Explain the ABCD rule of melanomas.

19. Explain how psychological hazards can adversely affect one's health.

20. Explain population growth using the S- and J-curves.

21. What percentage of the population growth is occurring in the more developed countries (MDCs)? In the less developed countries (LDCs)? What does such growth mean to all humans?

22. How close do you think the world is to reaching its carrying capacity?

23. Explain the role of the Federal Emergency Management Agency (FEMA) and contrast it with the role of the American Red Cross (ARC).

ACTIVITIES

1. Make arrangements to "shadow" a sanitarian from a local health department for at least half a day. Record and summarize the tasks in which he or she is involved and be sure to include in your notes all the tasks that were performed when you were with the sanitarian. Then, write a two-page paper answering the following:

   What professional training has the sanitarian completed to be qualified for this work?

   What role does this person play in protecting the community's health?

   What other tasks does the sanitarian routinely perform that he or she did not do on the day you visited?

   Would you like to be a sanitarian after you graduate? Why or why not?

2. Make arrangements to interview a director of environmental health in a local health department. Find answers to the following questions and summarize these answers in a two-page paper.

SCENARIO: ANALYSIS AND RESPONSE

Please take a moment to reread the scenario at the beginning of this chapter. Then reflect on the questions that follow.

1. At the present time, the U.S. government acknowledges that there is conclusive evidence that Agent Orange exposure is related to specific diseases, and it compensates Vietnam veterans who are affected. Those diseases include three types of cancer (Hodgkin's disease, non-Hodgkin's lymphoma, and soft tissue sarcoma) and two other types of disorders (chloracne—a disfiguring skin disorder—and a metabolic disorder called porphyria cutanea tarda). The government does not compensate for prostate cancer. Even though science cannot prove it, do you believe Agent Orange caused Gary's cancer? Why or why not?

2. Because of the adverse health conditions of many Vietnam veterans, a group of veterans filed suit against the seven U.S. chemical companies that produced Agent Orange. Before the case went to trial, the companies agreed to place $180 million into a fund that would be used to compensate victims and their families. The companies also denied any liability and stated they created the herbicide using the military's specifications. Do you feel these companies should be held responsible? Why or why not? Do you feel the U.S. government should be held responsible? Why or why not?

3. Do you feel that Gary was the victim of an environmental hazard (the chemical, Agent Orange), a sociological hazard (the war), neither, or both? Explain your response.

What are all the tasks this division of the health department carries out?

What is the primary environmental health problem of your community? Why is it a problem? How is it being dealt with?

If they inspect restaurants, which ones have the best sanitation practices?

What is an average day like for a health department sanitarian?

3. Interview at least three different farm workers. Ask if they know anyone who has ever been poisoned by a pesticide. Find out how each poisoning happened, ask if it could have been prevented, and find out what happened to the person who was poisoned. Write the results of your findings in a two-page paper.

4. Visit three different restaurants in your community. Ask to speak with the manager or assistant manager about the smoking policy in the restaurants. Find out what the policy is, who determined the policy, why it was created, and what happens if someone violates it. Write the results of your findings in a two-page paper.

5. Call your local health department and find out what kind of efforts have been made to eliminate lead poisoning. Ask about education programs and possible state or local laws. Also, find out if the health department will test for lead in the water and paint. If they will, ask about the procedures they use to do so. Write the results of your findings in a two-page paper.

6. Survey five of your friends by asking them the following questions. Once the interviews are complete, write a two-page paper summarizing their responses.

Do you lie out in the sun or go to tanning booths? If so, how often? Are you concerned about skin cancer?

What are the risk factors for skin cancer?

What is meant by the ABCD rule of melanoma?

Is tan skin more important to you than not getting cancer? If so, why?

7. Is radon gas a problem in your area of the country? If so, find out to what extent it is a problem and what percentage of the dwellings are contaminated. Also, obtain a home test kit and use it in the place where you live. In a two-page paper, report the extent of the problem in your community and the results of the test on your dwelling. Then project what your risk of disease from radon would be. (Note: If you are not sure where to get a radon test kit, contact your local health department.)

8. Go to the student union on your campus to conduct a survey of those who use the building. Ask the following questions of at least 25 people (do not interview people in only one part of the building; get responses from people in the food service areas, the lounges, bookstore, etc. Be sure to include students, faculty, and student union employees).

Are you a student, faculty member, or staff member?

Do you use tobacco in any form? If yes, what do you smoke or chew? How much?

Do you believe people should be allowed to smoke in this building? Why or why not?

Do you think smoking is a right or a privilege?

Are you in favor of a total ban on smoking on this campus? In all buildings? In offices? In residence halls?

After you have collected the data, summarize it in a written paper, and report any trends you find. Be sure to compare the answers of students to faculty and to staff.

9. Write a three-page position paper on one of the following questions. Make sure you cite references to support your position.

Should the United States be concerned with worldwide population growth?

Should the United States develop government policy to slow its population growth?

What is the best means for controlling population growth in any country?

10. Find an issue of a weekly news magazine (e.g., *Newsweek, Time*) or visit the FEMA Web site (www.fema .gov) to find information on a recent natural disaster. Read all the stories covering the disaster and then write a two-page paper identifying what you believe to be the major community health concerns that resulted from the disaster and why.

COMMUNITY HEALTH ON THE WEB

The Internet contains a wealth of information about community and public health. Increase your knowledge of some of the topics presented in this chapter by accessing the Jones and Bartlett Publishers Web site at **http://health.jbpub.com/book/communityhealth/6e** and follow the links to complete the following Web activities.

- National Center for Environmental Health
- The Foodborne Diseases Active Surveillance Network
- Population Connection

REFERENCES

1. Landrigan, P. J. (1992). "Commentary: Environmental Disease—A Preventable Epidemic." *American Journal of Public Health*, 82(7): 941-943.

2. Centers for Disease Control and Prevention (2006). "Surveillance for Waterborne-Disease Outbreaks Associated with Drinking Water and Water Not Intended for Drinking—United States, 2003–2004." *MMWR*, 55(SS12): 31-68.

3. Centers for Disease Control and Prevention (2006). "Surveillance for Waterborne-Disease Outbreaks Associated with Recreational Water—United States, 2003–2004." *MMWR*, 55(SS12): 1-23.

4. Centers for Disease Control and Prevention (1996). "Surveillance for Waterborne-Disease Outbreaks—United States, 1993–1994." *MMWR*, 45(SS-1): 1-33.

5. World Health Organization (2006). "Water Supply, Sanitation and Hygiene Development." Available at http://www.who.int/water_sanitation_health/hygiene/en/.

6. Centers for Disease Control and Prevention (1999). "Achievements in Public Health, 1900–1999: Fluoridation of Drinking Water to Prevent Dental Caries." *MMWR*, 48(41): 933-940.

7. Mead, P. S., L. Slutsker, V. Dietz, L. F. McCaig, J. S. Bresee, C. Shapiro, P. M. Griffin, and R. V. Tauxe (1999). "Food-Related Illness and Death in the United States." *Emerging Infectious Diseases*, 5(5): 607-621.

8. Centers for Disease Control and Prevention (1996). "Surveillance for Foodborne-Disease Outbreaks—United States, 1988–1992." *MMWR*, 45(SS-5): 1-66.

9. Centers for Disease Control and Prevention (2000). "Surveillance for Foodborne-Disease Outbreaks—United States, 1993–1997." *MMWR*, 49(SS-1): 1-62.

10. Centers for Disease Control and Prevention (6 October 2006). "Update on Multi-state Outbreak of *E. coli* 0157:H7 Infections from Fresh Spinach." Available at http://www.cdc.gov/foodborne/ecolispinach/100606.htm.

11. American Public Health Association (1999). "Food Safety [Fact sheet]." Available at http://www.apha.org/legislative/factsheets/fs.foodsafe.htm.

12. Centers for Disease Control and Prevention (2001). "Preliminary FoodNet Data on the Incidence of Foodborne Illnesses—Selected Sites, United States, 2000." *MMWR*, 50(13): 241-246.

13. Jones, T. F., B. Imhoff, M. Samuel, P. Mshar, K. G. McCombs, M. Hawkins, V. Deneen, M. Cambridge, and S. J. Olsen (2004). "Limitations to Successful Investigation and Reporting of Foodborne Outbreaks: An Analysis of Foodborne Disease Outbreaks in FoodNet Catchment Areas, 1998–1999." *Clinical Infectious Diseases*, 38(Suppl 3): S297-S302.

14. Centers for Disease Control and Prevention (1999). "Achievements in Public Health, 1900–1999: Safer and Healthier Foods." *MMWR*, 48(40): 905-913.

15. Centers for Disease Control and Prevention, Office of Communications (8 July 2003). "CDC Confirms Nation's First Human Case of West Nile in 2003 [Press release]." Available at http://www.cdc.gov/od/oc/media/pressrel/r030708.htm.

16. Centers for Disease Control and Prevention, Division of Vector-Borne Infectious Diseases (2004). "West Nile Virus: Background—Virus History and Distribution." Available at http://www.cdc.gov/ncidod/dvbid/westnile/background.htm.

17. Centers for Disease Control and Prevention, Division of Vector-Borne Infectious Diseases (2000). "Information on *Aedes albopictus*." Available at http://www.cdc.gov/ncidod/dvbid/arbor/albopic_new.htm.

18. Centers for Disease Control and Prevention, Division of Vector-Borne Infectious Diseases. "Information on *Aedes japonicus*." Available at http://www.cdc.gov/ncidod/dvbid/arbor/japonicus.htm.

19. Centers for Disease Control and Prevention (2005). "Lyme Disease: Statistics." Available at http://www.cdc.gov/ncidod/dvbid/lyme/ld_statistics.htm.

20. Miller, G. T. (2004). *Living in the Environment: Principles, Connections, and Solutions*, 13th ed. Pacific Grove, CA: Brooks/Cole-Thompson Learning.

21. Enger, E. D., and B. F. Smith (1992). *Environmental Science: A Study of Interrelationships*, 4th ed. Dubuque, IA: Wm. C. Brown.

22. U.S. Environmental Protection Agency (2000). *For Your Information: Pesticides and Child Safety. Prevention, Pesticides and Toxic Substances* (7506C 735-F-93-050). Washington, DC: Author.

23. Substance Abuse and Mental Health Administration (2006). *Results from the 2005 National Survey on Drug Use and Health: National Findings* (NSHUG Series H-30, HHS pub. no. SMA 06-4194). Rockville, MD: Author.

24. Overpeck, M. D., and A. J. Moss (1991). *Children's Exposure to Environmental Cigarette Smoke before and after Birth* (HHS pub. no. PHS-91-1250). Washington, DC: U.S. Government Printing Office.

25. U.S. Environmental Protection Agency (1993). *Respiratory Health Effects of Passive Smoking: Lung Cancer and Other Disorders* (EPA/600/6-90/006f). Washington, DC: U.S. Government Printing Office.

26. U.S. Department of Health and Human Services (1991). *Environmental Tobacco Smoke in the Workplace* (HHS [NIOSH] pub. no. 91-108). Washington, DC: U.S. Government Printing Office.

27. U.S. Environmental Protection Agency (1992). *Respiratory Health Effects of Passive Smoking: Lung Cancer and Other Disorders* (EPA/600/6-90/006). Washington, DC: U.S. Government Printing Office.

28. American Cancer Society (2006). *Cancer Facts and Figures—2006*. Atlanta, GA: Author.

29. California Environmental Protection Agency, Office of Environmental Health Hazard Assessment (September 1997). *Health Effects of Exposure to Environmental Tobacco Smoke*. Available at http://www.oehha.ca.gov/air/environmental_tobacco/finalets.html.

30. American Lung Association (2005). *State Legislated Actions on Tobacco Issues: 2005*. Washington, DC: Author. Available at http://slati.lungusa.org/reports/SLATI_05.pdf.

31. American Lung Association (2006). *State of Tobacco Control: 2006*. New York: Author. Available at http://www.lungusa.org/.

32. Chiras, D. D. (2001). *Environmental Science: Creating a Sustainable Future*, 6th ed. Sudbury, MA: Jones and Bartlett.

33. Silbergeld, E. K. (1997). "Preventing Lead Poisoning in Children." *Annual Review of Public Health*, 18: 187-210.

34. Centers for Disease Control and Prevention, National Center for Environmental Health (2004). "About Childhood Lead Poisoning." Available at http://www.cdc.gov/nceh/lead/about/about.htm.

35. U.S. Department of Health and Human Services (November 2000). *Healthy People 2010: Understanding and Improving Health*, 2nd ed. Washington, DC: U.S. Government Printing Office.

36. Centers for Disease Control and Prevention (1992). "Implementation of the Lead Contamination Control Act of 1988." *MMWR*, 41(17): 288-290.

37. Centers for Disease Control and Prevention (2000). "Elevated Blood Lead Levels among Internationally Adopted Children—United States, 1998." *MMWR*, 49(5): 97-100.

38. Centers for Disease Control and Prevention (2002). *National Center for Environmental Health Fact Book 2002*. Available at http://www.cdc.gov/nceh/publications/factbook/2002/default.htm.

39. U.S. Environmental Protection Agency (2006). "Radiation Protection: Radon." Available at http://www.epa.gov/radiation/radionuclides/radon.html.

40. Nichols, G. (1999). "The Ebb and Flow of Radon." *American Journal of Public Health*, 89(7): 993-994.

41. U.S. Environmental Protection Agency (2006). "Sunwise Program." Available at http://www.epa.gov/sunwise/uviscale.html.

42. New York City Department of Health and Mental Hygiene (7 April 2006). "Substantial Physical and Mental Health Effects Reported by WTC Building Survivors [Press release]." Available at http://www.nyc.gov/html/doh/html/pr2006/pr021-06.shtml.

43. Cunningham, W. P., M. A. Cunningham, and B. Saigo (2005). *Environmental Science: A Global Concern*, 8th ed. New York: McGraw-Hill.

44. U.S. Census Bureau (2004). *Global Population Profile: 2002* (International Population Reports WP/02). Washington, DC: U.S. Government Printing Office.

45. Hinrichsen, D., and B. Robey (Fall 2000). *Population and the Environment: The Global Challenge* (Population Reports, Series M, no. 15). Baltimore, MD: Johns Hopkins University School of Public Health, Population Information Program.

46. Kluger, J. (2000). "The Big Crunch." *Time* (Special Edition), Earth Day 2000: 44-47.

47. Manuel, J. (2006). "News Focus: In Katrina's Wake." *Environmental Health Perspectives*, 114 (1): A32-A39.

48. Centers for Disease Control and Prevention (2005). "Infectious Disease and Dermatological Conditions in Evacuees and Rescue Workers after Hurricane Katrina—Multiple States, August-September, 2005." *MMWR*, 54(Dispatch): 1-4.

49. Federal Emergency Management Agency (2006). "About FEMA." Available at http://www.fema.gov/about/history.shtm.

50. American Red Cross (2006). "Disaster Services." Available at http://www.redcross.org/.

Chapter 17

Injuries as a Community Health Problem

Chapter Objectives

After studying this chapter you will be able to:

1 Describe the importance of injuries as a
community health problem.

2 Explain why the terms *accidents* and *safety* have
been replaced by the currently more acceptable
terms *unintentional injuries, injury prevention,*
and *injury control* when dealing with such
occurrences.

3 Briefly explain the difference between intentional
and unintentional injuries and provide examples
of each.

4 List the four elements usually included in the
definition of the term *unintentional injury*.

5 Summarize the epidemiology of unintentional
injuries.

6 List strategies for the prevention and control of
unintentional injuries.

7 Explain how education, regulation, automatic
protection, and litigation can reduce the number
and seriousness of unintentional injuries.

8 Define the term *intentional injuries* and provide
examples of behavior that results in intentional
injuries.

9 Describe the scope of intentional injuries as a
community health problem in the United States.

10 List some contributing factors to domestic
violence and some strategies for reducing it.

11 List some of the contributing factors to the
increase in violence related to youth gangs and
explain what communities can do to reduce this
level of violence.

12 Discuss intervention approaches for preventing or
controlling intentional injuries.

SCENARIO

Peter decided to mow the lawn before his ball game. He felt he could complete the task in less than an hour. He checked and filled the gas tank, started the mower, and began mowing. In one corner of the yard, he found it easier to pull the lawnmower backward rather than to push it forward. Peter had done this many times, without incident. This time, he tripped over a stump and lost his balance. In attempting to regain his balance, he pulled harder on the mower, causing it to run over his foot. Instantly he experienced a severe sharp pain and automatically jerked his foot back, but it was too late; the mower blade had cut through Peter's shoe and big toe! Peter quickly turned off the mower and hobbled to the house. As he prepared to go to the emergency room at the local hospital, he was angry with himself as he thought about how his carelessness had caused his injury and might eventually lead to losing his toe.

INTRODUCTION

This chapter first defines and then examines the scope, causes, and effects on the community of both unintentional and intentional injuries. It also reviews approaches to the prevention and control of injuries and injury deaths.

Definitions

The word **injury** is derived from the Latin word for "not right."[1] Injuries result from "acute exposure to physical agents such as mechanical energy, heat, electricity, chemicals, and ionizing radiation interacting with the body in amounts or at rates that exceed the threshold of human tolerance."[2] In this chapter we discuss both **unintentional injuries,** injuries judged to have occurred without anyone intending that harm be done (such as those that result from car crashes, falls, drownings, and fires), and **intentional injuries,** injuries judged to have been purposely inflicted, either by another or oneself (such as assaults, intentional shootings and stabbings, and suicides).

The term *accident* has fallen into disfavor and disuse with many public health officials whose goal it is to reduce the number and seriousness of all injuries. The very word *accident* suggests a chance occurrence or an unpreventable mishap. Yet, we know that many, if not most, accidents are preventable. The term *unintentional injury* is now used in its place. Similarly, the rather vague term *safety* has largely been replaced by **injury prevention** or **injury control.** These terms are inclusive of all measures to prevent injuries, both unintentional and intentional, or to minimize their severity.

There are four significant characteristics of unintentional injuries: (1) they are unplanned events, (2) they usually are preceded by an unsafe act or condition (hazard), (3) they often are accompanied by economic loss, and (4) they interrupt the efficient completion of tasks.

An **unsafe act** is any *behavior* that would increase the probability of an unintentional injury. For example, driving an automobile while being impaired by alcohol or operating a power saw without eye protection is an unsafe act (see Figure 17.1). An **unsafe condition** is any *environmental factor* (physical or social) that would increase the probability of an unintentional injury. Icy streets are an example of an unsafe condition. Unsafe acts and unsafe conditions are **hazards.** While hazards do not actually *cause* unintentional injuries (an alcohol-impaired person may reach home uninjured, even over icy streets), they do increase the probability that an unintentional injury will occur.

injury
physical damage to the body resulting from mechanical, chemical, thermal, or other environmental energy

unintentional injury
an injury that occurred without anyone intending that harm be done

intentional injury
an injury that is purposely inflicted, either by the victim or by another

injury prevention (control)
an organized effort to prevent injuries or to minimize their severity

unsafe act
any behavior that would increase the probability of an injury occurring

FIGURE 17.1

An unsafe act is a behavior that increases the probability of an injury. Should this person be wearing eye protection?

unsafe condition
any environmental factor or set of factors (physical or social) that would increase the probability of an injury occurring

hazard
an unsafe act or condition

fatal injury
an injury that results in one or more deaths

disabling injury
an injury causing any restriction of normal activity beyond the day of the injury's occurrence

Cost of Injuries to Society

Injuries are costly to society in terms of both human suffering and economic loss. Injuries are a leading cause of death and disability in the world. An estimated 5.2 million people died from injuries in 2001.[3] This means that more than 14,000 people die each day in the world from injuries. Each year in the United States, more than 150,000 people die from **fatal injuries,** making this the fifth leading cause of death in this country. Specifically, in 2004, there were 161,808 injury deaths, which accounted for 6.7% of all deaths among residents of the United States.[4] Of these deaths, 112,012 (69%) were classified as unintentional injury deaths, 32,439 (20%) as suicides, and 16,611 (10%) as homicides. The remaining 746 deaths were either of undetermined intent or the result of legal intervention (see Figure 17.2).[4]

Deaths are only a small part of the total cost of injuries. Worldwide, 10.9% of the world's burden of disease can be attributed to injuries.[3] In the United States, there were 41.4 million injury-related visits to hospital emergency departments, 9.4 million injury-related visits to hospital ambulatory medical outpatient departments, and 105.2 million injury-related visits to physician offices, for a total of 156 million medically attended injury-related episodes in 2004.[5-7] Of these injuries, an estimated 23.2 million were **disabling injuries,** that is, injuries that restricted normal activity beyond the day of the injury (see Figure 17.3).[8]

In addition to the human suffering caused by injuries are the economic costs. These include the lifetime medical costs and the lifetime loss of productivity costs of the injuries. The most complete analysis of the cost of injuries recently published was based on 2000 figures: 149,000 fatalities, 1.9 million hospitalizations, and 48.1 million nonhospitalized treatment episodes. The combined economic burden of med-

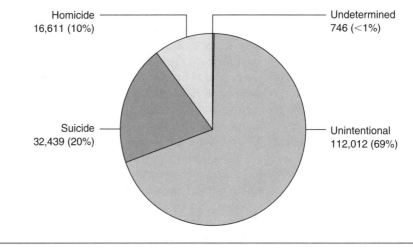

FIGURE 17.2

Injury deaths: United States, 2004.

Source: Miniño, A. M., M. Heron, S. L. Murphy, and K. D. Kochanek (2006). *Deaths: Final Data for 2004.* NCHS Health E-Stats. Available at http://www.cdc.gov/nchs/products/pubs/pubd/hestats/finaldeaths04/finaldeaths04.htm.

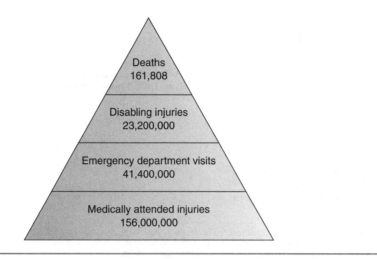

FIGURE 17.3

Burden of injury: United States, 2004.

Sources: Miniño, A. M., M. Heron, S. L. Murphy, and K. D. Kochanek (2006). *Deaths: Final Data for 2004*. NCHS Health E-Stats. Available at http://www.cdc.gov/nchs/products/pubs/pubd/hestats/finaldeaths04/finaldeaths04.htm; McCaig, L. F., and E. W. Nawar (2006). *National Ambulatory Medical Care Survey: 2004 Emergency Department Summary* (Advance Data from Vital and Health Statistics no. 372). Hyattsville, MD: National Center for Health Statistics; Middleton, K. R., and E. Hing (2006). *National Hospital Ambulatory Medical Care Survey: 2004 Outpatient Department Summary* (Advance Data from Vital and Health Statistics no. 373). Hyattsville, MD: National Center for Health Statistics; Hing, E., D. K. Cherry, and D. A. Woodall (2006). *National Ambulatory Medical Care Survey: 2004 Summary* (Advance Data from Vital and Health Statistics no. 374). Hyattsville, MD: National Center for Health Statistics; and National Safety Council (2006). *Injury Facts 2005–2006 Edition*. Itasca, IL: Author.

ical treatment and lost productivity totaled more than $406 billion. This figure comprises $143 billion (35%) for fatal injuries, $92 billion (23%) for hospitalized injuries, and nearly $171 billion (42%) for nonhospitalized injuries. The cost of lost productivity exceeds the cost of medical treatment for accidents in each of the categories of injuries just mentioned, but the difference is highest in fatal injuries, where loss of productivity makes up 99% of the economic burden.[9] The true economic burden of injuries is much greater than this estimate because it does not include value of life lost to premature mortality, loss of patient and caregiver time, and nonmedical expenditures such as insurance costs, property damage, litigation, decreased quality of life, and disability. In 2002, it was estimated that the economic impact of fatal and nonfatal unintentional injuries alone amounted to $575 billion, or approximately $2,000 per person in the United States.

Injuries contribute to premature deaths (deaths that occur before reaching the age of one's life expectancy) in the United States. In terms of years of potential life lost before 75 years of age (YPLL-75), unintentional injuries rank third. However, when one considers all injuries, both intentional and unintentional, then injuries are the leading cause of YPLL-75. Leading causes of YPLL-75 and number of deaths for various causes of death are shown in Table 17.1.[10,11]

It is important to understand that federal funding for health research is not allocated on a cost-per-death basis. The federal investment for injury research is only about one-seventh of that for cancer research and one-third of that for research on heart diseases and stroke (see Figure 17.4).[12]

Injuries place a special burden on our emergency departments because they are the leading cause of such visits, making up more than one-third of the total visits. There were an estimated 41.4 million injury-related emergency department (ED) visits during 2004, or 14.4 visits per 100 persons per year. This made up 37.3% of all ED visits in 2004. Included in

Table 17.1
Leading Causes of Years of Potential Life Lost (YPLL) and Number of Deaths for Leading Causes of Death: United States, 2003

Disease or Condition	Age-Adjusted YPLL before Age 75 (per 100,000 population)	Number of Deaths
Injury	1,602	163,988
Cancer	1,587	556,902
Heart disease	1,188	685,089
Stroke	204	157,689
Diabetes mellitus	185	74,219
Chronic lower respiratory diseases	184	126,382
Chronic liver disease and cirrhosis	160	27,503
Human immunodeficiency virus disease	153	13,658
Influenza and pneumonia	91	65,163

Sources: National Center for Health Statistics (2006). *Health, United States, 2006 with Chartbook on Trends in the Health of Americans with Special Feature on Pain.* Hyattsville, MD: National Center for Health Statistics; and Hoyert, E. L., M. P. Heron, S. L. Murphy, and H. Kung (2006). "Deaths: Final Data for 2003." *National Vital Statistics Reports,* 54(13): 1–120.

this total were 535,000 visits related to self-inflicted injuries. Sixty-seven percent of all ED injury visits are for unintentional injuries.[5]

UNINTENTIONAL INJURIES

Unintentional injuries are the cause of nearly two-thirds of all injury-related deaths in the United States and rank fifth as a leading cause of death (see Table 3.8). There were 112,012 unintentional injury deaths in 2004.[4] Accounting for those deaths were motor vehicle crashes (40%), followed by unintentional poisonings (18%) and falls (17%), along with other causes.[13] In addition to the human death toll were the economic costs, mentioned earlier, estimated at $574.8 billion, including $298 billion in lost wages and productivity, $99 billion in medical

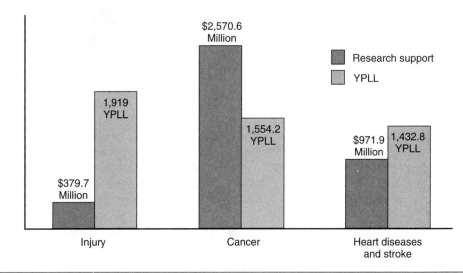

FIGURE 17.4
Average number of years of potential life lost (YPLL) versus the federal research investment.

Source: Bonnie, R. J., C. E. Fulco, and C. T. Liverman, eds. (1999). *Reducing the Burden of Injury: Advancing Prevention and Treatment.* Institute of Medicine, Committee on Injury Prevention and Control. Washington, DC: National Academies Press. Reprinted with permission.

expenses, $112 billion in insurance administration costs, and $65 billion in motor vehicle damage and other costs.[8] Clearly, unintentional injuries constitute one of America's major community health problems. One of the *Healthy People 2010* objectives is to reduce the rate of unintentional injuries from nearly 35 per 100,000 population to 17 per 100,000.[14]

Types of Unintentional Injuries

There are many types of unintentional injuries. The majority occur as a result of motor vehicle crashes, poisonings, falls, drownings, suffocation, fires and burns, and firearms. These are discussed briefly here.

Motor Vehicle Crashes

Road traffic crash victims can be found throughout the world. Worldwide, 1.26 million people were killed (3,000 each day) and 50 million were injured in road traffic crashes in 2000. An estimated 90% of deaths occurred in middle- or low-income countries as compared with just 10% in developed countries.[15]

In the United States, more people die from unintentional injuries associated with motor vehicle crashes than any other type of injury. In 2005 more than 6 million police-reported motor vehicle crashes occurred, including nearly 2 million crashes resulting in injuries. An estimated 1.9 million people were injured and 43,433 people were killed. Fatal injury rates per 100 million vehicle miles traveled (VMT), which had declined every year since 1995, rose slightly in 2005. A majority of those killed were drivers (64%), followed by passengers (28%), motorcycle riders (3%), pedestrians (3%), and pedalcyclists (2%).[16] One of the nation's *Healthy People 2010* objectives is to reduce the number of motor vehicle deaths per 100,000 population from the 1999 baseline of 14.7 to 9.2 by 2010. A second objective is to reduce the number of motor vehicle deaths per 100 million VMT from the 1998 baseline of 1.6 to 0.8 by 2010.[14] By 2005, only modest progress had been made on reaching these objectives (see Box 17.1).

Poisonings

Poisonings were the second leading cause of unintentional deaths in 2004, when unintentional poisoning deaths numbered 19,250.[13] These deaths resulted from unintentional ingestion of fatal doses of medicines and drugs, consumption of toxic foods such as mushrooms and

---

BOX 17.1 HEALTHY PEOPLE 2010 OBJECTIVE: REDUCE DEATHS CAUSED BY MOTOR VEHICLE CRASHES

Target and baseline:

Objective	Baseline Year	Baseline	1998	2005	Target 2010
15.15a Deaths from motor vehicle crashes (age-adjusted per 100,000 standard population)	1999	14.7	NA	14.66	8.0
15.15b Deaths from motor vehicle crashes (per 100 million vehicle miles traveled)	1998	1.6	BSL	1.47	0.8

For Further Thought

In 1999, drivers between 15 and 20 years old made up just 6.8% of the licensed drivers but were involved in 14.7% of fatal crashes. Do you think that issuing graduated driver's licenses to new drivers is a solution? If not, how would you suggest states respond to this problem?

Source: U.S. Department of Health and Human Services (2000). *Healthy People 2010: Understanding and Improving Health*, 2nd ed. Washington, DC: U.S. Government Printing Office.

shellfish, and from exposure to toxic substances in the workplace or elsewhere. Four-fifths of these poisonings occurred in homes, where poisonings are the leading cause of injury deaths.[8]

Falls

The third leading cause of unintentional fatal injuries is falls, which resulted in 18,535 deaths in 2004.[13] Falls were the leading cause of injury-related ED visits in 2004, with 8.5 million visits.[5] Falls can occur from one surface level to another—stairs or ladders, for example—or on the same level. More than half of the 17,000 or more deaths resulting from falls each year are from falls that occur at home, where falls account for one-third of all deaths from unintentional injuries.[8]

Falls disproportionately affect elders. Each year in the United States, falls affect approximately 30% of elders (adults 65 years of age and older).[17] Falls are the leading cause of both nonfatal and fatal injury among elders, and the Number 1 reason for ED visits among this population. Sixty-two percent of all nonfatal-injury ED visits by elders were attributed to falls.[18]

Other Types of Unintentional Injuries

Other leading causes of unintentional injury deaths in 2004 were fires and burns (3,223), drowning (3,180), all other transport deaths (2,986), and firearms (661). All other types of unintentional injury deaths numbered about 16,898 in 2004.[13]

Epidemiology of Unintentional Injuries

Unintentional injuries are a major community health concern because they account for a disproportionately large number of *early* deaths in our society. However, deaths are only a part of the human toll; incapacitation is another significant aspect of the problem. One in six hospital days can be attributed to unintentional injuries. As mentioned earlier, medical costs from unintentional injuries run into the billions of dollars annually. Many of these injuries, such as head and spinal cord injuries, result in long-term or permanent disabilities that can affect individuals and their families for years.

Some of the factors that describe where, when, and to whom unintentional injuries occur are discussed in the following sections. In addition to describing the occurrence of injuries by person, place, and time, we include a discussion of alcohol and other drugs as risk factors in unintentional injuries.

Person

Unintentional injuries resulting in death and disability occur in all age groups, genders, races, and socioeconomic groupings. However, certain groups are at greater risk for injury than others.

Age

After the first year of life, unintentional injuries become the leading cause of death in children. They are the leading cause of death in the following age groups: 1–4, 5–14, 15–24, 25–34, and 35–44 years of age. They are the third leading cause of death in the 45- to 54-year age group (after cancer and heart disease). Unintentional injuries account for 38% of the deaths in the 5- to 14-year age group; the percentage is higher for males (41%) than for females (32%).[19]

More than half of all deaths among older teenagers (15–19 years of age) are caused by unintentional injuries,[18] and 68% of the 18 million ED visits each year by adolescents are due to injuries. The highest rate of injury-related visits to EDs for all types of injuries is by 15- to 24-year-old males (see Figure 17.5).[5]

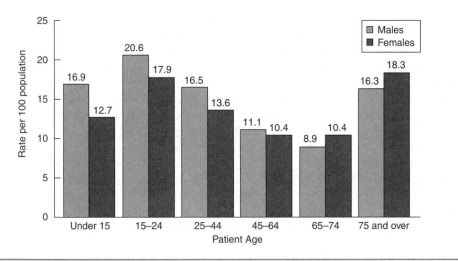

FIGURE 17.5

Rates of injury-related visits to emergency departments by age and sex, 2004.

Source: McCaig, L. F., and E. W. Nawar (2006). *National Ambulatory Medical Care Survey: 2004 Emergency Department Summary* (Advance Data from Vital and Health Statistics no. 372). Hyattsville, MD: National Center for Health Statistics.

Children and teenagers are at a higher than average risk of dying as a result of unintentional firearm injury. Unintentional nonfatal firearm-related injury rates are highest among persons aged 15 to 24 years, and these rates decrease with age[20] (see Figure 17.6). Nearly 10% of high school males carried a gun to school at least once in 2005.[21] Some people believe that childhood firearm deaths are a national tragedy in the United States. A child under 15

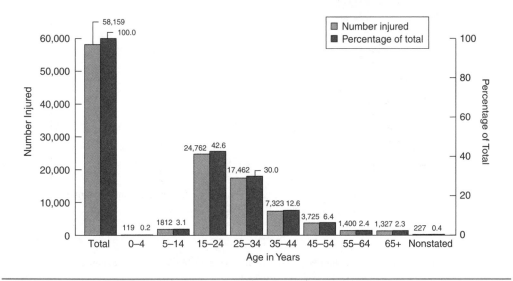

FIGURE 17.6

National estimates of the number and percentage of persons with nonfatal firearm injuries treated in hospital emergency departments, United States, 2004.

Source: U.S. Department of Health and Human Services, Centers for Disease Control and Prevention, National Center for Injury Prevention and Control (2006). *Firearm Injury Surveillance Study, 1993-2004* [Computer file] (ICPSR04595-V1). Atlanta, GA: Author. Available at http://webapp.icpsr.umich.edu/cocoon/ICPSR-STUDY/04595.xml.

years of age is nine times more likely to die of an unintentional firearm injury in the United States than in the other 25 industrialized nations (see Figure 17.7).[22] Unintentional firearm injuries constitute an important public health problem. Two states, California and Florida, have enacted legislation making adults legally responsible for the inappropriate storage of firearms.

For all age groups except persons 80 years and older, motor vehicle crashes are the leading cause of unintentional injury deaths.[2,11] However, rates of involvement in crashes resulting in fatal injuries in 2004 were the highest for drivers aged 16 to 20 (62 per 100,000 licensed drivers). This was twice the fatal injury involvement rate for all drivers (29 per 100,000 licensed drivers).[23]

Among elders (those 65 years and older), injuries are the eighth leading cause of death. Injury deaths would rank higher, but many elders die of other causes resulting from the aging process, such as heart disease, cancer, and stroke. An examination of the rates of death per 100,000 among elders reveals that elders have the highest unintentional injury death rate of

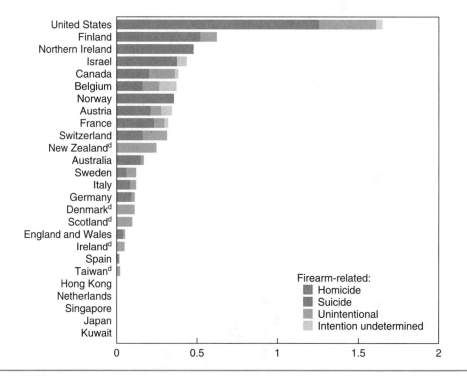

FIGURE 17.7

Rates[a] of firearm-related death[b] among children younger than 15 years in 26 industrialized countries.[c]

[a]Per 100,000 children aged < 15 years and for 1 year during 1990–1995.
[b]Homicides by firearm (*International Classification of Diseases,* 9th Rev., codes E965.0–E965.4), suicides by firearm (E955.0–E955.4), unintentional deaths caused by firearm (E922.0–E922.9), and firearm-related deaths for which intention was undetermined (E985.0–E985.4).
[c]All countries classified in the high-income group with population = 1 million (5) that provided complete data. In this analysis, Hong Kong, Northern Ireland, and Taiwan are considered as countries.
[d]Reported only unintentional firearm-related deaths.

Source: Centers for Disease Control and Prevention (1997). "Rates of Homicide, Suicide and Firearm-Related Deaths among Children—26 Industrial Countries." *MMWR,* 46(5): 101–105.

any age group (113 per 100,000). For those 85 years and older, the injury death rate climbs to 275 per 100,000.[2]

Falls are the leading cause of unintentional injury deaths for those 80 years and older. At age 80, the death rate from falls surpasses that for motor vehicle crashes and accounts for more than half of the unintentional injury-related deaths of this age group.

Elders are at age-increased risk of dying in car crashes, too. A report published by the AAA Foundation revealed that drivers 65 years and older are almost twice as likely to die in car crashes as drivers aged 55 to 64. Drivers 75 and older were two and one-half times as likely to die, and drivers 85 and over were almost four times as likely to die in car crashes compared with drivers aged 55 to 64.[24]

Elders also experience high rates of nonfatal injuries. In 2001, approximately 2.7 million elders (935,556 men and 1,731,640 women) were treated for nonfatal injuries in EDs. Elders are three times more likely to hospitalized following an injury than those younger than 65.[18]

Gender

Statistics indicate that, at every age level, males are much more likely to become involved in a fatal unintentional injury than females. Overall, the ratio of male deaths to female deaths is nearly 2:1. In the 15- to 24-year and 25- to 64-year age groups, males die from unintentional injuries at greater than three times the rate of their female counterparts. Although differences in unintentional injury death rates between the sexes decline with age, men retain a marginally higher rate even in the over-75-year age group. The type of unintentional fatality with the widest disparity in rates per 100,000 is firearm injuries (18.4 in males vs. 2.8 in females); the type with the narrowest is falls (6.4 in males vs. 5.5 in females).[2]

Minority Status

In 2002, unintentional injuries and adverse effects were the leading cause of death for all ages through the 25- to 34-year age group in all racial and ethnic groups except for blacks. In this racial group, homicide and legal intervention replaced unintentional injuries as the leading causes of injury deaths for the 15- to 24-year and 25- to 34-year age groups.[19] Age-adjusted death rates for unintentional injuries in 2002 were highest for the American Indian/Alaska Native population (48.4 per 100,000) and lowest for the Asian/Pacific Islander population (14.7 per 100,000). The white, non-Hispanic population had a rate of 37.0, while the Hispanic population had a slightly lower rate of 25.8 per 100,000 population.[19]

Place

Unintentional injuries occur wherever people are—at home, at work, or on the road. Although more injuries occur at home, more injury deaths occur on the road.

Home

People spend more time at home than any other place, so it is not surprising that 47.4% of all unintentional injuries and poisonings reported in the 2004 National Health Interview Survey were injuries that occurred in the home (see Figure 17.8).[25] Unintentional injuries in the home result from falls, burns, poisonings, accidental shootings and stabbings, and suffocation. Within the home, some areas are more dangerous than others. The presence of appliances (including stoves, toasters, mixers, and so on) and sharp knives in the kitchen makes this room one of the more dangerous in the house. Another location where many unintentional injuries occur, particularly to the very young and old, is on stairways. For children, the bathroom, garage, and basement are hazardous areas because of the drugs, cleaning agents, and other poisonous materials that are often stored in these areas. In the home, more people die in bedrooms, where they may be sleeping during a fire, than in any other room.

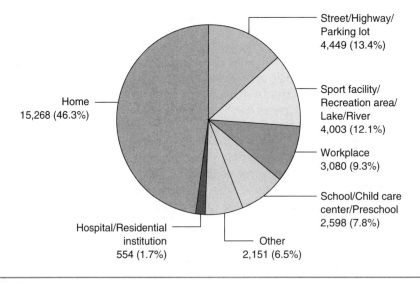

FIGURE 17.8

Number (in thousands) and percentage of injury episodes by place of occurrence: United States, 2004.

Source: Adams, P. F., and P. M. Barnes (2006). "Summary Health Statistics for the U.S. Population: National Health Interview Survey, 2004." *Vital and Health Statistics*, 10(229): 1–104.

Highway

More than 13% of all injuries reported in the National Health Interview Survey in 2004 were sustained on streets, highways, and parking lots.[25] Although these venues rank second to the home as places for nonfatal injuries, they rank first for fatal injuries. Approximately 40% of all unintentional injury deaths are motor vehicle deaths (see Figure 17.9). Significant progress has been made in reducing the rate of motor vehicle–related deaths, from 22.5 per 100,000 population in 1980 to 14.7 per 100,000 in 2005.[16] This has been achieved through effective interventions,

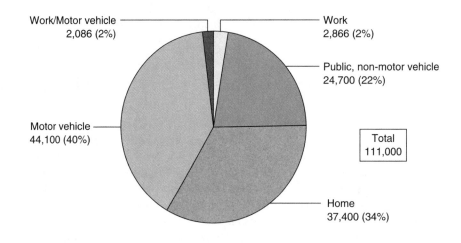

FIGURE 17.9

Unintentional injury deaths by class: United States, 2004. Note: Deaths for sections of chart add to more than the total because some deaths are included in more than one section.

Source: National Safety Council (2006). *Injury Facts 2005–2006 Edition.* Itasca, IL: Author. Reprinted with permission.

including increasing public awareness, education, legal proscriptions (such as child safety seats and safety belts), innovative vehicle and equipment designs, improved roadways, and enhanced medical systems.

Nonetheless, there are those who believe we could do a better job. One area of concern is the number of unlicensed or improperly licensed drivers on the highways. A five-year study (1993–1997) revealed that 20% of all fatal crashes—one in five—involve at least one improperly licensed driver. These are drivers with a license that is suspended, revoked, expired, cancelled, or denied. Nearly 4% of drivers involved in fatal crashes had no known license at all.[26]

Recreation/Sport Area

The third most likely place to sustain an injury that results in a visit to an ED is a recreation or sports area, such as a soccer field, baseball diamond, or basketball court. Approximately 12% of injuries reported in the 2004 National Health Interview Survey occurred in these settings.[25]

Workplace

The workplace ranks fourth as a location where unintentional injuries frequently occur. About 9.3% of reported injuries occurred in the workplace.[25] As one might imagine, the risk of injury varies widely among different occupations. Among the most dangerous occupations are mining, farming (including logging), and construction. (For more information about workplace injuries, see Chapter 18.)

Time

During the twentieth century, there were declines for some types of unintentional injuries and increases for others. For example, motor vehicle deaths fell from 53,543 in 1969 to 42,815 in 2005. This reduction occurred despite the fact that Americans drove 2.7 times more miles in 2005 than they did in 1980. The fatality rate per 100 million VMT declined from 3.35 to 1.47 during that 25-year period.[16] This reduction in the death rate from motor vehicle crashes in the United States is one of the ten most significant public health achievements of the twentieth century (see Box 17.2).

Since 1975, unintentional deaths from drowning, fires, and burns have declined by more than half, and from firearms by two-thirds. However, deaths from falls, which declined significantly from 1975 to 1986, have begun to increase in the past few years, as the U.S. population ages. Deaths from poisonings have also increased since the late 1970s,[8] and now rank second as a leading cause of unintentional injury deaths.[13]

There are seasonal variations in the incidence of some types of unintentional injuries, but these depend upon the types of injury. For example, 62% of all drownings occur in

---

BOX 17.2   TEN GREAT PUBLIC HEALTH ACHIEVEMENTS, 1900–1999: MOTOR VEHICLE SAFETY

**Bumper to Bumper and Curb to Curb . . .
Driving Is Safer Now Than in 1900**

Although more people are driving automobiles, traveling more miles, and driving at faster speeds than in 1900, driving is much safer now because of safer vehicles, highways, and drivers.

Since 1925, the annual death rate from motor vehicle travel has decreased 90%, despite the increase in miles traveled and the number of vehicles used per capita.

Approximately 85,000 American lives have been saved because of seat belts.

Using child safety seats has reduced the risk of infant death by 69% and of children aged 1 to 4 years by 47%.

Since 1987, community awareness and driving-while-intoxicated regulations have helped reduce alcohol-related traffic fatalities by 32%.

FIGURE 17.10
Nearly 40% of highway fatalities involve the use of alcohol.

four months—May, June, July, and August—when more people take part in water sports. Conversely, 65% of all deaths due to fires and burns are recorded during the six months from November through April, when furnaces, fireplaces, wood-burning stoves, and electric and kerosene space heaters are most often in use.[8]

Motor vehicle crash rates per 100 million VMT in 2002 were highest during November and December. Motor vehicle–related deaths increase markedly at night. Fatalities also occur at a higher rate on weekends (Friday through Sunday). Although more fatal crashes occur on Saturdays, more crashes of all types occur on Fridays. The hours between midnight and 3 A.M. Saturdays and Sundays are the most dangerous three-hour periods to travel by car (see Figure 17.10).[16]

Much publicity surrounds the number of motor vehicle deaths that occur during the following six major holiday periods: Memorial Day, Fourth of July, Labor Day, Thanksgiving, Christmas, and New Year. However, it has been shown that the number of crash-related deaths for these periods is not significantly different from the number occurring during nonholiday periods. However, the proportion of fatal crashes that are alcohol related is higher during holiday periods (about 50% for New Year's Day, Memorial Day, Fourth of July, and Labor Day; about 45% for Thanksgiving and Christmas) than during nonholiday periods (about 39%).[16]

Alcohol and Other Drugs as Risk Factors

An examination of the factors that contribute to intentional and unintentional injuries reveals that alcohol may be the single most important factor. This is certainly the case with fatal motor vehicle crashes, in which 39% of persons killed in traffic crashes in 2005 died in alcohol-related crashes. While 39% represents a significant decline from the 60% reported in 1982, it is still too high. There has also been a decline in the percentage of those killed in crashes who were intoxicated—that is, who had blood alcohol concentrations (BACs) that exceeded 0.08% (BAC > 0.08%)—from 53% in 1982 to 39% in 2005.[16]

The percentage of drivers in fatal crashes whose BAC exceeded the legal limit (0.08%) was 20% in 2005, but this percentage was four times higher at night than during the day. Alcohol was involved in 75% of the single-car crashes that occurred on a weekend night in which a 21-year-old or older driver or motorcycle operator was killed (see Figure 17.11). The percentage of drivers or motorcycle operators involved in fatal crashes whose BAC exceeded 0.08% was highest for drivers aged 21 to 24 years (37%) (see Figure 17.12), and twice as high for males as for females.[16] Forty-one percent of drivers and motorcycle operators involved in fatal crashes had a previous record of crashes, license suspension or revocation, DWI conviction, speeding conviction, or other harmful moving violation conviction.[16]

Unfortunately, drivers are not the only persons killed in alcohol-related motor vehicle crashes. Motor vehicle crashes are the leading cause of death among children aged 1 year and older in the United States, and one in four deaths of child passengers aged 14 years and older involves alcohol use. Of the 2,355 children who died in alcohol-related crashes during the period 1997 to 2002, 1,588 (68%) were riding with drinking drivers.[27]

Alcohol use often contributes to motor vehicle injuries and deaths in another way. Safety belt use by drinking drivers is lower than for their nondrinking counterparts, thus increasing the likelihood of a fatal outcome if there is a crash. In 1999, safety belts were used by only

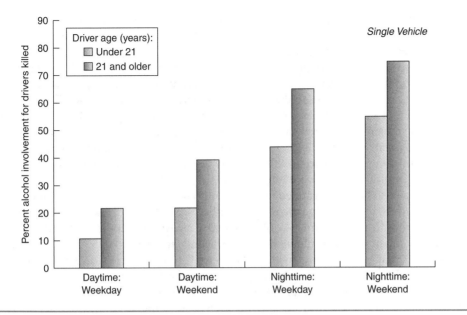

FIGURE 17.11

Alcohol involvement (BAC ≥ 0.01) for drivers or motorcycle operators killed, by driver age, time of day, and day of week.

Source: U.S. Department of Transportation, National Highway Traffic Safety Administration (2006). *Traffic Safety Facts 2006: A Compilation of Motor Vehicle Crash Data from the Fatality Analysis Reporting System and the General Estimates System* (DOT HS 810 631), Early ed. Washington, DC: Author. Available at http://www-nrd.nhtsa.dot.gov/pdf/nrd-30/NCSA/TSFAnn/TSF2005EE.

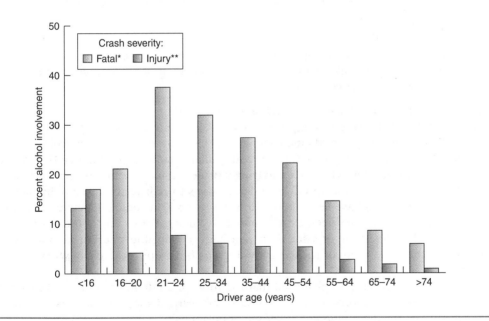

FIGURE 17.12

Percentage of driver or motorcycle operator alcohol involvement for fatal and injury crashes in 2002.

*For fatal crashes, alcohol involvement is a blood alcohol concentration (BAC) of 0.01 grams per deciliter or greater.
**For injury crashes, alcohol involvement is police-reported alcohol involvement.

Source: U.S. Department of Transportation, National Highway Traffic Safety Administration (2006). *Traffic Safety Facts 2006: A Compilation of Motor Vehicle Crash Data from the Fatality Analysis Reporting System and the General Estimates System* (DOT HS 810 631), Early ed. Washington, DC: Author. Available at http://www-nrd.nhtsa.dot.gov/pdf/nrd-30/NCSA/TSFAnn/TSF2005EE.

19% of fatally injured *intoxicated* drivers, compared with 30% of fatally injured impaired drivers (with BAC levels between 0.01% and 0.09%) and 48% of fatally injured sober drivers. Child passenger restraint use also decreases as the BAC of the driver increases. Of 1,409 child passengers with known restraint information who died while riding with drinking drivers (1997–2002), only 466 (32%) were restrained at the time of the crash. The likelihood that a child passenger restraint was used decreased with increases in drivers' BAC.[27] Passage of primary enforcement safety belt laws (laws that allow police to stop and ticket a driver solely because an occupant is unbelted) and stricter enforcement of these laws in all states could reduce child passenger deaths. Excessive drinking can also increase a pedestrian's chances of being killed by a motor vehicle. In 2005, nearly one-third (31%) of pedestrians 16 years or older killed by motor vehicles were intoxicated.[16]

Alcohol has also been determined to be an important factor in other types of unintentional injuries and deaths, including aquatic-related deaths. Nearly half of those who drown have evidence of alcohol in their blood. Alcohol is also a major risk factor for boating fatalities. Alcohol involvement was reported in 25% of all boating fatalities in 2005.[28] A U.S. Coast Guard study estimates that boat operators with a BAC above 0.10% are more than 10 times as likely to be killed in a boating accident than boat operators with zero BACs.[29] In another study, it was found that nearly half of all boating fatalities occurred when vessels were not under way. This implies that while it is dangerous when the person who is operating the boat is drinking, it is also dangerous when passengers have been drinking. Lastly, alcohol consumption lowers your chance of survival should you end up in the water. In a study conducted in Louisiana, alcohol and/or metabolites of an illicit drug were found in 60% of drowning victims aged 13 years or older.[30] Clearly, alcohol consumption and aquatic recreation are a dangerous combination.

Alcohol has also been shown to be a risk factor for bicyclists. More that one in three (36%) pedalcyclists killed in traffic crashes was killed in an alcohol-related crash.[16]

Prevention through Epidemiology

Sometimes it has been society's nature to wait until after a tragedy before correcting an existing hazard or dangerous situation. Most implementation of prevention activities related to injuries occurs only after costly disasters.

Early Contributors to Injury Prevention and Control

The first important efforts toward injury prevention and control began early in the twentieth century. Four of the most important contributors to early efforts at injury control were Hugh DeHaven, John E. Gordon, James Gibson, and William Haddon, Jr. Hugh DeHaven was a World War I combat pilot, who, after surviving a plane crash, dedicated his professional life to studying victims of falls in an effort to design ways to reduce the force of impact on a body. Many of his ideas have led to better design concepts, including structural adaptations to protect drivers and other occupants of moving vehicles. For example, today we have at our disposal the protection of safety belts, air bags, collapsible steering assemblies, and padded dashboards. Many of these safety devices built upon the early work of Hugh DeHaven.[31]

In 1949, John E. Gordon proposed that the tools of epidemiology be used to analyze injuries. Because of Gordon's work, a great deal was learned about risk factors, susceptible populations, and the distribution of injuries in populations.

In 1961, James Gibson proposed the idea that injury harm was caused by "energy interchange." Although this definition didn't fit well with certain injury deaths such as drowning and freezing, William Haddon, Jr., realized that in these cases, injury occurred because of the lack of necessary energy elements. Thus, the definition of injury supported by the National Center for Injury Prevention and Control (NCIPC) is "any intentional or unintentional damage to the body resulting from acute exposure to thermal, mechanical, electrical, or chemical energy or from the absence of such essentials as heat or oxygen."[31]

William Haddon, Jr., was both an engineer and a physician and is often considered the founding father of modern injury prevention research.[31] He was an unrelenting proponent of the epidemiological approach to injury control and insisted that the results of this work be used in the development of public policy. He was the foremost expert on highway safety in the 1960s and developed many successful countermeasures to reduce the number of unintentional highway injuries.

A Model for Unintentional Injuries

Until the 1950s, little progress occurred in the reduction of unintentional injuries and deaths. One reason for this was the failure to identify the causative agent associated with unintentional injuries. Chapter 4 discussed the public health model that describes communicable diseases in terms of the host, agent, and environment, arranged in a triangle. A similar **model for unintentional injuries** has been proposed. In this model, the injury-producing agent is *energy* (see Figure 17.13).

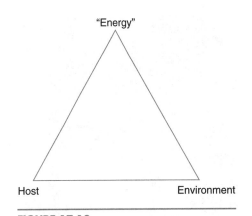

"Energy"

Host   Environment

FIGURE 17.13

The public health model for unintentional injuries.

model for unintentional injuries
the public health triangle (host, agent, and environment) modified to indicate energy as the causative agent of injuries

Examples of injury-producing energy are plentiful. A moving car, a falling object (or person), and a speeding bullet all have kinetic energy. When one of these moving objects strikes another object, energy is released, often resulting in injury or trauma. Similarly, a hot stove or pan contains energy in the form of heat. Contact with one of these objects results in the rapid transfer of heat. If the skin is unprotected, tissue damage (a burn) occurs. Electrical energy is all around us and represents a potential source of unintentional injuries. Even accidental poisonings fit nicely into the model that incorporates energy as the causative agent of injury. Cleansers, drugs, and medicines represent stored chemical energy which, when released inappropriately, can cause serious injury or death.

Prevention and Control Tactics Based upon the Model

Based upon the epidemiological model just described, there are four types of actions that can be taken to prevent or reduce the number and seriousness of unintentional injuries and deaths.[31] These four tactics are modified from those of Haddon. The first is to prevent the accumulation of the injury-producing agent, energy. Examples of implementing this principle include reducing speed limits to decrease motor vehicle injuries, lowering the height of children's high chairs and of diving boards to reduce fall injuries, and lowering the settings on hot water heaters to reduce the number and seriousness of burns. In our electrical example, circuit breakers in the home prevent the accumulation of excess electrical energy.

The second type of action is to prevent the inappropriate release of excess energy or to modify its release in some way. Flame-retardant fabric that will not ignite is an example of such a prevention. Currently, there is a law that requires that such a fabric be used in the manufacture of children's pajamas. The use of automobile safety belts is another example. In this case, excess energy (movement of a human body) is released into the safety belt instead of into the car's windshield (see Figure 17.14). In the prevention of fall injuries, hand rails, walkers, and nonslip surfaces in bathtubs prevent the inappropriate release of kinetic energy resulting from falls.

The third tactic involves placing a barrier between the host and agent. The insulation around electrical wires and the use of potholders and non–heat-transferring handles on cook-

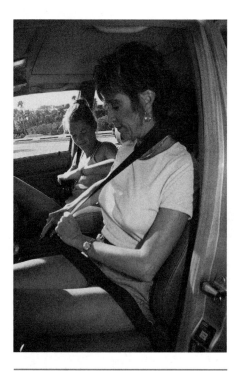

FIGURE 17.14
Safety belts prevent the inappropriate release of energy.

ware are examples of this preventive strategy. The use of sunscreen lotion and the wearing of a hat in the summer place a barrier between the sun's energy and you. Another example is the cable barriers being installed between opposing traffic lanes on many interstate highways. These installations not only serve as a barrier to protect oncoming traffic but also modify the release of energy and provide drivers and occupants with a relatively soft landing.

Finally, it is sometimes necessary or useful to completely separate the host from potentially dangerous sources of energy. Examples include the locked gates and high fences around electrical substations and swimming pools. At home, locking up guns and poisons provides protection against the likelihood of unintentional injury of young children.

Other Tactics

By viewing energy as the cause of unintentional injuries and deaths, it is possible to take positive steps in their prevention and control. There are still other actions that a community can take. First, injury-control education in the schools and in other public forums can be helpful. Second, improvements in the community's ability to respond to emergencies, such as encouraging the public to enroll in first aid and cardiopulmonary resuscitation (CPR) classes and expanding 911 telephone services, can limit disability and save lives. Third, communities can ensure that they have superior emergency and paramedic personnel by instituting the best possible training programs. The result will be improved emergency medical care and rehabilitation for the injured. Finally, communities can strengthen ordinances against high-risk behaviors, such as driving while impaired by alcohol, and then support their enforcement.

Community Approaches to the Prevention of Unintentional Injuries

There are four broad strategies for the prevention of unintentional injuries—education, regulation, automatic protection, and litigation.

Education

injury prevention education
the process of changing people's health-directed behavior so as to reduce unintentional injuries

Injury prevention education is the process of changing people's health-directed behavior in such a way as to reduce unintentional injuries. Education certainly has a place in injury prevention. Many of us remember the school fire drill, lessons on bicycle safety, and the school crossing guard. Undoubtedly, millions of injuries were prevented in these ways. However, injury prevention education has its limitations. Figure 17.15 illustrates both the inefficiency of public education and the difficulties of measuring a successful outcome.

Regulation

regulation
the enactment and enforcement of laws to control conduct

The former 55-mile-per-hour national speed limit is an example of the power of **regulation**—the enactment and enforcement of laws to control conduct—as a means of reducing the number and seriousness of unintentional injuries. For years, motorists were advised to drive more responsibly. Public service announcements in the 1960s and 1970s informed audiences that "speed kills," and advised motorists not to "drink and drive." However, the highway death toll continued to mount until 1974, when then President Gerald Ford issued the national 55-mile-per-hour speed limit. Although the primary purpose of the slower speed

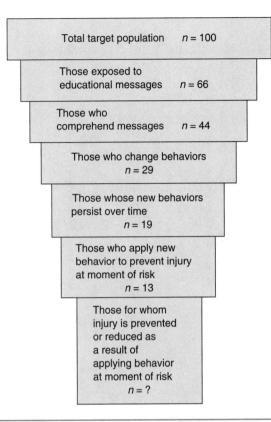

FIGURE 17.15

Attenuation of the effect of a public health education program.

Source: McLoughlin, E., C. J. Vince, A. M. Lee et al. (1982). "Project Burn Prevention: Outcome and Implications," *American Journal of Public Health,* 72(3): 241–247. As presented in U.S. Congress, Office of Technology Assessment (February, 1988). *Healthy Children: Investing in the Future* (pub. no. OTA-H-345). Washington, DC: U.S. Government Printing Office.

limit was to conserve gasoline during the Arab oil embargo, more than 9,000 lives were saved as the number of motor vehicle deaths dropped from 55,511 in 1973 to 46,200 in 1974 because of the slower speeds.

State laws requiring child safety seats and safety belt use are another example of regulation to reduce injuries. Beginning in the 1980s, automobile child restraint and safety belt legislation spread across the United States. All states now have child passenger safety seat or restraint requirements for children, and all states except for New Hampshire have safety belt use laws for adults.[16] There is quite a bit of variation in the provisions of these laws from state to state with regard to enforcement, level of fines, seats of the vehicle covered (front seat or all seats), and type of vehicle covered (see Table 17.2).[16] Passage and vigorous enforcement of safety belt regulations are one reason why motor vehicle fatalities have declined in recent years. Regulation is often aimed not at the consumer, but at the industry. For example, beginning with the 1990 models, car makers were required to equip all passenger cars with safety belts or air bags.

Another regulatory change that has helped reduce motor vehicle–related injuries is the lowering of the blood alcohol concentration at which a person is legally intoxicated to 0.08%. In 2004, Delaware became the final state to adopt this standard, which has now been adopted by all 50 states, Puerto Rico, and the District of Columbia. A systematic review of the

Table 17.2
Key Provisions of Occupant Restraint Laws

State	Enforcement	Belt Fine	Child Restraint Required[a]	Safety Belt Required[b]		Vehicles Exempted and Other Information[d]
				Seats	Ages[c]	
AL	Primary	$25	4 years and under and <40 lb	Front	Under 15, all seats	Designed for >10 passengers; model year <1965, rural mail carriers newspaper delivery, vehicles normally operating in reverse.
AK	Primary	$15	3 years and under	All	All	School bus, emergency vehicles, mail or newspaper delivery, non-highway vehicles generally.
AZ	Secondary	$10	4 years and under	Front	15 and under, all seats	Designed for >10 passengers; model year <1972, rural mail carriers.
AR	Secondary	$25	5 years and under and <60 lb	Front	14 and under, all seats	School, church, or public bus; model year <1968.
CA	Primary	$20	5 years and under or <60 lb; <60 lb in rear seat if available	All	All	Emergency vehicles, postal service vehicles, newspaper delivery vehicles.
CO	Secondary	$17	5 years and under and <55 inches tall	Front	All	Passenger bus, school bus, ambulance, postal service vehicles, delivery and pickup services.
CT	Primary	$15	1-6 years and <60 lb in child restraint system	Front	Under 16, all seats	Truck or bus >15,000 lb; public, emergency, and delivery vehicles; postal service vehicles; newspaper delivery vehicles.
DE	Primary	$25	6 years and under and <60 lb	All	All	Postal service vehicles, tractors, off-highway vehicles.
DC	Primary	$50	7 years and under	All	All	Seating >8 people.
FL	Secondary	$30	3 years and under	Front	Under 17, all seats	School bus purchased before 1/1/2001; farm tractors, trash trucks, newspaper delivery, living space of RVs, public bus, truck >5,000 lb. Number of passengers in pickup truck required to wear seat belt shall not exceed number of installed front seat belts (extra passengers exempted).
GA	Primary	$15–25	5 years and under and 57 inches tall or less	Front	17 and under, all seats	Designed for >10 passengers, pickups, off-road vehicles, vehicles used for frequent stops. Exemption for pickups applies to passengers 18 years and over.
HI	Primary	$55	7 years and under and <57 inches tall	Front	17 and under, all seats	Bus or school bus >10,000 lb, emergency vehicles, taxicabs. Exempts persons unable to use seat belt when all available seat belt assemblies are in use (in this case, unsecured children must sit in the back seat).
ID	Secondary	$10	6 years and under	All	All	>8,000 lb, mail carriers, implements of husbandry.
IL	Primary	$25	7 years and under	Front	15 and under, all seats	Emergency vehicles, vehicles making frequent stops. If driver is under 18, all passengers under 19 must be restrained. Children >40 lb may use lap belt in rear seat if no combination belt is available.
IN	Primary	$25	7 years and under	Front	15 and under, all seats	Truck, tractor, RV, pickup truck, SUV if registered as pickup truck, postal vehicles, delivery vehicles, taxi, bus, emergency vehicles, antique cars.
IA	Primary	$25	5 years and under	Front	10 and under, all seats	Delivery vehicles for that do not exceed 25 mph between stops, emergency vehicles, postal vehicles.
KS	Secondary	$10	7 years and under, < 80 lb, and <67 inches tall	Front	Under 14, all seats	Designed for >10 people; trucks >12,000 lb, off-road vehicles, postal vehicles, newspaper delivery vehicles.
KY	Primary	$25	<40 inches tall	All	All	Designed for >10 people, trucks >12,000 lb, farm trucks 2,000 lb or more, postal vehicles. Safety belt roadblocks prohibited. No points on driving record for belt violations.

State	Enforcement	Fine	Child restraint required	Seating position	Belt use required ages	Exemptions
LA	Primary	$25	5 years and under	Front	12 and under, all seats	Designed for >10 people, utility vehicles traveling <20 mph, model year <1981, postal vehicles, farm vehicles, persons delivering newspapers.
ME	Secondary	$25–$50	<40 lb in child restraint; 7 years and under and <80 lb in booster seat	All	All	Manufactured without safety belts, postal vehicles. Everyone in school bus equipped with safety belts must use them.
MD	Primary	$25	5 years and under or 40 lb or less	Outboard front	15 and under, all seats	"Historical" vehicles, for-hire vehicles, farm vehicles within 10 miles of farm, vanpool vehicles, ambulances, funeral limousines, modified vehicles 25+ years old.
MA	Secondary	$25	4 years and under and 40 lb or less	All	All	Truck >18,000 lb. buses and taxis, emergency vehicles, postal vehicles.
MI	Primary	$25	3 years and under	Front	15 and under, all seats	Taxi, bus, school bus, postal service vehicles, commercial vehicles making frequent stops.
MN	Secondary	$25	3 years and under	Front	10 and under, all seats	Farm pickup trucks, postal vehicles, commercial vehicles making frequent stops if not exceeding 25 mph between stops.
MS	Primary	$25	3 years and under	Front	Under 16, all seats	Farm vehicles, buses, postal vehicles, utility meter readers' vehicles, all-terrain vehicles, vehicles designed for > 15 people.
MO	Secondary	$10	Under 4 years and <40 lb in child restraint; 4–7 years, <80 lb, and <57 inches tall in booster seat	Front	Under 16, all seats	Designed for >10 people, truck <12,000 lb, postal service vehicles, vehicles being used for agriculture.
MT	Secondary	$20	5 years and under and <60 lb	All	All	Vehicles making frequent stops if exemption obtained from state; construction vehicles.
NE	Secondary	$25	5 years and under	Front	15 and under, all seats	Model year <1973, farm tractors and other agricultural equipment, buses, postal vehicles, ambulance or rescue service vehicles.
NV	Secondary	$25	5 years and under and 60 lb or less	All	All	Taxi, bus, school bus, postal service vehicles, emergency vehicles, delivery vehicles not exceeding 15 mph, any vehicle or seating position if the state determines compliance is impractical.
NH	No adult law	$25	5 years and under if <55 inches tall and <80 lb	All	Under 18 only (primary law)	School bus, vehicle for hire; model year <1968, antique cars, vehicles in parade traveling at 10 mph or less.
NC	Primary	$25	7 years and under if <55 inches tall and <80 lb	Front; all seats as of 7/1/07	15 and under, all seats; all ages as of 7/1/07	Designed for >11 people, farm vehicles, postal vehicles, designated commercial vehicles, emergency vehicles. If no lap and shoulder belt, children 40–80 lb may be in lap belt.
ND	Secondary	$20	6 years and under and <57 inches tall or <80 lb	Front	17 and under	Designed for >10 people, farm vehicles, rural mail carriers. When all seats or all front seat safety belts are used by other occupants.
NJ	Primary	$20	7 years and under and >80 lbs	Front	17 and under, all seats	Manufactured before 1966, rural letter carriers.
NM	Primary	$25	6 years and under or <60 lb	All	All	Vehicles >10,000 lb, rural letter carriers.
NY	Primary	$50–$100	6 years and under	Front	Under 16, all seats	Bus, school bus, taxi, emergency or delivery vehicle, rural letter carriers.
OH	Secondary	$30	3 years and under or <40 lb	Front	—	Postal service vehicles, vehicles delivering newspapers.
OK	Primary	$20	5 years and under	Front	12 and under, all seats	Farm vehicles, truck, truck tractor, RV, postal service vehicles, school buses, taxicabs, emergency vehicles.
OR	Primary	$75 or less	5 years and under and 60 lb or less	All	All	Newspaper, mail, meter, and transit vehicles; for-hire vehicles; trash trucks, emergency vehicles, taxicab operators.

(continues)

Table 17.2 (continued)

State	Enforcement	Belt Fine	Child Restraint Required[a]	Safety Belt Required[b] Seats	Safety Belt Required[b] Ages[c]	Vehicles Exempted and Other Information[d]
PA	Secondary	$10	7 years and under	Front	17 and under, all seats	Truck >7,000 lb, rural letter carriers, delivery vehicles traveling at 15 mph or less
RI	Secondary	$75	6 years and under, <54 inches tall, and <80 lb	All	All	Postal service vehicles.
SC	Primary	$25	1–6 years and 40–80 lb	All	All	Emergency vehicles, buses, postal service vehicles, delivery vehicles, vehicles carrying > 10 passengers, parade vehicles; vehicles in which all seating positions with safety belts are already occupied; persons occupying rear seat, unless the vehicle is equipped with a shoulder harness.
SD	Secondary	$20	4 years and under and <40 lb	Front	17 and under, all seats	Passenger bus, school bus, rural mail carriers, newspaper or periodical deliveries.
TN	Primary	$10	8 years and under and <57 inches tall	Front	Under 16, all seats	>8,500 lb, rural letter carriers, utility workers, newspaper delivery; vehicles in parades, hayrides, or crossing a highway from one field to another if operated at <15 mph.
TX	Primary	$25–$50	4 years and under and <36 inches tall	Front	16 and under, all seats	Designed for >10 people; truck >15,000 lb, farm vehicles, postal service vehicles, meter readers.
UT	Secondary	$45 or less	4 years and under	All	All	Passengers exempted if all seats occupied or if riding in seating positions not equipped with safety belts.
VT	Secondary	$25	6 years and under in child seat	All	All	Bus, taxi, rural mail carriers, delivery vehicles traveling at 15 mph or less, emergency vehicles, farm tractors.
VA	Secondary	$25	5 years and under	Front	Under 16, all seats	Designed for >10 people, taxi, police vehicles, rural mail carriers, newspaper delivery, utility meter readers, commercial vehicles making frequent stops.
WA	Primary	$35	7 years and under and <57 inches	All	All	Designed for >10 people; when all designated seating positions are occupied; vehicles exempted by state regulation, including farm, construction, or commercial vehicles making frequent stops.
WV	Secondary	$25	7 years and under and <57 inches	Front	Under 17, all seats	Designed for >10 people, rural mail carriers.
WI	Secondary	$10	7 years and under, 80 lb or less <57 inches	Front	All	Taxis, farm trucks engaged in farming, emergency vehicles required to make more than 10 stops per mile, rural mail carriers, land surveyors.
WY	Secondary	$25	8 years and under in rear seat, 80 lb or less in rear seat if available	All	All	Postal vehicles, emergency vehicles, buses. Excess passengers exempted if all seats are occupied.

[a]May include rear-facing child restraint seats, forward-facing child restraint seats, and booster seats.

[b]Virtually every state exempts persons who for medical reasons cannot use a safety belt and vehicles not originally required to be equipped with safety belts.

[c]The word "all" used in this category means that everyone in the vehicle must be restrained. For children, that may be a child restraint.

[d]Exemptions for emergency vehicles and buses generally do not apply to the driver.

Source: U.S. Department of Transportation, National Highway Traffic Safety Administration (2006). *Traffic Safety Facts 2005: A Compilation of Motor Vehicle Crash Data from the Fatality Analysis Reporting System and the General Estimates System* (DOT HS 810 631), Early ed. Washington, DC: Author. Available at http://www-nrd.nhtsa.dot.gov/pdf/nrd-30/NCSA/TSFAnn/TSF2005EE.

effectiveness of such laws has revealed that they decrease fatal alcohol-related motor vehicle crashes an average of 7%. This should save 400 to 600 lives per year nationally, and significantly decrease the number and seriousness of injuries.[32]

Inattention to the task of driving is the cause of many motor vehicle crashes. The authors of the report *Distraction in Everyday Driving* list the potentially distracting activities that drivers engage in while driving.[33] Drivers were found to be distracted 16% of the time with such activities as talking on a cell phone, eating, drinking, and adjusting the radio (see Table 17.3). Although there are local ordinances and some state restrictions, no state has completely banned all types of cell phones (handheld and hands-free) while driving. This continues to be an emerging highway safety issue, and some states are gathering data on the role of cell phones in motor vehicle crashes.[34] To check the cell phone use restrictions in your city or state, visit the Governors Highway Safety Association Web site: www.statehighwaysafety.org.

In a "free society," such as the one in which Americans live, there is a limit to how much can be accomplished through legislation. For example, it has been very difficult to reduce the number of firearm injuries in the United States through legislation because the National Rifle Association (NRA) has been able to lobby successfully against restrictions on gun ownership.

Another example of the difficulty of achieving a balance between personal freedoms and society's legitimate health interests is motorcycle helmet legislation. Studies show that helmet laws are associated with a 29% to 33% decrease in annual per capita motorcycle fatalities.[35] In 1975, all but two states required motorcyclists to use helmets. Beginning in 1976, states began to repeal these laws. By the end of 2006, only 20 states, Puerto Rico, and the District of Columbia required a helmet for all motorcyclists (see Table 17.4).[16]

The strategy of prevention through regulation can be difficult to implement. The idea of regulating health behavior grates against the individual freedom that Americans have come to expect. Why should someone be required to wear a safety belt? The answer to that is: For the

Table 17.3
Percentage of Drivers Engaging in Potentially Distracting Activities during 3 Hours of Driving, and Percentage Duration of These Activities When Their Vehicles Were Moving

Potential Distraction	% of Subjects	% of Total Driving Time
Talking on cell phone	30.0	
Answering cell phone	15.7	1.30*
Dialing cell phone	27.1	
Eating, drinking, spilling	71.4	1.45
Preparing to eat or drink	58.6	3.16
Manipulating music/audio controls	91.4	1.35
Smoking (includes lighting and extinguishing)	7.1	1.55
Reading or writing	40.0	0.67
Grooming	45.7	0.28
Baby distracting	8.6	0.38
Child distracting	12.9	0.29
Adult distracting	22.9	0.27
Conversing	77.1	15.32
Reaching, leaning, etc.	97.1	
Manipulating vehicle controls	100.0	3.78*
Other internal distraction	67.1	
External distraction	85.7	1.62

*Combined categories

Source: Stutts, J., J. Feaganes, E. Rodgman, C. Hamlett, T. Meadows, D. Reinfurt, K. Gish, M. Mercadante, and L. Staplin (2003). *Distractions in Everyday Driving.* Washington, DC: AAA Foundation for Traffic Safety. Used with permission of AAA Foundation.

Table 17.4
History of State Motorcycle Helmet Laws

State	Effective Date of Original Law[a]	Effective Date of Repeal/Amendment	
AL	11/06/67		
AK	01/01/71	6/23/76	Repealed for operators age 18 and over.
AZ	01/01/69	05/27/76	Repealed for age 18 and over.
AR	06/29/67	07/31/97	Repealed for age 21 and over.
CA	01/01/85[b]	01/01/92	Reinstated for all.
CO	07/01/69	05/23/77	Repealed.
CT	10/01/67	06/01/76	Repealed.
		01/01/90	Reinstated for under age 18.
DE	10/01/68	06/10/78	Repealed for age19 and older. All riders must have helmet in their possession.
		07/17/84	Helmet required for instruction permit holders.
DC	02/11/70		
FL	09/13/67	07/01/00	Repealed for age 21 and over if covered by insurance of at least $10,000 in medial benefits.
GA	07/01/69		
HI	06/04/67	06/07/77	Repealed for age 18 and over.
ID	01/01/68	03/29/78	Repealed for age 18 and over.
IL	07/01/67	05/28/69	Helmet law ruled unconstitutional by State Supreme Court.
IN	07/26/67	09/01/77	Repealed.
		01/01/84	Reinstated for under age 18.
IA	09/01/75	07/01/76	Repealed.
KS	07/01/67	07/01/70	Repealed for age 21 and over.
		07/01/72	Reinstated for all.
		07/01/76	Repealed for age 16 and over.
		07/01/79	Reinstated for ages 16 and 17.
KY	06/13/68	07/15/98	Repealed for age 21 and over provided operator has held motorcycle license for 1 year and has provided proof of health insurance when registering motorcycle.
		07/04/00	Health insurance requirement repealed.
LA	07/13/68	10/01/76	Repealed for age 18 and over.
		01/01/82	Reinstated for all.
		08/15/99	Repealed for age 18 and over with health insurance with $10,000 in medical benefits for bodily injuries.
		08/15/04	Reinstated for all.
ME	10/07/67	10/24/77	Repealed.
		07/03/80	Reinstated for under age 15.
		09/23/83	Required for holders of learners' permits and for licensees holding license for 1 year or less.
MD	07/01/68	07/01/79	Repealed for age 18 and over.
		10/01/92	Reinstated for all.
MA	05/22/67		
MI	03/10/67	06/12/68	All riders required to have helmet in their possession.
		07/29/69	Reinstated for all.
MN	05/01/68	04/06/77	Repealed for age 18 and over.
MS	03/28/74		
MO	09/28/67		

Table 17.4 Continued

State	Effective Date of Original Law[a]	Effective Date of Repeal/Amendment	
MT	07/01/73	07/01/77	Repealed for age 18 and over.
NE	05/29/67	09/01/77	Repealed (law was never enforced).
		01/01/89	Reinstated for all.
NV	01/01/72		
NH	09/05/67	08/07/77	Repealed for age 18 and over.
NJ	01/01/68		
NM	06/16/67	06/17/77	Repealed for age 18 and over.
NY	01/01/67		
NC	01/01/68		
ND	07/01/67	07/01/77	Repealed except for operators under age 18 and passengers, regardless of age, if required for operator.
OH	01/01/68	07/10/78	Repealed except for riders under age 18; operators having motorcycle license for less than 1 year; and passengers if required for operator.
OK	04/07/67	05/03/76	Repealed for age 18 and over.
OR	01/01/68	10/04/77	Repealed for age 18 and over.
		06/16/89	Reinstated for all (by voter referendum).
PA	07/01/68	09/04/03	Repealed for operator age 21 and over if operator has held motorcycle license for at least 2 years or has competed rider education. Repealed for passenger age 21 and over if operator is exempt.
RI	04/04/67	05/21/76	Repealed for all operators. Required for all passengers.
		07/01/92	Required for operators under 21, operators licensed for 1 year or less, and all passengers.
SC	07/01/67	06/18/80	Repealed for age 21 and older.
SD	07/01/67	07/01/77	Repealed for age 18 and over.
TN	06/01/67		
TX	08/28/67	05/20/77	Repealed for age 18 and over.
		09/01/89	Reinstated for all.
		09/01/97	Repealed for age 21 and over who have completed rider education or are covered by at least $10,000 in medical insurance.
UT	05/13/69	05/08/77	Repealed for age 18 and over.
VT	03/03/68		
VA	06/05/70		
WA	06/08/67	07/01/77	Repealed.
		07/26/87	Reinstated for under age 18.
		09/01/90	Reinstated for all.
WV	05/25/71		
WI	07/01/68	03/19/78	Repealed except for under age 18 and instruction permit holders.
WY	05/24/73	05/27/83	Repealed for age 18 and over.
PR	07/20/60		

[a]Original law applied to all motorcyclists, unless otherwise noted.
[b]Applied only to riders under age 15½.

Summary: Motorcycle helmets were required for all riders in 20 states, the District of Columbia, and Puerto Rico in 2005. Twenty-seven states had helmet requirements with exceptions (age, rider type, roadway type), and three states did not require helmets at all.

Source: U.S. Department of Transportation, National Highway Traffic Safety Administration (2006). *Traffic Safety Facts 2005: A Compilation of Motor Vehicle Crash Data from the Fatality Analysis Reporting System and the General Estimates System* (DOT HS 810 631), Early ed. Washington, DC: Author. Available at http://www-nrd.nhtsa.dot.gov/pdf/nrd-30/NCSA/TSFAnn/TSF2005EE.

FIGURE 17.16
Child safety caps are an example of automatic or passive protection.

automatic (passive) protection the modification of a product or environment so as to reduce unintentional injuries

litigation the process of seeking justice for injury through courts

good of the total public, to protect the resources, including human life, of the greater public. Others say, "It's my life, and if I choose to take the risk of dying by not wearing a safety belt, who should care?" That response is all well and good; but when life is lost, it affects many others, such as family members, friends, and co-workers, not just the deceased. This scenario would become worse if the person not wearing a safety belt does not die but becomes a paraplegic and a ward of the state. Many public resources then would have to be used.

At what point is some legislation enough? It is known that safety belts and air bags are good and effective, but so are helmets—at least they think so at the Indianapolis 500. So should people now work to pass a law that requires all automobile and truck drivers to wear helmets? How much legislated health behavior is enough?

Automatic Protection
When engineered changes are combined with regulatory efforts, remarkable results can sometimes be achieved. The technique of improving product or environmental design to reduce unintentional injuries is termed **automatic** (or **passive**) **protection**.[31] A good example is child-proof safety caps (see Figure 17.16). Child-proof safety caps on aspirin and other medicine were introduced in 1972. By 1977, deaths attributed to ingestion of analgesics and antipyretics had decreased 41%.[36] We are all familiar with automatic protection devices. Common examples include automatic shut-off mechanisms on power tools (such as lawn mowers), safety caps on toxic products, and the warning lights and sounds that remind us to buckle our safety belts in motor vehicles.

Litigation
When other methods fail, behavioral changes can sometimes come about through the courts. **Litigation**—lawsuits filed by injured victims or their families—has been successful in removing dangerous products from store shelves or otherwise influencing changes in dangerous behavior. Litigation against a manufacturer of unsafe automobile tires, for example, might result in safer tires. Lawsuits against bartenders and bar owners for serving alcohol to drunken customers, who have later injured other people, have produced more responsible server behavior at public bars. Alcohol-related deaths and injuries on college campuses have caused insurance companies to re-examine their liability insurance policies with fraternities and sororities. This has forced some of these organizations and the universities themselves to restrict the way alcohol is used. The outcome may be a drop in unintentional injuries on these campuses.

INTENTIONAL INJURIES

Intentional injuries, the outcome of self-directed and interpersonal violence, are a staggering community health problem in the United States. More than 50,000 people die, and millions of others receive nonfatal injuries each year, as a result of self-directed or interpersonal violence.[2,11] In 2004, an estimated 1.8 million persons were treated for nonfatal physical assault–related injuries in EDs.[5] Although the physical assault rate is higher for males than for females, the rate of ED visits for sexual assault–related injuries can be five times higher for females. The highest injury rates for both males and females was for the 20- to 24-year age group. The injury rate for black males was about 4.6 times higher than the rate for non-Hispanic white males.[37]

Types of Intentional Injuries

The spectrum of violence includes assaults, rapes, robberies, suicides, homicides, and the mal-treatment of children, elders, and intimate partners. In 2005, residents of the United States 12 years of age or older reported being victims in an estimated 5.2 million violent crimes. Stated another way, 21 of every 1,000 people in the United States were victims of violent crimes. This is a 58% decline from the 10.9 million violent crimes and victimization rate of 50 per 1,000 people recorded in 1993.[38]

In 2003, homicide and legal intervention ranked as the thirteenth leading cause of death in the United States, accounting for 17,732 deaths.[11] The homicide rate in the United States is significantly higher than in other industrialized nations. One of the *Healthy People 2010* objectives is to reduce the homicide rate from the 1999 baseline of 6.0 per 100,000 to 3.0 per 100,000 people (see Box 17.3). In the 15- to 24-year age group, deaths from homicide numbered 5,085, and homicide was the second leading cause of death in 2004.[39]

During that same year (2003), suicide ranked as the eleventh leading cause of death, accounting for 31,484 deaths.[11] Suicide accounts for about 20% of all injury deaths. Suicide among teenagers and young adults (15- to 24-year age group) numbered 4,316 and was the third leading cause of death in that age group in 2004.[39]

Interpersonal violence is a costly community health problem, not only because of the loss of life and productivity but also because of the economic cost to the community. Consider the community resources expended for each violent act. There are those of the police, the legal system, the penal system, emergency health care services, medical services, social workers, and many others. Clearly, this is a problem for which prevention is the most economic approach.

Epidemiology of Intentional Injuries

To better understand the problem of intentional injuries, it is instructive to look more closely at both the victims and the perpetrators of violence. Interpersonal violence disproportionately affects those who are frustrated and hopeless, those who are jobless and live in poverty, and those with low self-esteem. More violent acts, whether self-directed or directed at others, are committed by males. Firearms are increasingly involved in violent acts, with ever-increasing fatal consequences. Abuse of drugs, especially alcohol, also contributes to the number of intentional injuries. Additionally, perpetrators of violent acts are more likely to have been abused or neglected as children or exposed to violence and aggression earlier in their lives.

Homicide, Assault, and Rape

Between 1991 and 2004, the homicide rate declined from 9.8 to 5.5 per 100,000 people.[40] Both the upswing in the homicide rate prior to 1991 and the subsequent decline afterward resulted from large swings in the victimization rates of those less than 25 years of age. During that same period, the victimization rate for blacks was six times higher than for whites during some years.[41] Much of the increase in homicides could be traced to the use of handguns by juveniles involved in the distribution of crack cocaine.[41]

Research indicates a relationship between income level and risk for becoming a victim of violence. In 2004–2005, persons in households with annual incomes less than $7,500 were nearly twice as likely as persons in households with incomes of $75,000 or more to become victim of violent crime.[38]

Males and blacks as well as the poor are more vulnerable to violence. Except for rape and sexual assault, every violent crime victimization rate is higher for males than for females.

BOX
17.3
HEALTHY PEOPLE 2010 OBJECTIVE: REDUCE HOMICIDES

Objective 15-32: Reduce homicides.

Target: 3.0 homicides per 100,000 population.

Baseline: 6.0 homicides per 100,000 population occurred in 1999 (age adjusted to the year 2000 standard population).

Target setting method: Better than the best.

Objective	Baseline Year	Baseline	2003	Target 2010
	1999	6.0	6.0	2.8
Race and Ethnicity				
American Indian or Alaska Native	1999	9.1	7.3	2.8
Asian or Pacific Islander	1999	3.0	2.9	2.8
Asian	1999	DNC	DNA	2.8
Native Hawaiian or other Pacific Islander	1999	DNC	DNA	2.8
Black or African American	1999	20.1	21.0	2.8
White	1999	3.8	3.7	2.8
Hispanic or Latino	1999	7.6	7.7	2.8
Cuban	1999	5.8	5.4	2.8
Mexican American	1999	8.4	7.9	2.8
Puerto Rican	1999	9.0	7.9	2.8
Not Hispanic or Latino	1999	5.7	5.7	2.8
Black or African American, not Hispanic/Latino	1999	20.7	21.7	2.8
White, not Hispanic or Latino	1999	2.9	2.7	2.8
Gender				
Female	1999	2.9	2.6	2.8
Male	1999	9.1	9.4	2.8
Education level (persons aged 25 to 64 years)				
Less than high school	1999	16.4	17.4	NA
High school graduate	1999	9.7	10.2	NA
At least some college	1999	2.5	2.6	NA
Select Populations				
Children under 1 year (not age adjusted)	1999	8.3	8.2	NA
Children aged 1 to 4 years (not age adjusted)	1999	2.5	2.4	NA
Children aged 10 to 14 years (not age adjusted)	1999	1.2	1.0	NA
Adolescents aged 15 to 19 years (not age adjusted)	1999	10.4	9.5	NA
Persons aged 15 to 34 years (not age adjusted)	1999	11.7	12.2	NA
Intimate partners aged 14 to 45 years (spouse, ex-spouse, boyfriend, girlfriend) (not age adjusted)	1999	DNC	DNC	NA
Black or African Americans aged 15 to 34 years (not age adjusted):				
Females	1999	11.8	10.6	NA
Males	1999	77.4	83.6	NA
Hispanic males aged 15 to 34 years (not age adjusted)	1999	24.8	25.6	NA

DNC = Data are not collected. DNA = Data have not been analyzed. NA = Not applicable.

Note: Age-adjusted to the year 2000 standard population.

Sources: National Vital Statistics System (NVSS), CDC, NCHS; FBI Uniform Crime Reports, U.S. Department of Justice and http://wonder.cdc.gov.

For Further Thought

Homicide rates have declined since 1993. What are some of the reasons for this? Do you think they will continue to decline if the economy worsens and unemployment rises? What steps would you suggest to further lower homicide rates?

Sources: Healthy People 2010; CDC. Available at http://wonder.cdc.gov/.

Males experienced violent crime at rates 49% higher than females, and they account for about three-fourths of all murder victims.[38] However, females were victims of rape and sexual assault 12 times more often than males. In 2005, 27 blacks, 20 whites, and 13 persons of other races per 1,000 were victimized. In 2005 there were 7.6 aggravated assaults per 1,000 black persons, 3.8 per 1,000 white persons and 2.5 per 1,000 persons of other racial categories.[38]

Overall, it is estimated that less than half of all violent crimes committed in 2005 were reported to police. Furthermore, only 38% of rapes or sexual assaults were reported to police.[38] This makes the acquisition of accurate statistics on rape and attempted rape difficult. Although reported offenders are usually strangers, 78% of all rapes and sexual assaults are committed by someone acquainted with, known to, or related to the victim.[38]

Suicide and Attempted Suicide

As previously indicated, more than 30,000 suicides are reported each year in the United States, accounting for one-fifth of all injury mortality. In 2004, 32,439 suicide deaths were reported.[4] The suicide rate for men (17.6 per 100,000) was four times that for women (4.3 per 100,000) in 2003.[11] The rates of suicide in young people (15 to 24 years of age) nearly tripled between 1950 and 1995 but have since declined to 9.7 per 100,000.[10] Those for the elderly have also declined in recent years. Suicide rates in older men, however, remain quite high. Senior men (65 years old and older) are eight times more likely to commit suicide than senior women.[11]

Firearm Injuries and Injury Deaths

Statistics on fatal and nonfatal firearm injuries include data covering both intentional and unintentional incidents. When one considers all firearm deaths—those that result from both intentional and unintentional acts—firearms were the second leading cause of injury deaths after motor vehicles in 2002 and the leading cause of deaths due to traumatic brain injury.[2] In 2002, there were 30,242 firearm-related deaths. Of these, 17,108 (56.6%) were classified as suicide, 11,829 (39%) as homicide, 300 (1%) as resulting from legal intervention, and 243 (<1%) were of undetermined intent. Only 762 (2.5%) of all firearm fatalities were classified as unintentional deaths.[2] In 2002, firearms were used in 67% of all homicides, 54% of all suicides, and less than 1% of all unintentional injury deaths.[2] Males were six times more likely to die or be treated in a hospital emergency department for a gunshot wound than females.

At highest risk for homicide and suicide involving firearms are teenage boys and young men, aged 15 to 24 years. A national survey found that in 2005, nearly 10% of high school males had carried a handgun to school at least once in the past year.[21] The gun-toting behavior continues even in college. In a random sample of 10,000 undergraduate students, 4.3% reported that they had a working firearm at college, and 1.6% said they had been threatened with a gun while at college.[42] Despite these reports, death rates from firearms have declined in recent years. From 1993 to 2005, firearm death rates for 15- to 19-year-old males fell from 27.4 to 12.4 deaths per 100,000 people (a 62% drop), and for 20- to 24-year-old males, firearm death rates fell from 34.1 to 21.3 per 100,000 people (a 38% drop).[2,17]

When one compares the ratios of firearm-related fatalities to nonfatal injuries, the lethality of firearms becomes clear. When one looks at injuries from all causes, for each death, nine others are hospitalizations and 189 more are treated and released. When one looks at firearm-related injuries, for each death, only 1.2 people are hospitalized and one person is treated and released (Figure 17.17).[17]

One barrier to preventing firearm injuries and deaths is the absence of a detailed, federally supported reporting system. Unlike the highly developed reporting system for motor vehicle crashes and crash injuries, there is no such system for firearm-related injuries. Until a more comprehensive, national reporting system is in place, the Firearm Injury Surveillance

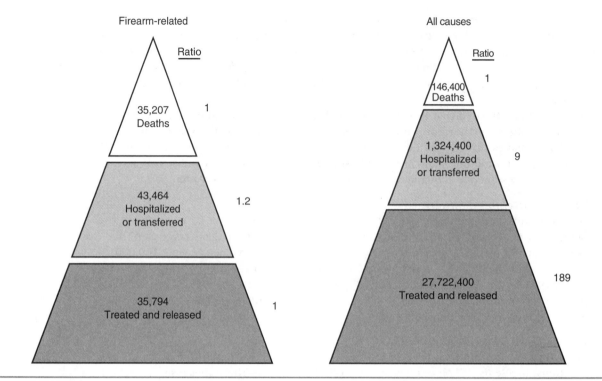

FIGURE 17.17

Injury pyramids for firearm-related injury versus all causes of injury: Firearm injuries are more deadly than other types of injuries.

Source: Centers for Disease Control and Prevention (2001). "Surveillance for Fatal and Nonfatal Firearm-Related Injuries—United States, 1993-1998." *MMWR,* 50(SS-2): 1-34.

Study, 1993–2004, is the single best source for nonfatal firearm injury data in the United States.[20]

Violence in Our Society and Resources for Prevention

A sixth-grade student brings a gun to school and kills a teacher and three students, a man is killed for "cutting" in line, and a child dies from punishment for breaking a rule at home. These are signs of the violent society in which Americans now find themselves living. Over the past few years, violence in America has increased. Many young people do not have the interest or skills to work out a solution to a conflict through verbal negotiation, and they resort to physical violence to resolve it. Some of these confrontations are gang-related, while others are simply individual actions. The availability of firearms in America makes violence all the more deadly, both for those in conflict and for innocent bystanders. In the next sections, we will discuss individual, family, and gang violence.

Individuals and Violence

A significant number of violent acts committed in the United States each year are committed by individuals who lack basic communication and problem-solving skills. Many of these people are not interested in resolving an argument through discussion or compromise. Instead, they are intent on "winning" their argument, by physical force if necessary. (After all, isn't that the way arguments are won in the movies?)

The availability and proliferation of firearms makes this approach particularly deadly. In 2001, homicide and legal intervention were the Number 1 cause of death for black Americans aged 15 to 24.[39] Unfortunately, violent confrontations often result in injuries and deaths not only for the victim, but also to others not directly involved in the confrontation.

Because of the level of violence, many schools and community organizations offer conflict resolution programs that teach youth alternative ways to resolve disagreements. These programs are designed for various grade levels and teach about the nature of conflicts, the harmful effects of violence, alternatives to violent behavior, and how to make safe decisions. Some of these programs, aimed specifically at reducing handgun-related violence, are listed in a report by the Office of Juvenile Justice and Delinquency Programs, United States Department of Justice. This report, *Promising Strategies to Reduce Gun Violence,* lists 60 of the more than 400 programs examined that were judged to be successful or "promising" at reducing gun violence.[43]

Family Violence and Abuse

One in every six homicides is the result of family violence. **Family violence** includes the maltreatment of children, intimate partner violence, sibling violence, and violence directed toward elder family members. Because children are our most important resources, and because being abused or neglected as a child increases one's risk for violent behavior as an adult, it is of paramount importance that society increase its efforts to intervene in cases of family violence. In recent years there has been increased attention paid to family violence, including violence against children and intimate partners. Between 1993 and 2001, the victimization rates for intimate partners and children declined. While some might credit this decline to improved efforts by the governmental and nongovernmental agencies involved with intervening and preventing violence among these groups, others would credit it to the strong economy during this period. Lower rates of unemployment mean better financial situations for families, lower levels of stress among family members, and fewer reports of domestic violence.

Child Maltreatment

Child maltreatment is an act or failure to act by a parent, caretaker, or other person as defined under state law that results in physical abuse, neglect, medical neglect, sexual abuse, emotional abuse, or an act or failure to act that presents an imminent risk of serious harm to a child. Also included are other forms of child maltreatment, such as child abandonment and congenital drug addiction. **Child abuse** can be physical, emotional, verbal, or sexual. Physical abuse is the intentional (nonaccidental) inflicting of injury on another person by shaking, throwing, beating, burning, or other means. Emotional abuse can take many forms, including showing no emotion and the failure to provide warmth, attention, supervision, or normal living experiences. Verbal abuse is the demeaning or teasing of another verbally. Sexual abuse includes the physical acts of fondling or intercourse, nonphysical acts such as indecent exposure or obscene phone calls, or violent physical acts such as rape and battery. **Child neglect** is a type of maltreatment that refers to the failure by the parent or legal caretaker to provide necessary, age-appropriate care when financially able to do so, or when offered financial or other means to do so. Neglect may be physical, such as the failure to provide food, clothing, medical care, shelter, or cleanliness. It also may be emotional, such as the failure to provide attention, supervision, or other support necessary for a child's well-being (see Figure 17.18). Or, it may be educational, such as the failure to ensure that a child attends school regularly. Educational neglect is one of the most common categories of neglect, followed by physical, and then emotional neglect.

family violence
the use of physical force by one family member against another, with the intent to hurt, injure, or cause death

child maltreatment
an act or failure to act by a parent, caretaker, or other person as defined under state law that results in physical abuse, neglect, medical neglect, sexual abuse, emotional abuse, or an act or failure to act that presents an imminent risk of serious harm to a child

child abuse
the intentional physical, emotional, verbal, or sexual mistreatment of a minor

child neglect
the failure of a parent or guardian to care for or otherwise provide the necessary subsistence for a child

FIGURE 17.18

Child neglect is the failure to provide care or other necessary subsistence for a child.

In 2004, 872,000 children under the age of 18 years were victims of abuse or neglect nationwide at a rate of 11.9 per 1,000 children. There has been a steady decline from the rate of reported child maltreatment since 1993, when the rate was 15.3 per 1,000 children (see Figure 17.19). Of the 872,000 children who were maltreated in 2004, 62% suffered neglect, 18% suffered physical abuse, 10% were sexually abused, 7% were psychologically abused, and 2% were medically neglected.[44] In 15% of all cases, other or additional types of maltreatment were reported, including abandonment, threats of harm to the child, and congenital drug addiction. The highest victimization rates were for the 0- to 3-year-old age group (16.1 maltreatments per 1,000 children), and these rates decline with age (see Figure 17.20). Rates of many types of maltreatment are the same for males and females, but the sexual abuse rate for female children was higher than the rate for male children. Victimization rates vary by race and ethnicity. In 2004, the lowest rates were for Asian children (3.7 children per 1,000), and the highest rates were for African American children (19.9 children per 1,000). Children who had been victimized prior to 2004 were almost three times more likely be victimized again in the first six months of 2004 than children without a prior history of victimization.[44]

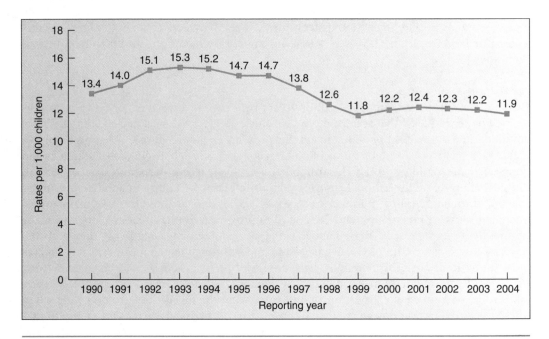

FIGURE 17.19

There has been a steady decline in the child maltreatment rates since 1993, when the rate was 15.3 victims per 1,000 children.

Source: U.S. Department of Health and Human Services, Administration on Children and Families (2004). *Child Maltreatment 2004.* Washington, DC: U.S. Government Printing Office. Available at http://www.acf.hhs.gov/programs/cb/pubs/cm04/cm04.pdf.

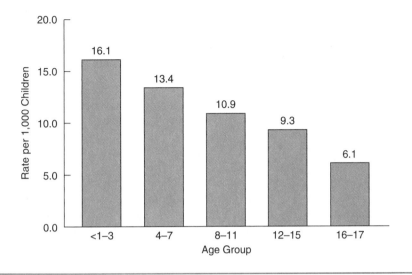

FIGURE 17.20

The highest victimization rates of child maltreatment occur in children of the youngest age groups (16.1 per 100,000 for children aged 3 and younger). Victimization rates decline with increasing age of the victim.

Source: U.S. Department of Health and Human Services, Administration on Children, Youth and Families (2004). *Child Maltreatment 2004.* Washington, DC: U.S. Government Printing Office. Available at http://www.acf.hhs.gov/programs/cb/pubs/cm04/cm04.pdf.

An estimated 1,490 children died of abuse or neglect in 2004, at a rate of approximately 2.03 deaths per 100,000 children. Four-fifths of the fatalities occurred in children under 4 years of age (see Figure 17.21). Maltreatment deaths were most often associated with neglect.[44]

Children who physically survive maltreatment may be scarred emotionally. "What happens to abused and neglected children after they grow up? Do the victims of violence and neglect later become criminals or violent offenders?"[45] In an attempt to answer these questions, researchers followed 1,575 child victims of abuse and neglect between 1967 and 1971. By the mid-1990s, 49% of the victims had been arrested for some type of nontraffic offense,

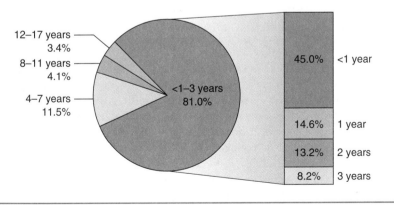

FIGURE 17.21

Percentage of child fatalities by age, 2004.

Source: U.S. Department of Health and Human Services, Administration on Children, Youth and Families (2004). *Child Maltreatment 2004.* Washington, DC: U.S. Government Printing Office. Available at http://www.acf.hhs.gov/programs/cb/pubs/cm04/cm04.pdf.

compared with 38% of the control group (who shared other risk factors such as poverty). Eighteen percent had been arrested for a violent crime, compared with 14% in the control group. These differences were regarded as significant by the researchers. A key finding of the study was that neglected children's rates of arrest for violence were almost as high as physically abused children's. Another key finding was that black individuals who had been abused or neglected as children were being arrested at much higher rates than white individuals with the same background.[45]

Prevention of Child Maltreatment

One of the keys to protecting children from maltreatment is a system of timely reporting and referral to one of the many state and local child protective service (CPS) agencies. Anyone may make such a report (e.g., relative, neighbor, or teacher). In 2004, 72.7% of child abuse and neglect reports were received from professionals—people who came into contact with the victim through their jobs.[44] Signs of neglect are apparent to the trained professional, such as a teacher, a school nurse, or another community health professional. Signs of neglect include extremes in behavior, an uncared-for appearance, evidence of a lack of supervision at home, or the lack of medical care.

"CPS agencies provide services to prevent future instances of child abuse or neglect and to remedy harm that has occurred as a result of child maltreatment."[44] These services are designed to increase the parents' child-rearing competence and knowledge of developmental stages of childhood. There may be an assessment of the family's strengths and weaknesses, the development of a plan based on the family's needs, and post-investigative follow-up services. Services might include respite care, parenting education, housing assistance, substance abuse treatment, day care, home visits, counseling, and other services. The goal is to ensure the safety of the child or children.[44]

There are many useful sources of information and support for those interested in preventing child abuse and neglect. The Child Welfare Information Gateway, sponsored by the Children's Bureau of the U.S. Department of Health and Human Services' Administration for Children and Families provides information, products, and technical assistance services to help professionals locate information related to child abuse and neglect and related child welfare issues (available at www.childwelfare.gov/). Another source of information is the *Committee for Children*. Its mission is to promote the safety, well-being, and social development of children (available at www.cfchildren.org). The *National Foundation for Abused and Neglected Children (NFANC),* created in 1992, is a nonprofit organization dedicated to the prevention of child abuse and neglect (available at www.gangfreekids.org/).

Elder Maltreatment

There are more than 36 million elders (persons 65 years of age and older) in the United States. Although elders experience violent crime and thefts at a lower rate than people of other age groups (2.4 per 1,000 population versus 21 per 1,000 for the population as a whole in 2005),[38] between 1 and 2 million of them have been abused, neglected, exploited, or otherwise mistreated.[46] Women over the age of 75 are particularly vulnerable, and elders over 80 are three times more likely to be abused as younger elders. Ninety percent of the known abusers are family members; two-thirds are adult children or their spouses.[47]

Abuse can be physical, sexual, psychological or emotional, or financial, or may involve abandonment, neglect, or self-neglect. Elders may be kicked, hit, denied food and medical care, or have their Social Security checks or other financial resources stolen or otherwise misappropriated. Most cases of elder abuse are not reported or only become apparent following other legal or medical proceedings; thus, accurate statistics on the incidence of elder abuse are unavailable. One source of information and assistance on elder abuse is the National Center on Elder Abuse (www.elderabusecenter.org/). As the American population ages, elder maltreatment is likely to become a community health problem of increasing importance.

Intimate Partner Violence

Intimate partner violence (IPV) can be defined as rape, physical assault, and stalking perpetrated by current and former dates, spouses, and cohabiting partners (cohabiting meaning living together at least some of the time as a couple).[48] Each year between 2 and 3 million women and men are victimized by their intimate partners. Sometimes intimate partner violence is deadly. In 2000 1,247 women and 440 men were murdered by an intimate partner.[49] Nearly two-thirds of women who reported being raped, physically assaulted, or stalked since age 18 were victimized by a current or former husband, cohabiting partner, boyfriend, or date.[50] Injuries to women from intimate partner physical violence are underreported, but more than 500,000 women injured as a result of IPV require medical treatment each year. Women spend more days in bed, miss more work, and suffer more from stress and depression than men. The health care costs of intimate partner rape, physical assault, and stalking exceed $5.8 billion each year.[50]

One in four women residing in the United States has been physically assaulted or raped by an intimate partner; one of 14 men has reported such an experience.[50] Women are also more likely than men to be murdered by an intimate partner. From 1993 to 2004, 30% of all women who were murdered were killed by an intimate partner, whereas only 5% of male murder victims were killed by an intimate partner.[51] Each year, thousands of American children witness IPV within their families. Witnessing such violence is a risk factor for developing long-term physical and mental health problems, including alcohol and substance abuse, becoming a victim of abuse, and perpetrating IPV.[50]

Despite the grim statistics just presented, the rates of victimization by an intimate partner have declined since 1993, when the rates were 9.8 per 1,000 for females and 1.6 per 1,000 for males. In 2004, these rates were 4 per 1,000 for females and 1 per 1,000 for males.[51]

Risk factors for women who are likely to experience IPV include having a family income below $10,000, being young (19–29 years of age), and living with an intimate partner who uses alcohol or other drugs. Another risk factor is a previous episode of abuse. In a dysfunctional relationship, the male intimate partner may seek to exert power and control over his female intimate partner, resulting in a cycle in which violence recurs (see Figure 17.22). The *cycle of violence* depicts the progression of steps leading up to an attack or episode of violence and the restoration of calm. It also lists the factors that produce stress or contribute to a stressful family environment and lead to a violent episode, along with some of the abuser's characteristics (see Figure 17.23). A violent episode may result from the loss of a job, a divorce, illness, death of a family member, or misbehavior (actual or perceived) of children or an intimate partner. The likelihood that abuse will occur is greatly increased if alcohol has been consumed. While selected interventions aimed at one factor (for example, the abuser) might mitigate against family violence, community efforts to reduce violence should be both comprehensive, involving a variety of approaches, and coordinated among all agencies involved in order to be effective.

Prevention of Intimate Partner Violence

Prevention of IPV involves improvements in identifying and documenting cases of IPV and increasing access to services for victims and perpetrators of IPV and their children. Coordinating community initiatives strengthens the safety networks for high-risk individuals and families. Some communities have established a "Violence Coordinating Council" that holds monthly meetings to set an agenda and action plans for the community and to determine and clarify the roles and responsibilities of agencies and individuals. It is important for communities to develop and implement a coordinated response with strong advocates from criminal justice, victim services, children's services, and allied professions.[52] One of the important groups of allied professionals are health care providers. A guide to training materials and programs on IPV and sexual assault has been published by the National Center for Injury Control and Prevention, CDC.[53]

intimate partner
violence (IPV)
rape, physical assault,
or stalking
perpetrated by
current or former
dates, spouses, or
cohabiting partners

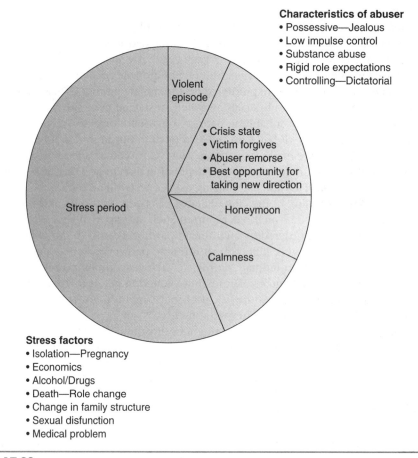

Characteristics of abuser
- Possessive—Jealous
- Low impulse control
- Substance abuse
- Rigid role expectations
- Controlling—Dictatorial

Violent episode

- Crisis state
- Victim forgives
- Abuser remorse
- Best opportunity for taking new direction

Stress period

Honeymoon

Calmness

Stress factors
- Isolation—Pregnancy
- Economics
- Alcohol/Drugs
- Death—Role change
- Change in family structure
- Sexual disfunction
- Medical problem

FIGURE 17.22

The need for power and control characterize the abusive intimate partner.

Source: Domestic Abuse Intervention Project in Duluth, Minnesota, as reported in the *AHEC NEWS,* a publication of the Area Health Education Centers of Oklahoma, *AHEC News* (February, 1994), 2(1): 9. Used with permission.

Violence in Schools

Although schools are one of the safest places for children to spend their time, even rare acts of violence strike terror into parents, teachers, and the children themselves. Highly publicized incidents of fatal shootings on school grounds have focused the nation's attention on the question of just how safe (or unsafe) our nation's schools are.

> Our nation's schools should be safe havens for teaching and learning, free of crime and violence. Any instance of crime or violence at school not only affects the individuals involved but also may disrupt the educational process and affect bystanders, the school itself, and the surrounding community.[54]

The National Center for Educational Statistics (NCES) collected data to determine the "frequency, seriousness, and incidence of violence in elementary and secondary schools."[55] The percentage of U.S. public schools experiencing one or more violent incidents increased between the 1999–2000 and the 2003–2004 school years from 71% to 81%. During the 2003–2004 school year, 77% of public schools reported instances of physical attacks or fights without a weapon, 53% reported threats of physical attacks without a weapon, 51% reported vandalism, 46% reported theft or larceny, and 15% reported possession of a knife or sharp

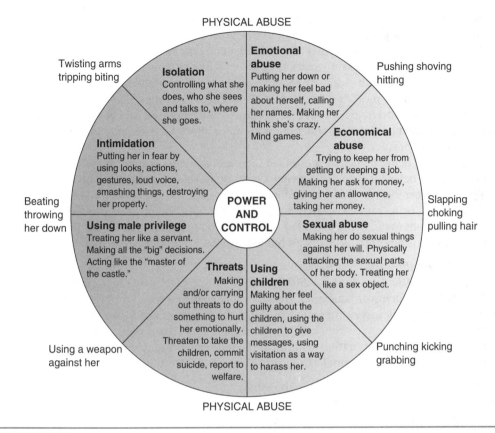

PHYSICAL ABUSE

FIGURE 17.23

Cycle of violence.

Source: Domestic Violence Intervention Services, Inc., Tulsa, Oklahoma, as published in *AHEC NEWS,* a publication of the Area Health Education Centers of Oklahoma, *AHEC News* (February, 1994), 2(1): 8. Used with permission.

object with intent to harm another. Six percent of public schools reported a student in possession of a firearm or explosive device, and 5% reported an attack or fight with a weapon. Only 3% reported sexual battery other than rape, and only 1% reported rape or attempted rape.[55] The incidence of violence is higher in middle and high schools than in elementary schools and higher in schools that report serious discipline problems than in schools that do not. While it seems as though the incidence of violent behavior in schools is high, the rates of some behaviors that contribute to violence, such as weapon carrying, actually declined from 11.8% in 1993 to 5.4% in 2005.[20,56]

Although multiple homicide events, such as those at Columbine High School and Virginia Tech, capture newspaper headlines and are lead stories on the evening news, the fact is that the odds of suffering a school-associated violent death are less than one in a million. Furthermore, only 19 of the more than 1,437 children nationwide who were murdered, and 3 of 1,285 children who committed suicide, in the 2003–2004 school year were at school (on school property, at a school-sponsored event, or on the way to or from school or a school-sponsored event).[55] The nature of crime away from school is far more serious than at school.

Most schools try to deal with violence problems by instituting zero tolerance policies toward serious student offenses. These policies, defined as school or district policy mandating predetermined consequences for various student offenses, have recently come under fire because administering such policies sometimes leads to somewhat ridiculous outcomes. In 2003–2004, almost all schools (98%) also utilized some type of security measures, such as visitor sign-ins, closed campuses (at lunch), drug sweeps, and random metal detectors. About 13% of public high schools had stringent security, such as daily or random metal detectors; 59% reported using one or more random dog sniffs to check for drugs, and 60% of high schools use security cameras to monitor the school. Most schools reported having some type of formal violence prevention or violence reduction program or effort. Sixty-six percent train staff in violence prevention practices.[57]

Bullying and being bullied at school are increasingly being recognized as associated with violence-related behavior (such as carrying a weapon to school, fighting, or becoming injured in a fight). Bullying includes being made fun of; being made the subject of rumors; being threatened with harm; being pushed, shoved, tripped, or spat upon; being pressured to do something one does not want to do; being excluded, or having one's property destroyed. In 2005, 28% of 12- to 18-year-olds reported having been bullied at school within the past six months.[55]

Safe Schools/Healthy Students Initiative

The *Safe Schools/Healthy Students Initiative* is a unique grant program jointly administered by the U.S. Departments of Education, Health and Human Services, and Justice. The program promotes a comprehensive, integrated problem-solving process for use by communities in addressing school violence. "Since 1999, more than 240 urban, rural, suburban, and tribal school districts—in collaboration with local mental health and juvenile justice providers—have received grants using a single application process."[58] Steps in the process are:

1. Establishing school–community partnerships
2. Identifying and measuring the problem
3. Setting measurable goals and objectives
4. Identifying appropriate research-based programs and strategies
5. Implementing programs and strategies in an integrated fashion
6. Evaluating the outcomes of programs and strategies
7. Revising the plan on the basis of evaluation information

The initiative requires comprehensive, integrated community-wide plans to address at least the following six elements:[58]

1. A safe school environment
2. Alcohol and other drugs and violence prevention and early intervention programs
3. School and community mental health preventive and treatment intervention services
4. Early childhood psychosocial and emotional development services
5. Supporting and connecting schools and communities (2004–present grantees); education reform (1999–2003 grantees)
6. Safe school policies

Youth Violence after School

Although violence in schools has grabbed the headlines, the real problem area is violence after school. Fewer and fewer children have a parent waiting for them at home after school. While many youths are able to supervise themselves and their younger siblings responsibly after school or are engaged in sports or other after-school activities, some are not. Statistics show that serious violent crime committed by juveniles peaks in the hours immediately after school (see Figure 17.24). Also, during these after-school hours, juveniles are most likely to become victims of crime, including violent crimes such as robberies and aggravated assaults. This is because at this unsupervised time, youth are more vulnerable to exploitation, injuries, and even death.[59]

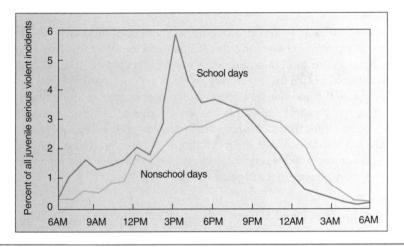

FIGURE 17.24

Serious violent crime committed by juveniles peaks in the hours immediately after school.

Source: United States Department of Justice, Office of Justice Programs, Office of Juvenile Justice and Delinquency Prevention (1999). *Violence after School. 1999 National Report Series, November 2000.* Washington, DC: Author.

For communities that want to become involved in reducing the problem of youth violence, the federal government has a variety of resources. One of these is *Best Practices of Youth Violence Prevention: A Sourcebook for Community Action.*[60] In addition, the federal government has established a Web site, www.afterschool.gov, that provides resources for communities that wish to develop after-school programs for youths. The Web site provides links to successful after-school programs, ideas for after-school activities, and Web sites for youths to visit after school. Additional information and resources are available at the National Center for Injury Prevention and Control's Web site.[61]

Violence in Our Communities

Youth gangs and gang violence contribute to the overall level of violence in the community and are a drain on community resources.

Youth Gang Violence

While most young women and men in the United States grow up subscribing to such American ideals as democracy, individualism, equality, and education, others do not. Many of those who do not are economically disadvantaged and have lost faith in society's capacity to work on their behalf. Some of these seek refuge and reward in organized subculture groups of youngsters who feel similarly disenfranchised.

One popular subculture structure is the **youth gang,** a self-formed association of peers bound together by mutual interests, with identifiable leadership and well-defined lines of authority. Youth gangs act in concert to achieve a specific purpose, and their acts generally include illegal activities and the control over a particular territory or enterprise. Types of illegal activities in which gang members participate include larceny/theft, aggravated assault, burglary/breaking and entering, and street drug sales.

A recent survey of a representative sample of 2,296 law enforcement agencies revealed youth gang activity in 29% of the districts under their jurisdiction. This is a significant decline since 1996, when 53% of jurisdictions reported youth gang activity. An estimated 24,000 gangs were active in 2,900 jurisdictions in the United States in 2004. Gang activity is more prevalent in cities with a population of 25,000 or greater. There were more than 760,000 active gang members in 2004.[62]

youth gang
an association of peers, bound by mutual interests and identifiable lines of authority, whose acts generally include illegal activity and control over a territory or an enterprise

Costs to the Community

Youth gangs and youth-gang-related violence present an enormous drain on the law enforcement resources of a community beyond the injuries and injury deaths that result from their activities. Pressured to "do something," field officers may be pulled from other duties and not replaced. If additional police are hired, it can cost the community $50,000 per year per officer. Next, there is the additional need to strengthen the prosecutor's office if the operation is to be effective. In short, the suppression of gangs by law enforcement is costly for communities, often depleting resources for other needed community improvements. Another problem is vandalism and the defacing of public and private buildings by gang-related graffiti. This money spent repairing damage and erasing graffiti could be used to hire teachers or to support educational activities.

Community Response

Many communities have responded effectively to the increased violence resulting from gang-related activity. Perhaps the best approach is a multifaceted effort involving law enforcement, education, diversion activities, and social services support. Suppression of gang activity by law enforcement is justified because many gang-related activities—such as selling illicit drugs, carrying and discharging weapons, and defacing property—are illegal. Education of children, teachers, parents, and community leaders is another facet of gang-related violence prevention. Just as there are drug abuse prevention curricula in schools, there are now anti-gang awareness programs in some schools. Diversion activities, including job opportunities and after-school activities such as enrichment programs, sports, and recreation, can reduce the attractiveness of less wholesome uses of free time. Sports and recreational activities have long been touted as a healthy outlet for pent-up physical energy. It seems logical to assume that young persons who participate in such activities would be less likely to become involved in destructive, violent behavior (see Figure 17.25).

FIGURE 17.25

Adequate recreational opportunities for youth can reduce violence in a community.

Federal Government's Response

In 1993, two important pieces of federal legislation were passed and signed into law: the Brady Handgun Violence Prevention Act and the National Child Protection Act of 1993. The "Brady Bill" was signed with great fanfare by then President Bill Clinton, who stated that "Americans are finally fed up with violence that cuts down another citizen with gunfire every 20 minutes" (see Figure 17.26). The Brady Handgun Violence Prevention Act (PL 103-159), implemented in February 1994, was aimed at reducing interstate gun trafficking and requires a five-day waiting period and a background check on all handgun buyers. One of the purposes of the waiting period is to allow time for state and local police to run background checks on the purchasers, some of whom might be legally barred from owning a handgun because of a criminal record.

In addition to the Brady Law, which established national restrictions on the acquisition of firearms and ammunition from federal firearms licensees, there are other laws that attempt to regulate firearms. At least 50 studies have been carried out to determine the effects of firearm laws on preventing violence. A task force report reviewed 51 such studies to determine whether there was sufficient evidence to determine that firearm laws do prevent violence in the community. The task force "found insufficient evidence to determine the effectiveness of any of the firearms laws or combinations of laws reviewed on violent outcomes."[63] The task force noted, however, that its finding did not mean there was evidence of ineffectiveness. Thus, it remains to be proven whether or not firearm laws can be effective in reducing firearm-related violence.

The National Child Protection Act, meanwhile, encourages states to require a fingerprint-based national background check on individuals seeking employment in the child care field. The Violent Crime Control and Law Enforcement Act of 1994 subsequently amended this act to also include those seeking employment with the elderly and disabled.

The Office of Justice Programs offers a variety of programs to state and local agencies aimed at reducing intentional violence. Included are programs to empower communities (Community Prosecution, Safe Schools Initiative, Safe Start, Weed and Seed, and Offender Reentry). There are also programs aimed at breaking the cycle of drug abuse and crime (the Drug Free Communities Program, the Drug Prevention Demonstration Program, and Enforcing Underage Drinking). Other programs combat family violence, violence against women, and violence on college campuses. Still others address youth violence and protect and support victims of crime. The purpose of these programs is to support communities in their efforts to reduce intentional violence and violence-related injuries.[64]

In conclusion, intentional injuries resulting from interpersonal violence remain a national as well as a community concern. Significant resources are available at the federal level (from the Departments of Health and Human Services and Justice) to help states and local communities reduce the number and seriousness of violence-related injuries. It is up to each concerned citizen to make sure that his or her own community is taking advantage of these resources.

FIGURE 17.26
On November 30, 1993, President Clinton signed into law the Brady Bill, as James Brady looked on. James Brady suffered a disabling firearm injury during an assassination attempt on President Reagan in 1981.

CHAPTER SUMMARY

- Injuries are the fifth leading cause of death in the United States.

- Unintentional and intentional injuries represent a major community health problem, not only because of the loss of life but also because of the lost productivity and the increase in the number of disabled Americans.

- Unintentional injuries are unplanned events that are usually preceded by an unsafe act or condition. They are often accompanied by economic loss, and they interrupt the efficient completion of a task.

- Most unintentional injuries occur in the home; most fatal unintentional injuries occur on the highway.

- Unintentional injuries occur across all age groups; however, they are the leading cause of death for younger Americans.

- Motor vehicle accidents are the leading cause of unintentional injury deaths, followed by poisonings, falls, fires and burns, and drownings.

- Males and minority groups suffer proportionately more unintentional injuries.

- Prevention and control of unintentional injuries and fatalities can be instituted based upon a model in which energy is the causative agent for injuries.

- There are also four broad strategies that can prevent unintentional injuries—education, regulation, automatic protection, and litigation. Together, these strategies may be used to reduce the numbers and seriousness of unintentional injuries in the community.

- Intentional injuries are the outcome of self-directed or interpersonal violence.

- The spectrum of violence includes assaults, rapes, robberies, suicides, homicides, and the maltreatment of children, elders, and intimate partners.

- Minorities and youths are at highest risk for injury or death from an intentional violent act.
- Family violence, including child and elder maltreatment, and intimate partner violence, is a serious and pervasive community health problem.
- Widely publicized fatal shootings in schools has once again focused national attention on violence in our schools. However, schools remain a relatively safe place for the nation's youth.
- Youth violence, including youth gang violence, grew in the 1990s but has since declined, in part because of federal, state, and local initiatives to address this problem.
- Significant resources are available at the federal level (from the Departments of Health and Human Services and Justice) to assist state and local community agencies in reducing the number and seriousness of violence-related injuries.

REVIEW QUESTIONS

1. List the ways in which injuries are costly to society and quantify the costs in terms of the United States.
2. Identify the leading types of unintentional injury deaths and the risk factors associated with each type of death.
3. Why have the terms *accident* and *safety* lost favor with injury prevention professionals?
4. What is a hazard? Do hazards cause accidents? Explain your answer.
5. What types of injuries are most likely to occur in the home, and in which rooms are they most likely to occur?
6. Characterize injuries from the following activities by time—motor vehicle driving, swimming, and heating the home.
7. How does alcohol consumption contribute to unintentional injuries?
8. Summarize the contributions of Hugh DeHaven, John E. Gordon, and William Hadden, Jr., to injury prevention and control.
9. Describe the epidemiological model for injuries and provide three examples of how energy causes injuries.
10. For each of your examples from Question 9, explain how the injury could have been prevented using prevention and control tactics.
11. List four broad strategies for the reduction of unintentional injuries and give an example of each.
12. Identify the different types of violent behavior that result in intentional injuries.
13. Describe the cost of intentional injuries to society.
14. Define *family violence* and give some examples.
15. Explain the difference between child abuse and child neglect. List some contributing factors to these phenomena. What is intimate partner violence?
16. How safe are our schools? How are schools responding to safety concerns?
17. What is a youth gang? Why are they attractive to some youths? How can communities compete for youths' attention?
18. Describe the best ways in which communities can respond to youth gang violence.
19. What is the Brady Law? Is it working?

ACTIVITIES

1. Obtain a copy of a local newspaper and find three stories dealing with unintentional injuries. Provide a two- or three-sentence summary of each article and then provide your best guess of (a) what the unsafe act or condition that preceded the event was, (b) what the resulting economic loss or injury was, and (c) what task was not completed.
2. Make an appointment and interview the director of safety on your campus. Find out what the most prevalent unintentional injuries are on campus, what strategies have been used to deal with them, and what could be done to eliminate them.
3. With guidance from your course instructor, conduct a random survey of safety belt use at your campus. Collect the data in such a manner that you can compare the results between school employees and students. Then, analyze your results and draw some conclusions.
4. Survey your home, apartment, or residence hall and create a room-by-room list of the unsafe conditions that may exist. Then, create a strategy for changing each condition.
5. Using a local newspaper, locate three articles that deal with violence. For each article, (a) provide a two-sentence summary, (b) identify and describe the victim and the perpetrator, (c) identify what you feel was the underlying cause of the violence, and (d) offer a suggestion as to how the violence could have been avoided or prevented.
6. Make an appointment with an officer of the local police department to interview him or her about violent crime in your hometown. Write a two-page summary of your interview and include answers to the following questions: (a) What is the Number 1 violent crime? (b) What is the law enforcement department doing to control violent crime? (c) Does the city have a comprehensive program against crime? (d) What can the typical citizen do to help reduce violence?

SCENARIO: ANALYSIS AND RESPONSE

Please take a moment to reread the scenario at the beginning of this chapter. Then reflect on the questions that follow.

1. How does the description of the unintentional injury fit the definition provided in the chapter? Can you identify each element of the definition as it pertains to this particular scenario?

2. Think about the four approaches to the prevention of unintentional injuries (education, regulation, automatic protection, and litigation). Provide an example of how each of these four approaches could prevent another similar injury from occurring.

---

7. Write a two-page paper on what the typical citizen can do about violence.

8. Think about the public health triangle model of disease (agent, host, and environment) and gang violence. Describe in writing who or what represents each of these factors. What steps can be taken to reduce gang-related violence using this public health model? List the steps explaining each one.

COMMUNITY HEALTH ON THE WEB

The Internet contains a wealth of information about community and public health. Increase your knowledge of some of the topics presented in this chapter by accessing the Jones and Bartlett Publishers Web site at **http://health.jbpub.com/book/communityhealth/6e** and follow the links to complete the following Web activities.

- National Center for Injury Prevention and Control
- Family Violence Prevention Fund
- Children's Safety Network

REFERENCES

1. Baker, S. P. (1989). "Injury Science Comes of Age." *Journal of the American Medical Association*, 262(16): 2284-2285.

2. Miniño, A. M., and R. N. Anderson (2006). "Deaths: Injuries, 2002." *National Vital Statistics Reports*, 54(10): 1-128.

3. Lopez, A. D., C. D. Mathers, M. Ezzati, D. T. Jamison, and C. Murray (2006). *Global Burden of Disease and Risk Factors*. New York: The World Bank and Oxford University Press.

4. Miniño, A. M., M. Heron, S. L. Murphy, and K. D. Kochanek (2006). *Deaths: Final Data for 2004*. NCHS Health E-Stats. Available at http://www.cdc.gov/nchs/products/pubs/pubd/hestats/finaldeaths04/finaldeaths04.htm.

5. McCaig, L. F., and E. W. Nawar (2006). *National Ambulatory Medical Care Survey: 2004 Emergency Department Summary* (Advance Data from Vital and Health Statistics no. 372). Hyattsville, MD: National Center for Health Statistics.

6. Middleton, K. R., and E. Hing (2006). *National Hospital Ambulatory Medical Care Survey: 2004 Outpatient Department Summary* (Advance Data from Vital and Health Statistics no. 373). Hyattsville, MD: National Center for Health Statistics.

7. Hing, E., D. K. Cherry, and D. A. Woodall (2006). *National Ambulatory Medical Care Survey: 2004 Summary* (Advance Data from Vital and Health Statistics no. 374). Hyattsville, MD: National Center for Health Statistics.

8. National Safety Council (2006). *Injury Facts 2005-2006 Edition*. Itasca, IL: Author.

9. Finkelstein, E. A., P. S. Corso, T. R. Miller et al. (2006). *The Incidence and Economic Burden of Injuries in the United States*. New York: Oxford University Press.

10. National Center for Health Statistics (2006). *Health, United States, 2006 with Chartbook on Trends in the Health of Americans with Special Feature on Pain*. Hyattsville, MD: National Center for Health Statistics.

11. Hoyert, E. L., M. P. Heron, S. L. Murphy, and H. Kung (2006). "Deaths: Final Data for 2003." *National Vital Statistics Reports*, 54(13): 1-120.

12. Bonnie, R. J., C. E. Fulco, and C. T. Liverman, eds. (1999). *Reducing the Burden of Injury: Advancing Prevention and Treatment*. Institute of Medicine, Committee on Injury Prevention and Control. Washington, DC: National Academy Press.

13. Miniño, A. M., M. P. Heron, and B. L. Smith (2006). "Deaths: Preliminary Data for 2004." *National Vital Statistics Reports*, 54(19): 1-52.

14. U.S. Department of Health and Human Services (2000). *Healthy People 2010: Understanding and Improving Health*, 2nd ed. Washington, DC: U.S. Government Printing Office.

15. Peden, M., R. Scurfield, D. A. Sleet, D. Hohan, A. A. Hyder, E. Jarawan, and C. Mathers, eds. (2004). *World Report on Road Traffic Injury and Prevention*. Geneva, Switzerland: World Health Organization.

16. U.S. Department of Transportation, National Highway Traffic Safety Administration (2006). *Traffic Safety Facts 2005: A Compilation of Motor Vehicle Crash Data from the Fatality Analysis Reporting System and the General Estimates System* (DOT HS 810 631), Early ed. Washington, DC: Author. Available at http://www-nrd.nhtsa.dot.gov/pdf/nrd-30/NCSA/TSFAnn/TSF2005EE.

17. Centers for Disease Control and Prevention (2006). "Fatalities and Injuries from Falls among Older Adults—United States, 1993-2003 and 2001-2005." *MMWR*, 55(45): 1221-1224.

18. Centers for Disease Control and Prevention (2003). "Public Health and Aging: Nonfatal Injuries among Older Adults Treated in Hospital Emergency Departments—United States, 2001." *MMWR*, 52(42): 1019-1022.

19. Anderson, R. H., and B. L. Smith (2005). "Deaths: Leading Causes for 2002." *National Vital Statistics Reports*, 53 (17): 1-92.

20. U.S. Department of Health and Human Services, Centers for Disease Control and Prevention, National Center for Injury Prevention and Control (2006). *Firearm Injury Surveillance Study, 1993–2004* [Computer file] (ICPSR04595-V1). Atlanta, GA: Author. Available at http://webapp.icpsr.umich.edu/cocoon/ICPSR-STUDY/04595.xml.

21. Centers for Disease Control and Prevention (2006). "Youth Risk Behavior Surveillance—United States, 2005." *MMWR*, 55(SS-5): 1–110.

22. Centers for Disease Control and Prevention (1997). "Rates of Homicide, Suicide and Firearm-Related Deaths among Children—26 Industrial Countries." *MMWR*, 46(5): 101–105.

23. U.S. Department of Transportation, National Highway Traffic Safety Administration (2005). *Traffic Safety Facts 2004: A Compilation of Motor Vehicle Crash Data from the Fatality Analysis Reporting System and the General Estimates System* (DOT HS 809 919), Early ed. Washington, DC: Author.

24. Griffin, L. I., III (2004). *Older Driver Involvement in Injury Crashes in Texas, 1975–1999*. Washington, DC: AAA Foundation for Traffic Safety. Available at www.AAAfoundation.org/.

25. Adams, P. F., and P. M. Barnes (2006). "Summary Health Statistics for the U.S. Population: National Health Interview Survey, 2004." *Vital and Health Statistics*, 10(229): 1–104.

26. Griffin, L. I., and S. DeLaZerda (2000). *Unlicensed to Kill*. Washington, DC: AAA Foundation for Traffic Safety. Available at http://www.aaafoundation.org/.

27. Centers for Disease Control and Prevention (2004). "Child Passenger Deaths Involving Drinking Drivers—United States, 1997–2002." *MMWR*, 53(4): 77–79.

28. U.S. Department of Homeland Security, U.S. Coast Guard (2005). *Boating Statistics—2005* (COMDTPUB P16754.19). Available at http://www.uscgboating.org/statistics/accident_stats.htm.

29. U.S. Department of Homeland Security, U.S. Coast Guard. *Boating Statistics—1999* (COMDTPUB P16754.16). Available at http://www.uscgboating.org/statistics/accident_stats.htm.

30. Centers for Disease Control and Prevention (2001). "Drowning—Louisiana, 1998." *MMWR*, 50(20): 413–414.

31. Christoffel, T., and S. S. Gallagher (2006). *Injury Prevention and Public Health: Practical Knowledge, Skills, and Strategies*, 2nd ed. Sudbury, MA: Jones and Bartlett.

32. Centers for Disease Control and Prevention (2006). "Effectiveness of 0.08% Blood Alcohol Concentration (BAC) Laws." In Task Force on Community Preventive Services, eds., *The Guide to Community Preventive Services*. Available at http://www.thecommunityguide.org/mvoi/mvoi-alc-08-laws.pdf.

33. Stutts, J., J. Feaganes, E. Rodgman, C. Hamlett, T. Meadows, D. Reinfurt, K. Gish, M. Mercadante, and L. Staplin (2003). *Distractions in Everyday Driving*. Washington, DC: AAA Foundation for Traffic Safety. Available at http://www.aaafoundation.org/.

34. Governors Highway Safety Association. "Cell Phone Restrictions—State and Local Jurisdictions." Available at http://www.statehighwaysafety.org/.

35. Waller, P. F. (2002). "Challenges in Motor Vehicle Safety." *Annual Review of Public Health*, 23: 93–113.

36. Centers for Disease Control (1982). "Unintentional and Intentional Injuries—United States." *MMWR*, 31(18): 240–248.

37. Centers for Disease Control and Prevention (2001). "Nonfatal Physical Assault Related Injuries Treated in Hospital Emergency Departments—United States, 2000." *MMWR*, 51(21): 460–463.

38. Catalano, S. M. (2006). *Criminal Victimization 2005* (NCJ 214644). Washington, DC: U.S. Department of Justice, Bureau of Justice Statistics. Available at http://www.ojp.usdoj.gov/bjs/pub/pdf/cv05.pdf.

39. Centers for Disease Control and Prevention, National Center for Injury Prevention and Control (2006). "WISQARS (Web-based Injury Statistics Query and Reporting System)." Available at http://www.cdc.gov/ncipc/wisqars/.

40. Fox, J.A., and M. W. Zawitz (2006). "Homicide Trends in the United States." Washington, DC: U.S. Department of Justice, Bureau of Justice Statistics. Available at http://www.ojp.gov/bjs/homicide/homtrnd.htm.

41. Blumstein, A., F. P. Rivara, and R. Rosenfeld (2000). "The Rise and Decline of Homicide—and Why." *Annual Review of Public Health*, 21: 505–541.

42. Miller, M., D. Hemenway, and H. Wechsler (2002). "Guns and Gun Threats at College." *Journal of American College Health*, 51(2): 57–65.

43. U.S. Department of Justice, Office of Juvenile Justice and Delinquency Programs. *Promising Strategies to Reduce Gun Violence*. Available at http://ojjdp.ncjrs.org/pubs/gun%5Fviolence/contents.html.

44. U.S. Department of Health and Human Services, Administration on Children, Youth and Families (2004). *Child Maltreatment 2004*. Washington, DC: U.S. Government Printing Office. Available at http://www.acf.hhs.gov/programs/cb/pubs/cm04/cm04.pdf.

45. National Institute of Justice (1996). *The Cycle of Violence Revisited*. Washington, DC: U.S. Department of Justice.

46. National Research Council (2003). *Elder Mistreatment: Abuse, Neglect, and Exploitation in an Aging America*. Washington, DC: National Academies Press.

47. National Center on Elder Abuse (1998). *The National Elder Abuse Incidence Study: Final Report*. Available at http://www.elderabusecenter.org/default.cfm?p=nis.cfm.

48. Tjaden, P., and N. Thoennes (2000). *Extent, Nature, and Consequences of Intimate Partner Violence: Findings from the National Violence Against Women Survey* (NCJ pub. no. 181867). Washington, DC: National Institute of Justice.

49. U.S. Department of Justice, Bureau of Justice Statistics (February 2003). *Crime Data Brief: Intimate Partner Violence, 1993–2001* (NCJ 197838). Available at http://www.ojp.usdoj.gov/bjs/.

50. Centers for Disease Control and Prevention, National Center for Injury Control and Prevention. "Intimate Partner Violence: Fact Sheet." Available at http://www.cdc.gov/ncipc/factsheets/ipvfacts.htm.

51. Catalano, S. (2006). "Intimate Partner Violence in the United States." Data from the Bureau of Justice Statistics, U.S. Department of Justice, Office of Justice Programs. Available at http://www.ojp.usdoj.gov/bjs/intimate/ipv.htm.

52. Meuer, T., A. Seymour, and H. Wallace (2001). "Domestic Violence." In A. Seymour, M. Murray, J. Sigmon, M. Hook, C. Edmunds, M. Gaboury, and G. Coleman, eds. (2001). *2000 National Victim Assistance Academy*. Washington, DC: Office for Victims of Crime.

53. Osattin, A., and L. M. Short (1998). *Intimate Partner Violence and Sexual Assault: A Guide to Training Materials and Programs for Health Care Providers*. Atlanta, GA: Centers for Disease Control and Prevention.

54. Henry, S. (2000). "What Is School Violence? An Integrated Definition." *Annals of the American Academy of Political and Social Science*, 567: 16–29. As cited in U.S. Department of Education, National Center for Education Statistics (2007). *Indicators of School Crime and Safety: 2006* (NCES pub. no. 2007-003). Washington, DC: Author. Available at http://nces.ed.gov/programs/crimeindicators/.

55. U.S. Department of Education, National Center for Education Statistics (2007). *Indicators of School Crime and Safety: 2006* (NCES pub. no. 2007-003). Washington, DC: Author. Available at http://nces.ed.gov/programs/crimeindicators/.

56. Centers for Disease Control and Prevention (1995). "Youth Risk Behavior Surveillance—United States, 1993." *MMWR CDC Surveillance Summaries*, 44(SS-1): 1–55.

57. U.S. Department of Education, National Center for Education Statistics (2004). *Crime and Safety in America's Public Schools: Select Findings from the School Survey on Crime and Safety* (NCES pub. no. 2004-370). Washington, DC: Author.

58. Substance Abuse and Mental Health Services Administration, U.S. Department of Health and Human Services (2006). "About the Safe Schools/Healthy Students (SS/HS) Initiative." Available at http://www.sshs.samhsa.gov/initiative/about.aspx.

59. U.S. Department of Justice, Office of Juvenile Justice and Delinquency Prevention (November 1999). *Violence after School* (1999 National Report Series). Washington, DC: Author.

60. Thornton, T. N., C. A. Craft, L. L. Dahlberg, B. S. Lynch, and K. Baer (2000). *Best Practices of Youth Violence Prevention: A Sourcebook for Community Action*. Atlanta, GA: Centers for Disease Control and Prevention.

61. Centers for Disease Control and Prevention, National Center for Injury Prevention and Control (2007). "Youth Violence: Prevention Strategies." Available at http://www.cdc.gov/ncipc/factsheets/yvprevention.htm.

62. Egley, A., Jr., and C. E. Ritz (April 2006). "Highlights of the 2004 National Youth Gang Survey." *OJJDP Fact Sheet*. U.S. Department of Justice, Office of Justice Programs, Office of Juvenile Justice and Delinquency Prevention. Available at http://www.iir.com/nygc/publications/fs200601.pdf.

63. Centers for Disease Control and Prevention (2003). "First Reports Evaluating the Effectiveness of Strategies for Preventing Violence: Firearm Laws—Findings from the Task Force on Community Preventive Services." *MMWR*, 52(RR-14): 11–20.

64. U.S. Department of Justice, Office of Justice Programs. "Welcome to OJP: Our Mission." Available at http://www.ojp.usdoj.gov/.

Chapter 18

Safety and Health in the Workplace

Chapter Outline

Scenario

Introduction
Scope of the Problem • Importance of Occupational Safety and Health to the Community

History of Occupational Safety and Health Problems
Occupational Safety and Health in the United States before 1970 • Occupational Safety and Health Act of 1970

Prevalence of Occupational Injuries, Diseases, and Deaths
Overview of Recent Trends in Workplace Injuries and Illnesses • Unintentional Injuries in the Workplace • Prevention and Control of Unintentional Injuries in the Workplace • Workplace Violence: Intentional Workplace Injuries • Occupational Illnesses and Disorders

Resources for the Prevention of Workplace Injuries and Diseases
Occupational Safety and Health Professionals • Occupational Safety and Health Programs

Chapter Summary

Review Questions

Scenario: Analysis and Response

Activities

Community Health on the Web

References

Chapter Objectives

After studying this chapter, you will be able to:

1 Describe the scope of the occupational safety and health problem in the United States and its importance to the community.

2 Identify some of the pioneers in the prevention of occupational injuries and disease.

3 Provide a short history of state and federal legislation on occupational safety and health.

4 Explain the difference between occupational injuries and occupational diseases and give several examples of each.

5 Discuss the types of injuries that frequently occur in the workplace and describe their occurrence with regard to person, place, and time.

6 Briefly describe broad strategies for preventing injuries in the workplace.

7 Identify the different types of occupational illnesses and disorders and list some of the causative agents.

8 Outline some general strategies for controlling these diseases.

9 List several occupational safety and health professions and describe what the professionals in each of these do.

10 List and briefly describe several occupational safety and health programs for the workplace.

SCENARIO

At first Jen was exited about her new job. Now that she had turned 21, she was permitted to work in the Terrace Lounge and Restaurant, where alcohol was served and the tips were excellent. She politely resigned from her job as a waitress at another restaurant where she had worked for more than two years. That restaurant, which enjoyed a clientele primarily of seniors, did not serve alcohol and had a no-smoking policy. She looked forward to working at the Terrace because she believed that she would make as much in tips in two nights as she made all week at her old job. This increase in earnings would help her buy many of the things she wanted for her baby, which was due in six months.

That was two months ago. Now she was wondering whether she really liked working at the Terrace. The problem was all the cigarette smoke. Her mother was the first to notice that her clothes smelled smoky. But Jen had also noticed the effects of working in the lounge. Her eyes always burned at the end of a night's work and lately her throat burned too. She had started to take her 10-minute breaks outside to enjoy a few breaths of clean air.

Then, she had begun to think about the effects of the inhaled cigarette smoke on the health of her baby. During her first checkup with the doctor after she realized she was pregnant, she had been asked whether she smoked. She had proudly answered, "No." But now she wondered, "Could working in such a smoky environment be harmful to my baby?" She hated the thought of having to quit this job because she was making good money, and her manager was very complimentary of her work.

INTRODUCTION

Globally, there are more than 2.6 billion workers, and the workforce is growing continuously. Approximately 85% of these workers are in developing countries, where workplace hazards are more severe. Each year there are as many as 270 million occupational injuries, resulting in 351,000 fatalities. If one includes occupational illnesses, an estimated 2.2 million people worldwide die each year. Annually, an estimated 160 million new cases of work-related diseases occur worldwide. Internationally, a large proportion of the unemployed, as many as 30%, suffer from injuries they received while at work.[1]

> **occupational disease**
> an abnormal condition, other than an occupational injury, caused by an exposure to environmental factors associated with employment

The number of civilian Americans employed in the labor force is approximately 149.3 million.[2] After home, Americans spend the next largest portion of their time at work; thus, safe and healthy workplaces are essential if America is to reach its health objectives by 2010. It is not always easy to distinguish between the terms *occupational injury* and *occupational illness* or *disease*. However, it is generally accepted that an **occupational disease** is any abnormal condition or disorder, other than one resulting from an occupational injury, caused by factors associated with employment. It includes acute or chronic illnesses or disease that may be caused by inhalation, absorption, ingestion, or direct contact. An **occupational injury** is any injury, such as a cut, fracture, sprain, amputation, etc., that results from a work-related event or from a single, instantaneous exposure in the work environment.[3]

> **occupational injury**
> an injury that results from exposure to a single incident in the work environment

Scope of the Problem

Each day in the United States, on average, 16 workers die from an injury sustained at work. Although even one worker death is one too many, it is instructive to note that the work-related fatality rates in America have declined significantly over the past 100 years. In 1912, an estimated 18,000 to 21,000 work-related unintentional injury deaths occurred, a death rate of 21 per 100,000 workers.[4] In 2005, there were 5,702 such deaths, and the death rate for occupational injury deaths had fallen to below 4 per 100,000 workers.[5]

A total of 4.2 million nonfatal injuries and illnesses were reported in private industry workplaces during 2005, resulting in a rate of 4.6 cases per 100 equivalent full-time workers. A total of 1.4 million injuries and illnesses in private industry required recuperation away from work beyond the day of the incident in 2002. The vast majority of these events, 4.4 million, were classified as injuries; about 294,500 were classified as illnesses.[6]

Even though more workplace injuries are reported than workplace illnesses, the estimated number of deaths is higher for workplace illnesses. For example, a 2000 study estimated that for each worker who died from a workplace injury in the United States, eight workers died from work-related diseases.[7] Worldwide, it is estimated that fewer than one in five work-related deaths is the result of an injury.[1]

Although significant progress has been made in reducing morbidity and mortality in the workplace in the United States, the U.S. occupational fatality rate is not the lowest among the highly developed nations. All but three members of the European Union—Austria, Portugal, and Spain—have lower occupational fatality rates than the United States.[8]

Occupational injuries and illnesses are an economic issue, too. It has been estimated that workplace injuries and deaths cost $142 billion in 2004, including $73 billion in lost wages and productivity, $26 billion in medical expenses, and $31 billion in administrative costs and other costs. Thus, each worker in America must produce $1,010 in goods or services just to offset the cost of work-related injuries.[4]

Importance of Occupational Safety and Health to the Community

Because of the grim statistics previously stated, it is important to recognize how occupational and community health problems are linked. The population of those working in industry is a subset of the population of the larger community in which the industry is located. Workers, usually the healthiest people in the community, are exposed in the course of their jobs to specific hazardous materials at the highest concentrations. It is in the factory that the most accurate exposure and health data are available for extrapolation to the general community. Most pollutants for which safe exposure levels have been adopted are workplace materials for which occupational exposures were studied first.

Hazardous agents in the workplace affect not only workers but also those outside the worksite. This can occur through soil and groundwater contamination with solids and liquids or air pollution with industrial gases and dusts. It can also occur through clothing and vehicle contamination, as in the case of asbestos workers whose wives and children became exposed to asbestos from these sources. It is important to note that the general population, which includes children, the elderly, and pregnant women, is more sensitive to exposure to pollutants than the workforce.

Another way that industries and their communities share health problems is in the instance of an industrial disaster. Examples include the Three Mile Island (Pennsylvania) nuclear reactor near-meltdown in the United States in 1979, the Bhopal tragedy in India in 1984, and the Chernobyl nuclear catastrophe in the Ukraine in 1986. In these cases, the risk of exposure to a chemical or nuclear energy source, which was originally limited to the workplace, became a community-wide risk.

Finally, it is important to recognize the workers themselves as a community, with common social problems and environmental risks. The failure to recognize the community nature of occupational groups and to monitor chronic conditions such as dermatitis, headaches, blood pressure, or blood chemistries has been a major weakness in our conventional approach to occupational health problems.

HISTORY OF OCCUPATIONAL SAFETY AND HEALTH PROBLEMS

Occupational risks undoubtedly occurred even in prehistoric times, not only during hunting and warfare, but also in more peaceful activities such as the preparation of flint by knapping. The discovery of flint heaps suggests that even these earliest of workers may have been at risk for silicosis (dust in the lungs).

An extensive historical review of occupational safety and health problems from early Egyptian times to the present day has been published.[9] The first of these milestones occurred in 1561 with George Agricola's treatise on mining, *De Re Metallica,* which emphasized the need for ventilation of mines. In 1567, the work of Philippus Aureolus Theophrastus Bombastus von Hohenheim, also known as Paracelsus, was published under the title *On the Miners' Sickness and Other Miners' Diseases*. These were the first significant works describing specific occupational diseases. The first work on occupational diseases in general was Ramazzini's *Discourse on the Diseases of Workers,* which appeared in 1700.[10,11] In this chapter, we will concentrate only on recent events in the United States and make only brief references to earlier milestones.

Occupational Safety and Health in the United States before 1970

The Industrial Revolution, which began in Britain in the eighteenth century, soon spread to continental Europe and then to the United States. Factors creating and driving the Industrial Revolution were the substitution of steam and coal for animal power, the substitution of machines for human skills, and other advances in industrial technology. These changes resulted in the rise of mass manufacturing, the organization of large work units such as mills and factories, and eventually the exposure of masses of workers to new hazards. Although mining remained the most dangerous form of work, there were soon other unsafe occupations, such as iron smelting and working in cotton mills and textile factories (see Figure 18.1).

workers' compensation laws
a set of federal laws designed to compensate those workers and their families who suffer injuries, disease, or death from workplace exposure

The recognition of the need to reduce workplace injuries began long before any attention was paid to workplace diseases. The earliest efforts of those responsible for inspecting workplaces were aimed primarily at the sanitation and cleanliness of workplaces. They soon became concerned with equipment safeguards and tending to those who had become injured or ill at work.[11] These efforts, while much needed and appreciated, did little to improve the overall health of the workforce.

State Legislation

The first official responses to new hazards in the workplace did not occur until 1835, when Massachusetts passed the first Child Labor Law, and later in 1867, when it created a Department of Factory Inspection to enforce it (see Figure 18.2). Under this law, factories were prohibited from hiring children younger than 10 years of age.[12] At this time the federal government was concerned only with working conditions of federal employees. In 1877, Massachusetts passed the first worker safety law, aimed at protecting textile workers from hazardous spinning machinery.[13]

In 1902, Maryland became the first state to pass any kind of workers' compensation legislation. In 1908, Congress, at the insistence of President Theodore Roosevelt, finally enacted the first of several **workers' compensation laws;** this first law covered certain federal employees. Over the next 40 years, all states and territories

FIGURE 18.1
Cotton mills in the late nineteenth century offered little protection from injuries.

FIGURE 18.2
Before child labor laws were passed, many children worked long hours at dangerous jobs such as mining.

Occupational Safety and Health Act of 1970 (OSHAct) comprehensive federal legislation aimed at ensuring safe and healthful working conditions for working men and women

eventually enacted some type of workers' compensation legislation, beginning with New York in 1910 and ending with Mississippi in 1948.[9] So ended the first wave of reform in occupational safety and health. With the exception of several other legislative efforts, little progress was achieved during the first half of the century in protecting workers from injuries in the workplace, and almost nothing was done about occupational illnesses.

There was one exception. Alice Hamilton (1869–1970) was a strong proponent of occupational health and a true pioneer in this field (see Figure 18.3). Over her 40-year career in occupational health, she led crusades to reduce poisonings from heavy metals such as lead and mercury. She investigated silicosis in Arizona copper mines, carbon disulfide poisoning in the viscose rayon industry, and many other industrial health problems.[12]

In spite of Hamilton's efforts, progress in occupational health legislation was slow in the first half of the twentieth century. Occupational diseases were by and large ignored. There was some safety legislation, such as the Coal Mine Safety Act of 1952. Beginning in the 1960s, some people began to take a closer look at the various state workers' safety and workers' compensation laws. It then was discovered that in most states, legislation was a fragmentary patchwork of laws; some states had good laws, but many had inadequate legislation. Many of the laws had failed to keep up with new technology or with inflation. Some groups of workers, including agricultural workers, were not covered at all by legislation. Other problems were the division of authority among various departments within state governments, fragmented record keeping, and inadequate administrative personnel.[14]

Federal Legislation

In 1884, the federal government created a Bureau of Labor, in 1910 the Federal Bureau of Mines, and in 1914 the Office of Industrial Hygiene and Sanitation in the Public Health Service. In 1916, Congress passed the Federal Employees' Compensation Act, which provided federal employees compensation if injured while on the job.[13] Quite a few important laws were passed between 1908 and 1970 (see Table 18.1), but the two most comprehensive laws were the Coal Mine Health and Safety Act of 1969 and the **Occupational Safety and Health Act of 1970 (OSHAct),** also known as the Williams-Steiger Act in honor of Senator Harrison A. Williams, Jr., and Congressman William A. Steiger, who worked for passage of the act. At the time the act was passed, 14,000 workers died each year on the job. Since its passage, the act has served to raise the consciousness of both management and labor to the problems of health and safety in the workplace.

Occupational Safety and Health Act of 1970

The purpose of the Occupational Safety and Health Act of 1970 is to ensure that employers in the private sector furnish each employee "employment and a place of employment which are free from recognized hazards that are causing or likely to cause death or serious

FIGURE 18.3
Alice Hamilton (1869–1970) was a pioneer in occupational safety and health in America.

Table 18.1
Highlights of Federal Occupational Safety and Health Legislation

Year	Legislation
1908	Federal Workmen's Compensation Act—limited coverage
1916	Federal Highway Aid Act
1926	Federal Workmen's Compensation Act—amended to include all workers
1927	Federal Longshoremen's and Harbor Workers' Compensation Act
1936	Walsh-Healey Public Contracts Act
1952	**Coal Mine Safety Act**
1958	Federal Longshoremen's and Harbor Workers' Compensation Act—amended to include rigid safety precautions
1959	Radiation Standards Act
1960	Federal Hazardous Substances Labeling Act
1966	National Traffic and Motor Vehicle Safety Act
1966	Child Protection Act—banned hazardous household substances
1967	National Commission on Product Safety created
1968	Natural Gas Pipeline Safety Act
1969	Construction Safety Act
1969	Child Protection Act—amended to broaden the coverage
1969	Coal Mine Health and Safety Act
1970	**Occupational Safety and Health Act**

physical harm."[13] Furthermore, employers were henceforth required to comply with all occupational safety and health standards promulgated and enforced under the act by the **Occupational Safety and Health Administration (OSHA),** which was established by the act.

Also established by the OSHAct was the **National Institute for Occupational Safety and Health (NIOSH),** a research body now located in the Centers for Disease Control and Prevention of the Department of Health and Human Services. NIOSH is responsible for recommending occupational safety and health standards to OSHA, which is located in the Department of Labor.

The OSHAct contains several noteworthy provisions. Perhaps the most important is the employee's right to request an OSHA inspection. Under this right, any employee or any employee representative may notify OSHA of violations of standards or of the general duty obligation (to provide a safe and healthy workplace) by the employer. Under the act, the employee's name must be withheld if desired, and the employee or a representative may accompany the OSHA inspectors in their inspection. By another provision of the OSHAct, individual states can regain local authority over occupational health and safety by submitting state laws that are and will continue to be as effective as the federal programs.[13]

PREVALENCE OF OCCUPATIONAL INJURIES, DISEASES, AND DEATHS

In this section, a brief overview of current trends in workplace injuries and illness is followed by a discussion of the occurrence and prevalence of work-related injuries and work-related diseases.

Overview of Recent Trends in Workplace Injuries and Illnesses

Since 1992, there has been a decline in the number of workplace injuries and illnesses reported in private industry. There were 4.2 million injuries and illnesses reported in 2005, resulting in a rate of 4.6 cases per 100 equivalent full-time workers per year. Approximately 2.4 million of these injuries and illnesses were cases with days away from work.[6] Ninety-four

Occupational Safety and Health Administration (OSHA)
the federal agency located within the Department of Labor and created by the OSHAct that is charged with the responsibility of administering the provisions of the OSHAct

National Institute for Occupational Safety and Health (NIOSH)
a research body within the Department of Health and Human Services that is responsible for developing and recommending occupational safety and health standards

percent of the 4.2 million injuries and illnesses (4.0 million) were injuries. About 242,500 new, nonfatal cases of occupational illnesses were reported in private industry in 2005. This figure does not include long-term latent illnesses, which are often difficult to relate to the workplace and therefore are underreported.[6]

The industries with the highest rates of nonfatal injuries and illnesses per 100 full-time workers in 2005 were manufacturing (6.3), construction (6.3), and agriculture, forestry, and fishing (6.1). Finance, insurance, and real estate had the lowest nonfatal injury and illness rates (see Figure 18.4).[6] Workplace injury and illness rates and cases with and without lost work-days have declined steadily since 1992 (see Figure 18.5).[6,15]

Unintentional Injuries in the Workplace

Unintentional injuries in the workplace include minor injuries (such as bruises, cuts, abrasions, and minor burns), and major injuries (such as amputations, fractures, severe lacerations, eye losses, acute poisonings, and severe burns). Statistics on injuries and injury deaths are available from several sources, including the National Center for Health Statistics (NCHS), the National Safety Council (NSC), the Bureau of Labor Statistics (BLS), and NIOSH. For this reason, estimates of the number of occupational injuries and injury deaths vary. However, beginning in 1992, the NSC adopted the figures published by BLS reports, including its *Census of Fatal Occupational Injuries (CFOI)* and its annual report on workplace injuries and illnesses. The BLS reports are the source of figures used in this text.[5,6]

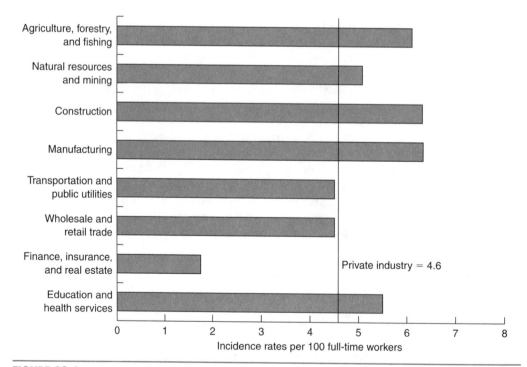

FIGURE 18.4

Nonfatal workplace injury and illness incidence rates by industry division, 2005.

Source: U.S. Department of Labor, Bureau of Labor Statistics (2006). *Workplace Injuries and Illnesses in 2005.* Available at http://www.bls.gov/iif/oshwc/osh/os/osnr0025.pdf.

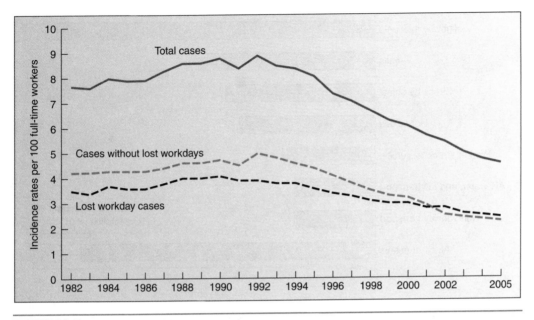

FIGURE 18.5

Workplace injury and illness incidence rates by type of case, 1982 to 2005.

Source: U.S. Department of Labor, Bureau of Labor Statistics (2006). *Workplace Injuries and Illnesses in 2005.* Available at
http://www.bls.gov/iif/oshwc/osh/os/osnr0025.pdf.

Fatal Work-Related Injuries

In 2005 there were 5,764 fatal work-related injuries, or about 16 per day.[5] This is a rate of 4.0
deaths per 100,000 workers, the lowest rate since the *CFOI* began in 1992. Highway incidents
continued to lead the way, with 1,428 deaths (25% of the total); followed by falls, with 767
fatal injuries (13%); worker struck by object or equipment, with 604 deaths (11%); homicides,
with 564 deaths (10%); worker struck by vehicle, with 390 deaths (7%); air, sea, and rail, with
372 deaths (6%); nonhighway transport deaths, with 340 deaths (6%); and other events, with
1,299 deaths (22%) (see Figure 18.6).[5]

Compared with 2004, fatal work injuries involving women were down 3%, but fatal work
injuries among workers younger than 20 years were up about 18%, and fatalities among agricultural workers were also 23% higher than in 2004. Also, in 2005, injuries attributable to hurricanes accounted for 29 fatal work injuries.[5]

The industries with the highest rates of fatal occupational injuries per 100,000 employees
in 2005 were agriculture, forestry, fishing, and hunting (32.5), mining (25.6), transportation
and warehousing (17.6), and construction (11.0). The industries with the lowest fatal injury
rates per 100,000 employees were education and health services (0.8) and financial activities
(1.0).[5]

Nonfatal Work-Related Injuries

In 2003, an estimated 3.4 million occupational injuries and illnesses were treated in emergency departments. Seventy-nine percent of these injuries and illnesses were in five diagnostic
categories. The most common types of injuries and illnesses were sprains and strains (27%);
lacerations, punctures, amputations, and avulsions (24%); contusions, abrasions, and
hematomas (18%); dislocations and fractures (7%); and burns (3%). The injury and illness rate
was twice as high for the 15- to 24-year age group (3.7 per 100 full-time equivalent [FTE]
workers) as it was for the 25- to 54-year age group (1.9 per 100 FTE workers). The highest

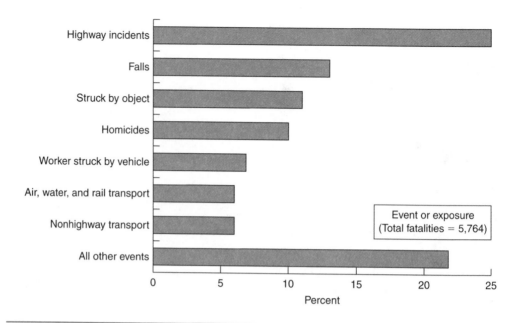

FIGURE 18.6

The manner in which workplace fatalities occurred, 2005.

Source: U.S. Department of Labor, Bureau of Labor Statistics (2006). *National Census of Fatal Occupational Injuries in 2005.* Available at http://www.bls.gov/news.release/pdf/cfoi.pdf.

nonfatal occupational injury and illness rates were among 18- to 19-year-olds. Males had higher injury rates than females in all age groups (see Figure 18.7). Workers with more serious injuries, about 2%, were hospitalized. Hospitalization rates were highest for workers 65 years and older.[16] The 2003 findings were comparable to earlier results from 1998.

Disabling injuries or illnesses are those in which the injured worker remains away from work because of the injury beyond the day in which the injury occurred. The most disabling type of injury or illness is carpal tunnel syndrome, which resulted in a median of 25 days away from work (see Figure 18.8).[17] Finally, the part of the body involved in the most cases with days away from work is the back, which accounted for almost one-fourth of all occupational injuries and illnesses.[17] The average cost of a disabling workplace injury was calculated at $34,000 in 2004.[4] One set of the *Healthy People 2010* objectives is to reduce work-related injuries that result in medical treatment, lost time from work, or restricted work activity (see Box 18.1).

Characteristics of Workers Involved in Work-Related Injuries

Differences in injury and injury death rates are often related to the age and gender of the worker. Injury death rate differences also occur between those of different income levels and races.

Age

Young workers aged 16 to 19 years accounted for 6.9 million (5.1%) of all employed workers in 2001, but accounted for just 3% of the 1.5 million injury and illness cases involving days away from work. Workers aged 16 to 17 and 18 to 19 years have the lowest workplace fatality rates of any age group (1.1 and 2.2 per 100,000 of workers, respectively). The lower injury, illness, and fatality rates for these groups may reflect the types of employment today's young

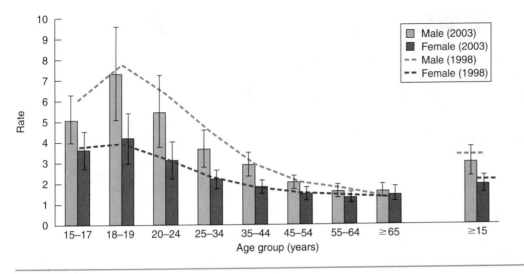

FIGURE 18.7

Estimated rates of nonfatal occupational injuries and illnesses among workers treated in hospital emergency departments, by age group and sex of worker—United States, 1998 and 2003. Rates are per 100 full-time equivalent (FTE) workers: one FTE equals 2,000 hours worked per year and includes hours for all jobs worked by a person.

Source: Centers for Disease Control and Prevention (2006). "Nonfatal Occupational Injuries and Illnesses among Workers Treated in Hospital Emergency Departments—United States, 2003." *MMWR*, 55(16): 449-452.

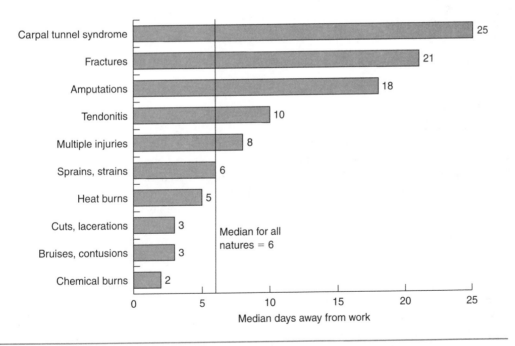

FIGURE 18.8

Characteristics of occupational injuries or illnesses. Median days away from work due to occupational injuries or illnesses in private industry by nature of injury or illness, 2001.

Source: National Institute for Occupational Safety and Health (2004). *Worker Health Chartbook, 2004.* Available at http://www.cdc.gov/niosh/pubs.html.

HEALTHY PEOPLE 2010: OBJECTIVES

Objective 20.2: Reduce work-related injuries resulting in medical treatment, lost time from work, or restricted work activities.

Target setting method: 30% improvement. (Better than the best will be used when data are available.)

Data sources: Annual Survey of Occupational Injuries and Illnesses, DOL, BLS; National Electronic Injury Surveillance System (NEISS), CPSC.

Target and baseline:

Objective	Reduction in Work-Related Injuries Resulting in Medical Treatment, Lost Time from Work, or Restricted Activity	1998 Baseline (unless noted)	2002* Status	2010 Target
		Injuries per 100 Full-Time Workers Aged 16 Years and Older		
20-2a.	All industry	6.2	5.0	4.3
20-2b.	Construction	8.7	6.9	6.1
20-2c.	Health services	7.9 (1997)	6.9	5.5
20-2d.	Agriculture, forestry, and fishing	7.6	6.0	5.3
20-2e.	Transportation	7.9 (1997)	5.8	5.5
20-2f.	Mining	4.7	3.4	3.3
20-2g.	Manufacturing	8.5	6.4	6.0
20-2h.	Adolescent workers	4.8 (1997)	—	3.4

*Due to revised OSHA reporting requirements, data are not comparable to those for previous years.

For Further Thought

The target is a 30% reduction in work-related injuries. What do you think the effect of a strong economy would have on reaching this goal? A weak economy? Do you think higher gasoline prices would make it easier or harder to achieve this objective?

Sources: U.S. Department of Health and Human Services (2000). *Healthy People 2010: Understanding and Improving Health,* 2nd ed. Washington, DC: U.S. Government Printing Office, November 2000; Centers for Disease Control and Prevention (2004). "Data 2010." Available at http://wonder.cdc.gov/data-2010/.

people find: Fewer are finding jobs in manufacturing and more are finding employment in the service industry.[17]

The service industry is also a major employer for older workers (workers aged 65 and older). However, older workers have the highest occupational fatality rates of any age group, 11.5 per 100,000 (see Figure 18.9). Older workers also have an increased burden of workplace injury and illness cases resulting in days away from work. The median number of days away from work following an injury was 14 for older workers, compared with 4 days for workers aged 16 to 19 years (see Figure 18.10).[17]

One group of workers that is of special concern is children. An estimated 70% to 80% of teens have worked for pay at some time during their high school years; 50% of employed youths work more than 15 hours during the school week. One in six works more than 25 hours during the school week. Although some level of employment may be desirable, studies show that teens who work more than 20 hours a week do worse academically and are more likely to abuse drugs and alcohol. There are other dangers, too. Every 30 seconds, a young worker under the age of 18 is injured in the workplace, and every five days a teenager dies because of a workplace injury.[18]

At particular risk are those youth who are employed in violation of child labor laws. An estimated 148,000 youth are illegally employed during an average week in the United States. This figure does not include the roughly 800,000 youth aged 6 to 17 years who are working as migrant and seasonal farmworkers.[18] A child labor survey found 4,059 child labor violations in

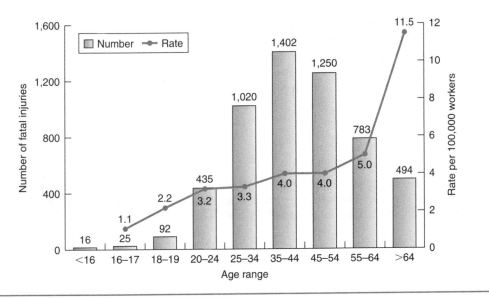

FIGURE 18.9

Number and rate of fatal occupational injuries by age of worker, 2002.

Source: U.S. Department of Health and Human Services, Centers for Disease Control and Prevention, National Institute for Occupational Safety and Health (2004). *Worker Health Chartbook, 2004* (HHS [NIOSH] pub. no. 2004-146). Cincinnati, OH: NIOSH Publications.

the 32 states reporting violations in 2004. The top five child labor violations related to minors engaged in prohibited hazardous work in 2004 involved working alone in a cash-based business, cooking, baking, serving alcohol, and working without adult supervision (in retail and restaurants); construction; power-driven machinery; driving on public roads or operating forklifts; and roofing.[19]

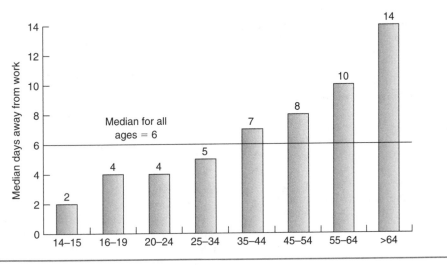

FIGURE 18.10

Median days away from work due to occupational injury or illness in private industry by age, 2001.

Source: U.S. Department of Health and Human Services, Centers for Disease Control and Prevention, National Institute for Occupational Safety and Health (2004). *Worker Health Chartbook, 2004* (HHS [NIOSH] pub. no. 2004-146). Cincinnati, OH: NIOSH Publications.

Youth employment peaks during summers, when an estimated 5.5 million youths find jobs. Young workers are at particular risk for injury because (1) they may not be trained to perform the assigned task, (2) they may not be adequately supervised, (3) they lack experience and maturity needed to perform assigned tasks and to recognize hazards, and (4) they may be unaware of child labor laws aimed at protecting them. The most dangerous types of work for youth are (1) agriculture, (2) retail trades, especially at night and handling cash, (3) transportation, and (4) construction. Box 18.2 provides recommendations for protecting the safety and health of young workers.[20]

BOX 18.2

HAZARDOUS WORK FOR ADOLESCENTS AND PRACTICAL STEPS FOR PROTECTING THEIR SAFETY AND HEALTH

Work Too Hazardous for Adolescents

- Working in or around motor vehicles
- Operating tractors and other heavy equipment
- Working in retail and service industries where there is a risk of robbery-related homicide
- Working on ladders, scaffolds, roofs, or construction sites
- Continuous manual lifting or lifting of heavy objects

Recommendations

Young Workers

Young workers should take the following steps to protect themselves:

1. *Know about and follow safe work practices.*
   - Recognize the potential for injury at work.
   - Follow safe work practices.
   - Seek information about safe work practices from employers, school counselors, parents, state labor departments, and the Department of Labor (DOL). Visit www.youthrules.dol.gov, or call 1-866-4-USWAGE.
2. *Ask about training:* Participate in training programs offered by your employer, or request training if none is offered.
3. *Ask about hazards:* Don't be afraid to ask questions if you are not sure about the task you are asked to do. Discuss your concerns with your supervisor or employer first.
4. *Know your rights:* Be aware that you have the right to work in a safe and healthful work environment free of recognized hazards. Visit www.osha.gov/sltc/teenworkers/index.html.
   - You have the right to refuse unsafe work tasks and conditions.
   - You have the right to file complaints with DOL when you feel your rights have been violated or your safety has been jeopardized.
   - You are entitled to workers' compensation for a work-related injury or illness.

5. *Know the laws:* Before you start work, learn what jobs young workers are prohibited from doing. State child labor laws may be more restrictive than federal laws, and they vary considerably from state to state. Visit www.youthrules.dol.gov or call 1-866-4-USWAGE.

Employers

Employers should take the following steps to protect young workers:

1. *Recognize the hazards.*
   - Reduce the potential for injury or illness in young workers by assessing and eliminating hazards in the workplace.
   - Make sure equipment used by young workers is safe and legal. Visit www.dol.gov/dol/topic/youthlabor/hazardousjobs.htm or call 1-866-4-USADOL.
2. *Supervise young workers.*
   - Make sure that young workers are appropriately supervised.
   - Make sure that supervisors and adult coworkers are aware of tasks young workers may or may not perform.
   - Label equipment that young workers cannot use, or color-code uniforms of young workers so that others will know they cannot perform certain jobs.
3. *Provide training.*
   - Provide training in hazard recognition and safe work practices.
   - Have young workers demonstrate that they can perform assigned tasks safely and correctly.
   - Ask young workers for feedback about the training.
4. *Know and comply with the laws:* Know and comply with child labor laws and occupational safety and health regulations that apply to your business. State laws may be more restrictive than federal laws, and they vary considerably from state to state. Post these

BOX
18.2   ᶜ(**CONTINUED**)

regulations for workers to read. For information about federal child labor laws, visit www.dol.gov/dol/topic/youthlabor/index.htm or call 1-866-4-USADOL. Links to state labor offices are available at www.iisa.net or www.youthrules.dol/gov/states.htm (1-866-4-USWAGE). Information about OSHA regulations that apply to workers of all age is available at www.osha.gov.

5. *Develop an injury and illness prevention program:* Involve supervisors and experienced workers in developing a comprehensive safety program that includes an injury and illness prevention program and a process for identifying and solving safety and health problems. OSHA consultation programs are available in every state to help employers identify hazards and improve their safety and health management programs. Visit www.osha.gov/oshprogs/consult.html.

Educators

Educators should take the following steps to protect young workers:

1. *Talk to students about work:* Talk to students about safety and health hazards in the workplace and students' rights and responsibilities as workers.

2. *Ensure the safety of school-based work experience programs:* Ensure that vocational education programs, school-to-work, or Workforce Investment Act partnerships offer students work that is allowed by law and is in safe and healthful environments free of recognized hazards. All such programs should include safety and health training.

3. *Include worker safety and health in the school curriculum:* Incorporate occupational safety and health topics into high school and junior high curricula (e.g., safety and health regulations, how to recognize hazards, how to communicate safety concerns, where to go for help). Information is available from NIOSH at www.cdc.gov/niosh/pdfs/99-141.pdf [NIOSH 1999] or 1-800-35-NIOSH.

4. *Know the laws:* If you are responsible for signing work permits or certificates, know the child labor

laws. State laws may be more restrictive than federal laws, and they vary considerably from state to state. Visit www.dol.gov/gol/topic/youthlabor/ResourcesforEducators.htm (or call 1-866-USADOL), www.youthrules.dol.gov (or call 1-866-4-USWAGE), or visit www.osha.gov/SLTC/teenworkers/index. html.

Parents

Parents should take the following steps to protect young workers:

1. *Take an active role in your child's employment.*
   - Know the name of your child's employer and your child's work address and phone number.
   - Ask your child about the types of work involved, work tasks, and equipment he or she uses at work.
   - Ask your child about training and supervision provided by the employer.
   - Be alert for signs of fatigue or stress as your child tries to balance demands of work, school, home, and extracurricular activities.

2. *Know the laws:* Be familiar with child labor laws. State laws may be more restrictive than federal laws, and they vary considerably from state to state. Don't assume that your child's employer knows about these laws. Visit www.dol.gov/dol/topic/youthlabor/ParentsofYoung.htm (or call 1-866-4-USADOL), www.youthrules.dol.gov (or call 1-866-4-USWAGE), or www.osha.gov/SLTC/teenworkers/index.html.

3. *Be aware of young workers' rights:* Report unsafe working conditions or employment in violation of child labor laws to DOL. Young workers are eligible for workers' compensation benefits if injured on the job.

4. *Share information with other parents:* Studies have shown that most young workers and parents are not aware of the laws and rights of young workers.

Source: U.S. Department of Health and Human Services, Centers for Disease Control and Prevention, National Institute for Occupational Safety and Health (2003). *NIOSH Alert: Preventing Deaths, Injuries, and Illnesses of Young Workers* (HHS [NIOSH] pub. no. 2003-128). Available at http://www.cdc.gov/ niosh/topics/youth.

Gender

More than 67 million women are part of the American labor force.[21] Since 1950, the labor force participation rate of women has nearly doubled, so that today more than half of all adult women work. In 2005, females made up 46% of the American workforce.[22] Although males made up 54% of the workforce, they worked 58.7% of all the hours worked. Because they work more hours and because there are still some dangerous jobs filled predominantly by males, males accounted for nearly two-thirds (66.1%) of all the injury and illness cases involving days away from work.[16] Women die of work-related injuries at much lower rates than men. In 2005, only 7% of those who died of an injury in the workplace were women (see Figure 18.11).[22] When figures are adjusted for the numbers of each sex in the workforce, the overall occupational death rate for men is over 9 times higher than for women (8.3 deaths per 100,000 for men, compared with 0.9 per 100,000 workers for women).[23] A significant portion of the difference results from men being employed in more dangerous jobs. Industries with the highest fatality rates are the same for both men and women—mining, agriculture, construction, and transportation. While the number of homicides is higher among men, proportionally homicides are greater for women, accounting for almost half of women's job-related fatalities.[23]

Like men, the most frequent job-related injury by body part injured by women was the hand, wrist, or fingers. However, when the injury resulted in one or more days away from work, the leading cause was back injuries. Nine million women had back pain, and one-third attributed this pain to the workplace. In fact, more that half of women in blue collar or service occupations attributed their back pain to the workplace.[23]

Working women are more likely than nonworking women to receive certain health benefits such as workplace prenatal education (offered in 9% of workplaces), weight control programs (24%), and cancer education (23%). Women in the workforce are more likely to be covered by health insurance than nonworking women (73% versus 46%) and were more likely to have a Pap test within the past three years (83% versus 73%).[23] One group of disorders in which females make up a higher proportion of cases with days away from work is anxiety, stress, and neurotic disorders. In 2001, female workers accounted for 64.9% of these cases.[17]

Poverty and Race

Studies show that those living in counties where income is lower have significantly higher occupational death rates than those living in higher-income counties. In general, death rates for nonwhites are about 12% higher than for whites (5.6 per 100,000 versus 5.0 per 100,000).[24] However, machinery injury death rates for whites are twice those of blacks. Hispanics, which make up 10.9% of the workforce, experience 15.2% of all occupational fatalities.[17] Native Americans are at highest risk for death from explosions and falling objects. Asians have very low death rates for occupational injuries. Although they make up 4.7% of the workforce, they experience only 2.5% of all occupational fatalities.[17] Occupational injury rates may reflect the types of employment in which workers find themselves.

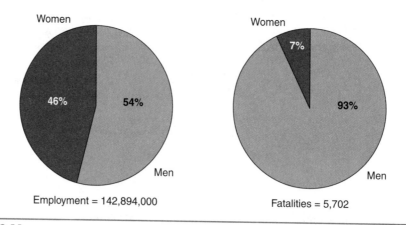

FIGURE 18.11

Employment and fatality profiles by gender of worker, 2005.

Source: U.S. Department of Labor, Bureau of Labor Statistics (2006). "Employment and Fatality Profiles by Gender of Worker, 2005." In *Census of Fatal Occupational Injuries Charts, 1992–2005.* Available at http://www.bls.gov/iif/oshcfoi1.htm#charts.

Geographic Differences in Workplace Injuries

During 2000, occupational injury death rates were highest in Alaska (20.9 per 100,000 workers), followed by Wyoming, Montana, Idaho, Mississippi, and West Virginia (see Figure 18.12).[17] Deaths from nonfarm machinery are higher in the mountain states, but deaths from farm machinery are higher in the north-central states. Work-related death rates from machinery, falling objects, electric current, and explosion are all higher in rural states. Within states, work-related deaths are higher in rural areas than in more urban areas.

Temporal Variations in Workplace Injuries

As mentioned previously, between 1912 and 2005 injury death rates among workers have declined 81% (from 21 per 100,000 workers to 4 per 100,000). During this period, the workforce in America has nearly quadrupled in size, and the amount of goods and services produced has increased ninefold.[4] These improvements in workplace safety have been considered one of the 10 greatest achievements in public health during the past century (see Box 18.3).

There is a seasonality to work-related deaths. Injury death rates from machinery, falling objects, electric current, and explosions are highest in the summer, when farming and construction work increase. Deaths from these causes are also more often reported during weekdays than on weekends, when, in general, more injury deaths occur.

Workplace Injuries by Industry and Occupation

Fatal and nonfatal occupational injury rates vary according to type of industry and type of occupation.

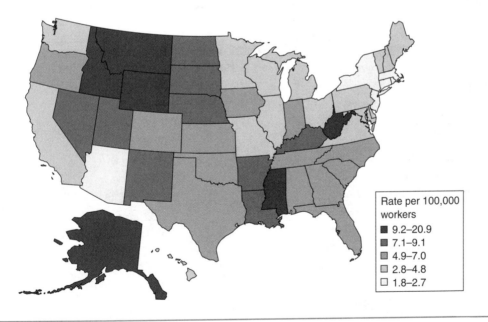

Rate per 100,000 workers
- 9.2–20.9
- 7.1–9.1
- 4.9–7.0
- 2.8–4.8
- 1.8–2.7

FIGURE 18.12

Average annual rate of fatal occupational injuries per 100,000 workers by state of death, 1980–2000. (All data for 1980–2000 exclude New York City.) The states with the highest fatality rates for occupational injury during 1980–2000 include Alaska (20.9 per 100,000 workers), Wyoming (14.9), Montana (11.1), Idaho (9.7), Mississippi (9.6), and West Virginia (9.6). The greatest number of fatal occupational injuries occurred in California (12,221), Texas (11,635), Florida (7,252), Illinois (5,145), and Pennsylvania (4,420).

Source: U.S. Department of Health and Human Services, Centers for Disease Control and Prevention, National Institute for Occupational Safety and Health (2004). *Worker Health Chartbook, 2004* (HHS [NIOSH] pub. no. 2004-146). Cincinnati, OH: NIOSH Publications.

BOX
18.3

TEN GREAT PUBLIC HEALTH ACHIEVEMENTS, 1900–1999: SAFER WORKPLACES

Saving Lives, Promoting Health, and Protecting Jobs

A Sharp Increase in the Workforce, but an Even Sharper Decline in Work-Related Deaths

At the beginning of the twentieth century, workers in the United States faced remarkably high risks to their health and safety. Today, despite a much larger workforce than ever before, work-related deaths have declined sharply. Identifying and correcting occupational health hazards has greatly reduced the health and safety risks for such occupations as construction workers, miners, and farmers.

From 1933 to 1997, according to the National Safety Council, work-related injuries declined 90%. And,

although the workforce tripled during those years, deaths declined from 37 per 100,000 to 4 per 100,000 workers.

If today's workforce of approximately 130 million were at the same risk for dying from injuries as workers in 1933, an additional 40,000 workers would have died in 1997 from preventable events.

In the coal mining industry, for example, improvements in workers' enviromental health and safety have resulted in lower rates of fatal injury, which were once common among miners.

Fatal Occupational Injuries by Industry

Injury death rates vary by type of industry and occupation. In 2005, fatality rates per 100,000 workers were highest for agriculture (32.5), followed by mining (25.6), transportation and warehousing (17.6), and then construction (11.0) (see Figure 18.13).[22] One of the *Healthy People 2010* objectives is to reduce deaths from work-related injuries for all industries. Mining,

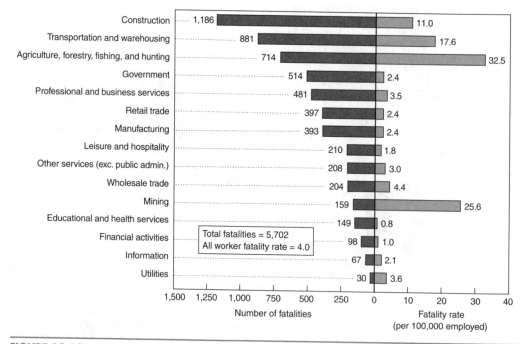

FIGURE 18.13

Number and rate of fatal occupational injuries by private industry sector, 2005. Although the construction sector recorded the highest number of fatal injuries, the highest fatality rates were in agriculture, forestry, fishing, and hunting and in mining. Rate = (Fatal work injuries/Employment) × 100,000.

Source: U.S. Department of Labor, Bureau of Labor Statistics (2006). "Employment and Fatality Profiles by Gender of Worker, 2005." In *Census of Fatal Occupational Injuries Charts, 1992–2005*. Available at http://www.bls.gov/iif/oshcfoi1.htm#charts.

BOX 18.4	HEALTHY PEOPLE 2010: OBJECTIVES

Objective 20.1: Reduce deaths from work–related injuries.

Target setting method: Better than the best for 20-1a; 30 percent improvement for 20-1b, 20-1c, 20-1d, and 20-1e. (Better than the best will be used when data are available.)

Data source: Census of Fatal Occupational Injuries (CFOI), DOL, BLS.

Target and baseline:

Objective	Reduction in Deaths from Work-Related Injuries	1998 Baseline	2002 Status	2010 Target
		Deaths per 100,000 Workers Aged 16 Years and Older		
20-1a.	All industry	4.5	4.0	3.2
20-1b.	Mining	23.6	23.5	16.5
20-1c.	Construction	14.6	12.2	10.2
20-1d.	Transportation	11.8	11.3	8.3
20-1e.	Agriculture, forestry, and fishing	24.1	22.7	16.9

For Further Thought

The targets call for reducing deaths from work-related injuries by 30%. In which industry do you think the target will be reached first? Why?

Sources: U.S. Department of Health and Human Services (2000). *Healthy People 2010: Understanding and Improving Health,* 2nd ed. Washington, DC: U.S. Government Printing Office; Centers for Disease Control and Prevention (2004). "Data 2010." Available at http://wonder.cdc.gov/data2010/.

agriculture, construction, and transportation offer the best opportunity for improvement, and specific objectives have been proposed for these industries (see Box 18.4). When these data are separated into more specific job categories, the highest job-related death rates for blue-collar workers in 2005 were found among fishermen, loggers, and pilots[25] (see Figure 18.14 and Table 18.2).

In the early 1990s, there was extensive media coverage of work-related homicides at U.S. Postal Service facilities. The phrase "Don't go postal on me," meaning don't become crazy or violent, is still heard occasionally. However, an examination of the occupational injury death rates for postal workers in the 1980s revealed that workplace injury death rates for postal workers were approximately 2.5 times lower than those for all workers combined.[26] A more recent study found that "'going postal' is a myth and a bad rap," and that postal workers are only one-third as likely as those in the national workforce to be victims of homicide at work. Some occupations are significantly more dangerous. For example, taxi drivers are 150 times likelier than letter carriers to be victims of homicide at work (31.54 versus 0.21 per 100,000).[27]

Nonfatal Occupational Injuries and Illnesses by Industry
A total of 4.2 million injuries and illnesses were reported in private industry workplaces during 2005, resulting in a rate of 4.6 cases per 100 equivalent full-time workers.[6] Goods-producing industries had higher rates than service-producing industries. Among goods-producing industries, manufacturing had the highest incidence rate in 2005 (6.3 cases per 100 full-time workers). In the service-producing industries, transportation and warehousing has the highest incidence rate (7.0 cases per 1,000 full-time workers). All 2005 incidence rates showed declines from 1998 levels.[6]

FIGURE 18.14
Among the jobs with the highest fatality rates is logging.

Table 18.2
Top Ten Most Dangerous Jobs in 2005

Rank	Occupation	Death Rate/ 100,000	Total Deaths
1	Fishers and fishing workers	118.4	48
2	Logging workers	92.9	80
3	Aircraft pilots	66.9	81
4	Structural iron and steel workers	55.6	35
5	Refuse and recylable material collectors	43.8	32
6	Farmers and ranchers	41.1	341
7	Electrical power line installers/repairers	32.7	36
8	Driver/sales workers and truck drivers	29.1	993
9	Miscellaneous agricultural workers	23.2	176
10	Construction laborers	22.7	339

Agricultural Safety and Health

One particularly hazardous occupation is farming. Those working on farms are at considerable risk not just for injuries, but for lung diseases, noise-induced hearing loss, skin diseases, and certain cancers associated with chemical use and sun exposure. About 3 million people are involved in farm operations and, if unpaid farm workers and family members are counted, the number is much higher. In 2005, 178 farm-related deaths were reported.[5] In 2005, agriculture (including forestry, fishing, and hunting) ranked first among major U.S. industries for work-related, unintentional injury fatality rates (see Figure 18.13).[5]

A major contribution to farm-related fatalities is farm machinery, particularly farm tractors. For more than two out of five farm worker deaths, the source of the fatal injury was a tractor, and more than half of these deaths resulted from tractor rollovers. Rollover incidents are those in which the tractor tips sideways or backwards (especially when the tractor is improperly hitched), crushing the operator (see Figure 18.15). While all tractors manufactured since 1985 are fitted with seat belts and **rollover protective structures (ROPS),** many tractors in use in the United States lack this equipment. The effectiveness of ROPS in protecting the tractor operator was demonstrated by statistics collected in Nebraska, where only 1 (2%) of 61 per-

rollover protective structures (ROPS) factory-installed or retrofitted reinforced framework on a cab to protect the operator of a tractor in case of a rollover

FIGURE 18.15

The timing of events during rear rollovers of farm tractors.

Source: Centers for Disease Control and Prevention (1996). "Fatalities Associated with Improper Hitching to Farm Tractors—New York, 1991–1995." *MMWR,* 45(15): 307–311.

sons operating ROPS-equipped tractors that rolled over died. These data compare favorably with a 40% death rate for the 250 persons involved in unprotected tractor rollover incidents. The single fatality in the ROPS-equipped tractor was not wearing a seat belt and was ejected from the ROPS-protected area.[28]

A 1997 report confirmed that farm tractor rollovers continue to account for about 130 work-related deaths every year.[29] It was estimated that in 1993 only 38% of all tractors in the United States were equipped with ROPS. A survey found that the mean age of 63 tractors purchased by Iowa farmers in 1995 was 18 years and that only 40% had ROPS. The OSHA standard requiring ROPS be installed on all tractors is not actively enforced on farms with fewer than 11 employees, and family farms without other employees are exempt from OSHA regulations. NIOSH can promote ROPS use but has no authority to require their use.[29]

FIGURE 18.16

It is not unusual for farm boys under the age of 12 to be seen driving tractors.

Another concern about farming is that it is one of the few industries in which the families of workers are also exposed to many of the same risks. More than 1 million youths 0 to 19 years of age reside in farm operator households, while another 800,000 children and adolescents live in households headed by hired farm workers. It is not unusual for farm boys under the age of 12 to be seen driving tractors (see Figure 18.16). Each year about 100 children are killed and 100,000 children and adolescents are injured in agriculture-related activities.[30] Many of those injured belong to the migrant workforce, where children as young as 12, 10, 8, and even 4 years of age can be found working in the fields. Testimony before the U.S. Senate Committee on Labor and Human Resources by Fernando Cuevas, Jr., paints a grim picture of migrant children (see Box 18.5).[31]

Of our 50 states, 48 rely heavily on migrant workers during the peak harvest season. These migrant workers have poor access to health care facilities; infant mortality is about 50 per 1,000 compared with the national average of about 7.2 per 1,000. In many cases, working conditions are hazardous, and water shortages require workers to drink water from irrigation ditches. Not only is such water unpurified, it is usually laden with agricultural chemicals and biological wastes. Migrant workers are also exposed to long hours in the sun, other unsanitary conditions, and numerous harmful pesticides from crop-dusting airplanes.

BOX
18.5

COMMENTS OF A YOUNG FARM WORKER

"When I was younger it was all a game to me. But as I started getting older it became a job, and at the age of about 7 and 8, I was competing with my parents and my older sisters. . . . I was able to get out of the fields permanently at the age of 15 to try and get a decent education. I also became an organizer for the Farm Labor Organizing Committee at the age of 16, and I continue to see many, many young children working out in the fields at the same age that I was—4-, 5-, 6-, 7-, and 8-year-olds. They are still working out in the fields. I see it every year, up in Ohio, I see it down in Texas, I see it in Florida, I see it anywhere that we go and organize."

Source: Committee on Labor and Human Resources (August 12, 1992). *Childhood Labor Amendments* (report no. 102-230, to accompany Senate Bill 600). Washington, DC.

Prevention and Control of Unintentional Injuries in the Workplace

Reducing the number and seriousness of injuries and illnesses in the workplace involves four fundamental tasks: anticipation, recognition, evaluation, and control.[32] *Anticipation* involves the foresight to envision future adverse events and take action to prevent them. A hazard inventory should be conducted to detect and record physical, ergonomic, chemical, biological, and psychological hazards in the workplace. *Recognition* involves surveillance and monitoring of the workforce for injuries and illnesses, including near misses. It includes inspections of the workplace for hazards, monitoring it for toxins, recording injuries, and conducting employee health screenings. All of the aforementioned activities include data collection. *Evaluation* is the assessment of the data that were collected during the recognition and monitoring activities. This includes toxicological, exposure, and clinical assessment as well as risk assessment. Epidemiology is part of the evaluation process. Risk assessment enables the translation of scientific information about hazards into decisions and policies that can improve workplace safety and health. Upon establishing the need for intervention, a decision concerning *control* can be made. The control may involve changes in the production process to make it safer, changes in the work environment to make it safer, or improvements in the use of personal protective equipment or apparel to protect individual workers. Finally, the education and training of workers can help to reduce workplace injuries and illnesses.[32]

National leadership in reducing the number and seriousness of workplace injuries and illnesses resides with OHSA and NIOSH. In an effort to chart the future course for research on workplace safety and health problems, NIOSH has developed a partnership with more than 500 public and private outside organizations and individuals. In 2006 the National Occupational Research Agenda (NORA), a framework to guide occupational safety and health research into the twenty-first century, marked ten years of achievement. A review of past accomplishments under NORA and the agenda for the future are available online.[33]

Workplace Violence: Intentional Workplace Injuries

Although only a small number of the incidents of workplace violence that occur each day make the news, some 1.7 million Americans are victims of workplace violence each year.[34] Many of us have heard about a teacher who was attacked by a student, a female worker who was sexually assaulted in the parking lot, a woman shot in her place of work by an irate boyfriend, or a pizza delivery man killed for a few dollars. In 2005, 564 homicides occurred in the workplace, making homicide the fourth leading cause of workplace fatalities behind highway incidents, being struck by an object, and falls, and the second leading cause of workplace deaths among women.[5]

There are many reasons for workplace homicides and violence. Researchers have divided workplace violence into four categories:[34]

Criminal intent (Type I): The perpetrator has no legitimate relationship to the business or its employees and is usually committing a crime, such as robbery, shoplifting, and trespassing. This category makes up 85% of the work-related homicides.

Customer/Client (Type II): The perpetrator has a legitimate relationship with the business and becomes violent while being served. This category includes customers, clients, patients, students, and inmates. This category represents 3% of the work-related homicides.

Worker-on-worker (Type III): The perpetrator is an employee or past employee of the business who attacks or threatens another employee or past employee of the workplace. Worker-on-worker violence accounts for 7% of workplace homicides.

Personal relationship (Type IV): The perpetrator usually does not have a relationship with the business but has a personal relationship with the intended victim. This category, which includes victims of domestic violence assaulted or threatened at work, makes up just 2% of workplace homicides.

Data on nonfatal workplace violence are more difficult to obtain than data on workplace homicides. One estimate is that about 1.7 million people are victims of nonfatal workplace violence each year.[34] Assaults occur almost equally among men and women. Most of these assaults occur in service settings such as hospitals, nursing homes, and social service agencies. Forty-eight percent of nonfatal assaults in the workplace are committed by health care patients.[34]

Risk Factors

Risk factors for encountering violence at work are listed in Box 18.6. They include working with the public, working around money or valuables, working alone, and working late at night. Additionally, there are certain industries and occupations that put workers at particular risk. For workplace homicides, the taxicab industry has the highest risk at 41.4 per 100,000, nearly 60 times the national average rate of 0.70 per 100,000. Other jobs that carry a higher than average risk for homicide are jobs in liquor stores (7.5), detective and protective services (7.0), gas service stations (4.8), and jewelry stores (4.7). The workplaces that have the highest risk of nonfatal assault (and the highest percentage of all assaults that occurred) are nursing homes (27%), social services (13%), hospitals (11%), grocery stores (6%), and restaurants or bars (5%).[34]

Prevention Strategies

Prevention strategies for workplace violence can be grouped into three categories—environmental designs, administrative controls, and behavior strategies. Before these strategies can be implemented, a workplace violence prevention policy should be in place. Such a policy should clearly indicate a zero tolerance of violence at work. Just as workplaces have mechanisms for reporting and dealing with sexual harassment, they must also have a policy in place to deal with violence. Such a policy must spell out how such incidents are to be reported, to whom, and how they are to be addressed.

Environmental designs to limit the risk of workplace violence might include implementing safer cash handling procedures, physically separating workers from customers, improving lighting, and installing better security systems at entrances and exits. Administrative controls include staffing policies (having more staff is generally safer than having fewer staff), procedures for opening and closing the workplace, and reviewing employee duties (such as han-

---

BOX 18.6	FACTORS THAT INCREASE A WORKER'S RISK FOR WORKPLACE ASSAULT

- Contact with the public
- Exchange of money
- Delivery of passengers, goods, or services
- Having a mobile workplace such as a taxicab or police cruiser
- Working with unstable or volatile persons in health care, social services, or criminal justice settings
- Working alone or in small numbers

- Working late at night or during early morning hours
- Working in high-crime areas
- Guarding valuable property or possessions
- Working in community-based settings

dling money) that may be especially risky. Behavior strategies include training employees in nonviolent response and conflict resolution and educating employees about risks associated with specific duties and about the importance of reporting incidents and adhering to administrative controls. Training should also include instruction on the appropriate use and maintenance of any protective equipment that may be provided.[34]

Occupational Illnesses and Disorders

Precise data on the number of cases of occupational illnesses are more difficult to acquire than data on injuries. It is more difficult to link illnesses to occupational exposure. Some illnesses that can result from occupational exposure (e.g., tuberculosis, cancer, and asthma) appear no different from those that result from exposure elsewhere. Also, there is usually a lengthy period of time between exposure and the appearance of disease, unlike injuries, which are usually evident immediately. Reported cases of illnesses in the workplace in 2005 accounted for fewer than 6% of the 4.2 million injury and illness cases. In private industry, 242,500 new cases of occupational illness were reported. Hearing loss accounted for 11% of the occupational illnesses in 2005. (Hearing loss was not reported as a separate category before 2004.) The illnesses reported in the figures are only the cases reported during 2005. Some conditions, such as various cancers, are slow to develop and are difficult to associate with the workplace. These diseases and conditions are often unrecognized and underreported in annual reports of injuries and illnesses.[6]

Types of Occupational Illnesses

Occupational diseases can be categorized by cause and by the organ or organ system affected. For example, repeated trauma is the cause, and the musculoskeletal system is the affected organ system. Exposure to asbestos is a cause of illness; the respiratory system, especially the lung, is the system affected.

Musculoskeletal Disorders

Musculoskeletal disorders are the most frequently reported occupational disorders. They include both acute and chronic injury to muscles, tendons, ligaments, nerves, joints, bones, and supporting vasculature. The leading type of musculoskeletal disorder was repeated trauma disorders (216,400), which made up 65% of all cases of nonfatal occupational illness in 2001.[17] Included in this category are carpal tunnel syndrome and noise-induced hearing loss. The Bureau of Labor Statistics reported an increase in rates for repeated trauma disorders from 5.1 per 10,000 full-time workers in 1984 to 41.1 in 1994. The rate then declined each year through 2001, when the rate was 23.8 per 10,000.[17]

Skin Diseases and Disorders

A total of 38,900 cases of occupational skin disorders were reported in 2001, less than half the number reported in 1974. Reported skin disorders included allergic and irritant dermatitis, eczema, rash, oil acne, chrome ulcers, and chemical burns. The highest incidences of occupational skin disorders were reported in agriculture, foresty, and fishing.[17] The skin may serve as the target organ for disease, or it may be the route through which toxic chemicals enter the worker's body.

Noise-Induced Hearing Loss

Noise-induced hearing loss is another form of repeated trauma. Approximately 30 million Americans are exposed to hazardous noise on the job, and an additional 9 million are at risk for hearing loss from other agents such as solvents and metals. Cases include workers with a permanent noise-induced hearing loss or with a standard threshold shift. Most of the cases were reported within manufacturing; within the manufacturing sector, 51% of the cases were associated with manufacturing.[17]

Respiratory Disorders

Occupational respiratory disorders are the result of the inhalation of toxic substances present in the workplace. The lungs, like the skin, can be both the target organ of disease and a portal of entry for toxic substances. Characteristic of occupational lung diseases are their chronic nature and the difficulty in early recognition (the latent period for such diseases may be 15 to 30 years). Also, there is the problem of multiple or mixed exposures in the home and the workplace.

Work-related asthma (WRA) is the most commonly reported occupational respiratory disease, even though estimates suggest that most cases are not recognized or reported as being work related. There is no estimate on how many cases of WRA occur nationwide. The highest percentage of cases occur among operators, fabricators, and laborers.[17]

One of the most important categories of lung diseases is **pneumoconiosis,** a fibrotic lung disease caused by the inhalation of dusts, especially mineral dusts. During the period 1968 through 1999, a total of 121,982 pneumoconiosis deaths were reported in U.S. residents.[17]

Types of pneumoconioses include coal workers' pneumoconiosis, asbestosis, silicosis, and byssinosis. The largest number of pneumoconiosis deaths were from coal workers' pneumoconiosis (CWP). **Coal workers' pneumoconiosis** (also called *black lung disease*), is an acute or chronic lung disease that is caused by inhaling coal dust (see Figure 18.17). Historically, deaths from CWP clearly outnumber all other types of pneumoconiosis deaths. During the period from 1987 to 1996, CWP made up 54% of all pneumoconiosis deaths.[35] However, deaths from CWP have declined during the last 30 years, from a high of 2,870 in 1972 to 858 in 2002.[17,36] No effective medical treatment is available for pneumoconiosis; therefore, primary prevention is essential.

Asbestos workers suffer from diseases that include **asbestosis** (an acute or chronic lung disease), lung cancer, and mesothelioma (cancer of the epithelial linings of the heart and other internal organs). In contrast to CWP, asbestosis deaths have increased from 77 in 1968 to nearly 1,473 in 2002. It now accounts for 34% of pneumoconiosis deaths.[17,36]

Workers in mines, stone quarries, sand and gravel operations, foundries, abrasive blasting operations, and glass manufacturing run the risk of **silicosis** (sometimes referred to as dust on the lungs) that is caused from inhaling crystalline silica. Silicosis deaths represent nearly 6% of all pneumoconiosis deaths in the United States. Mortality from silicosis has significantly declined in recent years from 1,157 in 1968 to 148 in 2002.[17,36]

Textile factory workers who inhale dusts from cotton, flax, or hemp often acquire **byssinosis** (sometimes called *brown lung disease*), an acute or chronic lung disease. In comparison with the other types of pneumoconiosis, byssinosis deaths are uncommon—10 or fewer cases were reported annually between 1996 and 2002.[36]

Other agents that can affect the lungs include metallic dusts, gases and fumes, and aerosols of biological agents (viruses, bacteria, and fungi). Health conditions that can result from exposure to these agents include occupational asthma, asphyxiation, pulmonary edema, histoplasmosis, and lung cancer.

Other Work-Related Diseases and Disorders

Other types of work-related illnesses and disorders are those that arise from poisonings and infections. Poisonings represented 1% of all nonfatal occupational illness cases in the **Survey of Occupational Injuries and Illnesses (SOII)** in 1997. Poisoning agents include heavy metals (including lead), toxic gases, organic solvents, pesticides, and other substances. Pesticides, when used properly, offer benefits to society, increasing crop production, preserving produce, and combating insect infestations. However, pesticides do represent a health risk, especially for agricultural workers. Approximately one billion pounds of pesticide active ingredients are used annually in the United States, where 16,000 separate pesticide products are

pneumoconiosis fibrotic lung disease caused by the inhalation of dusts, especially mineral dusts

coal workers' pneumoconiosis (CWP) acute and chronic lung disease caused by the inhalation of coal dust (black lung disease)

asbestosis acute or chronic lung disease caused by the deposition of asbestos fibers on lungs

silicosis acute or chronic lung disease caused by the inhalation of free crystalline silica

byssinosis acute or chronic lung disease caused by the inhalation of cotton, flax, or hemp dusts (brown lung disease)

Survey of Occupational Injuries and Illnesses (SOII) an annual survey of injuries and illnesses from a large sample of U.S. employers (approximately 250,000) maintained by the Bureau of Labor Statistics in the Department of Labor

FIGURE 18.17

Mining is a dangerous occupation due to exposure to both injuries and disease.

marketed. Each year, 10,000 to 20,000 physician-diagnosed pesticide poisonings occur among the approximately 3,380,000 agricultural workers.[37] During 1998–1999, 1,009 cases of acute pesticide-related occupational illness and three deaths were identified in just seven states: Arizona, California, Florida, Louisiana, New York, Oregon, and Texas. Among agricultural workers, the incidence rate was 18.2 cases per 100,000. The vast majority of these cases (72%) occurred in farm workers. Insecticides were responsible for the highest percentage of the poisoning cases (49%).[17]

In 2005, 14.5 million people were employed by hospitals or in the health care industry in the United States, making up 10.2% of the employed workforce.[2] More than 8 million of these workers are exposed to a variety of hazardous conditions, including infectious disease agents. Among the agents of concern are hepatitis B virus and human immunodeficiency virus (HIV). Health care workers are at risk if they become exposed to the blood or bodily fluids of patients or co-workers. The major route of exposure to these agents (82% of the cases) is percutaneous exposure (injuries through the skin) via contaminated sharp instruments such as needles and scalpels (see Figure 18.18). Exposure also occurs through contact with the mucous membranes of the eyes, nose, or mouth (14%), exposure to broken or abraded skin (3%), and through human bites (1%). Up to 800,000 percutaneous injuries occur annually, with an average risk of infection for HIV of 0.3% (3 per 1,000) and for hepatitis B of from 6% to 30%.[17] Health care workers are also at increased risk for acquiring other infectious diseases such as tuberculosis (TB); cases of TB in health care workers constitute about 3% of all TB cases.[35]

Another risk in health care settings is occupational exposure to antineoplastic drugs (drugs used in cancer treatment) and other hazardous drugs. Exposure to these substances can cause skin rashes, infertility, miscarriage, birth defects, and possibly leukemia or other cancers.[38] Exposure can occur while crushing tablets, reconstituting powdered drugs, expelling air from syringes filled with hazardous drugs, administering these drugs, or handling contaminated clothing, dressings, or body fluids. Currently, no statistics are available on the incidence of diseases and disorders resulting from these exposures, but NIOSH has issued an alert and guidelines for preventing exposure.[38]

FIGURE 18.18

Health care workers are exposed to a variety of workplace hazards, including infectious diseases.

In 2001, more than 5,000 cases of anxiety, stress, or neurotic disorders with time away from work were reported in the SOII. This is about 0.6 cases per 10,000 workers. Half of these cases required 25 or more days away from work, and women constituted 65% of the cases.[17] The exposures most frequently associated with anxiety, stress, or neurotic disorders were "harmful substances (30%) and assaults or violent acts (13%)."[35]

As stated previously, there are any number of health problems that, while prevalent and serious, could be the result of dual or multiple exposures (workplace and home). Among these are cardiovascular diseases, cancers, and reproductive disorders. Perhaps a million or more workers are exposed to agents that can produce cancer, for example. However, there are no reliable estimates on the actual number of cancer deaths that can be traced directly to occupational exposure. Thus, we have discussed here only conditions generally accepted to be solely or predominantly related to work.

Prevention and Control of Occupational Diseases and Disorders

Preventing and controlling occupational diseases requires the vigilance of employer and employee alike and the assistance of governmental agencies. The agent-host-environment disease model discussed earlier in this book is applicable to preventive strategies outlined here. Specific activities that should be employed to control occupational diseases include identification and evaluation of agents, standard setting for the handling of and exposure to causative agents, elimination or substitution of causative factors, engineering controls to provide for a safer work area, environmental monitoring, medical screenings, personal protective devices, health promotion, disease surveillance, therapeutic medical care and rehabilitation, and compliance activities.[39] In this regard, prevention and control of occupational diseases and disorders is similar to the prevention of occupational injuries.[32] Coordinated programs to monitor and reduce occupational hazards require professionally trained personnel. In a well-functioning program, these professionals work together as members of the occupational health and safety team.

RESOURCES FOR THE PREVENTION OF WORKPLACE INJURIES AND DISEASES

Community resources for the prevention of injuries and diseases attributable to the workplace include a variety of professional personnel and programs.

Occupational Safety and Health Professionals

The need for health professionals in the workplace is substantial. Among those with specialized training in their fields are safety engineers and certified safety professionals, health physicists, industrial hygienists, occupational physicians, and occupational health nurses.

Safety Engineers and Certified Safety Professionals

Approximately 400 academic institutions offer accredited programs that train occupational safety professionals. Many of these professionals will join the professional organization called the American Society of Safety Engineers (ASSE). "Founded in 1911, ASSE is the oldest and largest professional safety organization."[40] It has about 30,000 members who are involved in safety, health, and environmental issues in industry, insurance, government, and education. In spite of the name of this society, not all members are engineers. In fact, the background of the group is varied and includes a number of health educators.

Another recognizable group of trained professionals in this field is the Board of Certified Safety Professionals (BCSPs). This group is somewhat smaller; there are about 10,000 CSPs. "The Board of Certified Safety Professionals (BCSP) was organized as a peer certification board with the purpose of certifying practitioners in the safety profession."[41] Certification usually requires a bachelor's degree in engineering or in another scientific curriculum and the passing of two examinations.

Safety engineers and **certified safety professionals (CSPs)** design safety education programs, detect hazards in the workplace, and try to correct them (see Figure 18.19). Increased federal regulations have made the workload heavier for these occupational health professionals.

Health Physicists

Health physicists are concerned with radiation safety in the workplace. They monitor radiation within the work environment and develop plans for decontamination and coping with accidents involving radiation. It is estimated that there are approximately 11,000 health physicists in the United States. Many of these belong to the Health Physics Society, a 6,000-member,

safety engineer a safety professional employed by a company for the purpose of reducing unintentional injuries in the workplace

certified safety professional (CSP) a health and safety professional, trained in industrial and workplace safety, who has met specific requirements for board certification

health physicists safety professionals with responsibility for developing plans for coping with radiation accidents

FIGURE 18.19
Safety engineers prevent workplace injuries by detecting hazards.

industrial hygienists
health professionals concerned with health hazards in the workplace and with recommending plans for improving the healthiness of workplace environments

occupational physician (OP) or occupational medical practitioner (OMP)
a physician whose primary concern is preventive medicine in the workplace

occupational health nurse (OHN)
a registered nurse (RN) whose primary responsibilities include prevention of illness and promotion of health in the workplace

international scientific organization of professionals who are dedicated to promoting the practice of radiation safety.[42] An important certifying body of health physicists is the American Academy of Health Physics.[43]

Industrial Hygienists

Whereas the safety engineer or certified safety professional is primarily concerned with hazards in the workplace and injury control, the **industrial hygienist** is concerned with environmental factors that might cause illness. Examples of such factors might include poor ventilation, excessive noise, poor lighting, and the presence of hazardous substances.

It is estimated that there are 7,600 industrial hygienists practicing in the United States. Perhaps a third of them hold the title of Certified Industrial Hygienist (CIH), and many belong to the American Industrial Hygiene Association. To be certified requires a two-part written examination; the first part is given following one year of post-baccalaureate experience. The second is given after five years of professional activity. Many industrial hygienists belong to the American Conference of Governmental Industrial Hygienists (ACGIH). This 5,000-member organization advances worker health and safety through education and the development and dissemination of scientific and technical knowledge through their publications.[44]

Occupational Physicians

The **occupational physician (OP)** or **occupational medical practitioner (OMP)** is a medical practitioner whose primary concern is preventive medicine in the workplace. Many OPs or OMPs belong to the American College of Occupational and Environmental Medicine (ACOEM), which represents more than 6,000 physicians specializing in the field of occupational and environmental medicine (OEM). "The American Board of Preventive Medicine (ABPM) recognizes and certifies qualified physicians in the medical specialty of occupational medicine. Approximately 2,200 physicians have been 'board certified' in occupational medicine within the United States."[45]

Because physicians are highly skilled and highly salaried occupational health professionals, only the largest companies maintain full-time OPs. Smaller companies may hire OPs on a part-time basis or as consultants.

Occupational Health Nurses

The role of the **occupational health nurse (OHN)** has changed over the years from running the company's medical department and first aid station to one of greater emphasis on health promotion and illness prevention. Because the OHN may be the only health professional employed in smaller plants, it is clear that if injury prevention and health promotion programs are to be offered, the job will fall to this individual.

The OHN must be a registered nurse (RN) in the state in which he or she practices. It is unlikely that these persons will have had much formal training in occupational health nursing prior to receiving their baccalaureate degrees because most nursing curricula do not provide much training in this area. However, the American Board of Occupational Health Nurses, Inc., established in 1972, now offers certifications. Requirements include many hours of continuing-education credits and five years' experience in the field of occupational health nursing. ABOHN is the only certifying body for occupational health nurses in the United States. More than 8,500 occupational health nurses have been certified by ABOHN.[46] Many

OHNs belong to the American Association of Occupational Health Nurses (AAOHN), which was founded in 1942 and includes about 10,000 members.[47]

Occupational Safety and Health Programs

There are a number of programs that can be put in place in occupational settings to reduce injuries and diseases. These include preplacement examinations, health maintenance programs, safety awareness programs, health promotion programs, investigation of accidents, stress management programs, employee assistance programs, and rehabilitation programs.

Preplacement Examinations

The purpose of **preplacement examinations** is to make sure that the worker fits the job. By selecting the employee who is the best physically and mentally qualified for a specific job, probabilities of job-related injuries or illnesses are minimized. Periodic evaluations are necessary to ensure that the selected individual continues to be physically and mentally qualified to carry out the job assignment. Examinations are also recommended for transferred and return-to-work employees. Sometimes a phasing in of these employees is desirable.

Occupational Disease Prevention Programs and Safety Programs

Occupational health services that facilitate preventive activities in the workplace include disease prevention programs and safety programs.

Disease Prevention Programs

Originally, occupational disease programs focused on controlling occupational diseases that one might succumb to from exposure in the work environment. Agents of concern were chemicals, radiation, and perhaps even psychological and social factors that could lead to sickness or disability. Gradually, these disease prevention efforts broadened into health maintenance programs and included the early detection and treatment of such diseases as hypertension, diabetes, obesity, and heart disease in order to keep employees healthier and on the job longer.

Safety Programs

Safety programs are those portions of the workplace health and safety program aimed at reducing the number and seriousness of unintentional injuries on the job. Each company needs to have a policy statement, safe operating procedures, a disaster plan, policies for hazard control, and policies for the investigation of injuries in the workplace. Provisions must be made for regular safety inspections of the workplace and for the maintenance of accurate records for each injury and for analysis of such records. Each safety program should include safety orientation and training programs and programs on first aid and cardiopulmonary resuscitation.

Worksite Health Promotion Programs

Worksite health promotion (WHP) programs are workplace-based programs aimed at improving the health of employees through changes in behavior and lifestyle. The goals for the employer include reduction of absenteeism, lowering health insurance premiums, increasing productivity, and improving employee morale. Other reasons why employers might support WHP programs include reducing workers' compensation costs, increasing employee retention, and enhancing the company's image.[48]

In the United States, historically, health care insurance has come through one's employment. In 1965, the employers' share of the nation's health care bill was 18%; in 2006, it was 40%. In some companies the cost of providing health care for employees is equal to about 50% of the companies' profits.[48] Obviously, this upward trend in the cost of health care for employers cannot continue much longer. Until this system changes, however, employers are making serious efforts to reduce health care costs, and one effective way to do this is worksite health promotion.

---

preplacement examination a physical examination of a newly hired or transferred worker to determine medical suitability for placement in a specific position

safety programs those parts of the workplace safety and health program aimed at reducing unintentional injuries on the job

worksite health promotion (WHP) programs health promotion programs in the workplace that include health education, screening, and/or intervention designed to change employees' health behavior and reduce risks associated with disease or injury

Health promotion programs range in size from very modest programs that might include only hypertension screening to more comprehensive programs that offer cancer risk screening, nutrition and weight management, fitness, smoking cessation, stress management programs, and more. Generally, the objectives of these programs are to facilitate changes in behavior or lifestyle in order to prevent disease and to promote health.[48]

All indications are that WHP programs will continue to grow. Corporations not only see them as a means to control health care costs and show a concern for the employees, but also as a means by which to recruit new employees and to retain the ones currently in the organization. (See Chapter 5 for more information on health promotion programs.)

Employee Assistance Programs

employee assistance programs (EAPs) workplace-based programs that assist employees who have substance abuse, domestic, psychological, or social problems that interfere with their work performance

Employee assistance programs (EAPs) are programs that assist employees who have substance abuse, domestic, psychological, or social problems that interfere with their work performance. These programs, which arrived at many workplaces before WHP programs, originally arose in response to occupational alcohol problems. EAPs provide help to employees with a variety of problems that affect their work performance. Whereas WHP programs are primary prevention efforts, EAPs are secondary prevention or tertiary prevention efforts. They have as their goal the intervention and sometimes rehabilitation of employees with behavioral or other problems before such problems become costly for both the employer and employee.

CHAPTER SUMMARY

- After time spent at home, Americans spend the next largest portion of their time at work; thus, safe and healthy workplaces are essential if America is to reach its health potential.

- Every day approximately 16 people die from work-related injuries and many more people die of work-related diseases.

- Occupational health issues affect the quality of life economically as well as medically in communities in which workers live. Although occupational injuries and illnesses have been a long-standing concern of workers in America, rapid progress in reducing the number and seriousness of workplace injuries and illnesses became possible only after the passage of the Occupational Safety and Health Act (OSHAct) of 1970.

- The OSHAct established the Occupational Safety and Health Administration (OSHA) and the National Institute of Occupational Safety and Health (NIOSH) and required private industry to provide safe jobs and workplaces.

- The number and type of workplace injuries vary by person, place, time, and type of industry. Highway injuries are the leading cause of fatal work-related injuries. Falls and being struck by an object or equipment are the second and third leading causes of workplace deaths.

- Nonfatal work-related injuries cost both employees and employers in terms of lost wages and lost productivity.

- Workplace violence affects 1.7 million workers in the United States each year, and homicide is the fourth leading cause of workplace fatalities.

- Work-related injuries can be controlled by applying a variety of injury prevention strategies, including eliminating a dangerous job, changing the work environment, using safer machinery, and improving the selection and training of workers.

- Work-related illnesses and disorders kill thousands of workers and former workers each year.

- The types of illnesses and disorders that can be attributed to workplace exposure are many, including musculoskeletal conditions, dermatological conditions, lung diseases, and cancers, among many others.

- Repeated trauma is the leading cause of work-related nonfatal illnesses.

- There are numerous resources to aid in the prevention of occupational injuries and diseases, including occupational health professionals and workplace injury and illness prevention programs and worksite health promotion programs.

REVIEW QUESTIONS

1. Provide definitions of the terms *occupational injury* and *occupational disease* and give three examples of each.

2. In what ways are health problems in the workplace related to health problems in the general community?

3. How did the Industrial Revolution contribute to an increase in occupational health problems?

4. Who was Alice Hamilton? What did she do?

5. What were the deficiencies in state occupational safety and health laws in the early 1960s?

6. Discuss briefly the purpose of the Occupational Safety and Health Act of 1970 and outline its provisions.

7. What is OSHA and what does it do? What is NIOSH and what does it do?

8. What are some of the most frequently reported workplace injuries? Which are the leading causes of workplace injury deaths?

9. Which age group and gender of workers suffer the most occupational injuries? Which have the most fatal injuries?

10. Why is farming a particularly hazardous occupation? What are ROPS and how do they prevent deaths?

11. What are the risk factors for encountering violence in the workplace? Which occupation is at greatest risk for workplace homicides?

12. Outline some general control strategies that can reduce the number and seriousness of workplace injuries.

13. What is the most frequently reported occupational disorder?

14. What determines whether a musculoskeletal condition or skin condition should be considered an injury or a disease?

15. List four well-documented lung conditions that are related to occupational exposure. Name the occupations whose workers are at high risk for each of these conditions.

16. Why is it often difficult to prove that a disease or condition resulted from workplace exposure?

17. Outline some features of a workplace program to prevent or control occupational diseases. For each activity, indicate whether it is aimed at the agent, host, or environment aspect of the disease model.

18. List five health occupations that deal with worker safety and health. Describe their training and job assignments.

19. Name and describe four occupational safety and health programs.

20. What are some of the benefits of worksite health promotion programs for employers and employees?

ACTIVITIES

1. Examine your local newspaper every day for a week for articles dealing with occupational injury or illness. Find three articles and, after reading them, provide the following: A brief summary, the resulting injury or disease, the cause of the injury or disease, and a brief plan for how the organization could eliminate the cause.

2. Interview an individual who works in the profession you wish to enter after graduation. Ask him or her to describe what he or she feels are the most prevalent injuries and illnesses connected with his or her job. Also ask about specific preservice and in-service education the interviewee has had to protect against these problems. Finally, ask him or her to propose measures to limit future problems. Summarize your interview on paper in a two-page report.

3. If you have ever become injured or ill as a result of a job, explain what happened to you. In a two-page paper, identify the causative agent, how the injury could have been prevented, and what kind of training you had to prepare you for a safe working environment.

SCENARIO: ANALYSIS AND RESPONSE

Please take a moment to reread the scenario at the beginning of this chapter. Then reflect on the questions that follow.

1. If you were Jen, what would you do?

2. In 1998, California passed legislation protecting waitresses like Jen and bartenders by outlawing smoking in not only restaurants but also in bars. Do you support such legislation? How likely is it that your state legislature would pass a similar law?

3. Ambient smoke in a restaurant or bar is an example of situations that occur daily in the workplace.

Suppose you suspected that you were being exposed to a toxic agent where you worked. What would you do? Who would you contact? How could OSHA be of assistance?

4. Think about some of the jobs held by your fellow classmates. Do any of those jobs expose them to hazardous substances? Do any of the jobs students have put them at risk for injuries?

4. Go to the school library and research the injuries and diseases connected with your future profession. In a two-page paper, identify the major problems and what employers and employees should do about them and express concerns that you have about working in the profession due to these problems.

5. Visit any job site related to your future profession. At that site, find 10 things that employers and employees are doing to make it a safe work environment. List these 10 things briefly and explain the benefit of each one.

Community Health on the Web

The Internet contains a wealth of information about community and public health. Increase your knowledge of some of the topics presented in this chapter by accessing the Jones and Bartlett Publishers Web site at **http://health.jbpub .com/book/communityhealth/6e** and follow the links to complete the following Web activities.

- National Institute for Occupational Safety and Health
- Occupational Safety and Health Administration
- American Industrial Hygiene Association

References

1. International Labour Organization (2006). *World Day for Safety and Health at Work 2005: A Background Paper*. Geneva, Switzerland: Author. Available at http://www.ilo.org/public/english/bureau/inf/download/sh_background.pdf.

2. U.S. Bureau of the Census (2003). *Statistical Abstract of the United States—2003. The National Data Book*, 123rd ed. Available at http://www.census.gov/prod/www/statistical-abstract.html.

3. U.S. Department of Labor, Bureau of Labor Statistics. "BLS Glossary." Available at http://www.bls.gov/bls/glossary.htm.

4. National Safety Council (2006). *Injury Facts, 2005-2006 Edition*. Itasca, IL: Author.

5. U.S. Department of Labor, Bureau of Labor Statistics (2006). *National Census of Fatal Occupational Injuries in 2005*. Available at http://www.bls.gov/news.release/pdf/cfoi.pdf.

6. U.S. Department of Labor, Bureau of Labor Statistics (2006). *Workplace Injuries and Illnesses in 2005*. Available at http://www.bls.gov/iif/oshwc/osh/os/osnr0025.pdf.

7. National Institute for Occupational Safety and Health (2000). *Performance Highlights of the National Institute for Occupational Safety and Health* (HHS [NIOSH] pub. no. 2000-134). Cincinnati, OH: NIOSH Publications.

8. Health and Safety Executive (United Kingdom) (2006). "European Comparisons—Fatal Injuries." Available at http://www.hse.gov.uk/statistics/european/fatal.htm.

9. Felton, J. S. (1986). "History of Occupational Health and Safety." In J. LaDou, ed., *Introduction to Occupational Health and Safety*. Chicago: National Safety Council.

10. Rosen, G. (1958). *A History of Public Health*. New York: M.D. Publications.

11. LaDou, J., J. Olishifski, and C. Zenz (1986). "Occupational Health and Safety Today." In J. LaDou, ed., *Introduction to Occupational Health and Safety*. Chicago: National Safety Council.

12. Schilling, R. S. F. (1989). "Developments in Occupational Health." In H. A. Waldron, ed., *Occupational Health Practice*. Boston: Butterworths.

13. Ashford, N. A. (1976). *Crisis in the Workplace: Occupational Disease and Injury—A Report to the Ford Foundation*. Cambridge, MA: MIT Press.

14. Page, J. A., and M. W. O'Brien (1973). *Bitter Wages*. New York: Grossman.

15. U.S. Department of Labor, Bureau of Labor Statistics (2003). *Workplace Injuries and Illnesses in 2002*. Available at http://www.b9ls.gov/iif/home.htm.

16. Centers for Disease Control and Prevention (2006). "Nonfatal Occupational Injuries and Illnesses among Workers Treated in Hospital Emergency Departments—United States, 2003." *MMWR*, 55(16): 449-452.

17. U.S. Department of Health and Human Services, Centers for Disease Control and Prevention, National Institute for Occupational Safety and Health (2004). *Worker Health Chartbook, 2004* (HHS [NIOSH] pub. no. 2004-146). Cincinnati, OH: NIOSH Publications.

18. National Consumers' League (2003). "American Working Teens Fact Sheet." Available at http://nclnet.org/.

19. Child Labor Coalition (2005). "2004 Child Labor State Survey." Available at http://www.stopchildlabor.org/USchildlabor/2004_survey_results.htm.

20. U.S. Department of Health and Human Services, Centers for Disease Control and Prevention, National Institute for Occupational Safety and Health (2003). *NIOSH Alert: Preventing Deaths, Injuries, and Illnesses of Young Workers* (HHS [NIOSH] pub. no. 2003-128). Cincinnati, OH: NIOSH Publications. Available at http://www.cdc.gov/niosh/topics/youth/.

21. U.S. Department of Labor, Bureau of Labor Statistics (2007). *The Employment Situation: December 2006*. Available at http://www.bls.gov/news.release/pdf/empsit.pdf.

22. U.S. Department of Labor, Bureau of Labor Statistics (2006). "Employment and Fatality Profiles by Gender of Worker, 2005." In *Census of Fatal Occupational Injuries Charts, 1992-2005*. Available at http://www.bls.gov/iif/oshcfoi1.htm#charts.

23. Wagener, D. K., J. Walstedt, L. Jenkins, et al. (1997). *Women: Work and Health* (HHS pub. no. PHS 97-1415). Hyattsville, MD: National Center for Health Statistics.

24. Centers for Disease Control and Prevention (2001). "Fatal Occupational Injuries—United States, 1980-97." *MMWR*, 50(16): 317-320.

25. Christie, L. (17 August 2006). "America's Most Dangerous Jobs." CNNMoney.com. Available at http://money.cnn.com/2006/08/16/pf/2005_most_dangerous_jobs/index.htm.

26. Centers for Disease Control and Prevention (1994). "Occupational Injury Deaths of Postal Workers—United States, 1980-1989." *MMWR*, 43(32): 587-595.

27. The National Center on Addiction and Substance Abuse at Columbia University (2000). *The United States Postal Service Commission on a Safe and Secure Workplace*. New York: Author.

28. Centers for Disease Control and Prevention (1993). "Public Health Focus: Effectiveness of Rollover Protective Structures for Preventing Injuries Associated with Agricultural Tractors." *MMWR*, 42(3): 57-59.

29. Centers for Disease Control and Prevention (1997). "Use of Rollover Protective Structures—Iowa, Kentucky, New York, and Ohio, 1992-1997." *MMWR*, 46(36): 842-845.

30. U.S. Department of Health and Human Services, Centers for Disease Control and Prevention, National Institute for Occupational Safety and Health. "Injuries among Youth on Farms, 2001." Available at http://www.cdc.gov/niosh/docs/2004-172/pdfs/2004-172.pdf.

31. Novello, A. C. (1991). "A Charge to the Conference." Presented at the Surgeon General's Conference on Agricultural Safety and Health: Farm Safe 2000, Des Moines, IA.

32. Weeks, J. L., G. R. Wagner, K. M. Rest, and B. S. Levy (2005). "A Public Health Approach to Preventing Occupational Diseases and

Injuries" In B. S. Levy, G. R. Wagner, K. M. Rest, and J. L. Weeks, eds., *Preventing Occupational Disease and Injury*, 2nd ed. Washington, DC: American Public Health Association.

33. Centers for Disease Control and Prevention, National Institute of Occupational Safety and Health (2006). "The National Occupational Research Agenda (NORA)." Available at http://www.cdc.gov/niosh/nora/default.html.

34. Centers for Disease Control and Prevention, National Institute for Occupational Safety and Health (2004). *Violence on the Job* (NIOSH pub. no. 2004-100d). Available at http://www.cdc.gov/niosh/docs/video/violence.html.

35. National Institute for Occupational Safety and Health (2000). *Worker Health Chartbook, 2000* (HHS [NIOSH] pub. no. 2000-127). Cincinnati, OH: NIOSH Publications.

36. Centers for Disease Control and Prevention, National Institute for Occupational Safety and Health (2005). "Work-related Lung Disease (WoRLD) Surveillance System: December 2005 Updated Tables and Figures." Available at http://www2a.cdc.gov/drds/WorldReportData/.

37. Centers for Disease Control and Prevention, National Institute for Occupational Safety and Health (2005). "NIOSH Topic: Pesticide Illness and Injury Surveillance." Available at http://www.cdc.gov/niosh/topics/pesticides/.

38. Centers for Disease Control and Prevention, National Institute for Occupational Safety and Health (2004). *NIOSH Alert: Preventing Occupational Exposures to Antineoplastic and Other Hazardous Drugs in Health Care Settings* (HHS [NIOSH] pub. no. 2004-165). Cincinnati, OH: Author.

39. National Institute for Occupational Safety and Health (1986). *Proposed National Strategies for the Prevention of Leading Work-Related Diseases and Injury: Lung Diseases*. Cincinnati, OH: NIOSH Publications.

40. American Society of Safety Engineers (2007). Information on this organization is available at http://www.asse.org.

41. Board of Certified Safety Professionals (2007). Information on this organization is available at http://www.bcsp.org.

42. Health Physics Society (2007). Information on this organization is available at http://www.hps.org.

43. American Academy of Health Physics (2007). Information on this organization is available at http://www.hps1.org/aahp.

44. American Conference of Governmental Industrial Hygienists (2007). Information on this organization is available at http://www.acgih.org.

45. American College of Occupational and Environmental Medicine (2007). Information on this organization is available at http://www.acoem.org/home.htm.

46. American Board for Occupational Health Nurses, Inc. (2007). Information on this organization is available at http://www.abohn.org.

47. American Association of Occupational Health Nurses, Inc. (2007). Information on this organization is available at http://www.aaohn.org.

48. Chenoweth, D. H. (2007). *Worksite Health Promotion*, 2nd ed. Champaign, IL: Human Kinetics.

Appendix I

Case/Control Studies: How to Calculate an Odds Ratio

Let us assume that you selected 100 lung cancer cases and 1,000 controls of the same age, sex, and socioeconomic status as the cases. Suppose 90 of 100 cases of lung cancer had been regular smokers, but only 270 of 1,000 controls smoked. An odds ratio could be calculated by the formula $(A \times D) \div (B \times C)$, where cases and controls are designated as follows:

		Disease Present	
		Yes	No
Risk Factor Present	Yes	A	B
	No	C	D

In our example:

		Disease Present	
		Yes	No
Risk Factor Present	Yes	90	270
	No	10	730

Substituting our data into the formula:

$[(90 \times 730) \div (270 \times 10)] = 65,700 \div 2,700 = 24.33$. Thus, lung cancer victims have 24.33 times greater probability of having been a smoker.

COHORT STUDIES: HOW TO CALCULATE RELATIVE AND ATTRIBUTABLE RISK

Let us assume that in a cohort of 4,000 there were 1,000 smokers and 3,000 nonsmokers. If, after 20 years, cancer develops in 22 smokers (22 per 1,000) and in 6 nonsmokers (6 per 3,000 or 2 per 1,000), *relative risk* is the ratio of the incidence rates, 22 per thousand: 2 per thousand or 22:2 or 11 to 1.

Further, one can calculate an *attributable risk* by subtracting the deaths in the non-smoking group (2 deaths) from the number of lung cancer deaths in the smoking group (22 deaths). Thus, 20 deaths are attributable to smoking; the attributable risk is 20 per 1,000.

Appendix 2

Operational Definitions for the 1990 Census

American Indian, Eskimo, or Aleut Includes persons who classified themselves as such in one of the specific race categories identified below.

American Indian Includes persons who indicated their race as "American Indian," entered the name of an Indian tribe, or reported such entries as Canadian Indian, French-American Indian, or Spanish-American Indian.

Eskimo Includes persons who indicated their race as "Eskimo" or reported entries such as Arctic Slope, Inupiat, and Yupik.

Aleut Includes persons who indicated their race as "Aleut" or reported entries such as Alutiiq, Egegik, and Pribilovian.

Asian or Pacific Islander Includes persons who reported in one of the Asian or Pacific Islander groups listed on the questionnaire or who provided write-in responses such as Thai, Nepaili, or Tongan.

Asian Includes "Chinese," "Filipino," "Japanese," "Asian Indian," "Korean," "Vietnamese," and "Other Asian."

Chinese Includes persons who indicated their race as "Chinese" or who identified themselves as Cantonese, Tibetan, or Chinese American. In standard census reports, persons who reported as "Taiwanese" or "Formosan" are included here with Chinese. In special reports on the Asian or Pacific Islander population, information on persons who identified themselves as Taiwanese are shown separately.

Filipino Includes persons who indicated their race as "Filipino" or reported entries such as Philipino, Philipine, or Filipino-American.

Japanese Includes persons who indicated their race as "Japanese" and persons who identified themselves as Nipponese or Japanese-American.

Asian Indian Includes persons who indicated their race as "Asian Indian" and persons who identified themselves as Bengalese, Bharat, Dravidian, East Indian, or Goanese.

Korean Includes persons who indicated their race as "Korean" and persons who identified themselves as Korean-American.

Vietnamese Includes persons who indicated their race as "Vietnamese" and persons who identified themselves as Vietnamese-American.

Cambodian Includes persons who provided a write-in response such as Cambodian or Cambodia.

Hmong Includes persons who provided a write-in response such as Hmong, Laohmong, or Mong.

Laotian Includes persons who provided a write-in response such as Laotian, Laos, or Lao.

Thai Includes persons who provided a write-in response such as Thai, Thailand, or Siamese.

Other Asian Includes persons who provided a write-in response of Bangladeshi, Burmese, Indonesian, Pakistani, Sri Lankan, Amerasian, or Eurasian.

Pacific Islander Includes persons who indicated their race as "Pacific Islander" by classifying themselves into one of the following race categories or identifying themselves as one of the Pacific Islander cultural groups of Polynesian, Micronesian, or Melanesian.

Hawaiian Includes persons who indicated their race as "Hawaiian" as well as persons who identified themselves as Part Hawaiian or Native Hawaiian.

Samoan Includes persons who indicated their race as "Samoan" or persons who identified themselves as American-Samoan or Western Samoan.

Guamanian   Includes persons who indicated their race as "Guamanian" or persons who identified themselves as Chamorro or Guam.

Other Pacific Islander   Includes persons who provided a write-in response of a Pacific Islander group such as Tahitian, Northern Mariana Islander, Palauan, Fijiian, or a cultural group such as Polynesian, Micronesian, or Melanesian.

Black   Includes persons who indicated their race as "black or Negro" or reported entries such as African-American, Afro-American, black Puerto Rican, Jamaican, Nigerian, West Indian, or Haitian.

White   Includes persons who indicated their race as "white" or reported entries such as Canadian, German, Italian, Lebanese, Near Easterner, Arab, or Polish.

Other race   Includes all other persons not included in "white," "black," "American Indian, Eskimo, or Aleut," and "Asian or Pacific Islander" race categories described above. Persons reporting in the "Other race" category and providing write-in entries such as multiracial, multiethnic, mixed, interracial, Wesort, or a Spanish/Hispanic origin group (such as Mexican, Cuban, or Puerto Rican) are included here.

Hispanic origin   Of Hispanic origin are those who classified themselves in one of the specific Hispanic origin categories listed on the questionnaire—"Mexican," "Puerto Rican," or "Cuban"—as well as those who indicated that they were of "other Spanish/Hispanic" origin. Persons of "Other Spanish/Hispanic" origin are those whose origins are from Spain, the Spanish-speaking countries of Central or South America or the Dominican Republic, or they are persons of Hispanic origin identifying themselves generally as Spanish, Spanish-American, Hispanic, Hispano, Latino, and so on.

Note: These definitions were taken directly from U.S. Dept. of Commerce (1990). *Census of Population and Housing, Summary Population and Housing, Characteristics, United States.* Washington, DC: U.S. Government Printing Office.

Appendix 3

Revised Operational Definitions for 1997*

American Indian or Alaska Native A person having origins in any of the original peoples of North and South American (including Central America), and who maintains tribal affiliation or community attachment.

"Alaska Native" should replace the term "Alaskan Native."

Alaska Native should be used instead of Eskimo and Aleut.

Asian A person having origins in any of the original peoples of the Far East, Southeast Asia, or the Indian subcontinent including, for example, Cambodia, China, India, Japan, Korea, Malaysia, Pakistan, the Philippine Islands, Thailand, and Vietnam.

Native Hawaiian or Other Pacific Islander A person having origins in any of the original peoples of Hawaii, Guam, Samoa, or other Pacific Islands.

Hispanic or Latino A person of Cuban, Mexican, Puerto Rican, South or Central American, or other Spanish culture or origin, regardless of race. The term "Spanish origin" can be used in addition to "Hispanic or Latino."

*Federal programs had until January 1, 2003 to adopt these revised standards.

Source: Office of Management and Budget, *Revisions to the Standards for the Classification of Federal Data on Race and Ethnicity.* Available at http://www.whitehouse.gov/wh/eop/omb/html/fedreg/ombdir15.html.

Appendix 4

Self-Assessment Checklist Promoting Cultural Diversity and Cultural Competency

SELF-ASSESSMENT CHECKLIST FOR PERSONNEL PROVIDING SERVICES TO CHILDREN WITH SPECIAL HEALTH NEEDS AND THEIR FAMILIES

This checklist was developed by HRSA's Maternal and Child Health Bureau/Children with Special Health Needs component of the National Center for Cultural Competence. It is for personnel providing health services and supports to children with special health needs and their families and is intended to heighten the awareness and sensitivity of personnel to the importance of cultural diversity and cultural competence in human service settings. The checklist provides concrete examples of the kinds of values and practices that foster such an environment. *Directions: Select A, B, or C for each item listed below.*

A = Things I do frequently   B = Things I do occasionally   C = Things I do rarely or never

Physical environment, materials, and resources

___1. I display pictures, posters, and other materials that reflect the cultures and ethnic backgrounds of children and families served by my program or agency.

___2. I ensure that magazines, brochures, and other printed materials in reception areas are of interest to and reflect the different cultures of children and families served by my program or agency.

___3. When using videos, films, or other media resources for health education, treatment, or other interventions, I ensure that they reflect the cultures of children and families served by my program or agency.

___4. When using food during an assessment, I ensure that meals provided include foods that are unique to the cultural and ethnic backgrounds of children and families served by my program or agency.

___5. I ensure that toys and other play accessories in reception areas and those which are used during assessment are representative of the various cultural and ethnic groups within the local community and the society in general.

Communication styles

___6. For children who speak languages or dialects other than English, I attempt to learn and use key words in their language so that I am better able to communicate with them during assessment, treatment, or other interventions.

___7. I attempt to determine any familial colloquialisms used by children and families that may impact on assessment, treatment, or other interventions.

___8. I use visual aids, gestures, and physical prompts in my interactions with children who have limited English proficiency.

___9. I use bilingual staff or trained volunteers to serve as interpreters during assessment, meetings, or other events for parents who would require this level of assistance.

___10. When interacting with parents who have limited English proficiency I always keep in mind that:

___* limitations in English proficiency is in no way a reflection of their level of intellectual functioning.

___* their limited ability to speak the language of the dominant culture has no bearing on their ability to communicate effectively in their language of origin.

___* they may or may not be literate in their language of origin or English.

___11. When possible, I ensure that all notices and communiqués to parents are written in their language of origin.

___12. I understand that it may be necessary to use alternatives to written communications for some families, as word of mouth may be a preferred method of receiving information.

Values and attitudes

___13. I avoid imposing values that may conflict or be inconsistent with those of cultures or ethnic groups other than my own.

___14. In group therapy or treatment situations, I discourage children from using racial and ethnic slurs by helping them understand that certain words can hurt others.

___15. I screen books, movies, and other media resources for negative cultural, ethnic, or racial stereotypes before sharing them with children and their parents served by my program or agency.

___16. I intervene in an appropriate manner when I observe other staff or parents within my program or agency engaging in behaviors that show cultural insensitivity or prejudice.

___17. I understand and accept that family is defined differently by different cultures (e.g., extended family members, fictive kin, godparents).

___18. I recognize and accept that individuals from culturally diverse backgrounds may desire varying degrees of acculturation into the dominant culture.

___19. I accept and respect that male-female roles may vary significantly among different cultures (e.g., who makes major decisions for the family, play and social interactions expected of male and female children).

___20. I understand that age and life cycle factors must be considered in interactions with individuals and families (e.g., high value placed on the decisions of elders or the role of the eldest male in families).

___21. Even though my professional or moral viewpoints may differ, I accept the family/parents as the ultimate decision makers for services and supports for their children.

___22. I recognize that the meaning or value of medical treatment and health education may vary greatly among cultures.

___23. I accept that religion and other beliefs may influence how families respond to illnesses, disease, and death.

___24. I recognize and accept that folk and religious beliefs may influence a family's reaction and approach to a child born with a disability or later diagnosed with a disability or special health care needs.

___25. I understand that traditional approaches to disciplining children are influenced by culture.

___26. I understand that families from different cultures will have different expectations of their children for acquiring toileting, dressing, feeding, and other self-help skills.

___27. I accept and respect that customs and beliefs about food, its value, preparation, and use are different from culture to culture.

___28. Before visiting or providing services in the home setting, I seek information on acceptable behaviors, courtesies, customs, and expectations that are unique to families of specific cultures and ethnic groups served by my program or agency.

___29. I seek information from family members or other key community informants, which will assist in service adaptation to respond to the needs and preferences of culturally and ethnically diverse children and families served by my program or agency.

___30. I advocate for the review of my program's or agency's mission statement, goals, policies, and procedures to ensure that they incorporate principles and practices that promote cultural diversity and cultural competence.

There is no answer key. However, if you frequently responded "C", you may not necessarily demonstrate values and engage in practices that promote a culturally diverse and culturally competent service delivery system for children and families.

For more information contact: Tawara D. Goode, Georgetown University Child Development Center UAP. Adapted from "Promoting Cultural Competence and Cultural Diversity in Early Intervention and Early Childhood Settings" (Revised 1999).

Source: U.S. Department of Health and Human Services (2000). "Promoting Cultural Diversity and Culture Competency." Office of Minority Health, *Closing the Gap,* January, pp. 6–7.

Glossary Terms

absorption field The element of a septic system in which the liquid portion of waste is distributed.

accreditation The process by which an agency or organization evaluates and recognizes an institution as meeting certain predetermined standards.

acculturated The cultural modification of an individual or group by adapting to or borrowing traits from another culture.

acid rain Both wet and dry acidic deposits, which occur both within and downwind of areas that produce emissions containing sulfur dioxide and oxides of nitrogen (also called acid deposition).

Activities of Daily Living (ADLs) Eating, toileting, dressing, bathing, walking, getting in and out of a bed or chair, and getting outside.

acute disease A disease in which the peak severity of symptoms occurs and subsides within three months of onset, usually within days or weeks.

Administration on Aging An operating division of the Department of Health and Human Services designated to carry out the provisions of the Older Americans Act of 1965.

Administration for Children and Families An operating division of the Department of Health and Human Services that coordinates programs which promote the economic and social well-being of families, children, individuals, and communities.

adolescents and young adults Individuals between the ages of 15 and 24 years.

adult day care programs Daytime care provided to seniors who are unable to be left alone.

affective disorder Mental disorder characterized by a disturbance of mood, either depression or elation (mania); for example, bipolar disorder, major depression.

aftercare The continuing care provided to former drug abusers or drug-dependent persons.

age pyramid A conceptual model that illustrates the age distribution of a population.

age-adjusted rates Rates used to make comparisons of relative risks across groups and over time when groups differ by age structure.

aged The state of being old.

ageism Prejudice and discrimination against the aged.

Agency for Healthcare Research and Quality (AHRQ) An operating division of the Department of Health and Human Services that has the responsibility of overseeing health care research.

Agency for Toxic Substances and Disease Registry (ATSDR) An operating division of the Department of Health and Human Services created by Superfund legislation to prevent or mitigate adverse health effects and diminished quality of life resulting from exposure to hazardous substances in the environment.

agent (pathogenic agent) The cause of the disease or health problem; the factor that must be present in order for the disease to occur.

aging The physiological changes that occur normally in plants and animals as they grow older.

air pollution The contamination of the air by gases, liquids, or solids that interfere with the comfort, safety, or health of living organisms.

Air Quality Index (AQI) An index (number between 0–500) that indicates the level of pollution in the air and associated health risks.

airborne disease A communicable disease that is transmitted through the air (e.g., influenza).

Alcoholics Anonymous (AA) A fellowship of recovering alcoholics who offer support to anyone who desires to stop drinking.

alcoholism A disease characterized by impaired control over drinking, preoccupation with drinking, and continued use of alcohol despite adverse consequences.

alien A person born in and owing allegiance to a country other than the one in which he or she lives.

allied health care professionals Health care workers who provide services that assist, facilitate, and complement the work of physicians and other health care specialists.

allopathic providers Independent health care providers whose remedies for illnesses produce effects different from those of the disease. These people are doctors of medicine (MDs).

ambulatory care facilities Facilities that provide a wide array of outpatient services; these can range from hospital-based facilities to independently owned freestanding facilities.

American Cancer Society A voluntary health agency dedicated to fighting cancer and educating the public about cancer.

American Health Security Act of 1993 The comprehensive health care reform introduced by then President Clinton, but never enacted.

amotivational syndrome A pattern of behavior characterized by apathy, loss of effectiveness, and a more passive, introverted personality.

amphetamines A group of synthetic drugs that act as stimulants.

amplitude The loudness or intensity of sound measured in decibels.

anabolic drugs Compounds, structurally similar to the male hormone testosterone, that increase protein synthesis.

analytic study A type of epidemiological study aimed at testing hypotheses (e.g., observational, experimental).

anthroponosis A disease that infects only humans.

aquifer Underground soil formation that is saturated with water and available for human use by pumping.

asbestos A naturally occurring mineral fiber that has been identified as a class A carcinogen by the Environmental Protection Agency.

asbestosis Acute or chronic lung disease caused by the deposit of asbestos fibers on lungs.

assisted-living facility "A special combination of housing, personalized supportive services and health care designed to meet the needs—both scheduled and unscheduled—of those who need help with activities of daily living" (see Chapter 9, reference 33).

attack rate A special incidence rate calculated for a particular population for a single disease outbreak and expressed as a percent.

automatic (passive) protection The modification of a product or the environment in such a way as to reduce unintentional injuries.

bacteriological period The period in public health history from 1875 to 1900 during which the causes of many bacterial diseases were discovered.

barbiturates Depressant drugs based on the structure of barbituric acid; for example, phenobarbital.

behavioral health care services The managed care term for mental health and substance abuse/dependence care services.

benzodiazapines Nonbarbiturate depressant drugs; examples: Librium, Valium.

binge drinking Consuming five or more alcoholic drinks in a row for males, four or more for females.

biogenic pollutants Airborne biological organisms or their particles or gases or other toxic materials that can produce illness.

biological hazards Living organisms (and viruses), or their products, that increase the risk of disease or death in humans.

bioterrorism The threatened or intentional release of biological agents for the purpose of influencing the conduct of government or intimidating or coercing a civilian population to further political or social objectives.

bipolar disorder An affective mental disorder characterized by distinct periods of elevated mood alternating with periods of depression.

birth rate See *natality rate*.

blood alcohol concentration (BAC) The percentage of concentration of alcohol in the blood; a BAC of 0.08% or greater is regarded as the legal level of intoxication in all states.

Bloodborne Pathogen Standard A set of regulations promulgated by OSHA that sets forth the responsibilities of employers and employees with regard to precautions to be taken concerning bloodborne pathogens in the workplace.

bloodborne pathogens Disease agents, such as HIV, that are transmissible in blood and other body fluids.

body mass index (BMI) The ratio of weight (in kilograms) to height (in meters, squared). To calculate in pounds and inches, divide (weight in pounds)/2.20 by [(height in inches)/32.27]^2.

bottom-up community organization Organization efforts that begin with those who live within the community affected.

brownfield A property where the expansion, redevelopment, or reuse may be complicated by the presence or potential presence of a hazardous substance, pollutant, or contaminant (e.g., abandoned gas stations, industrial plants, and commercial worksites).

Bureau of Alcohol, Tobacco, Firearms and Explosives (ATF) The federal agency in the Department of Justice that regulates alcohol, tobacco, firearms, and explosives.

Bureau of Indian Affairs (BIA) The original federal government agency charged with the responsibility for the welfare of American Indians.

byssinosis Acute or chronic lung disease caused by the inhalation of cotton, flax, or hemp dusts; those affected include workers in cotton textile plants (sometimes called *brown lung disease*).

capitation See *prepaid health care.*

carcinogens Agents, usually chemicals, that cause cancer.

care manager One who helps identify the health care needs of an individual but does not actually provide the health care services.

care provider One who helps identify the health care needs of an individual and also personally performs the caregiving service.

carrier A person or animal that harbors a specific communicable disease agent in the absence of discernible clinical disease and serves as a potential source of infection to others.

carrying capacity The amount of resources (air, water, shelter, etc.) of a given environment necessary to support a certain-sized population.

case fatality rate (CFR) The percentage of cases of a particular disease that result in death.

case/control study An epidemiological study that seeks to compare those diagnosed with a disease (cases) with those who do not have the disease (controls) for prior exposure to specific risk factors.

cases People afflicted with a disease.

categorical programs Those programs available only to people who can be categorized into a specific group based on disease, age, family means, geography, or other variables.

cause-specific mortality rate (CSMR) An expression of the death rate due to a particular disease; the CSMR is calculated by dividing the number of deaths due to a particular disease by the total population and multiplying by 100,000.

census The enumeration of the population of the United States that is conducted every ten years; begun in 1790.

Center for Mental Health Services (CMHS) The federal agency, housed within the Department of Health and Human Service's Substance Abuse and Mental Health Services Administration, whose mission it is to conduct research on the causes and treatments for mental disorders.

Centers for Disease Control and Prevention (CDC) One of the operating divisions of the Public Health Service; charged with the responsibility for surveillance and control of diseases and other health problems in the United States.

Centers for Medicare and Medicaid Services (CMS) The federal agency responsible for overseeing Medicare, Medicaid, and the related quality assurance activities.

cerebrovascular disease (stroke) A disease in which the blood supply to the brain is interrupted.

certified safety professional (CSP) A health and safety professional, trained in industrial and workplace safety, who has met specific requirements for board certification.

chain of infection A model to conceptualize the transmission of a communicable disease from its source to a susceptible host.

chemical hazards Hazards caused by the mismanagement of chemicals.

chemical straitjacket The concept of a mental patient's behavior being restrained or subdued by a drug (chemical) such as Thorazine instead of by a physical straitjacket.

child abuse The intentional physical, emotional, verbal, or sexual mistreatment of a minor.

child maltreatment The act or failure to act by a parent, caretaker, or other person as defined under state law that results in physical abuse, neglect, medical neglect, sexual abuse, or emotional abuse, or an act or failure to act that presents an imminent risk of serious harm to the child.

child neglect The failure of a parent or guardian to care for or otherwise provide the necessary subsistence for a child.

childhood diseases Infectious diseases that normally affect people in their childhood (e.g., measles, mumps, rubella, and pertussis).

children Persons between 1 and 14 years of age.

chiropractor A nonallopathic, independent health care provider who treats health problems by adjusting the spinal column.

chlorofluorocarbons (CFCs) A family of chemical agents used in industry for such items as propellants, refrigeration, solvent cleaning, and insulation.

chlorpromazine The first and most famous antipsychotic drug, introduced in 1954 under the brand name Thorazine.

chronic disease A disease or health condition that lasts longer than three months, sometimes for the remainder of one's life.

citizen-initiated community organization See *bottom-up community organization.*

Clean Air Act (CAA) (P.L. 88-206) A 1963 law that provided the federal government with authority to address interstate air pollution problems.

Clean Water Act (CWA) (P.L. 92-500) A 1972 law that provided the federal government with authority to ensure water quality by controlling water pollution; first known as Federal Water Pollution Control Act Amendments.

club drugs A general term for those illicit drugs, primarily synthetic, that are most commonly encountered at night clubs and "raves." Examples include MDMA, LSD, GHB, GBL, PCP, ketamine, Rohypnol, and methamphetamines.

coal workers' pneumoconiosis (CWP) Acute and chronic lung disease caused by the inhalation of coal dust (sometimes called black lung disease).

coalition "Formal, long-term alliance among a group of individuals representing diverse organizations, factors, or constituencies within the community who agree to work together to achieve a common goal" (see Chapter 5, reference 13).

cocaine The psychoactive ingredient in the leaves of the coca plant, *Erythoxolyn coca.*

cognitive-behavioral therapy Treatment based on learning theory in which a patient learns adaptive skills through rewards and satisfaction.

cohort A group of people who share some important demographic characteristic—year of birth, for example.

cohort study An epidemiological study in which a cohort is selected, classified on the basis of exposure to one or more specific risk factors, and observed to determine the rates at which disease develops in each class.

co-insurance Portion of insurance company's approved amounts for covered services that the beneficiary is responsible for paying.

combustion (incineration) The burning of solid wastes.

combustion by-products Gases and other particles generated by burning.

communicable disease (infectious disease) An illness due to a specific communicable agent or its toxic products, which arises through transmission of that agent or its products from an infected person, animal, or inanimate reservoir to a susceptible host.

communicable disease model A visual representation of the interrelationships of agent, host, and environment—the three entities necessary for communicable disease transmission.

community A group of people who have common characteristics; communities can be defined by location, race, ethnicity, age, occupation, interest in particular problems or outcomes, or other common bonds.

community analysis A process by which community needs are identified.

community building "[A]n orientation to community that is strength based rather than need based and stresses the identification, nurturing, and celebration of community assets" (see Chapter 5, reference 14).

community capacity "The characteristics of communities that affect their ability to identify, mobilize, and address social and public health problems" (see Chapter 5, reference 3).

community diagnosis See *community analysis.*

community health The health status of a defined group of people and the actions and conditions to promote, protect and preserve their health.

community mental health centers Local agencies, initially built with federal funding, that provide the community members with mental health services.

community organizing "A process through which communities are helped to identify common problems or goals, mobilize resources, and in other ways develop and implement strategies for reaching their goals they have collectively set" (see Chapter 5, reference 1).

Community Support Program A federal program that offers financial incentives to communities to develop a social support system for the mentally ill.

complementary/alternative medicine (CAM) "A group of diverse medical and health care systems, practices, and products that are not presently considered to be a part of conventional medicine" (see Chapter 13, reference 32).

composting   The natural, aerobic biodegradation of organic plant and animal matter to compost.

Comprehensive Drug Abuse Control Act of 1970 (Controlled Substances Act)   The central piece of legislation that regulates controlled substances (drugs subject to abuse).

Comprehensive Environmental Response, Compensation, and Liability Act (CERCLA) (Superfund)   A 1980 law created by the federal government primarily to clean up abandoned hazardous waste sites.

congregate meal programs   Community-sponsored nutrition programs that provide meals at a central site, such as a senior center.

continuing care   Long-term care for chronic health problems, usually including personal care.

continuing-care retirement communities (CCRCs)   Planned communities for elders that guarantee a lifelong residence and health care.

controlled substances   Drugs regulated by the Comprehensive Drug Abuse Control Act of 1970, including all illegal drugs and many legal drugs that can produce dependence.

coordinated school health program   "An organized set of policies, procedures, and activities designed to protect and promote the health and well-being of students and staff which has traditionally included health services, healthful school environment, and health education. It should also include, but not be limited to, guidance and counseling, physical education, food service, social work, psychological services, and employee health promotion" (see Chapter 6, reference 3).

co-payment   A negotiated set amount the insured will pay for a certain service after paying the deductible.

core functions of public health   Health assessment, policy development, and health assurance.

coronary heart disease (CHD)   A noncommunicable disease characterized by damage to the coronary arteries, which supply blood to the heart.

cosmic radiation   That radiation which comes from outer space and the sun.

criteria pollutants   The most pervasive air pollutants in the United States.

crude birth rate   An expression of the number of live births per unit of population in a given period of time. For example, the crude birth rate in the United States in 1999 was 14.5 births per 1,000 population.

crude death rate (CDR)   An expression of the total number of deaths (from all causes) per unit of population in a given period of time. For example, the crude death rate in the United States in 2004 was 800.0 per 100,000 population.

crude rate   A rate in which the denominator includes the total population.

cultural and linguistic competency   A set of congruent behaviors, attitudes, and policies that come together in a system, agency, or among professionals that enables effective work in cross-cultural situations.

culturally sensitive   Having respect for cultures other than one's own.

curriculum   Written plan for instruction.

cycles per second (cps)   A measure of sound frequency.

death rate   See *mortality rate*.

decibels (dB)   A measure of sound amplitude.

deductible   The amount of expense that the beneficiary must incur before the insurance company begins to pay for covered services.

deinstitutionalization   The process of discharging, on a large scale, patients from state mental hospitals to less restrictive community settings.

demography (demographers)   The study of a population and those variables bringing about change in that population.

Department of Health and Human Services (HHS)   The largest federal department in the United States government, formed in 1980 and headed by a secretary who is a member of the president's cabinet.

dependency ratio   A ratio that compares the number of individuals whom society considers economically productive (the working population) to the number of those it considers economically unproductive (the nonworking or dependent population).

depressant   A psychoactive drug that slows down the central nervous system.

descriptive study   An epidemiological study that describes an epidemic with respect to person, place, and time.

designer drugs   Mind-altering drugs, synthesized in clandestine laboratories, that are similar to but structurally different from known controlled substances.

diagnosis-related groups (DRGs)   A procedure used to classify the health problems of all Medicare patients when they are admitted to a hospital.

direct transmission   The immediate transfer of an infectious agent by direct contact between infected and susceptible individuals.

disability-adjusted life years (DALYs)   A measure for the burden of disease that takes into account premature death and years lived with disability of specified severity and duration. One DALY is one lost year of healthy life.

disabling injury An injury causing any restriction of normal activity beyond the day of the injury's occurrence.

diseases of adaptation Diseases that result from chronic exposure to excess levels of stressors that elicit the General Adaptation Syndrome.

disinfection The killing of communicable disease agents outside the host, on counter tops, for example.

drug A substance other than food or vitamins that, upon entering the body in small amounts, alters one's physical, mental, or emotional state.

drug abuse Use of a drug despite the knowledge that continued use is detrimental to one's health or well-being.

drug abuse education Providing information about the dangers of drug abuse, changing attitudes and beliefs about drugs, providing skills necessary to abstain from drugs, and ultimately changing drug abuse behavior.

drug (chemical) dependence A psychological and sometimes physical state characterized by a craving for a drug.

Drug Enforcement Administration (DEA) The federal government's lead agency with the primary responsibility for enforcing the nation's drug laws, including the Controlled Substances Act of 1970.

drug misuse Inappropriate use of prescription or nonprescription drugs.

drug use A non-evaluative term referring to drug-taking behavior in general; any drug-taking behavior.

Earth Day Annual public observance for concerns about the environment; the first was held April 22, 1970.

elderhostel Education programs specifically for seniors, held on college campuses.

elderly (or elder) Individuals over 65 years of age.

elderly dependency ratio The dependency ratio that includes only the elderly.

electroconvulsive therapy (ECT) A method of treatment for mental disorders involving the administration of electric current to induce a coma or convulsions.

employee assistance programs (EAPs) Worksite-based, employer-sponsored programs that assist employees whose work performance suffers because of substance abuse or domestic, psychological, or social problems.

empowered community "One in which individuals and organizations apply their skills and resources in collective efforts to meet their respective needs" (see Chapter 5, reference 4).

end-of-life practice Health care services provided to individuals shortly before death.

endemic disease A disease that occurs regularly in a population as a matter of course.

environment All the external conditions, circumstances, and influences surrounding and affecting the growth and development of an organism or community of organisms.

environmental hazards Factors or conditions in the environment that increase the risk of disease or death in humans.

environmental health The study and management of environmental conditions that affect the health and well-being of humans.

Environmental Protection Agency (EPA) The federal agency primarily responsible for setting, maintaining, and enforcing environmental standards.

environmental sanitation The practice of establishing and maintaining healthy or hygienic conditions in the environment.

environmental tobacco smoke (ETS) Tobacco smoke in the ambient air.

epidemic An unexpectedly large number of cases of an illness, specific health-related behavior, or other health-related event.

epidemic curve A graphic display of the cases of disease according to the time or date of onset of symptoms.

epidemiologist An investigator who studies the occurrence of disease or other health-related conditions or events in defined populations.

epidemiology The study of the distribution and determinants of health-related states or events in specific populations, and the application of this study to control health problems.

equilibrium phase Last phase of the population growth S-curve, when the birth and death rates are equal.

eradication The complete elimination or uprooting of a disease (e.g., smallpox eradication).

etiology The cause of a disease (e.g., the etiology of mumps is the mumps virus).

evaluation Determining the value or worth of the objective of interest.

evidence-based practices Ways of delivering services to people using scientific evidence that shows that the services actually work.

exclusion A condition that is written into a health insurance policy indicating what is not covered by the policy.

exclusive provider organization (EPO) Similar to a preferred provider organization but with fewer providers and stronger financial incentives. See *preferred provider organization (PPO)*.

experimental study An analytic, epidemiological study in which investigators allocate exposure to the risk factor(s) and follow the subjects to observe disease development.

exponential phase Middle phase of the population growth S-curve, when the birth rate is greater than the death rate.

Family and Medical Leave Act (FMLA) Federal legislation that provides up to a 12-week unpaid leave to men and women after the birth of a child, an adoption, or an event of illness in the immediate family.

family planning The process of determining the preferred number and spacing of children in one's family and choosing the appropriate means to achieve this preference.

family violence The use of physical force by one family member against another, with the intent to hurt, injure, or cause death.

fatal injury An injury that results in one or more deaths.

fatality rate See *mortality rate*.

Federal Emergency Management Agency (FEMA) The nation's official emergency response agency.

Federal Water Pollution Control Act Amendments See *Clean Water Act*.

fee-for-service A method of paying for health care in which a bill (fee) is paid after the care (service) is rendered.

fertility rate The number of live births per 1,000 women of childbearing age (15–44 years).

fetal alcohol syndrome (FAS) A group of abnormalities that may include growth retardation, abnormal appearance of face and head, and deficits of central nervous system function including mental retardation in babies born to mothers who have consumed heavy amounts of alcohol during their pregnancies.

fetal deaths Deaths in utero with a gestational age of at least 20 weeks.

fight or flight reaction An alarm reaction that prepares one physiologically for sudden action (heart rate, blood pressure, and respiration increase).

fixed indemnity The maximum amount an insurer will pay for a certain service.

Food and Drug Administration (FDA) An operating division of the Department of Health and Human Services that regulates all food, over-the-counter and prescription drugs, medical devices, and cosmetics.

foodborne disease A disease transmitted through the contamination of food.

foodborne disease outbreak (FBDO) The occurrence of two or more cases of a similar illness resulting from the ingestion of food.

formaldehyde (CH_2O) A water-soluble gas used in aqueous solutions in hundreds of consumer products.

formative evaluation The evaluation that is conducted during the planning and implementing processes to improve or refine a program.

full-service hospitals Hospitals that offer services in all or most of the levels of care defined by the spectrum of health care.

functional limitations Difficulty in performing personal care and home management tasks.

gag rule Regulations that bar physicians and nurses in clinics receiving federal funds from counseling clients about abortions.

gatekeepers Those who control, both formally and informally, the political climate of the community.

General Adaptation Syndrome (GAS) The complex physiological responses resulting from exposure to stressors that can in time result in health deficits.

geriatrics The branch of medicine that deals with the structural changes, physiology, diseases, and other medical aspects of old age.

gerontology The study of aging, from the broadest perspective.

global warming The gradual increase in the earth's surface temperature.

government hospital A hospital that is supported and managed by governmental jurisdictions.

governmental health agency (or official health agencies) Health agencies that are part of the governmental structure (federal, state, or local) and that are funded primarily by tax dollars.

grass-roots community organizing A process that begins with those affected by the problem/concern.

greenhouse gases Atmosphere gases, principally carbon dioxide, the CFCs, methane, and nitrous oxide, that are transparent to visible light but absorb infrared radiation (heat).

groundwater Water located under the surface of the ground.

group model HMO An HMO that contracts with a multispecialty group practice.

hallucinogens Drugs that produce profound distortions of the senses.

hard-to-reach population Those in a priority population that are not easily reached by normal programming efforts.

hazard An unsafe act or condition.

hazardous waste "A solid waste or combination of solid wastes which—because of its quantity, concentration, or physical, chemical, or infectious characteristics—may (A) cause or significantly contribute to an increase in mortality or an increase in serious irreversible, or incapacitating reversible, illness; or (B) pose a substantial present or potential hazard to human health or the environment when improperly treated, stored, transported, or disposed of, or otherwise managed." (*Note:* This definition was taken from the Resource Conservation and Recovery Act of 1976.)

health A dynamic state or condition of the human organism that is multidimensional in nature, a resource for living, and results from a person's interactions with and adaptations to his or her environment; therefore, it can exist in varying degrees and is specific to each individual and his or her situation.

health education "Any combination of planned learning experiences based on sound theories that provide individuals, groups, and communities the opportunity to acquire information and the skills to make quality health decisions" (see Chapter 5, reference 25).

health maintenance organizations (HMOs) Groups that supply prepaid comprehensive health care with an emphasis on prevention.

health physicist A safety professional with responsibility for monitoring radiation within a plant environment, developing instrumentation for that purpose, and developing plans for coping with radiation accidents.

health promotion "Any planned combination of educational, political, environmental, regulatory, or organizational mechanisms that support actions and conditions of living conducive to the health of individuals, groups, and communities" (see Chapter 5, reference 25).

health resources development period The period in public health history from 1900 to 1960; a time of great growth in health care facilities.

Health Resources and Services Administration (HRSA) An operating division of the Department of Health and Human Services established in 1982 to improve the nation's health resources and services and their distribution to underserved populations.

health-adjusted life expectancy (HALE) The number of years of healthy life expected, on average, in a given population.

Healthy People 2010 The third set of health goals and objectives for the United States that defines the nation's health agenda and guides its health policy.

healthy school environment "The promotion, maintenance, and utilization of safe and wholesome surroundings, organization of day-by-day experiences and planned learning procedures to influence favorable emotional, physical and social health" (see Chapter 6, reference 31).

herbicide A pesticide designed specifically to kill plants.

herd immunity The resistance of a population to the spread of an infectious agent based on the immunity of a high portion of individuals.

home health care Care that is provided in the patient's residence for the purpose of promoting, maintaining, or restoring health.

home health care services Health care services provided in the patient's place of residence (home or apartment).

homebound A person unable to leave home for normal activities such as shopping, meals, or other activities.

hospice care A program of palliative and support care services providing physical, psychological, social, and spiritual care for dying persons, their families, and other loved ones by a hospice worker (see Chapter 13, reference 29).

Hospital Survey and Construction Act of 1946 (Hill-Burton Act) Federal legislation that provided substantial funds for hospital construction.

host A person or other living animal that affords subsistence or lodgment to a communicable agent under natural conditions.

hypercholesterolemia High levels of cholesterol in the blood.

hypertension A chronic condition characterized by a resting blood pressure reading of 140/90 mm of mercury or higher.

illegal alien An individual who entered this country without permission.

illicit (illegal) drugs Drugs that cannot be legally manufactured, distributed, bought, or sold, and that lack recognized medical value.

immigrant Individuals who migrate to this country from another country for the purpose of seeking permanent residence.

impairments Defects in the functioning of one's sense organs or limitations in one's mobility or range of motion.

implementation Putting a planned program into action.

incidence rate The number of new health-related events or cases of a disease in a population exposed to that risk during a particular period of time, divided by the total number in that same population.

incubation period   The period of time between exposure to an infectious agent and the onset of symptoms.

independent practice association (IPA) model HMO   An HMO in which individual physicians contract with the HMO to provide care for a certain number of enrollees; includes staff and network HMOs.

independent providers   Health care professionals with the education and legal authority to treat any health problem.

Indian Health Service (IHS)   An operating division of the Department of Health and Human Services whose goal is to raise the health status of the American Indian and Alaska Native to the highest possible level by providing a comprehensive health services delivery system.

indirect transmission   Communicable disease transmission involving an intermediate step; for example, airborne, vehicleborne, or vectorborne transmission.

indoor air pollution   The buildup of undesirable gases and particles in the air inside a building.

industrial hygienist   A health professional concerned with health hazards in the workplace, including such things as problems with ventilation, noise, and lighting; also responsible for measuring air quality and recommending plans for improving the healthiness of work environments.

infant death (infant mortality)   Death of a child under one year of age.

infant mortality rate   The number of deaths of children under one year of age per 1,000 live births.

infection   The lodgment and growth of a virus or microorganism in a host organism.

infectious disease   See *communicable disease*.

infectivity   The ability of a pathogen to lodge and grow in a host.

informal caregiver   One who provides unpaid care or assistance to one who has some physical, mental, emotional, or financial need that limits his or her independence.

inhalants   Breathable substances that produce mind-altering effects; for example, glue.

injury   Physical harm or damage to the body resulting from an exchange, usually acute, of mechanical, chemical, thermal, or other environmental energy that exceeds the body's tolerance.

injury prevention (control)   An organized effort to prevent injuries or to minimize their severity.

injury prevention education   The process of changing people's health-directed behavior in such a way as to reduce unintentional injuries.

insecticides   Pesticides designed specifically to kill insects.

Instrumental Activities of Daily Living (IADLs)   Measure of more complex tasks such as handling personal finances, preparing meals, shopping, doing homework, traveling, using the telephone, and taking medications.

intensity   Cardiovascular workload measured by heart rate.

intentional injury   An injury that is judged to have been purposely inflicted, either by the victim or another.

intern   A first-year resident.

internal radiation   Radiation in the human body that occurs as a result of ingesting food or inhaling air.

intervention   An activity or activities designed to create change in people.

intimate partner violence (IPV)   Rape, physical assault, or stalking perpetrated by current or former dates, spouses, or cohabiting partners, with cohabiting meaning living together at least some of the time as a couple.

isolation   The separation of infected persons from those who are susceptible.

Joint Commission   The predominant organization responsible for accrediting health care facilities.

labor-force ratio   A ratio of the total number of those individuals who are not working (regardless of age) to the number of those who are.

lag phase   Initial phase of the population growth S-curve, when growth is slow.

law enforcement   The application of federal, state, and local laws to arrest, jail, bring to trial, and sentence those who break drug laws or break laws because of drug use.

leachates   Liquids created when water mixes with wastes and removes soluble constituents from them by percolation.

lead   A naturally occurring mineral element found throughout the environment and produced in large quantities for industrial products.

licensed practical nurse (LPN)   Those prepared in one- to two-year programs to provide nontechnical bedside nursing care under the supervision of physicians or registered nurses.

life expectancy   The average number of years a person from a specific cohort is projected to live from a given point in time.

limited (restricted) care providers   Health care providers who provide care for a specific part of the body; for example, dentists.

limited-service hospitals   Hospitals that offer only the specific services needed by the population served.

litigation   The process of seeking justice for injury through courts.

lobotomy Surgical severance of nerve fibers of the brain by incision.

long-term care Different kinds of help that people with chronic illnesses, disabilities, or other conditions need to deal with the circumstances that limit them physically or mentally.

low-birth-weight infant An infant that weighs less than 2,500 grams, or 5.5 pounds, at birth.

Lyme disease A systematic, bacterial, tickborne disease with symptoms that include dermatologic, arthritic, neurologic, and cardiac abnormalities.

mainstream tobacco smoke The smoke of burning tobacco inhaled and exhaled by the smoker.

major depression An affective disorder characterized by a dysphoric mood, usually depression, or loss of interest or pleasure in almost all usual activities or pastimes.

majority Those with characteristics that are found in over 50% of a population.

malignant neoplasm Uncontrolled new tissue growth resulting from cells that have lost control over their growth and division.

managed behavioral health care organizations (MBHOs) Managed care providers who specialize in providing mental health care services.

managed care Health plans that integrate the financing and delivery of health care services to covered individuals by means of arrangements with selected providers to furnish comprehensive services to members; explicit criteria for the selection of health care providers; significant financial incentives for members to use providers and procedures associated with the plan; and formal programs for quality assurance and utilization review.

marijuana Dried plant parts of *Cannabis sativa*.

maternal, infant, and child health The health of women of childbearing age from pre-pregnancy, through pregnancy, labor and delivery, and the postpartum period and the health of the child prior to birth through adolescence.

maternal mortality The death of a woman while pregnant or within 42 days of termination of pregnancy, irrespective of the duration and the site of the pregnancy, from any cause related to or aggravated by the pregnancy or its management but not from accidental or incidental causes.

maternal mortality rate Number of mothers dying per 100,000 live births in a given year.

Meals on Wheels program A community-supported nutrition program in which prepared meals are delivered to elders in their homes, usually by volunteers.

median age The age at which half of the population is older and half is younger.

Medicaid A national federal-state health insurance program for the poor.

medically indigent Those lacking the financial ability to pay for their own medical care.

Medicare A national health insurance program for people 65 years of age and older, certain younger disabled people, and people with permanent kidney failure.

Medigap Private health insurance to supplement Medicare benefits—that is, to fill in the gaps of Medicare.

mental disorder Deficiency in one's psychological resources for dealing with everyday life, usually characterized by distress or impairment of one or more areas of functioning.

mental health Emotional and social well-being, including one's psychological resources for dealing with the day-to-day problems of life.

mental hygiene movement A movement by those who believed that mental illness could be cured if identified and treated at an early stage; proponents were Adolph Meyer and Clifford Beers.

mental illness A collective term for all mental disorders.

Mental Retardation Facilities and Community Mental Health Centers (CMHC) Act of 1963 (Community Mental Health Act of 1963) A law that provided federal funds directly to communities to assist in the building and funding of community mental health centers.

metastasis The spread of a disease, such as cancer, by the transfer of cells by means of the blood or lymphatics.

methamphetamine The amphetamine drug most widely abused.

methaqualone An illicit depressant drug.

methcathinone (cat) An illicit, synthetic drug, similar to the amphetamines, that first appeared in the United States in 1991.

middle old Those 75 to 84 years of age.

migration Movement of people from one country to another.

minority groups Subgroups of the population that consist of less than 50% of the population.

minority health The morbidity and mortality of American Indians/Alaska Natives, Asian Americans and Pacific Islanders, black Americans, and Americans of Hispanic origin in the United States.

mixed model HMO A hybrid form of a health maintenance organization.

model for unintentional injuries The public health triangle (host, agent, and environment) modified to indicate energy as the causative agent of injuries.

modern era of public health The era of American public health that began in 1850 and continues today.

modifiable risk factor Factors contributing to the development of a noncommunicable disease that can be altered by modifying one's behavior or environment; for example, cigarette smoking is a modifiable risk factor for coronary heart disease.

moral treatment Treatment for mental illness in eighteenth and nineteenth centuries, based on belief that mental illness was caused by moral deterioration.

morbidity rate The rate of illness in a population.

mortality (fatality) rate The rate of deaths in a population.

multicausation disease model A visual representation of the host, together with various internal and external factors that promote and protect against disease.

municipal solid waste (MSW) Waste generated by individual households, businesses, and institutions located within municipalities.

narcotics Drugs similar to morphine that reduce pain and induce a stuporous state.

natality (birth) rate The rate of births in a population.

National Alliance for the Mentally Ill (NAMI) A national voluntary health agency that advocates for the mentally ill.

National Ambient Air Quality Standards (NAAQSs) Standards created by the EPA for allowable concentration levels of outdoor air pollutants.

National Electronic Telecommunications System (NETS) The electronic reporting system by which state health departments send health records to the Centers for Disease Control and Prevention (CDC).

National Institute of Mental Health (NIMH) The agency of the National Institutes of Health whose mission is to conduct research on the causes of and treatments for mental disorders.

National Institute for Occupational Safety and Health (NIOSH) A research body within the Centers for Disease Control and Prevention, Department of Health and Human Services, that is responsible for developing and recommending occupational safety and health standards.

National Institute on Drug Abuse (NIDA) The federal government's lead agency for drug abuse research; part of the National Institutes of Health.

National Institutes of Health (NIH) The research division of the Department of Health and Human Services. It is part of the Public Health Service.

National Mental Health Association (NMHA) A national voluntary health association that advocates for mental health and for those with mental illnesses; it has 600 affiliates in 43 states.

natural hazards Events of nature that increase the probability of disease, injury, or death of humans.

needs assessment The process of collecting and analyzing information to develop an understanding of the issues, resources, and constraints of the priority population, as related to the development of health promotion programs.

neonatal deaths (neonatal mortality) Deaths occurring during the first 28 days after birth.

neonatologist A medical doctor who specializes in the care of newborns from birth to two months of age.

net migration The population gain or loss resulting from migration.

network model HMO A type of IPA HMO that contracts with more than one medical group practice.

neuroleptic drug A drug that reduces nervous activity; another term for antipsychotic drug.

noise pollution Excessive sound; unwanted sound.

nonallopathic providers Independent providers who provide nontraditional forms of health care.

noncommunicable disease (noninfectious disease) A disease not caused by a communicable agent, and that thus cannot be transmitted from infected host to susceptible host.

nonphysician practitioners (NPPs) Clinical professionals who practice in many of the areas similar to those in which physicians practice, but who do not have an MD or DO degree (see Chapter 13, reference 1).

nonpoint source pollution All pollution that occurs through the runoff, seepage, or falling of pollutants into the water.

nontarget organisms All other susceptible organisms in the environment, for which a pesticide was not intended.

notifiable diseases Infectious diseases for which health officials request or require reporting for public health reasons.

observational study An analytic, epidemiological study in which an investigator or investigators observe the natural course of events, noting exposed and unexposed subjects and disease development.

occupational disease Any abnormal condition or disorder, other than one resulting from an occupational injury, caused by an exposure to environmental factors associated with employment.

occupational health nurse (OHN) A registered nurse whose primary responsibilities include prevention of illness and promotion of health in the workplace.

occupational injury An injury that results from exposure to a single incident in the work environment (e.g., cut, fracture, sprain, amputation).

occupational physician (OP) or occupational medical practitioner (OMP) A medical practitioner (doctor) whose primary concern is preventive medicine in the workplace.

Occupational Safety and Health Act of 1970 (OSHAct) Comprehensive federal legislation aimed at assuring safe and healthful working conditions for working men and women.

Occupational Safety and Health Administration (OSHA) The federal agency located within the Department of Labor and created by the OSHAct that is charged with the responsibility of administering the provisions of the OSHAct.

odds ratio A probability statement about the association between a particular disease and a specific risk factor, often the outcome of a retrospective (case/ control) study.

Office of National Drug Control Policy (ONDCP) The headquarters of America's drug control effort, located in the executive branch of the federal government, and headed by a director appointed by the president.

official health agency See *governmental health agency*.

old Those 65 years of age and older.

old old Those 85 years of age and older.

Older Americans Act of 1965 Federal legislation to improve the lives of elders.

operationalize (operational definition) To provide working definitions.

osteopathic providers Independent health care providers whose remedies emphasize the interrelationships of the body's systems in prevention, diagnosis, and treatment.

over-the-counter (OTC) drugs (nonprescription drugs) Drugs (except tobacco and alcohol) that can be legally purchased without a physician's prescription (e.g., aspirin).

ownership A feeling that one has a stake in or "owns" the object of interest.

ozone layer Ozone gas (O_3) found in the stratosphere.

pandemic An outbreak of disease over a wide geographical area, such as a continent.

parity The concept of equality in health care coverage for people with mental illness and those with other medical illnesses or injuries.

passive smoking The inhalation of environmental tobacco smoke by nonsmokers.

pathogenicity The capability of a communicable agent to cause disease in a susceptible host.

peer counseling programs School-based drug education programs in which students discuss alcohol and other drug-related problems with other students.

pest Any organism—multicelled animal or plant, or microbe—that has an adverse effect on human interests.

pesticides Synthetic chemicals developed and manufactured for the purpose of killing pests.

phasing in Implementation of an intervention with small groups prior to its implementation with the entire priority population.

philanthropic foundation An endowed institution that donates money for the good of humankind.

photochemical smog A secondary air pollutant created when primary pollutants react with oxygen and sunlight.

physical dependence Drug dependence in which discontinued use results in the onset of physical illness.

physician-hospital organizations (PHOs) Various agreements between physicians and hospitals to form units to negotiate with insurers as managed care organizations.

pilot test Presentation of the intervention to just a few individuals, who are either from the intended priority population or from a very similar population.

placebo A blank treatment (e.g., a sugar pill).

pneumoconiosis Fibrotic lung disease caused by the inhalation of dusts, especially mineral dusts.

point-of-service (POS) option An option of a health maintenance organization plan that allows enrollees to be at least partially reimbursed for selecting a health care provider outside the plan.

point source epidemic curve An epidemic curve depicting a distribution of cases that can all be traced to a single source of exposure.

point source pollution Pollution that can be traced to a single identifiable source.

polydrug use Concurrent use of multiple drugs.

population at risk Those in the population who are susceptible to a particular disease or condition.

population health The health status of people who are not organized and have no identity as a group or locality and the actions and conditions to promote, protect, and preserve their health.

population-based public health practice Incorporates interventions aimed at disease prevention and health promotion, specific protection, and case findings.

postneonatal deaths (postneonatal mortality) Deaths that occur between 28 days and 365 days after birth.

pre-existing condition   A medical condition that had been diagnosed or treated usually within six months before the date a health insurance policy goes into effect.

preferred provider organization (PPO)   An organization that buys fixed-rate (discount) health services from providers and sells them (via premiums) to consumers.

premature infant   One born following a gestation period of 38 weeks or less, or one born at a low birth weight.

prenatal health care (prenatal care)   One of the fundamentals of a safe motherhood program, which includes three major components: risk assessment, treatment for medical conditions or risk reduction, and education. Prenatal health care should begin before pregnancy when a couple is considering having a child and continue throughout pregnancy.

prepaid health care   A method of paying for covered health care services on a per-person premium basis for a specific period of time prior to service being rendered. Also referred to as capitation.

preplacement examination   A physical examination of a newly hired or transferred worker to determine medical suitability for placement in a specific position.

prevalence rate   The number of new and old cases of a disease in a population in a given period of time, divided by the total number of that population.

prevention   The planning for and taking of action to forestall the onset of a disease or other health problem before the occurrence of undesirable health events.

preventive care   Care given to healthy people to keep them healthy.

priority population (audience)   Those whom a program is intended to serve.

primary medical care   The provision of integrated, accessible health care services by clinicians who are accountable for addressing a large majority of personal health care needs, developing a sustained partnership with patients, and practicing in the context of family and community.

primary prevention   Preventive measures that forestall the onset of illness or injury during the prepathogenesis period.

private (proprietary) or investor-owned hospitals   For-profit hospitals.

pro-choice   A medical/ethical position that holds that women have a right to reproductive freedom.

pro-life   A medical/ethical position that holds that performing an abortion is an act of murder.

problem drinker   One for whom alcohol consumption results in personal, economic, medical, social, or any other type of problem.

professional nurse   A registered nurse holding a bachelor of science degree in nursing (BSN).

program planning   A process by which an intervention is planned to help meet the needs of a priority population.

propagated epidemic curve   An epidemic curve depicting a distribution of cases traceable to multiple sources of exposure over time.

proportionate mortality ratio (PMR)   The percentage of overall mortality in a population that can be assigned to a particular cause or disease.

prospective pricing system (PPS)   One in which providers are paid predetermined amounts of money per procedure for services provided.

prospective study   An epidemiological study that begins in the present and continues into the future for the purpose of observing the development of disease (e.g., cohort study).

providers   Health care facilities or health professionals that provide health care services.

psychoactive drugs   Mind-altering drugs; drugs that affect the central nervous system.

psychological dependence   A psychological state characterized by an overwhelming desire to continue use of a drug.

psychopharmacological therapy   Treatment for mental illness that involves medications.

psychotherapy   A treatment methodology based on the Freudian concept of emotional release (catharsis), sexual conflict resolution, and subconscious drives.

public health   Things that society does collectively to assure the conditions in which people can be healthy.

public health professional   A health care worker who works in a public health organization.

Public Health Service (PHS)   An agency in the Department of Health and Human Services (HHS) that is comprised of eight of the 11 operating divisions of HHS.

public health system   The organizational mechanism of those activities undertaken within the formal structure of government and the associated efforts of private and voluntary organizations and individuals.

public hospitals   Hospitals that are supported and managed by governmental jurisdictions.

public policy   The guiding principles and courses of action pursued by governments to solve practical problems affecting society.

quality management and utilization review   The analysis of provided health care for its appropriateness by someone other than the patient and provider.

quarantine Limitation of freedom of movement of those who have been exposed to a disease and may be incubating it.

quasi-governmental health organizations Organizations that have some responsibilities assigned by the government but operate more like voluntary agencies; for example, the American Red Cross.

radiation Energy released when an atom is split or naturally decays from a less stable to a more stable form.

radon A naturally occurring radioactive gas that cannot be seen, smelled, or tasted; it is formed by the radioactive decay of uranium-238.

rate The number of events (cases of disease) that occur in a given period of time.

recycling The collection and sorting of materials that would otherwise be considered waste, processing these into raw materials for manufacturing new products, and subsequent use of those new products.

reform phase of public health The period of public health from 1900 to 1920, characterized by social movements to improve health conditions in cities and in the workplace.

refugee A person who flees one area or country to seek shelter or protection from danger in another.

registered nurse (RN) An appropriately prepared nurse who has passed the state RN licensing examination.

regulation The enactment and enforcement of laws to control conduct.

rehabilitation center A facility in which restorative care is provided following injury, disease, or surgery.

relative risk A statement of the relationship between the risk of acquiring a disease when a specific risk factor is present and the risk of acquiring that same disease when the risk factor is not present.

resident A physician who is training in a specialty.

residues and wastes Unwanted by-products of human activities.

Resource Conservation and Recovery Act of 1976 (RCRA) A federal law that sets forth guidelines for the proper handling and disposal of solid and hazardous wastes.

respite care Planned short-term care, usually for the purpose of relieving a full-time informal caregiver.

restorative care Care provided to patients after a successful treatment or when the progress of a incurable disease has been arrested.

retirement communities Residential communities that have been specifically developed for those in their retirement years.

retrospective study An epidemiological study that looks into the past for clues to explain the present distribution of disease.

risk factors Factors that increase the probability of disease, injury, or death.

Roe v. Wade A 1973 Supreme Court decision that made it unconstitutional for state laws to prohibit abortions.

Rohypnol (flunitrazepam) A depressant in the benzodiazepine group that has achieved notoriety as a date rape drug.

rollover protective structures (ROPS) Factory-installed or retrofitted reinforced framework on a cab to protect the operator of a tractor in case of a rollover.

runoff Flow of water over land surfaces (including paved surfaces), typically from precipitation.

Safe Drinking Water Act (SDWA) A 1974 federal law that instructed the EPA to set maximum contaminant levels for specific pollutants in drinking water.

safety engineer A health and safety professional, sometimes with an engineering background, employed by a company for the purpose of reducing unintentional injuries in the workplace.

safety programs Those parts of the workplace health and safety program aimed at reducing unintentional injuries on the job.

sanitarians Environmental workers responsible for inspection of restaurants, retail food outlets, public housing, and other facilities to assure compliance with public health codes.

sanitary landfill A municipal waste disposal site located on land suited for this purpose and upon which solid waste is spread in thin layers and covered with a fresh layer of soil.

sanitation The promotion of hygiene and prevention of disease by maintenance of clean conditions through hygienic disposal or recycling of waste material, such as human fecal waste.

school health coordinator A professional at the district (or school) level responsible for management and coordination of all school health policies, activities, and resources.

school health council Individuals from a school or school district and its community who work together to provide advice on aspects of the school health program.

school health education The development, delivery, and evaluation of a planned curriculum, kindergarten through grade 12.

school health policies Written statements that describe the nature and procedures of a school health program.

school health services Health services provided by school health workers to appraise, protect, and promote the health of students and school personnel.

scope Part of the curriculum that outlines what will be taught.

secondary medical care Specialized attention and ongoing management for common and less frequently encountered medical conditions, including support services for people with special challenges due to chronic or long-term conditions.

secondary prevention Preventive measures that lead to early diagnosis and prompt treatment of a disease or injury to limit disability and prevent more severe pathogenesis.

secondhand smoke Environmental tobacco smoke (ETS); tobacco smoke in the ambient air that can be inhaled.

self-help support groups Groups of concerned citizens who are united by a shared interest, concern, or deficit not shared by other members of the community; Alcoholics Anonymous, for example.

self-insured organization One that pays the health care costs of its employees with the premiums collected from the employees and the contributions made by the employer.

senior centers Facilities where elders can congregate for fellowship, meals, education, and recreation.

septic tank A watertight concrete or fiberglass tank that holds sewage; one of two main parts of a septic system.

sequence Part of the curriculum that states in what order the content will be taught.

sick building syndrome A term to describe a situation in which the air quality in a building produces generalized signs and symptoms of ill health in the building's occupants.

sidestream tobacco smoke The smoke that comes off the end of burning tobacco products.

silicosis Acute or chronic lung disease caused by the inhalation of free crystalline silica; those affected include workers in mines, stone quarries, sand and gravel operations, and abrasive blasting operations.

sliding scale fee A fee based on ability to pay.

sludge A semisolid mixture of solid waste that includes bacteria, viruses, organic matter, toxic metals, synthetic organic chemicals, and solid chemicals.

smokeless tobacco (spit tobacco) Snuff and chewing tobacco.

social capital "Relationships and structures within a community that promote cooperation for mutual benefit" (see Chapter 5, reference 1).

Social Security Administration (SSA) An independent federal agency that administers programs that provide financial support to special groups of Americans.

socioeconomic status A demographic term which takes into consideration the combination of social and economic factors.

solid waste Garbage, refuse, sludges, and other discarded solid materials, including solid waste materials resulting from industrial, commercial, and agricultural operations and from community activities; not included are solid or dissolved materials in domestic sewage or other significant pollutants in water resources, such as silt, dissolved or suspended solids in industrial wastewater effluents, dissolved materials in irrigation return flows, or other common water pollutants.

solid waste management The process of waste reduction, product reuse and recycling, and disposal.

sound-level meter Instrument used to measure sound.

source reduction A waste management approach entailing the reduction or elimination of use of materials that produce an accumulation of solid waste.

Special Supplemental Food Program for Women, Infants, and Children See *WIC*.

specialty hospital A hospital that provides mainly one type of medical service, is for-profit, and is owned at least in part by the physicians who practice in it.

specific rate A rate of a specific disease in a population or the rate of events in a specific population (e.g., cause-specific death rate, age-specific death rate).

spectrum of health care delivery The array of types of care—from preventive to continuing, or long-term, care. It comprises four levels of care.

spiritual era of public health A time during the Middle Ages when the causation of communicable disease was linked to spiritual forces.

staff model HMO A health maintenance organization that hires its own staff of health care providers.

standard of acceptability A comparative mandate, value, norm, or group.

State Children's Health Insurance Program (SCHIP) A title insurance program under the Social Security Act that provides health insurance to uninsured children.

stimulant A drug that increases the activity of the central nervous system; for example, methamphetamine.

student assistance programs (SAPs) School-based drug education programs to assist students who have alcohol or other drug problems.

Substance Abuse and Mental Health Services Administration (SAMHSA) An operating division of the Department of Health and Human Services whose stated mission is the reduction of the incidence and prevalence of alcohol and other drug abuse and mental disorders, the improvement of treatment outcomes, and the curtailment of the consequences of mental health problems for families and communities.

sudden infant death syndrome (SIDS) Sudden unanticipated death of an infant in whom, after examination, there is no recognized cause of death.

summative evaluation The evaluation that determines the impact of a program on the priority population.

Superfund legislation See *Comprehensive Environmental Response, Compensation, and Liability Act.*

Supplemental Security Program of the Social Security Administration that provides cash benefits to elderly, blind, and disabled Americans with minimal resources.

surface water Water that is found on the earth's surface (e.g., oceans, rivers, streams, ponds, lakes, etc.).

Survey of Occupational Injuries and Illnesses (SOII) An annual survey of injuries and illnesses from a large sample of U.S. employees (approximately 250,000) maintained by the Bureau of Labor Statistics in the Department of Labor.

Synar Amendment A federal law that requires states to set the minimum legal age for purchasing tobacco products at 18 years and that requires states to enforce this law.

synesthesia Impairment of mind (by hallucinogens) characterized by a sensation that senses are mixed (e.g., seeing sounds and hearing images).

tardive dyskinesia Irreversible, involuntary, and abnormal movements of the tongue, mouth, arms, and legs which can result from long-term use of certain antipsychotic drugs such as chlorpromazine.

target organism (target pest) The organism for which a pesticide is applied.

terrestrial radiation Radiation that comes from radioactive minerals within the earth.

tertiary medical care Specialized and technologically sophisticated medical and surgical care for those with unusual or complex conditions (generally no more than a few percent of the need in any service category).

tertiary prevention Measures aimed at rehabilitation following significant pathogenesis.

thermal inversion Condition that occurs when warm air traps cooler air at the surface of the earth.

third-party payment system A health insurance term indicating that bills will be paid by the insurer (the government or private insurance company) and not the patient (first party) or the health care provider (the second party).

Thorazine See *chlorpromazine.*

Title X A portion of the Public Health Service Act of 1970 that provides funds for family planning services for low-income people.

tolerance Physiological and enzymatic adjustments that occur in response to the chronic presence of drugs, reflected in the need for ever-increasing doses to achieve a previous level of effect.

top-down funding A method of funding in which funds are transmitted from the federal or state government to the local level.

total dependency ratio The dependency ratio that includes both youth and elderly.

transinstitutionalization The process by which patients from one type of public institution, a mental hospital for example, end up in a different institution, such as a nursing home or jail, because of changes in federal policy.

treatment An activity or activities designed to create change in people.

ultraviolet (UV) radiation Radiation energy with wavelengths ranging from 0 to 400 nm.

unintentional injury An injury judged to have occurred without anyone intending that harm be done.

unmodifiable risk factors Factors contributing to the development of a noncommunicable disease that cannot be altered by modifying one's behavior or environment.

unsafe act Any behavior that would increase the probability of an injury occurring.

unsafe condition Any environmental factor or set of factors (physical or social) that would increase the probability of an injury occurring.

urbanization The process by which cities develop and grow and a country's population changes from primarily rural to urban. It is caused by the migration of people from the countryside to the city in search of better jobs and living conditions.

U.S. Census The enumeration of the population of the United States that is conducted every 10 years; begun in 1790.

vector A living organism, usually an arthropod, that can transmit a communicable disease agent to a susceptible host (e.g., mosquitoes, ticks, lice, fleas).

vectorborne disease A communicable disease transmitted by insects or other arthropods; for example, St. Louis encephalitis.

vectorborne disease outbreak (VBDO) The occurrence of two or more cases of a vectorborne disease.

vehicle Inanimate materials or objects, such as clothes, bedding, toys, hypodermic needles; or nonliving biological materials such as food, milk, water, blood, serum or plasma, tissues or organs, that can serve as a source of infection.

vehicleborne disease A communicable disease transmitted by nonliving objects; for example, typhoid fever can be transmitted by water.

visitor services A community social service involving one individual taking time to visit with another who is unable to leave his or her residence.

vital statistics Statistical summaries of vital records—records of major life events, such as births, deaths, marriages, divorces, and infant deaths.

volatile organic compounds (VOCs) Compounds that exist as vapors over the normal range of air pressures and temperatures.

voluntary health agency A nonprofit organization created by concerned citizens to deal with health needs not met by governmental health agencies.

voluntary hospital A nonprofit hospital administered by a religious, fraternal, or other charitable community organization.

wastewater The aqueous mixture that remains after water has been used or contaminated by humans.

water pollution Any physical or chemical change in water that can harm living organisms or make the water unfit for other uses.

waterborne disease A disease that is transmitted through contamination of water.

waterborne disease outbreak (WBDO) The occurrence of two or more cases of a similar illness resulting from the ingestion of drinking water or after exposure to water used for recreational purposes and epidemiological evidence that implicates water as the probable source of illness.

watershed The area of land from which all of the water that is under it or drains from it goes into the same place and drains in one point; for example, the Mississippi River watershed drains and collects all the water from the land extending from east of the Rocky Mountains to the Appalachian Mountains and from the upper Midwest all the way south to the Gulf of Mexico.

WIC (also known as the Special Supplemental Food Program for Women, Infants, and Children) A federal program sponsored by the United States Department of Agriculture designed to provide supplemental foods, nutrition and health education, and referrals for health and social services to improve the health of at-risk, economically disadvantaged women who are pregnant or are caring for infants and children under age five.

workers' compensation laws A set of federal laws designed to compensate those workers and their families who suffer injuries, disease, or death from workplace exposure.

worksite health promotion (WHP) programs Workplace-based, employer-sponsored programs provided to employees and aimed at improving the health of employees through changes in behavior and lifestyle.

World Health Assembly Body of delegates of the member nations of the World Health Organization.

World Health Organization (WHO) Most widely recognized international governmental health organization today. Created in 1948 by representatives of United Nations countries.

years of potential life lost (YPLL) The number of years lost when death occurs before the age of 65 or 75.

young old Those 65 to 74 years of age.

youth dependency ratio The dependency ratio that includes only youth.

youth gang A self-formed association of peers, bound together by mutual interests, with identifiable leadership and well-defined lines of authority, who act in concert to achieve a specific purpose and whose acts generally include illegal activity and control over a territory or an enterprise.

zero population growth (ZPG) A state in which the birth and death rates for a given population are equal.

zoonosis A communicable disease transmissible under natural conditions from vertebrate animals to humans.

Index

Skin diseases/disorders, 588
Sliding scale, 51
Sludge, 478
Smallpox, 13, 14, 23, 66, 107
Smog, photochemical, 468
Smokeless tobacco, 221
Smoking, 5
    adolescents/young adults and, 221-222, 224-226, 351
    during pregnancy, 194
    factors that contribute to, 345-347
    pollution from, 472
    secondhand (environmental tobacco), 351, 470, 471-472, 502-504, 505
    social norms and, 10
    statistics on, 351-352
Snow, John, 15, 66, 490
Social action, 123
Social ecology, 347
Social engineering, period of, 19
Social factors, 9-11
Social Marketing Assessment and Response Tool (SMART), 134
Social norms, affects on community health, 10
Social organizations, work of, 58-59
Social planning, 123
Social Security Act (1935), 19, 203
Society of State Directors of Health, Physical Education, and Recreation, 160-161
Socioeconomic status (SES)
    affects on community health, 10-11
    defined, 298
    minorities and disparities in health due to, 298-304
Sociological hazards, 512-515
Solid waste
    defined, 451
    management, 453-459
    sources of, 451-453
Source reduction, 454
Specialty hospital, 400-401
Specific rates, 69-70
Spiritual era of public health, 13
Spontaneous generation, 16
Staff model HMOs, 432
Standard of acceptability, 141
State Children's Health Insurance Program (SCHIP), 47, 206, 383, 418-419
State health agencies, 48-50
State hospitals, 324
Statistical Abstract of the United States, 82
Steiger, William A., 570
Steroids, 354-355
Stimulants, 359-360
Stormwater runoff, 474
Strep throat, 19
Stress, 321-323, 511-512
Strokes, 5, 103-104
Student assistance programs (SAPs), 367
Studies, epidemiology, 85-90
Subacute care, 387

Substance Abuse and Mental Health Services Administration (SAMHSA), 48, 162, 229, 318, 335, 363
Sudden infant death syndrome (SIDS), 196-197
Suicide
    adolescents and, 218-219
    statistics on, 318-320, 549
Summative evaluation, 141
Superfund legislation, 45, 462
Surface water, 473
Survey of Occupational Injuries and Illnesses (SOII), 589-590
Synar Amendment, 351
Synesthesia, 357
Syphilis, 13, 19, 66, 101

Tardive dyskinesia, 327
Target pest/organism, 501
Teachers, school health programs and role of, 150
Terrestrial radiation, 481
Terrorism, 24-25, 511-512
    bioterrorism, 23, 25
Tertiary medical care, 388
Tertiary prevention, 109, 360-361
Tetanus, 16
Thermal inversion, 468
Third-party payment system, 380-381, 416
Thomas, William, 256
Thorazine (chlorpromazine), 326, 327
Thurmond, Strom, 78
Title V, 203-204
Title X, 184-185, 186
Tobacco, use of. *See* Smoking
Tolerance, 356
Top-down funding, 38
Total dependency ratio, 247
Toxic shock syndrome, 23, 64
Trachoma, 13
Traditions, affects on community health, 9
Transinstitutionalized, 328
Transmission modes, for communicable diseases, 101-102
Transportation, for elders, 262-263
Treatment, drug abuse, 361
Treatment group, 89
Trench fever, 102
Truman, Harry, 434
Trust for America's Health (TFAH), 25
Tuberculosis, 13, 16, 18, 23, 55, 101
Tuke, William, 323
Turfism, 129
Typhoid fever, 14, 16, 101, 102, 490
Typhus, 13
    epidemic, 102
    murine, 102, 499

Ultraviolet radiation, 509-511
Unintentional injuries. *See* Injuries, unintentional
UN Children's Fund (UN International Children's Emergency Fund) (UNICEF), 25, 39, 209
United Nations Millennium Declaration, 28, 40-41

PHOTO CREDITS

p. 9, © Rubberball Productions/Getty Images; p. 10, © Weldon Schloneger/ShutterStock, Inc.; p. 11, © Styve Reineck/ShutterStock, Inc.; p. 12, © Visual Arts Library (London)/Alamy Images; p. 14t, Courtesy of CDC; p. 17, Courtesy of Library of Congress, Prints & Photographs Division, [reproduction number LC-USZ62-7386]; p. 23, © Xinhua/Landov; p. 24, © Reuters/Kai Pfaffenbach/Landov; p. 45, Courtesy of James Gathany/CDC; p. 53, © National Library of Medicine; p. 54, © Keystone/Laurent Gillieron/AP Photos; p. 56, © EMPICS/Landov; p. 58, Courtesy of James F. McKenzie; p. 65, Courtesy of The National Archives; p. 82, Photographed by Lloyd Wolf for the U.S. Census Bureau, Public Information Office (PIO); p. 84, Courtesy of CDC; p. 99, Photographed by Lloyd Wolf for the U.S. Census Bureau, Public Information Office (PIO); p. 101, © Custom Medical Stock Photo; p. 102, © Dr. Jeremy Burgess/Photo Researchers, Inc.; p. 115, © Photodisc; p. 122, © AbleStock; p. 127, Courtesy of James Gathany/CDC; p. 133, Courtesy of US Surgeon General's Office; p. 135b, © Kimberly Hall/ShutterStock, Inc.; p. 149, © David Young-Wolff/PhotoEdit; p. 150, © ImageSource/age fotostock; p. 157, © Mary Kate Denny/PhotoEdit; p. 158, © Don Tremain/age fotostock; p. 159, © Comstock Images/Alamy Images; p. 165, © Chitose Suzuki/AP Photos; p. 177t, © LiquidLibrary; p. 188b, © Joe Marquette/AP Photos; p. 189, © Photodisc; p. 199, © Photodisc; p. 206, © A. Ramey/PhotoEdit; p. 221, © VStock LLC/age fotostock; p. 234, © LiquidLibrary; p. 241, Courtesy of James F. McKenzie; p. 242, © AP Photos; p. 244t, © Gregory Kendall/ShutterStock, Inc.; p. 249, © Comstock Images/Getty Images; p. 250b, © marilyn barbone/ShutterStock, Inc.; p. 257, © Stock Connection Distribution/Alamy Images; p. 260, © Dennis MacDonald/age fotostock; p. 261, © The Centers for Medicare & Medicaid Services; p. 265, © Dennis MacDonald/PhotoEdit; p. 270, © SuperStock/age fotostock; p. 317t, © Gerald Bernard/ShutterStock, Inc.; p. 323, © National Library of Medicine; p. 324t, © National Library of Medicine; p. 324b, Courtesy of Department of Social and Health Services, Washington State; p. 325, © National

Library of Medicine; p. 326, © AP Photos; p. 328, © James Shaffer/PhotoEdit; p. 329, © Photos.com; p. 331t, © Tim Harman/ShutterStock, Inc.; p. 331b, Courtesy of Cpl. Brian Reimers/U.S. Marines; p. 333, © David Buffington/Photodisc/Getty Images; p. 345, © www.imagesource.com/Jupiterimages; p. 347, © BananaStock/age fotostock; p. 349, © Mark Humphrey/AP Photos; p. 355, © Pictor International/ImageState/Alamy Images; p. 359t, © The Meridian Star, Kyle Carter/AP Photos; p. 360, © Netea Mircea Valentin/ShutterStock, Inc.; p. 364, Courtesy of Gerald L. Nino/U.S. Customs and Border Protection; p. 366, © Lisa C. McDonald/ShutterStock, Inc.; p. 367, Courtesy of D.A.R.E. America; p. 379, © Reuters/Brian Snyder/Landov; p. 381, © Kimberly White/Bloomberg News/Landov; p. 389, © Reuters/Jason Reed/Landov; p. 394, © Stuart Pearce/Pixtal/age fotostock; p. 397, © Creatas/Alamy Images; p. 399, © Susan Van Etten/PhotoEdit; p. 402, Courtesy of James F. McKenzie; p. 410, © Photos.com; p. 423, © SuperStock/age fotostock; p. 35, © Jim West/Alamy Images; p. 449, © Photodisc; p. 450, © Aaron Kohr/ShutterStock, Inc.; p. 451, © Comstock Images/age fotostock; p. 454b, © David R. Frazier Photolibrary, Inc./Alamy Images; p. 455, © Visions of America, LLC/Alamy Images; p. 460, © michael ledray/ShutterStock, Inc.; p. 467t, © Photos.com; p. 478, © Wade H. Massie/ShutterStock, Inc.; p. 498, Courtesy of USGS; p. 504, © Bill Aron/PhotoEdit; p. 505, © Tony Freeman/PhotoEdit, Inc.; p. 510, © Photos.com; p. 512, © Gulnara Samoilova/AP Photos; p. 517, Courtesy of Andrea Booher/FEMA; p. 524t, © DigitalVues/Alamy Images; p. 534, © Pixtal/age fotostock; p. 538, © Photodisc/Getty Images; p. 552t, © Julie Plasencia/AP Photos; p. 560, © Photos.com; p. 561, © AP Photos; p. 569, © Omikron/Photo Researchers, Inc. ; p. 570t, © Photo Researchers, Inc. ; p. 570b, © National Library of Medicine; p. 583, © Photodisc; p. 585, © David R. Photolibrary, Inc./Alamy Images; p. 590t, © Rubberball Productions/Creatas; p. 590b, © Photos.com; p. 592, © ImageSource/age fotostock.